Register Now for Online Access to Your Book!

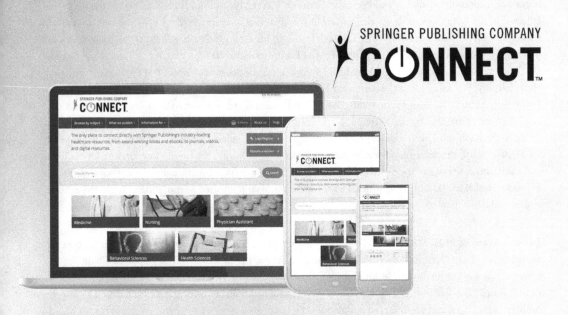

SPRINGER PUBLISHING COMPANY
CONNECT.™

Your print purchase of *Health Equity* **includes online access to the contents of your book**—increasing accessibility, portability, and searchability!

Access today at:

**http://connect.springerpub.com/content/book/978-0-8261-7724-7
or scan the QR code at the right with your smartphone
and enter the access code below.**

668GA4MP

D1224368

SPRINGER PUBLISHING COMPANY

View all our products at springerpub.com

K. Bryant Smalley, PhD, PsyD, MBA, is a licensed clinical psychologist and health equity researcher. He serves as the Associate Dean for Research in the Mercer University School of Medicine, where he is also Professor of Community Medicine and Psychiatry. Prior to Mercer, he co-founded and served as the Executive Director of the Rural Health Research Institute at Georgia Southern University. He also served in multiple leadership roles (including Director of Clinical Training) for Georgia Southern's PsyD program, a clinical psychology program focused on preparing mental health practitioners for practice in underserved areas. Dr. Smalley is the past chair of the American Psychological Association's Committee on Rural Health, is a Health Equity Ambassador for the American Psychological Association, has previously been invited to discuss health disparity issues with the White House Rural Council, and was named both Researcher of the Year and Educator of the Year by the National Rural Health Association. Dr. Smalley's work has been supported by more than $12 million in federal grants from organizations including the National Institutes of Health (NIH), the Health Resources and Services Administration (HRSA), and the federal Corporation for National and Community Service (CNCS), including Center of Excellence funding through the National Institute on Minority Health and Health Disparities. His research has been published in more than 70 journal articles, books, and book chapters.

Jacob C. Warren, PhD, MBA, CRA, is a behavioral epidemiologist specializing in health equity research. He is the Associate Dean for Diversity, Equity, and Inclusion, the Rufus C. Harris Endowed Chair, the Director of the Center for Rural Health and Health Disparities, the Vice Chair for Research, and Professor of Community Medicine in the Mercer University School of Medicine, which is dedicated to meeting the health needs of rural and underserved populations. He has served in a variety of academic and research leadership positions and has been PI of more than $12 million in federally funded research and service grants focused on the study and elimination of health inequities in various groups. His work has been supported by NIH, CNCS, and HRSA, including Center of Excellence funding through the National Institute on Minority Health and Health Disparities. He is a health equity ambassador for the American Psychological Association, is chair of the State of Georgia's Migrant Farmworker Advisory Board, and was named Researcher of the Year by the National Rural Health Association. Dr. Warren has published over 70 journal articles, books, and book chapters.

M. Isabel Fernández, PhD, is a community psychologist whose health equity work focuses on substance abuse and HIV prevention and treatment in African American and Hispanic populations. She is the Director of the Behavioral Health Promotion Program in the Nova Southeastern University College of Osteopathic Medicine, where she also serves as the Associate Dean of Faculty Research, the Director of the Student Research Fellowship Program, and Professor of Public Health. Dr. Fernández has received more than $15 million in funding from NIH, the Centers for Disease Control and Prevention (CDC), and the Substance Abuse and Mental Health Services Administration (SAMHSA) to support her health equity–focused work, published more than 100 peer-reviewed journal articles, and served as senior advisor to multiple NIH Centers of Excellence and national working groups focused on health equity issues. Prior to her academic career, she served as a Health Scientist Administrator for the National Institute on Mental Health (NIMH) within NIH, as a Senior Policy Analyst within the U.S. Public Health Service, and as both a Behavioral Scientist and an AIDS Information Specialist within the CDC. In these roles, she served as a national expert in the development and implementation of ground-level health equity–focused substance use and HIV prevention efforts, advised senior administration regarding policy issues, developed testimony and other briefing materials for use in congressional hearings and committees, and coordinated NIMH's participation in collaborative AIDS research and prevention projects.

HEALTH EQUITY

A Solutions-Focused Approach

K. Bryant Smalley, PhD, PsyD, MBA

Jacob C. Warren, PhD, MBA, CRA

M. Isabel Fernández, PhD

Editors

SPRINGER PUBLISHING COMPANY

First Springer Publishing edition 2021

No part of this publication may be reproduced, stored in a retrieval system, or transmitted in any form or by any means, electronic, mechanical, photocopying, recording, or otherwise, without the prior permission of Springer Publishing Company, LLC, or authorization through payment of the appropriate fees to the Copyright Clearance Center, Inc., 222 Rosewood Drive, Danvers, MA 01923, 978-750-8400, fax 978-646-8600, info@copyright.com or on the Web at www.copyright.com.

Springer Publishing Company, LLC
11 West 42nd Street, New York, NY 10036
www.springerpub.com
connect.springerpub.com/

Acquisitions Editor: David D'Addona
Compositor: S4Carlisle Publishing Services

ISBN: 978-0-8261-7723-0
ebook ISBN: 978-0-8261-7724-7
DOI: 10.1891/9780826177247

Qualified instructors may request supplements by emailing textbook@springerpub.com

Instructor's Manual: 978-0-8261-6936-5
Test Bank: 978-0-8261-6938-9 (Available in Respondus 4.0®)
PowerPoint Slides: 978-0-8261-6937-2
Sample Syllabus: 978-0-8261-6947-1

20 21 22 23 / 5 4 3 2 1

The author and the publisher of this Work have made every effort to use sources believed to be reliable to provide information that is accurate and compatible with the standards generally accepted at the time of publication. The author and publisher shall not be liable for any special, consequential, or exemplary damages resulting, in whole or in part, from the readers' use of, or reliance on, the information contained in this book. The publisher has no responsibility for the persistence or accuracy of URLs for external or third-party Internet websites referred to in this publication and does not guarantee that any content on such websites is, or will remain, accurate or appropriate.

Library of Congress Cataloging-in-Publication Data

Names: Smalley, K. Bryant, editor. | Warren, Jacob C., editor. |
  Fernández, M. Isabel, PhD, editor.
Title: Health equity : a solutions-focused approach / [edited by] K. Bryant
  Smalley, Jacob C. Warren, M. Isabel Fernández.
Other titles: Health equity (Smalley)
Description: First Springer Publishing edition. | New York : Springer
  Publishing Company, 2021. | Includes bibliographical references and
  index.
Identifiers: LCCN 2020018438 (print) | LCCN 2020018439 (ebook) | ISBN
  9780826177230 (paperback) | ISBN 9780826177247 (ebook)
Subjects: MESH: Health Equity | United States
Classification: LCC RA427.8 (print) | LCC RA427.8 (ebook) | NLM W 76 AA1
  | DDC 362.1--dc23
LC record available at https://lccn.loc.gov/2020018438
LC ebook record available at https://lccn.loc.gov/2020018439

Contact us to receive discount rates on bulk purchases.
We can also customize our books to meet your needs.
For more information please contact: sales@springerpub.com

Publisher's Note: New and used products purchased from third-party sellers are not guaranteed for quality, authenticity, or access to any included digital components.

Printed in the United States of America.

For all of the brave members of the communities discussed throughout this book who fought for recognition, respect, and equality.

We are all in your debt.

—Bryant, Jacob, and Isa

CONTENTS

CONTRIBUTORS

Jasmine A. Abrams, PhD　Assistant Professor, Department of Community Health Sciences, Boston University, Boston, Massachusetts

Momi Akana　Executive Director, Keiki O Ka 'Āina Family Learning Centers, Hawai'i

Faye Z. Belgrave, PhD　Professor, Department of Psychology, Virginia Commonwealth University, Richmond, Virginia

Shannon Brownlee, MPH　Lecturer, Public Health and Health Sciences, University of Michigan, Flint, Michigan

Cleopatra Caldwell, PhD　Professor, Health Behavior and Health Education, Director, Center for Research on Ethnicity, Culture, and Health, School of Public Health, University of Michigan, Ann Arbor, Michigan

Denise C. Carty, PhD　Affiliate, Center for Research on Ethnicity, Culture, and Health, School of Public Health, University of Michigan, Ann Arbor, Michigan

E. Hill De Loney, MA　Director, Flint Odyssey House Awareness Center, Flint, Michigan

Mark Edberg, PhD, MA　Director, Avance Center for the Advancement of Immigrant/Refugee Health, Associate Professor, Department of Prevention and Community Health, Milken Institute School of Public Health, The George Washington University, Washington, DC

M. Isabel Fernández, PhD　Director, Behavioral Health Promotion Program, Professor of Public Health, Nova Southeastern University, Fort Lauderdale, Florida

Tonya French-Turner, MBA　Co-Director, Community Core, Healthy Flint Research Coordinating Center, Flint, Michigan

Deliana Garcia, MA　Director, International Projects and Emerging Issues, Migrant Clinicians Network, Austin, Texas

Lauren R. Gilbert, PhD, MPH　Assistant Professor, Department of Community Medicine, Mercer University School of Medicine, Macon, Georgia

Emily Graybill, PhD, NCSP   Clinical Assistant Professor and Associate Director, Center for Leadership in Disability, School of Public Health, Georgia State University, Atlanta, Georgia

Iva GreyWolf, PhD   Psychologist and Cultural Consultant, President, Society of Indian Psychologists, Roseburg, Oregon

Derek M. Griffith, PhD   Professor, Medicine, Health, and Society, Founder and Director, Center for Research on Men's Health, Vanderbilt University, Nashville, Tennessee

Christina E. Harris, MD   Attending Physician, VA Greater Los Angeles Healthcare System, Health Sciences Associate Clinical Professor, Department of Medicine, UCLA David Geffen School of Medicine, Los Angeles, California

Ifeoma Stella Izuchukwu, MD, MPH   Attending Physician, VA Greater Los Angeles Healthcare System, Health Sciences Clinical Professor, Department of Medicine, UCLA David Geffen School of Medicine, Los Angeles, California, Colonel and Squadron Commander, U.S. Air Force Reserve Command, March Air Reserve Base, California

Joseph Keawe'aimoku Kaholokula, PhD   Professor, Department of Native Hawaiian Health, John A. Burns School of Medicine, University of Hawai'i at Mānoa, Honolulu, Hawai'i

Earl Kawa'a, MSW   Cultural Practitioner, Hawai'i

Kent D. Key, PhD   Director, Office of Community Scholars and Partnerships, Division of Public Health, Michigan State University College of Human Medicine, Flint, Michigan

Simona C. Kwon, DrPH, MPH   Associate Professor, Department of Population Health, NYU School of Medicine, New York, New York

Sahnah Lim, PhD   Assistant Professor, Department of Population Health, NYU School of Medicine, New York, New York

Mele A. Look, MBA   Director of Community Engagement, Department of Native Hawaiian Health, John A. Burns School of Medicine, University of Hawai'i at Mānoa, Honolulu, Hawai'i

Margaret Murray   Project Assistant, Center for Leadership in Disability, School of Public Health, Georgia State University, Atlanta, Georgia

Jennifer L. Nguyễn, PhD, MPH   Assistant Professor, Department of Pharmacy Practice, Mercer University College of Pharmacy, Atlanta, Georgia

Judith Palfrey, MD   Senior Associate in Pediatrics, Boston Children's Hospital, Boston, Massachusetts

Shilpa Patel, PhD   Senior Program Officer, Center for Health Care Strategies, Hamilton, New Jersey

Liana Petruzzi, MSW   Doctoral Candidate, Steve Hicks School of Social Work, The University of Texas at Austin, Austin, Texas

Miguel Pinedo, PhD   Assistant Professor, Department of Kinesiology and Health Education, The University of Texas at Austin, Austin, Texas

Royleen J. Ross, PhD   Consultant, Secretary, Society of Indian Psychologists, Nome, Alaska

Mary (Dicey) Jackson Scroggins, MA   Director of Global Outreach and Engagement, International Gynecologic Cancer Society, Washington, DC

Eric K. Shaw, PhD   Associate Professor, Department of Community Medicine, Mercer University School of Medicine, Savannah, Georgia

K. Bryant Smalley, PhD, PsyD, MBA   Associate Dean for Research, Professor of Community Medicine and Psychiatry, Mercer University School of Medicine, Macon, Georgia

Shelley Soong, PhD   Research Associate, Department of Native Hawaiian Health, John A. Burns School of Medicine, University of Hawai'i at Mānoa, Honolulu, Hawai'i

Jean R. Sumner, MD, FACP   Dean, School of Medicine, Professor, Department of Internal Medicine, Mercer University School of Medicine, Macon, Georgia

Edward Tepporn, BA   Executive Vice President, Asian & Pacific Islander American Health Forum, Oakland, California, Executive Director, Angel Island Immigration Station Foundation, San Francisco, California

Erin Vinoski Thomas, PhD, MPH, CHES   Research Assistant Professor and Director of Health and Wellness, Center for Leadership in Disability, School of Public Health, Georgia State University, Atlanta, Georgia

Carmen R. Valdez, PhD   Associate Professor, Department of Population Health, Dell Medical School, and Steve Hicks School of Social Work, The University of Texas at Austin, Austin, Texas

Monique Vasquez, MSSW, MPH   Project Coordinator, Department of Population Health, Dell Medical School, The University of Texas at Austin, Austin, Texas

Jacob C. Warren, PhD, MBA, CRA   Associate Dean for Diversity, Equity, and Inclusion, Endowed Chair and Director, Center for Rural Health and Health Disparities, Professor of Community Medicine, Mercer University School of Medicine, Macon, Georgia

Donna L. Washington, MD, MPH   Director, VHA Health Equity–Quality Enhancement Research Initiative National Partnered Evaluation Center, Women's Health-Focused Research Area Lead, VA HSR&D Center for the Study of Healthcare Innovation, Implementation & Policy (CSHIIP), Department of Medicine, VA Greater Los Angeles Healthcare System, Professor, Department of Medicine, UCLA David Geffen School of Medicine, Los Angeles, California

PREFACE

We all should know that diversity makes for a rich tapestry, and we must understand that all the threads of the tapestry are equal in value no matter what their color.

—Maya Angelou

It feels as though the field of health equity has finally come into its time. Conversations about the presence of health disparities have evolved into discussions of how to eliminate them, which have in turn evolved into a broader movement to truly achieve equity in health predictors, statuses, and outcomes. The field of health equity is at its core a branch of social justice, and the movement has clearly begun. The road is long, however, and the issues that drive the underlying presence of health disparities remain firmly in place. The field also remains very new, particularly in investigating the unique health and healthcare needs of groups that are not only marginalized in society, but also largely neglected in the scientific literature.

Despite its relative youth, however, the field has produced critical knowledge about the origins of health equity issues and has also produced resounding successes in promoting equity itself. This book is a manifestation of that knowledge. Our hope for this textbook is that it serves for students of public health and other health disciplines as not only a comprehensive guide to the historical origins of health inequities and the predominant health issues for diverse groups, but also more importantly that it serves as a guide to developing and implementing solutions to achieve health equity developed by and for the communities affected. This solutions-focused and community-affirming approach permeates the book's philosophy—each chapter focused on a specific health equity community includes authorship from members of that specific community and an illustrative case example of how equity-focused efforts have been successfully implemented.

We begin the book with an overview of the major dynamics of health equity for both the experienced and the new student, focusing on historical perspectives, the role of prejudice and discrimination, an overview of cross-cutting health equity frameworks and theories, and a summary of three major methods of implementing health equity research and collaboration. We then present 13 community-specific chapters that summarize current needs and applied solutions for groups ranging from Native Hawaiians to individuals with disabilities, each authored or coauthored by one or more members of the community being discussed. We then conclude the book with a discussion of the importance of cultural humility and a summary of where the field of health equity is poised to go from here. An intersectionality perspective is interwoven throughout the text to help affirm that all people are an assemblage of multiple cultural identities, each of which may be subject to health equity concerns. **Instructor resources for this text include an Instructor's Manual, chapter PowerPoint presentations, Test Bank, and a Sample Syllabus, which may be requested by emailing textbook@springerpub.com.** The book has been specifically designed for courses in health disparities, health equity, social determinants of health, social epidemiology, and multicultural health. The combination of integrative chapters (e.g., racism and discrimination) and population-specific chapters (e.g., immigrant populations) allows learners to see both the commonalities and the individualities that exist across populations striving to achieve health equity. In addition, the book's continuous focus on intersectionality ensures that—even in chapters focused on specific populations—the reader continues to understand the interconnected nature of all aspects of identity and the dynamics of health equity.

Because of its focus on issues that are sometimes deemed too complex or intractable to meaningfully change, the quest to achieve health equity for all people can seem overwhelming, but these problems are no match for the determination, spirit, and compassion of those who enter the field. We hope this book helps you in your quest.

K. Bryant Smalley, PhD, PsyD, MBA
Jacob C. Warren, PhD, MBA, CRA
M. Isabel Fernández, PhD

I

INTRODUCTION AND OVERVIEW

HEALTH EQUITY: OVERVIEW, HISTORY, AND KEY CONCEPTS

K. BRYANT SMALLEY ■ JACOB C. WARREN ■ M. ISABEL FERNÁNDEZ

LEARNING OBJECTIVES

- Describe how health is not treated as a fundamental right within the United States
- Discuss the meaning and interrelated nature of health disparities, health equity, and social justice
- Describe how the Healthy People initiative helped to frame the approach to achieving health equity in the United States
- Summarize the ways in which historical factors impact the ability of groups impacted by health disparities to trust the healthcare industry
- Contrast the concepts of equality, equity, and justice

INTRODUCTION

The field of health equity is broad and ever-expanding. It challenges us all to think about the fundamental nature of health, of society, and ultimately of human rights. Is having equal access to live a healthy life a right or a privilege? Unfortunately, in the United States health is a privilege afforded most readily to those with sufficient socioeconomic status to afford it and enough socio-demographic standing to have equal access to the resources necessary to attain and maintain it. While several states have taken it upon themselves to ensure all residents have access to health-care, the very patchwork nature of such access proves that health is not considered a right in our country.

Those working in health equity, however, reject this notion, instead believing that all people—regardless of their cultural and demographic background—should have equal opportunity to live a life of health. As with other rights, however—for example the right to vote or the right to marry—society has intentionally and unintentionally placed and reinforced barriers to health that disproportionately impact minority and other marginalized populations. As discussed in Chapter 2, Prejudice, Discrimination, and Health, issues of discrimination and unequal distribution of resources plague our health system and have significant long-term effects on the health of several subpopulations in the United States discussed throughout this text. In attempts to combat these effects, researchers and practitioners have developed a number of models, frameworks, and strategies that are also described in these pages that strive to not only eliminate health disparities, but also to change the fundamental systems such that they create equity in health.

To provide broader context for the remainder of the text's content, in this first chapter we briefly summarize the field at large, provide an abbreviated history of the field of health equity, and conclude with a discussion of the complexities of even naming solutions to these issues.

HEALTH DISPARITIES, HEALTH EQUITY, AND SOCIAL JUSTICE

Definitions and Origins

One of the major complexities with the field of health equity is a lack of consistency of definitions, and at times contention among practitioners and researchers regarding terminology. Most agree that, while the concept certainly predated this time, the term "health disparity" came into use in the early 1990s (Braveman, 2014). While there is ongoing debate regarding the definition of the term, it is etymologically drawn from the Latin "dis," meaning "not," and "paritas," meaning "equal." In its purest sense, then, the word "disparity" refers to simple inequality. However, the English word "disparity" is a cognate of the French *disparité*, meaning unequal in rank or status. This reveals the truer sense typically meant when referring to a health disparity: an inequality in health status or outcomes related to some kind of injustice, oppression, or difference in sociodemographic status. This is in contrast to a simple inequality, which is a difference between groups that may or may not be related to social injustice (e.g., the incidence of skin cancer is higher in Caucasian individuals, but this is attributable to biology rather than injustice; most would not consider this a "true" health disparity).

While generally keeping within that theme, there remain competing definitions that incorporate varying factors under the umbrella of "health disparity." The Centers for Disease Control and Prevention (CDC) has defined "health disparities" as "differences in health outcomes between groups that reflect social inequalities" (Frieden, 2011, p. 1). This definition emphasizes the social nature of disparities, but focuses primarily on outcomes, failing to take into account broader health status (e.g., functioning). The American Public Health Association (APHA, n.d.) has a broader definition of "differences in health status between people that are related to social or demographic factors such as race, gender, income, or geographic region." This definition makes more explicit the relationship with membership in specific demographic groups and broadens the scope to have a focus on health status rather than just health outcomes. While the U.S. Department of Health and Human Services (DHHS) has numerous definitions (e.g., the CDC has its own just described), in its Healthy People 2010 initiative, the agency defined "health disparities" to be "differences that occur by gender, race or ethnicity, education or income, disability, living in rural localities, or sexual orientation" (DHHS, 2000, p. 11). The selection of these specific categories has been criticized as largely arbitrary (Braveman et al., 2011) but has shaped which groups are typically considered when we use the phrase "health disparities." Another criticism is, unlike CDC's definition, both APHA's and Healthy People's definitions remove the focus from the underlying inequities driving the process, instead relating it most directly to the demographic group itself (rather than the injustices associated with being a member of that group). In essence, the APHA and Healthy People are focused on the difference—the health disparity—rather than the fundamental processes driving those differences—the issues in health equity. The definition of disparities was subsequently revised in Healthy People 2020 (DHHS, 2010), which used a very in-clusive and equity-focused definition of "a particular type of health difference that is closely linked with economic, social, or environmental disadvantage" and explicitly stating that it is related to "characteristics historically linked to discrimination or exclusion" (p. 46). Such definitions—while more inclusive and typically viewed as preferable to the more specific ones just described—still make it somewhat arbitrary as to what someone considers a health disparity. While definitions clearly vary and evolve over time, the core consideration in health disparities is the link to some kind of injustice—the premise being that there is nothing "essential" about the differences, and we as a society are responsible for both their presence and their elimination. To further clarify this distinction, recent movements have embraced the term *health inequities* rather than health disparities, defined by the American Public Health Association as being "created when barriers prevent individuals and communities from accessing [health] and reaching their full potential" (APHA, n.d.).

SICKLE CELL DISEASE—SIMPLE INEQUALITY OR HEALTH DISPARITY?

The example of sickle cell disease is often discussed within the context of health disparities, as it is one of very few outcomes whose racial differences can be explained biologically. Sickle cell disease occurs when an individual is homozygous for a gene affecting the production of hemoglobin, which in turn distorts the shape of red blood cells. To be born with sickle cell dis-ease, both of a baby's parents must have had either sickle cell disease (homozygous) or sickle cell trait (heterozygous carriers). Persons of African descent are nearly 25 times as likely to be born with sickle cell trait (Ojodu, Hulihan, Pope, & Grant, 2014; typically attributed to evolution-ary advantages of the anti-malarial properties of sickle cells), creating a direct link between race and the disease. However, does this truly represent a disparity if the difference is related purely to genetics, and not to social inequality? Many argue that sickle cell disease itself is not a disparity; however, there is evidence that there are disparities within sickle cell disease. While it is often thought of as a "Black" disease, sickle cell disease does occur in patients of all races and ethnicities. Studies have shown that when presenting to an emergency room for sickle cell–related emergency, African American patients with sickle cell disease wait 25% longer to receive services than other patients (Haywood, Tanabe, Naik, Beach, & Lanzkron, 2013), and half of youth with sickle cell disease report experiencing racist events in medical care settings (Wakefield et al., 2018). Thus, while the presence of sickle cell disease may not be a disparity, there are still disparities and social justice issues within sickle cell disease treatment in need of intervention.

The Emergence of Health Equity

The field of health disparities has grown tremendously in the past several decades, but in more recent years has been criticized for its focus on outcomes and differences—in essence, dwelling in the problem rather than the solution. The health equity movement grew from this burgeoning desire to change the situation itself—in trying to eliminate health disparities, our goal is to achieve health equity. Interestingly, even the concept of health equity has since been broadened. As discussed throughout this text, and in detail in Chapter 3, Health Equity Frameworks and Theories, the vast majority of health disparity issues are now viewed through the lens of social determinants of health—that is, differences in outcomes are rarely accurately attributable to uninfluenced individual behavior (e.g., choosing to smoke), and are more precisely related to differences in factors related to that behavior (e.g., stress levels, poverty, educational attainment, neighborhood environment). To truly eliminate health disparities and thereby achieve health equity, many solutions require a social justice lens. Changing the societal discrimination that elevates baseline stress levels in African Americans would impact much more than just health, but is still essential in achieving health equity for African American populations—thus the path to health equity in many cases lies in social justice. Figure 1.1 illustrates how these three concepts—health disparities, health equity, and social justice—represent different facets of a continuum of concepts.

While historically the field of health equity focused mainly on racial/ethnic differences in health, more recently other groups have been incorporated into the field, such as individuals with diverse sexual orientations and gender identities, individuals with disabilities, and individuals of varying geographic backgrounds (e.g., rural). This expansion has also opened the door for overarching frameworks such as Intersectionality Theory (see Chapter 3, Health Equity Frameworks and Theories), which have begun to explore the ways in which overlapping identities come together to influence health outcomes (e.g., how do the experiences of a straight transgender Latinx woman compare to a bisexual cisgender Asian man, and how do those identities intersect in determining their health?). At the same time, this diversity of focus has led to a literature that is at times fragmented. While the experiences of each group impacted by disparities is unique and worthy of individual study, there are themes that also repeat—for example, the effects of discrimination impact nearly all health disparity groups. One goal of our text is to examine health equity through both lenses—the unique lessons of the experiences of individual health disparity groups (e.g., migrant health), and the broader strategies and convergence of approaches demonstrated to be impactful across multiple populations affected by health disparities (e.g., the importance of cultural humility).

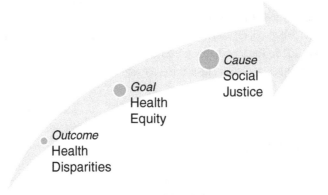

FIGURE 1.1 Relationship between health disparities, health equity, and social justice.

HISTORICAL CONTEXT OF HEALTH DISPARITIES

The history of discrimination, marginalization, and direct victimization of minority groups within the medical profession is deep and dark, and is described in more detail in Chapter 2, Prejudice, Discrimination, and Health. Many "modern" medical treatments and even devices can trace their roots to experiments conducted on slaves. In an example summarized by Kathleen Bachynski (2018), in 1894 the *Journal of the American Medical Association* published a commentary describing how "for the first time in the history of the United States, a public statue has been erected to the memory of a member of the medical profession" ("The statue of Dr. J. Marion Sims in Bryant Park," 1894, p. 689). That physician was Dr. J. Marion Sims, whose likeness initially rested in Bryant Park and was subsequently moved to Central Park (directly across from the New York Academy of Medicine). Sims was lauded in the 1894 article for being elected to the presidency of the American Medical Association in 1875, for founding the first women's hospital in the United States, and for being designated as a Chevalier of the Legion of Honor by Napoleon. Sims additionally invented the precursor of the modern speculum and developed a method to cure vesico-vaginal fistula. What the article fails to mention is the method whereby his techniques were developed—experimentation on slave women without anesthesia in order to increase their ability to both return to "work" in the fields more quickly and to preserve their ability to have more children and thereby grow the slave population in America. Despite its clear reverence for a man who literally took ownership of slave women so he could experiment on them, the statue dedicated to his "brilliant achievements" and "services in the cause of … mankind" retained its prominent location until it was removed in early 2018.

The story of Sims is emblematic of the ways in which inequities in healthcare itself are deeply rooted and still affecting us today. These stories are not all remote, however. The Tuskegee Syphilis Study, in which the precursor agency to the CDC conducted unconsented research on African American men in which they actively withheld effective treatment for decades, is often cited as a source of modern mistrust of the medical community. Similarly, the oft-ignored history of American eugenics—in which mostly minority patients were sterilized against their will and often even without their knowledge—contributes to the reality that for the majority of our history, the healthcare system has failed to even recognize the fundamental humanity and autonomy of marginalized groups, much less worked to meet their unique health needs in a way to achieve health equity.

While there are many other dark chapters of this history that could be written, there are also shining examples of ways in which people have made substantial contributions to end these injustices and their long-term effects. Dr. John Ruffin, a renowned biologist, took his quest for health equity to the federal government when he became the National Institutes of Health's (NIH's) first Associate Director for Minority programs in 1990. From there, he led the transition of the Office of Minority Programs first into the Office of Research on Minority Health in 1993, then into the National Center on Minority Health and Health Disparities in 2000, and ultimately into the National Institute on Minority Health and Health Disparities in 2010 (NIMHD, 2019), charged with coordinating and overseeing the NIH's investments in minority health and health disparities research. The impact of his work to institutionalize the importance of health disparities throughout not only the NIH, but also the federal government at large, is incalculable and laid the groundwork for much of the research described throughout this text.

TABLE 1.1 Evolution of Equity-Focused Goals in the Healthy People Initiative

ITERATION	STATED EQUITY-FOCUSED GOAL(S)
Healthy People 2000	None
Healthy People 2010	Two goals, including: ■ Eliminate health disparities
Healthy People 2020	Four goals, including: ■ Achieve health equity, eliminate disparities, and improve the health of all groups
Healthy People 2030	Five goals, including: ■ Eliminate health disparities, achieve health equity, and attain health literacy to improve the health and well-being of all ■ Create social, physical, and economic environments that promote attaining full potential for health and well-being for all

Another important turning point in the federal recognition of health disparities was the second iteration of the Healthy People initiative. First launched in 1990, Healthy People 2000 laid out the U.S. Department of Health and Human Services' roadmap for improving the health of Americans by the turn of the century. The plan consisted of 22 priority areas determined to be the most important components of achieving a healthy America. This helped to shape HHS policies and funding decisions for a decade, until it was revised and updated into Healthy People 2010 in the year 2000. Healthy People 2010 marked an important turning point in the field of health disparities, as the initiative had two overarching goals, one of which was to eliminate health disparities. This directed much-needed federal attention to the emerging field of health disparities research, and provided the impetus for federal agencies to begin prioritizing health disparities research in ways not previously done. Reflecting the growth within the field, Healthy People 2020 (released in 2010) incorporated into its four overarching goals the target of achieving health equity, partially shifting the national attention from just eliminating disparities to truly focusing on achieving equity itself. While Healthy People 2030 was still in the process of being finalized at the time of publication of this book, preliminary draft goals include not only a statement of the need to achieve health equity, but also the specific prioritization of methods to do so: a focus both on health literacy and on creating "social, physical, and economic environments that promote attaining full potential for health and well-being for all." The evolution of these goals is summarized in Table 1.1.

EQUALITY, EQUITY, AND JUSTICE

As we discuss the overarching goal for this body of work—to achieve health equity—there remains an issue with consistency of message. Part of this has to deal with the related, but distinct nature of equality, equity, and justice. While often used interchangeably, "equality" and "equity" are not the same. The concept of equality is ensuring that everyone is allocated equal access to a certain resource, whereas the concept of equity is ensuring that everyone has an equal outcome. Consider an example of the allocation of resources to public health districts. Equality would hold that funding should be apportioned based upon population size—for instance, an urban center of 250,000 residents should receive $25 million in the same way that a rural area of 250,000 residents should receive $25 million—each resident resulting in a $100 budgetary allocation. Such an approach, however, ignores the structural realities that urban and rural areas are different. The catchment area for the 250,000 urban residents may be less than 100 square miles, whereas the rural catchment area may be thousands of square miles. This geographic factor alone is enough to highlight that the increased need of rural residents (in this case based just upon staff travel distances) merits an increase in allocation of funds if the goal truly is to reach comparable outcomes (i.e., equity). In essence, achieving equity requires providing strategic support where it is most needed, which may involve "unequal" distribution of resources in order to actually achieve an equitable outcome.

A final perspective focuses on justice. Fundamentally, one major reason that rural residents would need additional transportation support to reach services is the lack of public transportation available in rural areas. If public transportation were to be put into place, then the additional allocation of resources would no longer be needed. This is the work of justice—to remove whatever fundamental barrier exists that is leading to the inequity in the first place. This is often easier said than done, of course, but the work of social justice counteracts the need to provide unequal resources (which often makes taxpayers and legislators very uncomfortable, despite its essential nature to achieve equity).

A popular visual representation of the interplay of equality, equity, and justice depicts three individuals attempting to see over a fence at a baseball game (see Figure 1.2). The three individuals are of differing heights (representing different levels of need), yet all three are being treated equally in panel 1—each has received one box to help them see over the fence. At this level, one individual has more than adequate clearance, but one remains unable to see the game. In the second panel, equity has been achieved by reassigning one box from the first person to the third; to have equal *outcomes*, it was necessary to have strategic, albeit unequal, distribution of resources to overcome the higher level of need. A justice lens, however, does not focus on how to get everyone where they can see over the fence, but rather focuses on removing the barrier itself. In the third panel, the fence itself has been removed, allowing for the boxes to metaphorically be moved to a new issue that needs resolution. Equality therefore treats everyone the same, equity treats

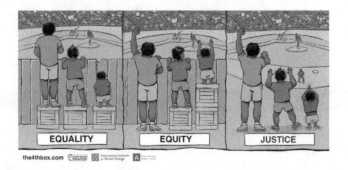

FIGURE 1.2 Common representation of equality, equity, and justice.

SOURCE: Reproduced with permission from Center for Story-Based Strategy. (n.d.). *#the4thBox*. Retrieved from https://www.storybasedstrategy.org/the4thbox

individuals in a way necessary to achieve equal outcomes, and justice removes the fundamental barriers in place that led to the disparity in the first place.

While variations of this image are very commonly used to facilitate discussions of equality, equity, and justice, there are problems with the way it visually depicts the differences in needs between groups. As drawn, there is a fundamental difference between the individuals that is leading to the need for equity and justice—the height of the individual. In reality, the differences we see in health disparities are not the product of individual characteristics of the group, but rather relate to the sociocultural context in which individuals find themselves. An alternate version has been developed that more fully depicts the reality of inequities—that different groups do not start from the same position of advantage, and equity efforts are required to counteract these situational differences (Kuttner, 2016). In these alternate versions, the concept of equality and equity are depicted by showing three individuals of equal height but standing upon unequal ground and blocked by an uneven fence. This places some individuals at higher ground with a lower fence, and some individuals at lower ground with a higher fence. These variations help to reinforce that issues with equity are not due to something fundamentally different in the people themselves; rather, it is related to the situation and environment in which they find themselves.

CONCLUSION

The fundamental inequities in health that occur between sociodemographic groups in the U.S. represent some of the darkest aspects of our culture, and yet the field of health equity is strikingly new. Ultimately grounded in a historical context of racism, discrimination, injustice, disadvantage, and privilege, it is easy to become overwhelmed with the systemic nature of the issues that must be addressed to truly achieve health equity. Despite this, every day an army of community members and professionals work to do just that—change a system that has so deeply entrenched inequities into our daily lives that it was not until the 1990s that the federal government began to acknowledge the need for change. The work is hard, and at times feels painfully slow, but at the same time, it is some of the most important work being done in our nation.

Our hope for this text is that it will provide not only a historical and descriptive perspective on how we have reached this point, but also clear examples of successes and strategies that can be implemented to address the many concerns identified in its pages. This solutions-focused approach permeates the text, and we hope will inspire you to begin or continue critical work in these areas.

DISCUSSION QUESTIONS

- How would a movement toward universal health insurance (e.g., Medicare-for-All) not fully solve issues related to inequities in access to healthcare?

- Consider the case of deaths due to diabetes, which are more common among African American women than other demographic groups. How would you describe the disparity, the health equity goal, and a related social justice issue critical in achieving equity in this area?

- How have the evolving Healthy People goals mirrored the evolving field of health disparities and health equity?

- It is well established that minority groups are under-represented in clinical trials research. Describe structural and historical issues that contribute to this underrepresentation.

- Does inequality necessarily translate into inequity? What are the ways to achieve equity even without achieving equality?

REFERENCES

American Public Health Association. (n.d.). *Health equity*. Retrieved from https://www.apha.org/topics-and-issues/health-equity

Bachynski, K. (2018, June 4). American medicine was built on the backs of slaves. And it still affects how doctors treat patients today. *Washington Post*. Retrieved from https://www.washingtonpost.com/news/made-by-history/wp/2018/06/04/american-medicine-was-built-on-the-backs-of-slaves-and-it-still-affects-how-doctors-treat-patients-today

Braveman, P. (2014). What are health disparities and health equity? We need to be clear. *Public Health Reports*, *129*(1 Suppl. 2), 5–8. doi:10.1177/00333549141291S203

Braveman, P. A., Kumanyika, S., Fielding, J., LaVeist, T., Borrell, L. N., Manderscheid, R., & Troutman, A. (2011). Health disparities and health equity: The issue is justice. *American Journal of Public Health*, *101*(S1), S149–S155. doi:10.2105/AJPH.2010.300062

Center for Story-Based Strategy. (n.d.). *#the4thBox*. Retrieved from https://www.storybasedstrategy.org/the4thbox

Frieden, T. R. (2011). Foreword to CDC Health Disparities and Inequalities Report—United States, 2011. *Morbidity and Mortality Weekly Report*, *60*(S1), 1. Retrieved from https://www.cdc.gov/mmwr/pdf/other/su6001.pdf

Haywood, C., Jr., Tanabe, P., Naik, R., Beach, M. C., & Lanzkron, S. (2013). The impact of race and disease on sickle cell patient wait times in the emergency department. *American Journal of Emergency Medicine*, *31*(4), 651–656. doi:10.1016/j.ajem.2012.11.005

Kuttner, P. (2016). *The problem with that equity vs. equality graphic you're using*. Retrieved from http://culturalorganizing.org/the-problem-with-that-equity-vs-equality-graphic

National Institute on Minority Health and Health Disparities. (2019). *History*. Retrieved from https://www.nimhd.nih.gov/about/overview/history

Ojodu, J., Hulihan, M. M., Pope, S. N., & Grant, A. M. (2014). Incidence of sickle cell trait—United States, 2010. *Morbidity and Mortality Weekly Report*, *63*(49), 1155–1158. Retrieved from https://www.cdc.gov/mmWr/preview/mmwrhtml/mm6349a3.htm

The statue of Dr. J. Marion Sims in Bryant Park. (1894). *Journal of the American Medical Association*, *23*(18), 689–690. doi:10.1001/jama.1894.02421230029003

U.S. Department of Health and Human Services. (2000). *Healthy People 2010: Understanding and improving health*. Washington, DC: US Government Printing Office. Retrieved from https://www.healthypeople.gov/2010/Document/pdf/uih/2010uih.pdf

U.S. Department of Health and Human Services. (2010). *Phase I report: Recommendations for the framework and format of Healthy People 2020*. Retrieved from http://www.healthypeople.gov/sites/default/files/PhaseI_0.pdf

Wakefield, E. O., Pantaleao, A., Popp, J. M., Dale, L. P., Santanelli, J. P., Litt, M. D., & Zempsky, W. T. (2018). Describing perceived racial bias among youth with sickle cell disease. *Journal of Pediatric Psychology*, *43*(7), 779–788. doi:10.1093/jpepsy/jsy015

PREJUDICE, DISCRIMINATION, AND HEALTH

DENISE C. CARTY ▪ KENT D. KEY ▪ CLEOPATRA CALDWELL ▪
TONYA FRENCH-TURNER ▪ SHANNON BROWNLEE ▪ E. HILL DE LONEY

LEARNING OBJECTIVES

- Define racism, prejudice, and discrimination, and identify the levels at which they operate
- Describe the ways in which racism directly impacts health
- Discuss the ways in which racism affects different racial/ethnic groups
- Identify strategies that can be used to address racism and health
- Describe how community-based interventions can be designed to impact racism at multiple levels

INTRODUCTION

In this chapter, we describe racism and summarize its impact on health inequities for African Americans and other racial and ethnic groups in the U.S. We use "racism" as an umbrella term that encompasses racial ideology, racial prejudice, internalized racism, racial discrimination, and racism-related structures in institutions and society. After describing key dimensions of racism, we explain mechanisms through which each dimension of racism is associated with health inequities. Next, drawing from the public health literature, we highlight empirical support for how racism is associated with health outcomes in racialized population groups in the U.S. We end with a case study of what one community has done to address racism as a fundamental determinant of racial disparities in infant mortality. Throughout this chapter, we use "inequities" and "disparities" interchangeably. We prefer the term "inequities" to connote that health differences fueled by racism are inherently unjust, unfair, and avoidable.

Definitions of Racism

Racism is a system of beliefs and structures that denigrate and disadvantage members of racial groups who are categorized and regarded as inferior. A definition of racism is "beliefs, attitudes, institutional arrangements, and acts that tend to denigrate individuals or groups because of phenotypic characteristics or ethnic group affiliation" (Clark, Anderson, Clark, & Williams, 1999, p. 805). Racism has been operationalized at intrapersonal, interpersonal, and structural levels (Bonilla-Silva, 1997; Jones, 2000; Williams, Lawrence, & Davis, 2019).

The major components or levels of racism can be visualized as intersecting circles rather than discrete classifications. Intrapersonal racism is the ideology of racism internalized in people's thoughts, and it consists of both prejudice and internalized racism. Racial prejudice is operationalized as racist beliefs and attitudes, and it is often subtle or unconscious (Dovidio, 2001; Quillian, 2006), whereas internalized racism is acceptance of negative stereotypes about one's racial group (Jones, 2000). Interpersonal racism, indicated as discrimination, refers to actions or behaviors that unfairly target individuals based on their race. Discrimination can occur between individuals or across institutions, and the differential impact by race can be deliberate or unintentional (Williams et al., 2019). Institutional and structural racism are often described interchangeably. Institutional racism refers to discriminatory policies and practices within institutions such as healthcare, education, and housing (Bailey et al., 2017). Structural racism refers to totality of ways that stratified social systems result in differential opportunities and distribution of societal resources by race (Bonilla-Silva, 1997).

Regardless of the definitions or conceptualizations used, it is essential to understand that racism is multidimensional and systemic. The different levels or dimensions of racism represent differences in the actors, victims, settings, or mechanisms through which each dimension contributes to health inequities. However, each dimension has interactional components. Racism is a pervasive phenomenon that negatively impacts marginalized groups even in the absence of explicitly perceived or reported acts of racism. Individual "acts" of racism rarely operate in isolation, but are driven, often unthinkingly, by ideologies of racial superiority and inferiority and a self-replicating system of disadvantage and oppression for subordinated populations (Bonilla-Silva, 1997).

Four key concepts illustrate racism: (a) prejudice; (b) discrimination; (c) structural racism; and (d) internalized racism. Each concept is listed and described based on the degree to which the concept has been discussed and studied in the medical and public health literature.

Racial prejudice. Racial prejudice refers to negative beliefs, attitudes, or assumptions held about individuals or groups based on their race. Racial prejudice is rooted in ideology and reflects collective biases and misunderstandings that are perpetuated in societies. Hence, prejudice is both an individual and collective phenomenon (Blair & Brondolo, 2017). More nuanced descriptions of prejudice include aversive racism which refers to prejudice at the hands of liberal actors who are not viewed as ostensibly racist (Pearson, Dovidio, & Gaertner, 2009). Racial prejudice perpetuates stigma, which can be a major source of stress for individuals in racially-stigmatized groups (Meyer, Schwartz, & Frost, 2008). Consequences of this stigmatization include stereotype threat and internalized racism that are negative psychological responses to pervading stereotypes about one's racial group (Aronson, Burgess, Phelan, & Juarez, 2013). Prejudice can occur based on race, sex, disability, and other stigmatized social statuses, and prejudice can ultimately lead to interpersonal and systemic discrimination and violence against people in stigmatized social groups (Stuber, Meyer, & Link, 2008). Acknowledging prejudice in multiple forms is important to understanding additional burdens and disadvantages due to the intersections of race and gender, race and class, or race and sexual orientation, for example (Schulz & Mullings, 2006).

Discrimination. Racial discrimination is "differential treatment on the basis of race that disadvantages a racial group" (Blank, Dabady, & Citro, 2004, p. 4); similar definitions apply to discrimination based on sex, sexual orientation, gender identity, and other factors. Discrimination is often studied in public health based on retrospective, self-reported experiences of discrimination (Paradies et al., 2015; Williams & Mohammed, 2009). However, discrimination does not have to be personally recognized nor intentional to have negative consequences for health. Several studies show that implicit bias among health professionals contributes to biased decision-making and lower quality of care (Fitzgerald & Hurst, 2017). Neither the actors nor the targets are likely to perceive or articulate this bias. Institutionalized forms of racial discrimination such as housing discrimination and unequal treatment in healthcare impact individual and population health regardless of conscious perception or reporting.

Structural racism. Structural racism is a social system rooted in racial ideologies that maintains unequal distribution of and access to power and societal resources (Bonilla-Silva, 1997). Structural racism results in systemic racial group inequities that can impact health (Gee & Ford, 2011). Racism is manifested structurally via racial residential segregation (Williams & Collins, 2001), environmental injustice (Morello-Frosch, Zuk, Jerrett, Shamasunder, & Kyle, 2011), political disenfranchisement (Rodriguez, Geronimus, Bound, & Dorling, 2015), mass incarceration (Wildeman & Wang, 2017), and immigration policies (Martinez et al., 2015).

Structural racism is also represented by historical traumas such as African American enslavement (Gaskin, Headen, & White-Means, 2005; Prather et al., 2018), colonization and forced removal of Native Americans from their lands (Dunbar-Ortiz, 2014), internment of Japanese Americans (Gee, Ro, Shariff-Marco, & Chae, 2009), and social marginalization and criminalization of undocumented immigrants (LeBrón & Viruell-Fuentes, 2019). These historical experiences can have intergenerational effects on health (Brave Heart & DeBruyn, 1998; Gee & Ford, 2011). Racism, particularly its structural components, is viewed as a fundamental cause of health inequities (Phelan & Link, 2015).

Internalized racism, cultural racism, and implicit bias. A less frequently researched area in health is internalized racism, whereby members of stigmatized races accept negative stereotypes about their individual or group abilities and self-worth (Jones, 2000). Internalized racism can result in negative self-concepts, depression, and psychological distress for persons who internalize stereotypes of racial inferiority (Mouzon & McLean, 2017). A related concept is "cultural racism," which highlights the ideological and cultural systems that propagate false notions of the superiority of Whites and "white" culture (Cogburn, 2019).

A consequence of cultural racism that has garnered attention in health disparities literature is the notion of implicit or unconscious bias. Implicit bias results from internalized perceptions about group inferiority that are subconsciously acted upon, often to the detriment of the stigmatized groups (van Ryn et al., 2011). Implicit bias among health professionals is associated with poor patient–provider communication and biased treatment recommendations (Fitzgerald & Hurst, 2017). A correlate of implicit bias is aversive racism, which refers to subtle biases in social interactions and decision-making, even among well-intentioned individuals, that contributes to disparities (Pearson et al., 2009).

Genetics, Race, and Racism

A sophisticated understanding of race and racism precludes genetic explanations for racial inequities in health. Science confirms that no genes exclusively or consistently map onto Black or White races, therefore it is misguided to attribute genetics as a primary explanation for racial disparities

(Foster & Sharp, 2004; Goodman, 2000). Race is not real in the biogenetic sense. Rather, race is a social construct that categorizes groups based on ideologies of group superiority and inferiority relative to phenotype, group affiliation, and socially ascribed characteristics (Harawa & Ford, 2009). Racial classification in the U.S. maintains systems of power and privilege for persons racialized and socially accepted as White relative to all other racial/ethnic classes (Omi & Winant, 2015). Despite its genetic irrelevance, race remains an important social factor to consider when describing health inequities due to the close correlations between race and health. However, race is inappropriate to explain health inequities without discussion of co-occurring factors that systematically map onto race to produce differential health outcomes (LaVeist, 1996).

Racism is a peculiar system that both reifies and contradicts the notion of race. Racial classifications and group membership have shifted throughout U.S. history and are still evolving. For example, former Polish and other immigrants who were marginalized because of their ethnicity ultimately became accepted as White (Roediger, 2005). Ethno-religious groups such as Arab or Muslim are normatively racialized as non-White, although Arabs are classified as White in the U.S. Census (Garner & Selod, 2014). Many Latinos/Latinas of Mexican origin, although officially classified as White, are designated foremost as an ethnic group and routinely differentiated from non-Hispanic Whites (Viruell-Fuentes, Miranda, & Abdulrahim, 2012).

In this chapter, we acknowledge the primacy of racism, which transcends fluid conceptualizations of race. We use the terms African American, Black, Asian American, American Indian/Alaska Native, Native American, Latino/Latina/Latinx, and White as relevant to the sociopolitical or scientific context discussed. Racism in the U.S. has particular relevance for African Americans in terms of the intensity and scale of impact, and most studies of racism and health inequities focus on African Americans. Much of our discussion refers to African Americans to reflect the prevailing social, historical, and academic focus on this population. We also refer to Latinos/Latinas and Arab Americans during our discussion in light of the emergent racialization of these groups in the U.S. We acknowledge that there is vast heterogeneity within these broad racial categorizations. However, in-depth coverage of how racism impacts all of these groups is beyond the scope of this chapter. We contend that racism is a system that negatively impacts all groups who are conferred a subordinate racial status; hence, the definitions and discussions about racism in this chapter can be applied broadly to multiple racial groups and even further extended into constructs such as heterosexism and transphobia.

HOW RACISM HARMS HEALTH

Racism operates through multiple pathways and has been associated with multiple health outcomes (Dominguez, 2008; Harrell et al., 2011; Phelan & Link, 2015; Williams & Mohammed, 2013). In this section, we present selected findings that support how racism impacts health for varying population groups. We highlight stress, racial residential segregation, and immigration policy as key pathways through which racism harms health. An emphasis on racism as a determinant of health does not negate interacting factors such as socioeconomic status that remain important drivers of health inequity. However, studies that have analyzed associations between various measures of racism and health have observed sustained effects of racism independent of socioeconomic, demographic, and other health risk factors. Most studies are cross-sectional, and therefore a cause-and-effect relationship between racism and the studied outcome cannot be established. Hence, we report associations. Each reported association implies that higher levels of racism are linearly and significantly associated with health in an unfavorable direction.

Perceived Racism and Health Outcomes

Racism has received considerable attention in public health research as a contributing cause of adverse health outcomes. Overall, racism is associated with poor mental and physical health, although studies are most frequent and the effects are more robust for measures of perceived or self-reported discrimination and mental health outcomes (Paradies et al., 2015; Williams & Mohammed, 2013). Racism has been linked to mental distress and psychiatric disorders in African American, Asian, and Latino/Latina populations (Lewis, Cogburn, & Williams, 2015). A meta-analysis of racism and mental health outcomes that included over 300 studies indicated that self-reported racism was associated with depression, psychological distress, anxiety, post-traumatic stress disorder, and other negative mental health outcomes in addition to decreased positive mental health indicators such as self-esteem, life satisfaction, and overall well-being (Paradies et al., 2015).

Racism is associated with overall physical health, but the association with discrete health outcomes is mixed. Cardiovascular disease risk factors are commonly studied in research that examines racism and physical health. Perceived racism has a positive association with ambulatory blood pressure across multiple studies (Brondolo, Love, Pencille, Schoenthaler, & Ogedegbe, 2011; Dolezsar, McGrath, Herzig, & Miller, 2014), but the relationship to hypertension and other cardiovascular disease risk factors is mixed (Lewis, Williams, Tamene, & Clark, 2014; Paradies et al., 2015). A meta-analysis of perceived racism and physical health outcomes in 50 studies found consistent associations with perceived racism and overweight measures (Paradies et al., 2015). National studies have found that self-reported racism is associated with obesity in Black women (Cozier et al., 2014) and men (Thorpe, Parker, Cobb, Dillard, & Bowie, 2017). Perceived racial discrimination has also been associated with smoking (Borrell et al., 2007; Corral & Landrine, 2012; Landrine & Klonoff, 2000) and alcohol use (Borrell, Kiefe, Diez-Roux, Williams, & Gordon-Larsen, 2013) in African Americans. Most studies of racism and health have examined African American populations, but there is growing attention to documenting how perceived racism influences health in other racial and ethnic groups. Additional discussion of health equity among African American populations can be found in Chapter 5, African American Health Equity.

Asian Americans. Although Asian Americans may be stereotyped as a "model minority," they are not immune to the effects of racism. In a nationwide survey, Asian Americans (including Filipino, Chinese, and Vietnamese subpopulations) were more likely to report discrimination due to race, ethnicity, or skin color than discrimination due to other causes such as gender, age, or income (Gee, Spencer, Chen, & Takeuchi, 2007). In addition, perceived discrimination among Asian Americans was positively associated with the number of reported chronic health conditions including cardiovascular and respiratory diseases, other chronic illnesses, and chronic pain (Gee, Spencer, Chen, & Takeuchi, 2007). Asian Americans who self-reported discrimination were two to three times more likely to have a mental health disorder, including depression and anxiety, controlling for sociodemographic, cultural, and co-occurring health factors (Gee, Spencer, Chen, Yip, & Takeuchi, 2007).

Some studies have highlighted coping styles used by Asians to buffer discrimination experiences. Perceived racial discrimination was associated with depression among Southeast Asian refugees (Noh, Beiser, Kaspar, Hou, & Rummens, 1999) and Korean immigrants (Noh & Kaspar, 2003) in Canada. Passive coping and high ethnic identity among Southeast Asians and active, problem-focused coping among more established Korean immigrants moderated the effect of perceived racism on depression. In another study, Asian Americans who reported high levels of racial/ethnic discrimination were less likely to be current smokers if they had high levels of ethnic identity (Chae et al., 2008). These studies demonstrate variation by national origin, refugee or immigrant status, and ethnic identity, and suggest that culturally-concordant coping may help to buffer the deleterious health effects of racism at the individual level.

Additional discussion of health equity among Asian populations can be found in Chapter 7, Asian American Health Equity.

Latinos/Latinas. In the U.S., Latinos/Latinas are designated as an ethnic group, and they are primarily enumerated in the White racial category according to the U.S. Census (U.S. Census Bureau, 2019). However, Latinos/Latinas hold a subordinate racial position relative to non-Hispanic Whites, and they are often viewed as "foreigners" regardless of nativity or immigration status (LeBrón & Viruell-Fuentes, 2019). This marginalization makes Latinos/Latinas subject to racial/ethnic discrimination, and there is a growing body of work examining racism and health among Latinos/Latinas (Viruell-Fuentes et al., 2012). In a multi-site study, perceived ethnic discrimination was prevalent among Central Americans, Cubans, Dominicans, Mexicans, Puerto Ricans, South Americans, and Other Latino/Latinas (Arellano-Morales et al., 2015). Perceived racial discrimination has also been associated with self-reported mental health (Stuber, Galea, Ahern, Blaney, & Fuller, 2003) and physical health (Finch, Hummer, Kolody, & Vega, 2001) in Latino/Latina populations. Among Puerto Ricans in Boston, Massachusetts, perceived discrimination due to ethnicity, race, or language was associated with more reported chronic medical conditions, past smoking, and higher diastolic blood pressure (Todorova, Falcon, Lincoln, & Price, 2010). Oza-Frank and Cunningham (2010) observed that increasing body mass index (BMI) was associated with longer duration of U.S. residence for Latino/Latina immigrants. Additional discussion of health equity among Latinx populations can be found in Chapter 6, Health Equity in U.S. Latinx Populations.

Arab Americans. Arab Americans are at heightened risk of experiencing racial hostility due to the social and political climate that associates Arabs and Muslims with terrorism. Arab Americans who are of Middle Eastern descent are formally classified as White (Office of Management and Budget, 1997). However, for many Arab Americans, the racialization of Islam ascribes to them a marginalized social position and they are subject to significant discrimination and associated health effects (Abuelezam, El-Sayed, & Galea, 2017; Samari, Alcala, & Sharif, 2018). California and Michigan have the largest populations of Arab Americans in the U.S., and most population health studies of Arab Americans are based in those states. In a Detroit study, Arab Americans were more likely to report perceived discrimination if they identified as non-White, but they were more likely to experience psychological distress associated with discrimination if they identified as White (Abdulrahim, James, Yamout, & Baker, 2012). In a population-based study in Michigan, Arab Americans who perceived ethnic discrimination and individual or family abuse after 9/11 reported higher levels of psychological distress and worse self-reported health status (Padela & Heisler, 2010). In California, women who had Arab surnames had increased rates of preterm birth and low birth weight 6 months after 9/11 compared to baseline rates in the previous year (Lauderdale, 2006). Similar results were not replicated among Arab American women in Michigan who experienced no change in preterm birth or low birth weight before and after 9/11

(El-Sayed, Hadley, & Galea, 2008). A number of studies have documented increased psychological distress for Muslim populations related to discrimination based on their religious or ethnic identity (Samari et al., 2018). Finally, Arab Americans are increasingly the victims of hate crimes and hence subject to direct physical and psychological trauma which impact their health (Arab American Institute Foundation, 2018).

Native Americans. There is a well-documented history of racial inequities experienced by Native Americans in the U.S. (Brave Heart & DeBruyn, 1998; Jones, 2006). Much of the public health literature addresses how social disadvantage and psychological trauma influence health behaviors such as alcohol and substance use (Skewes & Blume, 2019). There is also a large literature on health conditions such as cardiovascular diseases, diabetes, and other chronic diseases and risk factors (Hutchinson & Shin, 2014). Published research on measured racism or racial discrimination in relation to specific health outcomes for Native Americans is less common. In a small sample of American Indians in the Northern Plains, perceived racial discrimination was associated with elevated diastolic blood pressure (Thayer, Blair, Buchwald, & Manson, 2017). Perceived racial discrimination was also associated with smoking in a multi-site urban American Indian/Alaska Native LGBT population (Johnson-Jennings, Belcourt, Town, Walls, & Walters, 2014). Reported racial discrimination was also associated with illicit substance use in a sample of American Indian youth residing in the Cherokee Nation (Garrett, Livingston, Livingston, & Komro, 2017). Greater availability of public health data on American Indian/Alaska Native populations (Bauer & Plescia, 2014) and expanded use of standardized self-report measures of discrimination with this population may improve findings on perceived discrimination and health among Native Americans (Gonzales et al., 2016). Additional discussion of health equity among Native American populations can be found in Chapter 8, American Indian and Alaska Native Health Equity.

Racism and Stress

Stress is an important mechanism through which racism harms health. As a chronic stressor, racism can cause biological dysfunction at the cellular level and health deterioration over the life course (Gee, Walsemann, & Brondolo, 2012; Harrell et al., 2011). One marker of chronic stress is allostatic load, a maladaptive biological response to frequent and cumulative stress which impairs normal neuroendocrine and inflammatory mechanisms and results in accelerated wear-and-tear on body systems (McEwen & Wingfield, 2003). Racial discrimination has been shown to affect stress pathways by dysregulating the hypothalamic-pituitary-adrenal (HPA) axis and producing elevated stress hormones such as cortisol, which causes inflammation and precipitates disease (Berger & Sarnyai, 2015). Another stress-related mechanism is the shortening of cellular telomeres—an indicator of premature aging (Liu & Kawachi, 2017).

Although findings are mixed, there is plausible support that racism-related stress is associated with physiologic changes that precipitate poor health. Studies indicate greater cardioreactivity in African American women in response to simulated stressors (Lepore et al., 2006; McNeilly et al., 1995) as well as greater allostatic load (Chyu & Upchurch, 2011) and hypertension prevalence (Hicken, Lee, Morenoff, House, & Williams, 2014) in relation to stress. Other studies have found associations with racial discrimination and shortened telomeres in African American men and women (Chae et al., 2014; Lu et al., 2019). Alternatively, studies have also demonstrated no direct association between racism-related stress and adverse physiologic responses (Albert et al., 2008; Krieger et al., 2013).

Racism is one of multiple "stressors" that humans can experience, alongside other stressors such as death of a family member, divorce, job loss, and other stressful events. Nonetheless, racism is not merely a life event, but a total lived experience. The pervasiveness of racism makes it a particularly noxious stressor that impacts health over the life course (Gee et al., 2012). Racism operates as microaggressions (Lewis, Williams, Peppers, & Gadson, 2017), unfair treatment (Chae et al., 2008), and major events (DeVylder et al., 2018; Lopez et al., 2017; Padela & Heisler, 2010). Racism can be direct or vicarious (Heard-Garris, Cale, Camaj, Hamati, & Dominguez, 2018). Structural racism produces inequities in education, employment, housing, and healthcare (Gee & Ford, 2011). All of these experiences contribute to chronic, cumulative stress for racially marginalized individuals and communities. Racism is thus a "mega" stressor that encapsulates multiple stressful experiences.

Actions employed by individuals to counter racism-related stress can also harm health. One such mechanism is high-effort coping, whereby individuals persist doggedly to counteract social stereotypes and resist social and structural barriers. James (1994) coined the term "John Henryism" to describe this phenomenon with reference to African American or Black populations. Other researchers have described this concept as "vigilance" (Himmelstein, Young, Sanchez, & Jackson, 2015) with applicability to diverse racial/ethnic groups. Overall, the findings on vigilant, high-effort coping are mixed, with evidence of limited effect or differential impact on health across populations by race, sex, and socioeconomic status (Felix et al., 2019; Subramanyam et al., 2013).

Social–psychological responses such as internalized racism have been associated with major depression and psychological distress in African Americans (James, 2017; Mouzon & McLean, 2017). Internalized racism has also been linked to adverse birth outcomes (Chae et al., 2018) and hypertension (Chae, Nuru-Jeter, & Adler, 2012) in Blacks.

Stress-induced unhealthy behaviors can be a potential pathway through which racism influences health outcomes. Perceived racial discrimination has been associated with smoking and alcohol consumption in African Americans (Borrell et al., 2013) and heavy drinking in Latinos/Latinas (Borrell et al., 2010). Race-related stress was also associated with emotional eating in Black women (Longmire-Avital & McQueen, 2019). However, in a longitudinal analysis, racial discrimination did not predict unhealthy eating behaviors over time in a cohort of Black Americans monitored for hypertension and related risk factors (Forsyth, Schoenthaler, Ogedegbe, & Ravenell, 2014).

Residential Segregation

Racial residential segregation refers to the relative concentration and geographic separation of racial groups in residential areas (Massey & Denton, 1988). Historical policies and practices such as redlining and mortgage discrimination helped to create the current conditions of racially segregated communities with concentrated neighborhood disadvantage (Massey & Denton, 1993; Williams & Collins, 2001). Residential segregation dictates the quality of schools (Kozol, 1991) and employment opportunities (Dickerson, 2007), which are known predictors of health via educational attainment and income.

Racial segregation also influences the built environment in ways that lessen or promote health risks. Neighborhood factors that promote obesogenic environments in Black and Latino/Latina communities are low availability of supermarkets, parks, and exercise facilities, and safety issues related to crime and traffic which deter physical activity (Lovasi, Hutson, Guerra, & Neckerman, 2009). Kwate (2008) conceptualized that concentrated poverty, permissive zoning regulations, commercial targeting, and relative lack of political power promoted the proliferation of fast food establishments in predominantly Black neighborhoods and consequential risks for obesity. Racial inequities in poverty, unemployment, and home ownership at the county level were also associated with a higher prevalence of obesity in communities (Bell, Kerr, & Young, 2019).

Racially segregated neighborhoods have increased exposure to environmental toxins (Morello-Frosch et al., 2011) and lack structural supports for health-promoting activities such as walking and other recreational activities (Kramer & Hogue, 2009; Williams & Collins, 2001). Residents of racially-segregated neighborhoods may also have limited access to quality healthcare facilities and less use of health services (Gaskin, Price, Brandon, & LaVeist, 2009). In terms of measurable effects, racial segregation has been associated with preterm birth and low birth weight (Mehra et al., 2017), cancer disparities (Landrine et al., 2017), and cardiovascular disease risks (Kershaw & Albrecht, 2015).

Immigration Policy

Immigration policy can be conceptualized as structural racism to the extent that it negatively targets and disadvantages racialized groups. Historically, immigration and citizenship-related policies gave preference to White populations and European-origin nationalities, to the exclusion of non-European immigrants, including persons from Asian countries, the Pacific Islands, Africa, the Caribbean, and South and Central America (Gee & Ford, 2011). Racist theories about non-White people as diseased, unclean, morally corrupt, and inferior contributed to these policies (Gee & Ford, 2011). Although the 1965 Immigration and Naturalization Act repealed many of the explicit national-origin restrictions, there has been a resurgence of exclusionary immigration policies targeting immigrants from Central and South America and from Arab countries in the Middle East (Abuelezam et al., 2017; Gee & Ford, 2011).

The process of social stratification of immigrant groups impacted by immigration policies contributes to the "racialization" of these groups. Racialization refers to the construction of race in the larger society (Omi & Winant, 2015). Inherent in the racialization process is not just the assigning of a racial category, but the social ranking ascribed to that category. In the U.S. context, White is presumed to be racially dominant, and all other groups are ranked lower in the racial hierarchy. The racialization process would render Mexican immigrants and Arabs as non-White despite their official categorization as White by federal standards (Office of Management and Budget, 1997). Although Latinos/Latinas are considered an ethnic group by federal standards, in practice they are marginalized along racial/ethnic lines (LeBrón & Viruell-Fuentes, 2019; Omi & Winant, 2015).

The marginalization and exclusion of immigrant groups as a result of immigration policy constricts opportunities for immigrant groups, in turn creating health inequities. Documented and undocumented immigrants have restricted access to safety nets such as Medicaid, housing and education subsidies, and other public support programs (Gee & Ford, 2011). The barring of undocumented workers from legal employment increases the chances for inequitable pay and working conditions. These conditions can help to concentrate poverty and have other indirect and direct effects on health.

Other consequences of racialization and "othering" of immigrant groups include social stress in relation to discrimination and immigration policies. The threat of deportation can create heightened vigilance and chronic stress in immigrant communities. Latinos/Latinas in states and communities with more exclusionary immigrant policies have reported more perceived discrimination (Almeida, Biello, Pedraza, Wintner, & Viruell-Fuentes, 2016), poorer self-rated health (Vargas, Sanchez, & Juarez, 2017), and more frequent poor mental health days (Hatzenbuehler et al., 2017) than their counterparts in communities with less restrictive immigration policies. Immigration raids have also been associated with lower self-rated health and increased risk of low birth weight among Latinos/Latinas in affected communities, regardless of immigration status (Novak, Geronimus, & Martinez-Cardoso, 2017; Vargas et al., 2017). Moreover, enforcement of federal immigration laws by local authorities have resulted in greater mistrust of health services and delayed healthcare seeking among immigrant Latinos/Latinas (Rhodes et al., 2015).

Other racial/ethnic groups are not immune to the deleterious effects of anti-immigration policies or public sentiment on health. In theory, racialization would be a normative experience for all migrant groups to the U.S. with varying impact by immigration cohort period, national origin, and racial phenotype together with moderators such as socioeconomic status, time in the U.S., and psychosocial orientations such as ethnic identity. However, studies are mixed with no generalized pattern of positive or negative adaptation and related health effects across immigrant groups to the racialization process in the U.S. (Cobb et al., 2019; Gee et al., 2009; Landale & Oropesa, 2002; Mouzon & McLean, 2017; Read & Emerson, 2005; Samari et al., 2018).

Healthcare

A 2003 Institute of Medicine Report and subsequent federal reports on inequalities in healthcare have documented differences in the access to, and quality of, care for racial and ethnic minorities that are associated with poorer health outcomes (Agency for Healthcare Research and Quality, 2019; Smedley, Stith, & Nelson, 2003). In general, African Americans receive lower quality healthcare (Fiscella & Sanders, 2016) and report more racial discrimination in health encounters (Smedley et al., 2003) than Whites. It has been shown that implicit bias in the healthcare system results in healthcare that is perceived more negatively by African Americans than Whites (Johnson, Saha, Arbelaez, Beach, & Cooper, 2004; van Ryn & Burke, 2000). Implicit bias and perceived racism are associated with less patient-centered communication, patient mistrust of the healthcare system, delayed entry into care, and lower adherence to prescribed treatment (Ben, Cormack, Harris, & Paradies, 2017; Blair et al., 2013). However, the weight of the evidence does not associate implicit bias with differential medical treatment or patient health outcomes (Hall et al., 2015). Feagin and Bennefield (2014) argue that the individual-level assessments and provider–patient interactions are insufficient to capture the effect of racism on health or healthcare inequalities, and they advocate for a more historical and structural analysis of how racism has structured ideology and healthcare institutions and left a legacy of extensive health inequities in communities.

STRATEGIES TO ADDRESS RACISM AND HEALTH

Public health practitioners may be less likely to view structural factors, including racism, within the purview of professional intervention. However, addressing fundamental causes has been articulated as necessary for reducing health inequities (Ford & Airhihenbuwa, 2010; Link & Phelan, 1995). Accordingly, addressing racism is a critical approach to advancing health equity (Bailey et al., 2017). The public health literature is replete with observational studies testing various associations of racism (particularly self-reported discrimination) with health, but the field is lacking in interventions to remedy structural and other forms of racism (Carty et al., 2011; Castle, Wendel, Kerr, Brooms, & Rollins, 2019; Hardeman, Murphy, Karbeah, & Kozhimannil, 2018). In this section, we explore specific tools and interventions to address racism to reduce health inequities.

On an intrapersonal level, there are some orientations that people use, consciously or subconsciously, to counter the effects of racism. James (1993) offered a unique cultural perspective that highlighted indigenous cultural strengths within communities that could be employed to buffer against racism. Another orientation is racial or ethnic identity (Caldwell, Kohn-Wood, Schmeelk-Cone, Chavous, & Zimmerman, 2004). The interaction of racial/ethnic identity with other social identities (i.e., gender, age, economic status) highlights the intersectional approach to understanding and working with racially identified groups.

To delineate the meaning of racialized experiences for the mental health of ethnically diverse Black adolescents, Caldwell, Guthrie, and Jackson (2006) examined the intersectional nature of ethnicity and gender as social identities in the face of racial discrimination. They found that African American and Caribbean Black youth shared a number of characteristics related to discriminatory experiences, the meaning of racial identity, and mental health, regardless of ethnicity or gender, perhaps because of the strong ethnic homogenizing forces that are prevalent in American society. There were, however, unique findings that demonstrated the complexity of race/ethnicity and gender as embedded social identities. Multiple aspects of racial identity (e.g., centrality of race, public regard or the views of others, racial pride) were protective factors, but in different ways. Centrality of race to identity was associated with fewer depressive symptoms for Caribbean Black females, while believing that other groups had favorable views about Blacks related to fewer depressive symptoms for Caribbean Black males. Less racial pride was associated with more depressive symptoms for females, regardless of ethnicity. Further, African American and Caribbean Black females who reported more experiences with racial discrimination also reported higher levels of depressive symptoms, while discriminatory experiences were associated with lower self-esteem for all youth.

Seaton, Caldwell, Sellers, and Jackson (2010) also used an intersectional approach to examine ethnicity, gender, and age as moderators of perceived discrimination and mental health. They determined that older Caribbean Black female adolescents exhibited higher depressive symptoms and lower life satisfaction when faced with higher levels of discrimination compared with older African American male adolescents.

These nuanced findings are essential for developing services for ethnically diverse Black youth for whom different racial identity attitudes are critical to consider in efforts to reduce intrapersonal distress due to racial discrimination. For example, Miller and colleagues conducted a review of psychological practice recommendations to address racism (Miller et al., 2018). They categorized eight general approaches that counselors used. Approaches included psychoeducation, validation, critical consciousness, examination of privilege and racial attitudes, culturally responsive social support, developing a positive identity, minimizing self-blame, and outreach/advocacy. Framed with an intersectionality lens, approaches to intervention should incorporate multiple social identities to reflect the meaning of racialized experiences for ethnically diverse Black populations (Caldwell et al., 2006).

Community-Based Approaches

Socio Ecological Model and Undoing Racism

The Genesee County/Flint, MI Racial and Ethnic Approaches to Community Health (REACH) team was guided by the Socio-Ecological Model (SEM) that recognizes the need for engagement at all levels (individual, interpersonal, organizations/institutions, community, providers/healthcare systems, and policy). This model provided a broad platform for addressing social determinants of health associated with racial disparities in infant mortality. Guided by the SEM, the REACH team, comprised of public health, community, academic, and other institutional partners, developed and implemented interventions with a focus on "undoing" racism at the individual, institutional, and systems levels. In addition, REACH adopted principles of the People's Institute for Survival and Beyond (PISAB), which holds that racism has been consciously and systematically erected, and it can be undone only if people understand what it is, where it comes from, how it functions, and why it is perpetuated (PISAB, n.d.). The REACH team adopted the PISAB working

---

CASE STUDY | **UNDOING RACISM TO REDUCE RACIAL DISPARITIES IN INFANT MORTALITY**

Racism is a stressor on multiple levels for African Americans and other racial and ethnic minorities. Racism has been shown to negatively impact one's health, including depressive symptoms, serious psychological distress, decreased self-esteem, and poorer overall physical and mental health (Williams & Mohammed, 2013). More specifically, the health impacts of racism on African American women of childbearing age include maternal stress, low birth weight, preterm delivery, and damaging effects on women's reproductive health and that of their unborn infants (Dominguez, 2011; Giurgescu, McFarlin, Lomax, Craddock, & Albrecht, 2011).

To address these health disparities, multiple community-based interventions working simultaneously can be effective in reducing racial and ethnic health inequities and improving health outcomes for affected individuals and populations. Racial and Ethnic Approaches to Community Health (REACH) in Flint, Michigan was one such program (Carty et al., 2011; Kannan, Sparks, Webster, Krishnakumar, & Lumeng, 2010; Kruger, Carty, Turbeville, French-Turner, & Brownlee, 2015; Kruger, French-Turner, & Brownlee, 2013; Pestronk & Franks, 2003; Selig, Tropiano, & Greene-Moton, 2006). An overarching strategy for the program was the adoption of the socio-ecological model (SEM), which allowed the Flint REACH team to address racism on multiple levels.

This case study will describe a community's (Flint/Genesee County, MI) efforts to address racism and its effects on health disparities in maternal and infant health. Quotes from REACH program participants, general community residents, and REACH program coordinators are highlighted as we share what we did and what we learned.

definition of racism, "racism = racial prejudice + power," which was easy to adopt and understand among various stakeholders (PISAB, n.d.). Clear distinctions between racism, prejudice, bigotry, and associated terms were also necessary to move the work forward. The REACH team developed a shared understanding of racism, acknowledged its multi-faceted manifestations and health impacts, and worked collaboratively to mitigate those negative effects to reduce disparities in African American infant mortality.

Table 2.1 illustrates interventions that were created and strategically aligned with all levels of the SEM using PISAB principles and describes the impact at each level.

Community Voices

Individual/interpersonal level

Just hearing a different perspective probably opened a door to me wanting to learn even more about the physical impacts of racism and the impact that can have on a pregnancy and on the infant.

Organizational/institutional level

It has been difficult for organizations to get involved because everyone has their own agenda. But focusing on those shared issues that affect infant mortality is a way to bring some of those organizations into this forum. It's about highlighting how infant mortality is connected to violence, to the community, to unity, to familial responsibility.

Health system/providers level

REACH is one of the unique places where the community actually gets to talk to the people in healthcare. Oftentimes, healthcare is just thrown at us without our input. But this is a place where we actually get to talk to those people who were in charge of it, and who were making some decisions and also voice our opinions and concerns.

Societal/policy level

I think it's strategically important that REACH is housed in the health department, which is a policy-making agency within the community for healthcare and health service delivery. As it relates to mortality and other health-related issues, you have the community people who help make policy as part of the process, as opposed to institutions making policy before engaging the community.

Community-Based and Community-Engaged Approaches

Community engagement (CE) is defined as the process of working collaboratively with groups of people who are affiliated by geographic proximity, special interests, or similar situations with respect to issues affecting their well-being (CDC, 1997). The CE approach involves improving population health by building trust, utilizing effective communication strategies, creating long-standing collaborations, and enlisting new allies and resources. Community-based participatory approaches (CBPA) fall on the spectrum of CE, and necessitate CE throughout the process (Key et al., 2019).

The REACH team adopted CBPA/CE principles to guide the project approach in engaging community-based organizations, faith-based organizations, and other institutions within the

TABLE 2.1 Socio-Ecological Model and Related Interventions and Impact for Genesee County/Flint, MI Racial and Ethnic Approaches to Community Health (REACH) Program

SOCIO-ECOLOGICAL LEVEL	REACH INTERVENTIONS	FOCUS AREAS	IMPACT
Individual/ Interpersonal	▪ Undoing Racism Workshops ▪ Birth Brothers and Birth Sisters ▪ Black Men for Social Change ▪ Women Taking Charge of Their Health Destiny ▪ African Culture Education Development Center ▪ Middle Passage Experience ▪ African American Healthy Eating Curriculum ▪ African Health Navigators ▪ Maternal and Infant Health Advocacy Service	▪ Undoing internalized racial oppression ▪ Teaching African history and culture; promoting cultural pride; self-love ▪ Individual and family advocacy and support ▪ Peer mentorship ▪ Promoting healthy behaviors	▪ Engaged, educated, and empowered community residents concerning racism, health disparities, and infant mortality. ▪ Interventions provided self- and cultural empowerment to inform health consciousness and decision-making.
Organizational/ Institutional	▪ Windshield Bus Tours ▪ Undoing Racism Workshops ▪ Middle Passage Experience ▪ African Culture Education Development Center	▪ Interactive community driving tours with students, professionals, and executive leaders to highlight social determinants influencing maternal and infant health ▪ Educating and reforming institutional "gatekeepers"	▪ Raised awareness of historical, cultural, social, and environmental barriers that negatively affect the health outcomes of African Americans in Flint/Genesee County.
Healthcare Systems and Providers	▪ Undoing Racism Workshops ▪ Windshield Tours ▪ African Culture Education Development Center	▪ Undoing institutionalized racism	▪ Explored the role of "unconscious racism" within institutions and systems.

(continued)

TABLE 2.1 Socio-Ecological Model and Related Interventions and Impact for Genesee County/Flint, MI Racial and Ethnic Approaches to Community Health (REACH) Program *(continued)*

SOCIO-ECOLOGICAL LEVEL	REACH INTERVENTIONS	FOCUS AREAS	IMPACT
Healthcare Systems and Providers (cont.)	▓ Cultural Competence Training ▓ Programs to Reduce Infant Death Effectively ▓ Fetal-Infant Mortality Review	▓ Provider bias ▓ Quality healthcare	▓ Highlighted the role providers and systems play in perpetuating racism and understanding how it can be "undone" to provide those services necessary to reduce racial disparities in infant mortality. ▓ Provided the services necessary to optimize maternal health and reduce infant mortality risks.
Community	▓ Billboard Media Campaign ▓ Community Outreach and Engagement	▓ Advocate for improvements in social and built environment ▓ Engagement and outreach to communities ▓ Foster community strengths and resources ▓ Community-based participatory approaches	▓ Successfully advocated to improve the built environment by adding a new bus stop in an underserved community to improve transportation access to community resources such as clinics and grocery stores.
Societal/Policies	▓ Community Outreach and Engagement ▓ Community Leadership Strategies	▓ SWOT analysis ▓ Identify priority systemic changes needed to improve health equity	▓ Identified systemic changes needed in education, healthcare, and social service institutions. ▓ Transformed the role of gatekeepers.

SWOT, strengths, weaknesses, opportunities, and threats.

African American community in creating culturally specific interventions. This provided the opportunity to utilize community expertise in the design and implementation of these interventions. In addition, these principles framed the project's work by bringing to bear the value the community partners' knowledge of knowing what will and will not work within the community's context. This model was a true representation of community being an equal and equitable partner.

Community Voices

In order to address any disparity – and I'm talking disparities across the board, across all races – you really have to involve the community. The community has to be top priority. They have to be equal players at the table, and I mean equal in their voice, equal in the resources, equal in the implementation, in the decision-making and everything. They have to be equal partners. We can't just rely on our specialties, our public health training, and think that we know what works for the people out in the community. We need to talk to the people and have them on board with us every step of the way.

Community Outreach and Engagement

Utilizing multiple engagement strategies, the REACH team was able to garner community buy-in and provide education through outreach events. Through citywide media campaigns (i.e., billboards, educational information on city buses) and numerous events, the REACH project was well-received by the community. REACH also held annual events to report on the progress of the project and gain valuable feedback and input from community residents. This feedback was collected and integrated into the work plans.

Community Voices

We went out to a selective area that had most of the infant mortality cases in the neighborhood, and we canvassed the whole area with information and resources. We passed out bags for people with cleansing supplies and information letting women know how to connect to one of the major hospitals. We addressed food issues and directed them to fresh fruit that they could pick up at a church around the corner. It was really informative. We did that four years in a row.

Lessons Learned

Addressing Racism Using the Socio-Ecological Model

Addressing racial and ethnic infant mortality from an "undoing" racism perspective is complex. There is no "one size fits all" model to do this type of work. The impact that racism has on racial and ethnic health disparities is multi-faceted. Therefore, multi-faceted approaches were most effective in addressing the issue. The SEM worked well for the Genesee County REACH project. This approach allowed for community participation on multiple levels to address the impact of racism on health disparities. Specifically-tailored work plans with activities and expected outcomes were developed at each SEM level to gauge effectiveness. Most importantly, community partners were extensively involved with the design and adaptation of the work and ongoing community engagement at all levels was a key component to the success of the project.

Community Voices

One of the things that appeals to us is looking at all of the different variables that go into infant mortality. It really is about the big picture.

Bidirectional Education

Early in the development of the REACH project, it was clear that bidirectional education was warranted given the diversity of the REACH team. Trust and transparency were of the utmost importance. In order to achieve this, communication was crucial in ensuring equal and equitable contributions to the processes. Health department, academic, and institutional partners also understood the necessity of being culturally sensitive to the needs, beliefs, and approaches for effectively engaging community residents. In turn, community residents and REACH program participants often remarked on bidirectional transfer of information to and from their households and neighborhoods as central to creating the capacity for community to discuss the multi-levels of racism, its impact on community health, and REACH program interventions designed to undo racism. Engaging in dialogues on multiple levels in the community was a strength for the project.

Community Voices

The REACH program involves people of African descent, people who look like me. And they show how we can work together in the community to help us with our own health and environment and how to live comfortably and engage my children and my grandchildren. So, I'm learning and teaching at the same time.

Community-Developed Interventions

Interventions that were co-developed and co-created by the African American community were most effective in garnering community buy-in. This bolstered the confidence of community members, which was particularly important when they needed to engage with powerful systems such as governmental bodies and healthcare systems. This sense of co-ownership generated community buy-in and provided a sustainable model for many of the REACH project interventions.

For example, character development and mentorship strategies were employed to enhance mental and physical health and promote pregnancy prevention among youth. Character development began with fostering an understanding of the history and culture of African Americans and Ancient Africans (how the village model worked, how they ate, how they lived, and what they believed). Next, the program explored how African Americans value themselves and others who look like them. This was followed by instilling an understanding of cultural pride and identity which began with an individual focus and expanded to embrace the family and broader community.

Community Voices

Character development teaches young men and women that they are valuable because they're intelligent, because they have character, because they have purpose, and because their life has meaning. How does this connect to infant mortality? If I can get young ladies and young men to start to value who they are, then sex is not the only thing that they think they have of value. Each sees themselves as a full, complete person who has inner value, as opposed to only seeing their value to someone else. And so that's where we see that connection and we feel very strongly that is a valid connection.

CONCLUSION

As described previously, racism is a system of beliefs, actions, and structures that oppresses members of minority racial groups. The impact that historical and current racism has upon the health of minority groups within the United States is profound, and operates on intrapersonal, interpersonal, and structural levels. Each level has similar but also unique elements impacting health that require multiple levels of intervention to adequately address. Increasing evidence directly connects experiences of racism to biological processes in the body (such as allostatic load), providing new avenues for quantifying its effects on health. Multiple frameworks for addressing the effects of racism exist, and approaches that address health equity from an intersectional lens are particularly important.

DISCUSSION QUESTIONS

- Why is it important to distinguish between prejudice and discrimination? Which is related more closely to implicit bias, and why?

- How do social and biological bases for health inequities (e.g., racism, allostatic load) help to counter erroneous assertions regarding a genetic basis for inequities?

- Why is it important to take an intersectional lens when examining the effects of racism on different racial/ethnic groups?

- Consider the case of the role of healthcare discrimination in receipt of needed painkiller medication. What are intervention targets at each level of the socio-ecological model?

- Why is it important to have the voice of communities affected by racism at the heart of efforts to ameliorate its effects?

REFERENCES

Abdulrahim, S., James, S. A., Yamout, R., & Baker, W. (2012). Discrimination and psychological distress: Does Whiteness matter for Arab Americans? *Social Science and Medicine, 75*, 2116–2123. doi:10.1016/j.socscimed.2012.07.030

Abuelezam, N. N., El-Sayed, A. M., & Galea, S. (2017). Arab American health in a racially charged U.S. *American Journal of Preventive Medicine, 52*, 810–812. doi:10.1016/j.amepre.2017.02.021

Agency for Healthcare Research and Quality. (2019, September). *2018 National Healthcare Quality and Disparities Report*. Retrieved from https://www.ahrq.gov/research/findings/nhqrdr/nhqdr18/index.html

Albert, M. A., Ravenell, J., Glynn, R. J., Khera, A., Halevy, N., & de Lemos, J. A. (2008). Cardiovascular risk indicators and perceived race/ethnic discrimination in the Dallas Heart Study. *American Heart Journal, 156*, 1103–1109. doi:10.1016/j.ahj.2008.07.027

Almeida, J., Biello, K. B., Pedraza, F., Wintner, S., & Viruell-Fuentes, E. (2016). The association between anti-immigrant policies and perceived discrimination among Latinos in the US: A multilevel analysis. *Social Science and Medicine Population Health, 2,* 897–903. doi:10.1016/j.ssmph.2016.11.003

Arab American Institute Foundation. (2018). *Underreported, under threat: Hate crime in the United States and the targeting of Arab Americans 1991-2016.* Retrieved from https://d3n8a8pro7vhmx.cloudfront.net/aai/pages/14141/attachments/original/1534353696/Underreported_Under_Threat.pdf?1534353696

Arellano-Morales, L., Roesch, S. C., Gallo, L. C., Emory, K. T., Molina, K. M., Gonzalez, P., … Brondolo, E. (2015). Prevalence and correlates of perceived ethnic discrimination in the Hispanic Community Health Study/Study of Latinos Sociocultural Ancillary Study. *Journal of Latina/o Psychology, 3,* 160–176. doi:10.1037/lat0000040

Aronson, J., Burgess, D., Phelan, S. M., & Juarez, L. (2013). Unhealthy interactions: The role of stereotype threat in health disparities. *American Journal of Public Health, 103,* 50–56. doi:10.2105/AJPH.2012.300828

Bailey, Z. D., Krieger, N., Agenor, M., Graves, J., Linos, N., & Bassett, M. T. (2017). Structural racism and health inequities in the USA: Evidence and interventions. *Lancet, 389,* 1453–1463. doi:10.1016/S0140-6736(17)30569-X

Bauer, U. E., & Plescia, M. (2014). Addressing disparities in the health of American Indian and Alaska Native people: The importance of improved public health data. *American Journal of Public Health, 104*(Suppl. 3), S255–S257. doi:10.2105/AJPH.2013.301602

Bell, C. N., Kerr, J., & Young, J. L. (2019). Associations between obesity, obesogenic environments, and structural racism vary by county-level racial composition. *International Journal of Environmental Research and Public Health, 16,* 861. doi:10.3390/ijerph16050861

Ben, J., Cormack, D., Harris, R., & Paradies, Y. (2017). Racism and health service utilisation: A systematic review and meta-analysis. *PLoS One, 12,* e0189900. doi:10.1371/journal.pone.0189900

Berger, M., & Sarnyai, Z. (2015). "More than skin deep": Stress neurobiology and mental health consequences of racial discrimination. *Stress, 18,* 1–10. doi:10.3109/10253890.2014.989204

Blair, I. V., & Brondolo, E. (2017). Moving beyond the individual: Community-level prejudice and health. *Social Science and Medicine, 183,* 169–172. doi:10.1016/j.socscimed.2017.04.041

Blair, I. V., Steiner, J. F., Fairclough, D. L., Hanratty, R., Price, D. W., Hirsh, H. K., … Havranek, E. P. (2013). Clinicians' implicit ethnic/racial bias and perceptions of care among Black and Latino patients. *Annals of Family Medicine, 11,* 43–52. doi:10.1370/afm.1442

Blank, R. M., Dabady, M., & Citro, C. F. (Eds.) (2004). *Measuring racial discrimination: Panel on methods for assessing discrimination.* Washington, DC: National Academies Press. Retrieved from https://www.nap.edu/read/10887/chapter/1

Bonilla-Silva, E. (1997). Rethinking racism: Toward a structural interpretation. *American Sociological Review, 62,* 465–480. doi:10.2307/2657316

Borrell, L. N., Diez Roux, A. V., Jacobs, D. R., Jr., Shea, S., Jackson, S. A., Shrager, S., & Blumenthal, R. S. (2010). Perceived racial/ethnic discrimination, smoking and alcohol consumption in the Multi-Ethnic Study of Atherosclerosis (MESA). *Preventive Medicine, 51,* 307–312. doi:10.1016/j.ypmed.2010.05.017

Borrell, L. N., Jacobs, D. R., Jr., Williams, D. R., Pletcher, M. J., Houston, T. K., & Kiefe, C. I. (2007). Self-reported racial discrimination and substance use in the coronary artery risk development in adults study. *American Journal of Epidemiology, 166,* 1068–1079. doi:10.1093/aje/kwm180

Borrell, L. N., Kiefe, C. I., Diez-Roux, A. V., Williams, D. R., & Gordon-Larsen, P. (2013). Racial discrimination, racial/ethnic segregation, and health behaviors in the CARDIA study. *Ethnicity and Health, 18,* 227–243. doi:10.1080/13557858.2012.713092

Brave Heart, M. Y., & DeBruyn, L. M. (1998). The American Indian holocaust: Healing historical unresolved grief. *American Indian and Alaska Native Mental Health Research, 8*(2), 60–82. doi:10.5820/aian.0802.1998.60

Brondolo, E., Love, E. E., Pencille, M., Schoenthaler, A., & Ogedegbe, G. (2011). Racism and hypertension: A review of the empirical evidence and implications for clinical practice. *American Journal of Hypertension, 24,* 518–529. doi:10.1038/ajh.2011.9

Caldwell, C. H., Guthrie, B. J., & Jackson, J. S. (2006). Identity development, discrimination, and psychological well-being among African American and Caribbean Black adolescents. In A. J. Schulz & L. Mullings (Eds.), *Gender, race, class, & health: Intersectional approaches* (pp. 163–191). San Francisco, CA: Jossey Bass.

Caldwell, C. H., Kohn-Wood, L. P., Schmeelk-Cone, K. H., Chavous, T. M., & Zimmerman, M. A. (2004). Racial discrimination and racial identity as risk or protective factors for violent behaviors in African American young adults. *American Journal of Community Psychology*, 33, 91–105. doi:10.1023/B:AJCP.0000014321.02367.dd

Carty, D. C., Kruger, D. J., Turner, T. M., Campbell, B., DeLoney, E. H., & Lewis, E. Y. (2011). Racism, health status, and birth outcomes: Results of a participatory community-based intervention and health survey. *Journal of Urban Health*, 88, 84–97. doi:10.1007/s11524-010-9530-9

Castle, B., Wendel, M., Kerr, J., Brooms, D., & Rollins, A. (2019). Public health's approach to systemic racism: A systematic literature review. *Journal of Racial and Ethnic Health Disparities*, 6, 27–36. doi:10.1007/s40615-018-0494-x

Centers for Disease Control and Prevention. (1997). *Principles of community engagement*. Atlanta, GA: CDC/ATSDR Committee on Community Engagement.

Chae, D. H., Clouston, S., Martz, C. D., Hatzenbuehler, M. L., Cooper, H. L. F., Turpin, R., … Kramer, M. R. (2018). Area racism and birth outcomes among Blacks in the United States. *Social Science and Medicine*, 199, 49–55. doi:10.1016/j.socscimed.2017.04.019

Chae, D. H., Nuru-Jeter, A. M., & Adler, N. E. (2012). Implicit racial bias as a moderator of the association between racial discrimination and hypertension: A study of midlife African American men. *Psychosomatic Medicine*, 74, 961–964. doi:10.1097/PSY.0b013e3182733665

Chae, D. H., Nuru-Jeter, A. M., Adler, N. E., Brody, G. H., Lin, J., Blackburn, E. H., & Epel, E. S. (2014). Discrimination, racial bias, and telomere length in African-American men. *American Journal of Preventive Medicine*, 46, 103–111. doi:10.1016/j.amepre.2013.10.020

Chae, D. H., Takeuchi, D. T., Barbeau, E. M., Bennett, G. G., Lindsey, J., & Krieger, N. (2008). Unfair treatment, racial/ethnic discrimination, ethnic identification, and smoking among Asian Americans in the National Latino and Asian American Study. *American Journal of Public Health*, 98, 485–492. doi:10.2105/AJPH.2006.102012

Chyu, L., & Upchurch, D. M. (2011). Racial and ethnic patterns of allostatic load among adult women in the United States: Findings from the National Health and Nutrition Examination Survey 1999-2004. *Journal of Women's Health*, 20, 575–583. doi:10.1089/jwh.2010.2170

Clark, R., Anderson, N. B., Clark, V. R., & Williams, D. R. (1999). Racism as a stressor for African Americans. *The American Psychologist*, 54, 805–816. doi:10.1037/0003-066X.54.10.805

Cobb, C. L., Meca, A., Branscombe, N. R., Schwartz, S. J., Xie, D., Zea, M. C., … Sanders, G. L. (2019). Perceived discrimination and well-being among unauthorized Hispanic immigrants: The moderating role of ethnic/racial group identity centrality. *Cultural Diversity and Ethnic Minority Psychology*, 25, 280–287. doi:10.1037/cdp0000227

Cogburn, C. D. (2019). Culture, race, and health: Implications for racial inequities and population health. *Milbank Quarterly*, 97, 736–761. doi:10.1111/1468-0009.12411

Corral, I., & Landrine, H. (2012). Racial discrimination and health-promoting vs damaging behaviors among African-American adults. *Journal of Health Psychology*, 17, 1176–1182. doi:10.1177/1359105311435429

Cozier, Y. C., Yu, J., Coogan, P. F., Bethea, T. N., Rosenberg, L., & Palmer, J. R. (2014). Racism, segregation, and risk of obesity in the Black Women's Health Study. *American Journal of Epidemiology*, 179, 875–883. doi:10.1093/aje/kwu004

DeVylder, J. E., Jun, H. J., Fedina, L., Coleman, D., Anglin, D., Cogburn, C., … Barth, R. P. (2018). Association of exposure to police violence with prevalence of mental health symptoms among urban residents in the United States. *JAMA Network Open*, 1, e184945. doi:10.1001/jamanetworkopen.2018.4945

Dickerson, N. T. (2007). Black employment, segregation, and the social organization of metropolitan labor markets. *Economic Geography*, 83(3), 283–307. doi:10.1111/j.1944-8287.2007.tb00355.x

Dolezsar, C. M., McGrath, J. J., Herzig, A. J., & Miller, S. B. (2014). Perceived racial discrimination and hypertension: A comprehensive systematic review. *Health Psychology*, 33, 20–34. doi:10.1037/a0033718

Dominguez, T. P. (2008). Race, racism, and racial disparities in adverse birth outcomes. *Clinical Obstetrics and Gynecology, 51*, 360–370. doi:10.1097/GRF.0b013e31816f28de

Dominguez, T. P. (2011). Adverse birth outcomes in African American women: The social context of persistent reproductive disadvantage. *Social Work in Public Health, 26*, 3–16. doi:10.1080/10911350902986880

Dovidio, J. F. (2001). On the nature of contemporary prejudice: The third wave. *Journal of Social Issues, 57*, 829–849. doi:10.1111/0022-4537.00244

Dunbar-Ortiz, R. (2014). *An indigenous peoples' history of the United States.* Boston, MA: Beacon Press.

El-Sayed, A., Hadley, C., & Galea, S. (2008). Birth outcomes among Arab Americans in Michigan before and after the terrorist attacks of September 11, 2001. *Ethnicity and Disease, 18*, 348–356.

Feagin, J., & Bennefield, Z. (2014). Systemic racism and U.S. health care. *Social Science and Medicine, 103*, 7–14. doi:10.1016/j.socscimed.2013.09.006

Felix, A. S., Shisler, R., Nolan, T. S., Warren, B. J., Rhoades, J., Barnett, K. S., & Williams, K. P. (2019). High-effort coping and cardiovascular disease among women: A systematic review of the John Henryism hypothesis. *Journal of Urban Health, 96*, 12–22. doi:10.1007/s11524-018-00333-1

Finch, B. K., Hummer, R. A., Kolody, B., & Vega, W. A. (2001). The role of discrimination and acculturative stress in the physical health of Mexican-origin adults. *Hispanic Journal of Behavioral Sciences, 23*, 399–429. doi:10.1177/0739986301234004

Fiscella, K., & Sanders, M. R. (2016). Racial and ethnic disparities in the quality of health care. *Annual Review of Public Health, 37*, 375–394. doi:10.1146/annurev-publhealth-032315-021439

Fitzgerald, C., & Hurst, S. (2017). Implicit bias in healthcare professionals: A systematic review. *BMC Medical Ethics, 18*, 19. doi:10.1186/s12910-017-0179-8

Ford, C. L., & Airhihenbuwa, C. O. (2010). Critical race theory, race equity, and public health: Toward antiracism praxis. *American Journal of Public Health, 100*(Suppl. 1), S30–S35. doi:10.2105/AJPH.2009.171058

Forsyth, J. M., Schoenthaler, A., Ogedegbe, G., & Ravenell, J. (2014). Perceived racial discrimination and adoption of health behaviors in hypertensive Black Americans: The CAATCH trial. *Journal of Health Care for the Poor and Underserved, 25*, 276–291. doi:10.1353/hpu.2014.0053

Foster, M. W., & Sharp, R. R. (2004). Beyond race: Towards a whole-genome perspective on human populations and genetic variation. *Nature Reviews Genetics, 5*, 790–796. doi:10.1038/nrg1452

Garner, S., & Selod, S. (2014). The racialization of Muslims: Empirical studies of Islamophobia. *Critical Sociology, 41*, 9–19. doi:10.1177/0896920514531606

Garrett, B. A., Livingston, B. J., Livingston, M. D., & Komro, K. A. (2017). The effects of perceived racial/ethnic discrimination on substance use among youths living in the Cherokee Nation. *Journal of Child & Adolescent Substance Abuse, 26*, 242–249. doi:10.1080/1067828X.2017.1299656

Gaskin, D. J., Headen, A. E., Jr., & White-Means, S. I. (2005). Racial disparities in health and wealth: The effects of slavery and past discrimination. *The Review of Black Political Economy, 32*, 95–110. doi:10.1007/s12114-005-1007-9

Gaskin, D. J., Price, A., Brandon, D. T., & LaVeist, T. A. (2009). Segregation and disparities in health services use. *Medical Care Research and Review, 66*, 578–589. doi:10.1177/1077558709336445

Gee, G. C., & Ford, C. L. (2011). Structural racism and health inequities: Old issues, new directions. *Du Bois Review: Social Science Research on Race, 8*, 115–132. doi:10.1017/S1742058X11000130

Gee, G. C., Ro, A., Shariff-Marco, S., & Chae, D. (2009). Racial discrimination and health among Asian Americans: Evidence, assessment, and directions for future research. *Epidemiologic Reviews, 31*, 130–151. doi:10.1093/epirev/mxp009

Gee, G. C., Spencer, M. S., Chen, J., & Takeuchi, D. (2007). A nationwide study of discrimination and chronic health conditions among Asian Americans. *American Journal of Public Health, 97*, 1275–1282. doi:10.2105/AJPH.2006.091827

Gee, G. C., Spencer, M., Chen, J., Yip, T., & Takeuchi, D. T. (2007). The association between self-reported racial discrimination and 12-month DSM-IV mental disorders among Asian Americans nationwide. *Social Science and Medicine, 64*, 1984–1996. doi:10.1016/j.socscimed.2007.02.013

Gee, G. C., Walsemann, K. M., & Brondolo, E. (2012). A life course perspective on how racism may be related to health inequities. *American Journal of Public Health, 102*, 967–974. doi:10.2105/AJPH.2012.300666

Giurgescu, C., McFarlin, B. L., Lomax, J., Craddock, C., & Albrecht, A. (2011). Racial discrimination and the Black-White gap in adverse birth outcomes: A review. *The Journal of Midwifery & Women's Health, 56,* 362–370. doi:10.1111/j.1542-2011.2011.00034.x

Gonzales, K. L., Noonan, C., Goins, R. T., Henderson, W. G., Beals, J., Manson, S. M., … Roubideaux, Y. (2016). Assessing the everyday discrimination scale among American Indians and Alaska natives. *Psychological Assessment, 28,* 51–58. doi:10.1037/a0039337

Goodman, A. H. (2000). Why genes don't count (for racial differences in health). *American Journal of Public Health, 90,* 1699–1702. doi:10.2105/AJPH.90.11.1699

Hall, W. J., Chapman, M. V., Lee, K. M., Merino, Y. M., Thomas, T. W., Payne, B. K., … Coyne-Beasley, T. (2015). Implicit racial/ethnic bias among health care professionals and its influence on health care outcomes: A systematic review. *American Journal of Public Health, 105,* e60–e76. doi:10.2105/AJPH.2015.302903a

Harawa, N. T., & Ford, C. L. (2009). The foundation of modern racial categories and implications for research on Black/White disparities in health. *Ethnicity and Disease, 19,* 209–217. Retrieved from https://www.ethndis.org

Hardeman, R. R., Murphy, K. A., Karbeah, J., & Kozhimannil, K. B. (2018). Naming institutionalized racism in the public health literature: A systematic literature review. *Public Health Reports, 133,* 240–249. doi:10.1177/0033354918760574

Harrell, C. J. P., Burford, T. I., Cage, B. N., Nelson, T. M., Shearon, S., Thompson, A., & Green, S. (2011). Multiple pathways linking racism to health outcomes. *Du Bois Review: Social Science Research on Race, 8,* 143–157. doi:10.1017/S1742058X11000178

Hatzenbuehler, M. L., Prins, S. J., Flake, M., Philbin, M., Frazer, M. S., Hagen, D., & Hirsch, J. (2017). Immigration policies and mental health morbidity among Latinos: A state-level analysis. *Social Science and Medicine, 174,* 169–178. doi:10.1016/j.socscimed.2016.11.040

Heard-Garris, N. J., Cale, M., Camaj, L., Hamati, M. C., & Dominguez, T. P. (2018). Transmitting trauma: A systematic review of vicarious racism and child health. *Social Science and Medicine, 199,* 230–240. doi:10.1016/j.socscimed.2017.04.018

Hicken, M. T., Lee, H., Morenoff, J., House, J. S., & Williams, D. R. (2014). Racial/ethnic disparities in hypertension prevalence: Reconsidering the role of chronic stress. *American Journal of Public Health, 104,* 117–123. doi:10.2105/AJPH.2013.301395

Himmelstein, M. S., Young, D. M., Sanchez, D. T., & Jackson, J. S. (2015). Vigilance in the discrimination-stress model for Black Americans. *Psychology & Health, 30,* 253–267. doi:10.1080/08870446.2014.966104

Hutchinson, R. N., & Shin, S. (2014). Systematic review of health disparities for cardiovascular diseases and associated factors among American Indian and Alaska native populations. *PLoS One, 9,* e80973. doi:10.1371/journal.pone.0080973

James, D. (2017). Internalized racism and past-year major depressive disorder among African-Americans: The role of ethnic identity and self-esteem. *Journal of Racial Ethnic Health Disparities, 4,* 659–670. doi:10.1007/s40615-016-0269-1

James, S. A. (1993). Racial and ethnic differences in infant mortality and low birth weight: A psychosocial critique. *Annals of Epidemiology, 3,* 130–136. doi:10.1016/1047-2797(93)90125-N

James, S. A. (1994). John Henryism and the health of African-Americans. *Culture, Medicine and Psychiatry, 18,* 163–182. doi:10.1007/BF01379448

Johnson, R. L., Saha, S., Arbelaez, J. J., Beach, M. C., & Cooper, L. A. (2004). Racial and ethnic differences in patient perceptions of bias and cultural competence in health care. *Journal of General Internal Medicine, 19,* 101–110. doi:10.1111/j.1525-1497.2004.30262.x

Johnson-Jennings, M. D., Belcourt, A., Town, M., Walls, M. L., & Walters, K. L. (2014). Racial discrimination's influence on smoking rates among American Indian Alaska Native two-spirit individuals: Does pain play a role? *Journal of Health Care for the Poor and Underserved, 25,* 1667–1678. doi:10.1353/hpu.2014.0193

Jones, C. P. (2000). Levels of racism: A theoretic framework and a gardener's tale. *American Journal of Public Health, 90,* 1212–1215. doi:10.2105/AJPH.90.8.1212

Jones, D. S. (2006). The persistence of American Indian health disparities. *American Journal of Public Health, 96,* 2122–2134. doi:10.2105/AJPH.2004.054262

Kannan, S., Sparks, A. V., Webster, J. D., Krishnakumar, A., & Lumeng, J. (2010). Healthy eating and harambee: Curriculum development for a culturally-centered bio-medically oriented nutrition education program to reach African American women of childbearing age. *Maternal Child Health Journal, 14*, 535–547. doi:10.1007/s10995-009-0507-9

Kershaw, K. N., & Albrecht, S. S. (2015). Racial/ethnic residential segregation and cardiovascular disease risk. *Current Cardiovascular Risk Reports, 9*, 10. doi:10.1007/s12170-015-0436-7

Key, K. D., Furr-Holden, D., Lewis, E. Y., Cunningham, R., Zimmermann, M., Johnson-Lawrence, V., & Selig, S. (2019). The continuum of community engagement in research: A roadmap for understanding and addressing progress. *Progress in Community Health Partnerships, 13*, 427–434. doi:10.1353/cpr.2019.0064

Kozol, J. (1991). *Savage inequalities*. New York, NY: Crown Publishers.

Kramer, M. R., & Hogue, C. R. (2009). Is segregation bad for your health? *Epidemiologic Reviews, 31*, 178–194. doi:10.1093/epirev/mxp001

Krieger, N., Waterman, P. D., Kosheleva, A., Chen, J. T., Smith, K. W., Carney, D. R., … Freeman, E. R. (2013). Racial discrimination & cardiovascular disease risk: My body my story study of 1005 US-born Black and White community health center participants (US). *PLoS One, 8*, e77174. doi:10.1371/journal .pone.0077174

Kruger, D. J., Carty, D. C., Turbeville, A. R., French-Turner, T. M., & Brownlee, S. (2015). Undoing racism through Genesee county's REACH infant mortality reduction initiative. *Progress in Community Health Partnerships, 9*, 57–63. doi:10.1353/cpr.2015.0004

Kruger, D. J., French-Turner, T., & Brownlee, S. (2013). Genesee County REACH windshield tours: Enhancing health professionals understanding of community conditions that influence infant mortality. *Journal of Primary Prevention, 34*, 163–172. doi:10.1007/s10935-013-0301-8

Kwate, N. O. (2008). Fried chicken and fresh apples: Racial segregation as a fundamental cause of fast food density in Black neighborhoods. *Health and Place, 14*, 32–44. doi:10.1016/j.healthplace.2007.04.001

Landale, N. S., & Oropesa, R. S. (2002). White, Black or Puerto Rican? Racial self-identification among mainland and island Puerto Ricans. *Social Forces, 81*, 231–254. doi:10.1353/sof.2002.0052

Landrine, H., Corral, I., Lee, J. G. L., Efird, J. T., Hall, M. B., & Bess, J. J. (2017). Residential segregation and racial cancer disparities: A systematic review. *Journal of Racial Ethnic Health Disparities, 4*, 1195–1205. doi:10.1007/s40615-016-0326-9

Landrine, H., & Klonoff, E. A. (2000). Racial discrimination and cigarette smoking among Blacks: Findings from two studies. *Ethnicity and Disease, 10*, 195–202.

Lauderdale, D. S. (2006). Birth outcomes for Arabic-named women in California before and after September 11. *Demography, 43*, 185–201. doi:10.1353/dem.2006.0008

LaVeist, T. A. (1996). Why we should continue to study race...But do a better job: An essay on race, racism and health. *Ethnicity and Disease, 6*, 21–29.

LeBrón, A. M. W., & Viruell-Fuentes, E. A. (2019). Racism and the health of Latina/Latino communities. In C. L. Ford, D. M. Griffith, M. A. Bruce, & K. L. Gilbert (Eds.), *Racism: Science & tools for the public health professional*. Washington, DC: American Public Health Association. doi:10.2105/9780875533049ch21

Lepore, S. J., Revenson, T. A., Weinberger, S. L., Weston, P., Frisina, P. G., Robertson, R., … Cross, W. (2006). Effects of social stressors on cardiovascular reactivity in Black and White women. *Annals of Behavioral Medicine, 31*, 120–127. doi:10.1207/s15324796abm3102_3

Lewis, J. A., Williams, M. G., Peppers, E. J., & Gadson, C. A. (2017). Applying intersectionality to explore the relations between gendered racism and health among Black women. *Journal of Counseling Psychology, 64*, 475–486. doi:10.1037/cou0000231

Lewis, T. T., Cogburn, C. D., & Williams, D. R. (2015). Self-reported experiences of discrimination and health: Scientific advances, ongoing controversies, and emerging issues. *Annual Review of Clinical Psychology, 11*, 407–440. doi:10.1146/annurev-clinpsy-032814-112728

Lewis, T. T., Williams, D. R., Tamene, M., & Clark, C. R. (2014). Self-reported experiences of discrimination and cardiovascular disease. *Current Cardiovascular Risk Reports, 8*, 365. doi:10.1007/s12170-013 -0365-2

Link, B. G., & Phelan, J. C. (1995). Social conditions as fundamental causes of disease. *Journal of Health and Social Behavior, 35*, 80–94. doi:10.2307/2626958

Liu, S. Y., & Kawachi, I. (2017). Discrimination and telomere length among older adults in the United States. *Public Health Reports, 132,* 220–230. doi:10.1177/0033354916689613

Longmire-Avital, B., & McQueen, C. (2019). Exploring a relationship between race-related stress and emotional eating for collegiate Black American women. *Women and Health, 59,* 240–251. doi:10.1080/03630242.2018.1478361

Lopez, W. D., Kruger, D. J., Delva, J., Llanes, M., Ledon, C., Waller, A., ... Israel, B. (2017). Health implications of an immigration raid: Findings from a Latino community in the midwestern United States. *Journal of Immigrant and Minority Health, 19,* 702–708. doi:10.1007/s10903-016-0390-6

Lovasi, G. S., Hutson, M. A., Guerra, M., & Neckerman, K. M. (2009). Built environments and obesity in disadvantaged populations. *Epidemiologic Reviews, 31,* 7–20. doi:10.1093/epirev/mxp005

Lu, D., Palmer, J. R., Rosenberg, L., Shields, A. E., Orr, E. H., DeVivo, I., & Cozier, Y. C. (2019). Perceived racism in relation to telomere length among African American women in the Black Women's Health Study. *Annals of Epidemiology, 36,* 33–39. doi:10.1016/j.annepidem.2019.06.003

Martinez, O., Wu, E., Sandfort, T., Dodge, B., Carballo-Dieguez, A., Pinto, R., ... Chavez-Baray, S. (2015). Evaluating the impact of immigration policies on health status among undocumented immigrants: A systematic review. *Journal of Immigrant and Minority Health, 17,* 947–970. doi:10.1007/s10903-013-9968-4

Massey, D. S., & Denton, N. A. (1988). The dimensions of residential segregation. *Social Forces, 67,* 281–315. doi:10.2307/2579183

Massey, D. S., & Denton, N. A. (1993). *American apartheid: Segregation and the making of the underclass.* Cambridge, MA: Harvard University Press.

McEwen, B. S., & Wingfield, J. C. (2003). The concept of allostasis in biology and biomedicine. *Hormones and Behavior, 43,* 2–15. doi:10.1016/S0018-506X(02)00024-7

McNeilly, M. D., Robinson, E. L., Anderson, N. B., Pieper, C. F., Shah, A., Toth, P. S., ... Gerin, W. (1995). Effects of racist provocation and social support on cardiovascular reactivity in African American women. *International Journal of Behavioral Medicine, 2,* 321–338. doi:10.1207/s15327558ijbm0204_3

Mehra, R., Boyd, L. M., & Ickovics, J. R. (2017). Racial residential segregation and adverse birth outcomes: A systematic review and meta-analysis. *Social Science and Medicine, 191,* 237–250. doi:10.1016/j.socscimed.2017.09.018

Meyer, I. H., Schwartz, S., & Frost, D. M. (2008). Social patterning of stress and coping: Does disadvantaged social statuses confer more stress and fewer coping resources? *Social Science and Medicine, 67,* 368–379. doi:10.1016/j.socscimed.2008.03.012

Miller, M. J., Keum, B. T., Thai, C. J., Lu, Y., Truong, N. N., Huh, G. A., ... Ahn, L. H. (2018). Practice recommendations for addressing racism: A content analysis of the counseling psychology literature. *Journal of Counseling Psychology, 65,* 669–680. doi:10.1037/cou0000306

Morello-Frosch, R., Zuk, M., Jerrett, M., Shamasunder, B., & Kyle, A. D. (2011). Understanding the cumulative impacts of inequalities in environmental health: Implications for policy. *Health Affairs, 30,* 879–887. doi:10.1377/hlthaff.2011.0153

Mouzon, D. M., & McLean, J. S. (2017). Internalized racism and mental health among African-Americans, US-born Caribbean Blacks, and foreign-born Caribbean Blacks. *Ethnicity and Health, 22,* 36–48. doi:10.1080/13557858.2016.1196652

Noh, S., Beiser, M., Kaspar, V., Hou, F., & Rummens, J. (1999). Perceived racial discrimination, depression, and coping: A study of Southeast Asian refugees in Canada. *Journal of Health and Social Behavior, 40,* 193–207. doi:10.2307/2676348

Noh, S., & Kaspar, V. (2003). Perceived discrimination and depression: Moderating effects of coping, acculturation, and ethnic support. *American Journal of Public Health, 93,* 232–238. doi:10.2105/AJPH.93.2.232

Novak, N. L., Geronimus, A. T., & Martinez-Cardoso, A. M. (2017). Change in birth outcomes among infants born to Latina mothers after a major immigration raid. *International Journal of Epidemiology, 46,* 839–849. doi:10.1093/ije/dyw346

Office of Management and Budget. (1997). Revisions to the standards for the classification of federal data on race and ethnicity. *Federal Register, 62,* 58782–58790. Retrieved from https://www.govinfo.gov/content/pkg/FR-1997-10-30/pdf/97-28653.pdf

Omi, M., & Winant, H. (2015). *Racial formation in the United States* (3rd ed.). New York, NY: Routledge.

Oza-Frank, R., & Cunningham, S. A. (2010). The weight of US residence among immigrants: A systematic review. *Obesity Reviews, 11*, 271–280. doi:10.1111/j.1467-789X.2009.00610.x

Padela, A. I., & Heisler, M. (2010). The association of perceived abuse and discrimination after September 11, 2001, with psychological distress, level of happiness, and health status among Arab Americans. *American Journal of Public Health, 100*, 284–291. doi:10.2105/AJPH.2009.164954

Paradies, Y., Ben, J., Denson, N., Elias, A., Priest, N., Pieterse, A., … Gee, G. (2015). Racism as a determinant of health: A systematic review and meta-analysis. *PLoS One, 10*, e0138511. doi:10.1371/journal.pone.0138511

Pearson, A. R., Dovidio, J. F., & Gaertner, S. L. (2009). The nature of contemporary prejudice: Insights from aversive racism. *Social and Personality Psychology Compass, 3*, 314–338. doi:10.1111/j.1751-9004.2009.00183.x

People's Institute for Survival and Beyond. (n.d.). *Undoing racism.* Retrieved from http://www.pisab.org/

Pestronk, R. M., & Franks, M. L. (2003). A partnership to reduce African American infant mortality in Genesee County, Michigan. *Public Health Reports, 118*, 324–335. doi:10.1016/S0033-3549(04)50256-X

Phelan, J. C., & Link, B. G. (2015). Is racism a fundamental cause of inequalities in health? *Annual Review of Sociology, 41*, 311–330. doi:10.1146/annurev-soc-073014-112305

Prather, C., Fuller, T. R., Jeffries, W. L. T., Marshall, K. J., Howell, A. V., Belyue-Umole, A., & King, W. (2018). Racism, African American women, and their sexual and reproductive health: A review of historical and contemporary evidence and implications for health equity. *Health Equity, 2*, 249–259. doi:10.1089/heq.2017.0045

Quillian, L. (2006). New approaches to understanding racial prejudice and discrimination. *Annual Review of Sociology, 32*, 299–328. doi:10.1146/annurev.soc.32.061604.123132

Read, J. G., & Emerson, M. O. (2005). Racial context, Black immigration and the U.S. Black/White health disparity. *Social Forces, 84*, 181–199. doi:10.1353/sof.2005.0120

Rhodes, S. D., Mann, L., Siman, F. M., Song, E., Alonzo, J., Downs, M., … Hall, M. A. (2015). The impact of local immigration enforcement policies on the health of immigrant Hispanics/Latinos in the United States. *American Journal of Public Health, 105*, 329–337. doi:10.2105/AJPH.2014.302218

Rodriguez, J. M., Geronimus, A. T., Bound, J., & Dorling, D. (2015). Black lives matter: Differential mortality and the racial composition of the U.S. Electorate, 1970–2004. *Social Science and Medicine, 136–137*, 193–199. doi:10.1016/j.socscimed.2015.04.014

Roediger, D. R. (2005). *Working toward Whiteness: How America's immigrants became White: The strange journey from Ellis Island to the suburbs.* New York, NY: Basic Books.

Samari, G., Alcala, H. E., & Sharif, M. Z. (2018). Islamophobia, health, and public health: A systematic literature review. *American Journal of Public Health, 108*, e1–e9. doi:10.2105/AJPH.2018.304402

Schulz, A. J., & Mullings, L. (Eds.). (2006). *Gender, race, class, and health: Intersectional approaches.* San Francisco, CA: Jossey Bass.

Seaton, E., Caldwell, C. H., Sellers, R. M., & Jacson, J. S. (2010). An intersectional approach for understanding perceived discrimination and psychological well-being among African American and caribbean black youth. *Developmental Psychology, 46*(5), 1372–1379. doi:10.1037/a0019869

Selig, S., Tropiano, E., & Greene-Moton, E. (2006). Teaching cultural competence to reduce health disparities. *Health Promotion Practice, 7*, 247S–255S. doi:10.1177/1524839906288697

Skewes, M. C., & Blume, A. W. (2019). Understanding the link between racial trauma and substance use among American Indians. *American Psychologist, 74*, 88–100. doi:10.1037/amp0000331

Smedley, B. D., Stith, A. Y., & Nelson, A. R. (Eds.). (2003). *Unequal treatment: Confronting racial and ethnic disparities in health care.* Washington, DC: National Academies Press.

Stuber, J., Galea, S., Ahern, J., Blaney, S., & Fuller, C. (2003). The association between multiple domains of discrimination and self-assessed health: A multilevel analysis of Latinos and Blacks in four low-income New York City neighborhoods. *Health Services Research, 38*, 1735–1759. doi:10.1111/j.1475-6773.2003.00200.x

Stuber, J., Meyer, I., & Link, B. (2008). Stigma, prejudice, discrimination and health. *Social Science and Medicine, 67*, 351–357. doi:10.1016/j.socscimed.2008.03.023

Subramanyam, M. A., James, S. A., Diez-Roux, A. V., Hickson, D. A., Sarpong, D., Sims, M., … Wyatt, S. B. (2013). Socioeconomic status, John Henryism and blood pressure among African-Americans in the Jackson Heart Study. *Social Science and Medicine, 93*, 139–146. doi:10.1016/j.socscimed.2013.06.016

Thayer, Z. M., Blair, I. V., Buchwald, D. S., & Manson, S. M. (2017). Racial discrimination associated with higher diastolic blood pressure in a sample of American Indian adults. *American Journal of Physical Anthropology, 163*, 122–128. doi:10.1002/ajpa.23190

Thorpe, R. J., Jr., Parker, L. J., Cobb, R. J., Dillard, F., & Bowie, J. (2017). Association between discrimination and obesity in African-American men. *Biodemography and Social Biology, 63*, 253–261. doi:10.1080/19485565.2017.1353406

Todorova, I. L., Falcon, L. M., Lincoln, A. K., & Price, L. L. (2010). Perceived discrimination, psychological distress and health. *Sociology of Health and Illness, 32*, 843–861. doi:10.1111/j.1467-9566.2010.01257.x

U.S. Census Bureau. (2019, June). *Annual estimates of the resident population by sex, age, race, and Hispanic origin for the United States and States: April 1, 2010 to July 1, 2018*. Retrieved from https://factfinder.census.gov/faces/tableservices/jsf/pages/productview.xhtml?src=bkmk

van Ryn, M., Burgess, D. J., Dovidio, J. F., Phelan, S. M., Saha, S., Malat, J., ... Perry, S. (2011). The impact of racism on clinician cognition, behavior, and clinical decision making. *Du Bois Review: Social Science Research on Race, 8*, 199–218. doi:10.1017/S1742058X11000191

van Ryn, M., & Burke, J. (2000). The effect of patient race and socio-economic status on physicians' perceptions of patients. *Social Science and Medicine, 50*, 813–828. doi:10.1016/S0277-9536(99)00338-X

Vargas, E. D., Sanchez, G. R., & Juarez, M. (2017). Fear by association: Perceptions of anti-immigrant policy and health outcomes. *Journal of Health Politics, Policy and Law, 42*, 459–483. doi:10.1215/03616878-3802940

Viruell-Fuentes, E. A., Miranda, P. Y., & Abdulrahim, S. (2012). More than culture: Structural racism, intersectionality theory, and immigrant health. *Social Science and Medicine, 75*, 2099–2106. doi:10.1016/j.socscimed.2011.12.037

Wildeman, C., & Wang, E. A. (2017). Mass incarceration, public health, and widening inequality in the USA. *Lancet, 389*, 1464–1474. doi:10.1016/S0140-6736(17)30259-3

Williams, D. R., & Collins, C. A. (2001). Racial residential segregation: A fundamental cause of racial disparities in health. *Public Health Reports, 116*, 404–416. doi:10.1016/S0033-3549(04)50068-7

Williams, D. R., Lawrence, J. A., & Davis, B. A. (2019). Racism and health: Evidence and needed research. *Annual Review of Public Health, 40*, 105–125. doi:10.1146/annurev-publhealth-040218-043750

Williams, D. R., & Mohammed, S. A. (2009). Discrimination and racial disparities in health: Evidence and needed research. *Journal of Behavioral Medicine, 32*, 20–47. doi:10.1007/s10865-008-9185-0

Williams, D. R., & Mohammed, S. A. (2013). Racism and health I: Pathways and scientific evidence. *American Behavioral Scientist, 57*, 1152–1173. doi:10.1177/0002764213487340

HEALTH EQUITY FRAMEWORKS AND THEORIES

JACOB C. WARREN ■ K. BRYANT SMALLEY

LEARNING OBJECTIVES

- Describe the five domains of Social Determinants of Health
- Define Intersectionality Theory and discuss the ways in which it impacts health equity
- Discuss how Minority Stress Theory helps to explain higher rates of health risk behaviors in populations affected by prejudice and discrimination
- Apply Maslow's Hierarchy of Needs to the field of health equity
- Describe how the Social Ecological Model provides a framework for developing multilevel health equity interventions

INTRODUCTION

Over the years, a number of frameworks, models, and theories have been developed that have become integral to understanding the field of health equity. Some are used to understand the ways in which health disparities develop, some help to expand our thinking about the identities that are so often discussed as a part of the health equity field, and still others help us understand the ways in which we can target programs and interventions in a way to combat the systemic nature of inequities. These models do not compete with each other—rather, they each help to explain a different dimension of health equity.

We begin with an overview of Social Determinants of Health, which helps to crystallize the ways in which a person's context and lived experiences shape their health and form the basis from which health decisions and actions are made. We then summarize Intersectionality Theory, which focuses on the ways in which multiple identities combine within an individual in ways that can have a profound impact on health. Next, we explore the Minority Stress Theory, used to explain how daily exposure to discrimination increases risk for a number of health risk behaviors and, in turn, health outcomes. We then explore a fundamental psychological theory, Maslow's Hierarchy of Needs, which provides context to the struggle many individuals face as they prioritize their own self-care and growth. We then conclude with the sociological Social Ecological Model, which helps provide a framework for understanding the complex interplay of personal and contextual factors that influence people's everyday lives and ways in which interventions and programs can take this full context into account. Our goal is to demonstrate how each of these theories and frameworks can be used to understand and intervene in issues related to health equity.

SOCIAL DETERMINANTS OF HEALTH

While now a core framework through which health equity is examined, focusing on the social determinants of health (SDOH) is a relatively new endeavor. Defined by the World Health Organization (WHO) as "the conditions in which people are born, grow, live, work, and age" (WHO, 2019), the phrase does not appear to have come into play in its current usage until the 1990s, and even then took decades to reach the prominence it has today (see Figure 3.1 for a graph of the use of the phrase "social determinants of health" in the research literature).

While it may seem common sense and common knowledge today, the idea that factors outside of an individual affect not only their health outcomes, but also their underlying health behaviors, was revolutionary within the field. This has become even more so the case as we have learned that a substantial component of the origin of health disparities lies not in individual behavior, but in the sociocultural context individuals find themselves in. With the popularization of the Social Determinants of Health Framework, for the first time there was a true model through which to conceptualize the impact of factors such as discrimination, and thereby justify the argument that these factors play a critical role in health disparities.

Healthy People 2020 conceptualized Social Determinants of Health into five categories: Economic Stability, Education, Social and Community Context, Health and Health Care, and Neighborhood and Built Environment. They also identified "key issues" within each category "that make up the underlying factors in the arena of social determinants of health" (Office of Disease Prevention and Health Promotion, n.d., "Approach to Social Determinants of Health") These are presented in Table 3.1.

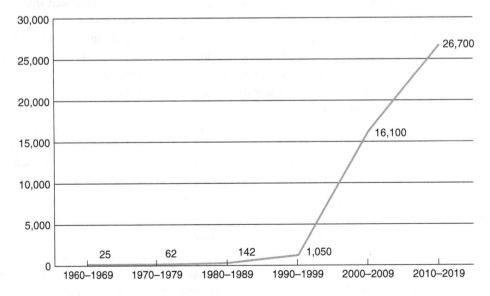

FIGURE 3.1 Google Scholar search results for "Social Determinants of Health."

TABLE 3.1 Categories and Key Issues of Healthy People 2020's Social Determinants of Health Framework

ECONOMIC STABILITY	EDUCATION	SOCIAL AND COMMUNITY CONTEXT	HEALTH AND HEALTH CARE	NEIGHBORHOOD AND BUILT ENVIRONMENT
Employment Food insecurity Housing instability Poverty	Early childhood education and development Enrollment in higher education High school graduation Language and literacy	Civic participation Discrimination Incarceration Social cohesion	Access to healthcare Access to primary care Health literacy	Access to foods that support healthy eating patterns Crime and violence Environmental conditions Quality of housing

The literature surrounding the effects of each of these social determinants—and more—is robust and ever-growing. A summary is beyond the scope of the current chapter, but readers are encouraged to draw upon the resources of the WHO's division of Social Determinants (www.who.int/social_determinants/themes/en), the Healthy People initiative (www.HealthyPeople.gov), and the Centers' for Disease Control and Prevention (CDC) Social Determinants division (http://cdc.gov/socialdeterminants).

It is important to avoid the temptation to conclude that the source of disparities is variations in the socioeconomic aspects of the social determinants of health. For instance, it is well-known that education level is strongly correlated with employability, and that members of racial and ethnic minority groups are less likely to receive higher education degrees. It is easy to (incorrectly) conclude that differences seen in employment rates are explained by differences in education attainment. A granular look at Bureau of Labor Statistics data, however, reveals this to be far from the case. As shown in Figure 3.2, African Americans face a higher unemployment rate than all other racial/ethnic groups even at each level of education—in some instances, nearly triple the rate. In fact, the unemployment rate for Caucasians with only a high school diploma is lower than the unemployment rate for African Americans at all but the highest level of education. The effects of discrimination and other societal barriers to employment thus extend well beyond the effect of any individual social determinant of health such as education level. This is not to say that increasing the opportunity for minority youth and young adults to achieve higher education goals is not important; it is simply to point out that the role that social determinants play in health disparities and health equity should not be oversimplified.

INTERSECTIONALITY THEORY

Intersectionality Theory traces its roots to a 1989 article by Kimberlé Crenshaw entitled "Demarginalizing the Intersection of Race and Sex: A Black Feminist Critique of Antidiscrimination Doctrine, Feminist Theory, and Antiracist Policies." In this seminal article, she coins the term "intersectionality" in the context of the lived experiences of African American women in particular. In her critique, she artfully makes the case that ignoring either the race or the gender of African American women is commonplace, yet fails to recognize the interconnected and complex

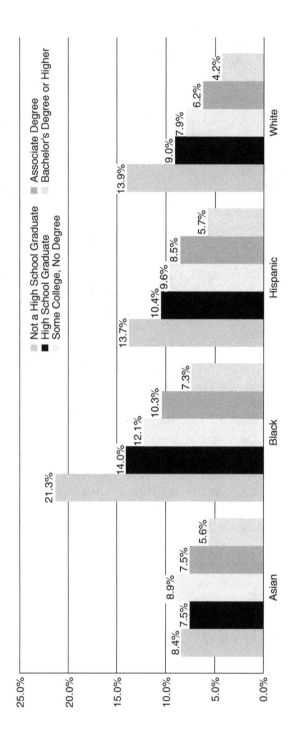

FIGURE 3.2 Unemployment rates by education level and race/ethnicity.

SOURCE: Bureau of Labor Statistics, 2010, as presented by the College Board. (2019). *Unemployment rates by education level and race/ethnicity, 2009.* Retrieved from https://trends.collegeboard.org/education-pays/figures-tables/unemployment-rates-education-level-and-race-ethnicity-2009

nature of their two oppressed identities. In brief, she argues that to truly understand injustice, one cannot ignore the presence of either identity. Applying what is known about discrimination experienced by African Americans as a community and what is by women as a gender cannot adequately capture the unique experience of living at the juncture of these two identities. As she states:

> *If any real efforts are to be made to free Black people of the constraints and conditions that character-ize racial subordination, then theories and strategies purporting to reflect the Black community's needs must include an analysis of sexism and patriarchy. Similarly, feminism must include an analysis of race if it hopes to express the aspirations of non-white women…. In order to include Black women, both movements must distance themselves from earlier approaches in which experiences are relevant only when they are related to certain clearly identifiable causes (for example, the oppression of Blacks is sig-nificant when based on race, of women when based on gender). (p. 166)*

Since the publication of her article, Intersectionality Theory's initial focus on race and gender has been expanded to include all dimensions of an individual's identity, most frequently including race, gender, sexual orientation, gender identity, and geographic origin (see Figure 3.3), although the model is flexible to any number of examined identities.

Intersectionality Theory has become one of the most important guiding principles in the field of health equity because of its ability to incorporate an individual's multiple identities in a way that traditional health disparities work did not. For instance, given the inherent population focus of health disparities research, the literature largely has focused on differences between African American and Caucasian individuals, or LGBTQ and non-LGBTQ individuals, for instance. In developing solutions, however, one cannot ignore the race and gender of an LGBTQ person if hoping to have any chance at real-world impact. Solutions that examine the overlap of these iden-tities have the greatest chance at success, scalability, and acceptability. At the same time, the lens

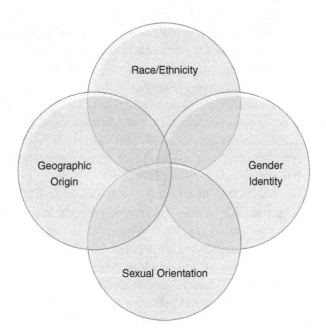

FIGURE 3.3 The intersecting nature of multiple identities.

of intersectionality provides the opportunity to realize that work focused on a specific group has much broader implications. For example, a properly-designed focus on the income inequality experienced by women as a whole will help to improve the lives of minority women as well (and potentially in even greater ways than for non-minority women).

It is critical to always keep intersectionality in mind when discussing groups impacted by health disparities, because everyone is made of multiple identities. Failing to recognize this, and drawing conclusions about an entire population without regard to the subgroup diversity that exists, borders on the kind of stereotyping that underlies much of the existence of health disparities in the first place. For this reason, we are emphasizing intersectionality throughout this entire text—all of Section II's chapters, which focus on specific populations, include specific discussion of intersectionality within that group to highlight what is known. A major limitation, though, remains the limited literature that truly examines issues with an intersectional lens—in part due to a lack of understanding of its importance, and in part due to methodological complications that arise (e.g., recruiting a sufficiently diverse sample to allow for examination of intersecting identities; see Chapter 4, Health Equity Research and Collaboration Approaches, for additional discussion).

MINORITY STRESS

Minority Stress Theory was developed initially to describe how the oppressive climate experienced by LGBTQ individuals contributes to their increased levels of engagement in a number of health risk behaviors. Specifically, Minority Stress Theory holds that the continual and lifetime experiences of discrimination, victimization, and harassment that result from heterosexism, cisgenderism, homophobia, and transphobia directly impact the ability of LGBTQ individuals to maintain both mental and physical health at the same levels seen in non-LGBTQ groups (Hendricks & Testa, 2012; Meyer, 1995, 2003, 2013). The model was a critical step in understanding LGBTQ health, as it helped to refocus intervention targets away from the individual behaviors of LGBTQ individuals and more on the broader social reasons for those behaviors. For example, rather than focusing on the higher rates of substance abuse among gay men in comparison to heterosexual men, Minority Stress Theory refocuses the conversation on the increased likelihood of, for instance, a history of victimization and trauma, which are well-established risk factors for substance abuse. By refocusing the conversation on the origins of the behavior, more effective interventions can be developed, and researchers and practitioners can help to overcome the inherent victim-blaming that often accompanies behaviors such as substance abuse. Because of its flexibility to multiple identities and its focus on the process whereby individuals experience discrimination, Minority Stress Theory has also been used as a model for minority oppression in other groups as well (e.g., racial/ethnic minorities).

Minority Stress Theory holds that the stressors experienced by LGBTQ individuals (and by extension, other minority groups) have three aspects that uniquely drive health risks (Dentato, 2012). First, these stressors are unique, in that individuals who are not a part of minority groups do not experience them. For example, while all populations experience financial stress, such a stress is not a part of minority stress. Instead, minority stress specifically focuses on experiences such as prejudice, microaggressions, identity rejection, internalized homophobia, and hate-based victimization. Given its unique effect upon members of minority groups, the minority stress model helps to explain why such experiences are a critical underlying source of disparities. Second, minority stress is chronic due to its integration into the very fabric of society. Stereotyping, prejudice, and discrimination are not transient experiences and follow individuals wherever they may go physically and socially, and the stress related to these experiences therefore constantly affects the lived experience of members of minority groups. Finally, minority stress is socially-based in that it is derived entirely from social origins. For example, the stress related to raising a child is universal and largely drawn from within. In contrast, the minority stress related to being African American in an oppressive society is not essential and exists only because of the sociocultural inequalities that exist in our society. Minority stress is therefore a created, non-essential stress that presents a unique opportunity for intervention and larger social justice focus. However, at the same time, the social nature of minority stress can lead to a sense of powerlessness and despair, while also promoting concealment and social isolation to avoid related experiences.

MASLOW'S HIERARCHY OF NEEDS

Although traditionally considered a motivational psychology model, Maslow's Hierarchy of Needs (Maslow, 1943, 1954) has also been applied to understanding the ways in which people make decisions about their health-related behaviors. Maslow's theory holds that the degree of motivation for a certain behavior is driven by the level of needs that a person has already met. Maslow proposed five levels of needs of decreasing importance to survival: physiological, safety, love and belonging, esteem, and self-actualization. These needs are often presented as a pyramid, as in Figure 3.4, with examples of each level presented in Table 3.2. Maslow's theory argues that until a more basic level of needs is met, an individual will not be motivated to engage in activities related to a higher level of need. Maslow originally proposed his framework as a discrete process, wherein an individual met their physiological needs, then worked to meet their safety needs, and so on until reaching self-actualization. Subsequent expansions of the model have argued that there is a natural ebb and flow between the levels, and even a "reset" effect should something happen to threaten a lower level of need (e.g., the loss of a job might move someone from focusing on self-actualization back to focusing on physiological).

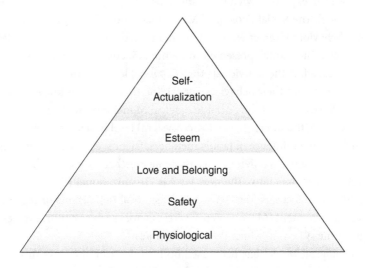

FIGURE 3.4 Maslow's Hierarchy of Needs.

TABLE 3.2 **Examples of Each Level of Maslow's Hierarchy of Needs**

LEVEL	EXAMPLES
Physiological	Food, water, shelter, sleep, clothing
Safety	Security, stability
Love and belonging	Friendships, intimacy, family
Esteem	Legacy, accomplishment
Self-actualization	Leisure goals, talent acquisition

Maslow's hierarchy has been used throughout nearly every field that touches on human behavior, but its relevance to health equity comes in its ability to help explain how sociocultural disadvantage prevents individuals from pursuing certain behaviors (e.g., health-related) and from achieving their full potential in society. For an individual that experiences workplace discrimination, for instance, their ability to meet both their safety and even their physiological needs is jeopardized. According to Maslow's theory, this person then feels sufficient threat to their basic survival that behaviors related to health and well-being may readily be ignored in preference to those that help to ensure more basic needs. In essence, the increased fragility of safety and physiological needs for marginalized groups continually impedes an individual's ability to pursue items such as esteem and self-actualization, which in turn will impact not only physical health, but also mental health. Despite predating it by decades, Maslow's framework intersects quite well with the Social Determinants of Health Framework because of its ability to explain why the continued threat of losing access to basic needs (e.g., physiological) has such a systemic impact on an individual.

SOCIAL ECOLOGICAL MODEL

The final model we will explore is what has come to be referred to as Bronfenbrenner's (1989) Social Ecological Model. The Social Ecological Model focuses on the ways in which an individual's own beliefs and behaviors interact with and are influenced by their broader social, geographic, and cultural context. The model, presented in Figure 3.5, consists of four levels of increasingly complex systems that affect the individual. The Individual level focuses on those particular traits of the person that influence their behaviors—including things such as knowledge, attitudes, and beliefs. Each progressive level of the Social Ecological Model represents interactions of the level one step below. As such, the Interpersonal (Microsystem) level is made of the interactions of individuals. This includes the influence of family members, friends, etc. The next level is Community (Mesosystem), which connects different microsystems together—for example, schools, churches, organized sports, and social clubs. The next level is Organizational (Exosystem), comprised of factors that influence collections of mesosystems (e.g., local politics, major regional employers). The final level is Environment (Macrosystem), where factors such as cultural values, norms, laws, and policies affect the system in which everyone operates.

The Social Ecological Model has been used both to describe the ways in which health disparities are created and sustained, and to develop multilevel interventions to address the inherently complex nature of solutions. As an example, African American women are more likely

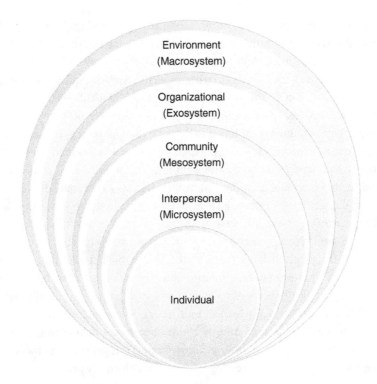

FIGURE 3.5 Social Ecological Model.

to have diabetes (both diagnosed and undiagnosed) and have higher diabetes-specific mortality rates (Chow, Foster, Gonzalez, & McIver, 2012). Examining this disparity across the levels of the Social Ecological Model reveals the following potential factors: (a) Individual (motivation for self-management; health literacy regarding diabetes self-care); (b) Interpersonal (family pressures regarding changing dietary habits); (c) Community (church groups promoting healthy behaviors); (d) Organizational (availability of employer-sponsored wellness classes); and (e) Environment (state-level decision not to expand Medicaid). Similarly, developing potential intervention strategies across multiple social ecological levels could include: (a) Individual (increasing individual health literacy regarding diabetes); (b) Interpersonal (developing family-level interventions to promote social support); (c) Community (connecting family-level interventions together through group-based psychoeducation at churches); (d) Organizational (raising awareness among self-insured companies of the financial benefits of supporting diabetes self-management); and (e) Environment (working with legislators to understand the state-level financial effects of uncontrolled diabetes). The creation of multilevel interventions is discussed in more detail in Chapter 4, Health Equity Research and Collaboration Approaches.

CONCLUSION

There are several frameworks, models, and theories that are applied within the field of health equity, ranging from individual behavior models through explanatory systems for the origins of disparities themselves. The Social Determinants of Health Framework—defined by the WHO (2019) as "the conditions in which people are born, grow, live, work, and age"—extends the common perception of health as solely an individual-level issue by framing health within the broader socio-environmental context in which people live. Intersectionality Theory focuses on recognizing that identity is complex and multifaceted, and to truly understand health equity one must examine not just a single identity (e.g., racial, ethnic), but the constellation of identities that shape one's health behaviors and outcomes (e.g., race, ethnicity, gender identity, sexual orientation, geography). Minority Stress Theory, originally developed to describe the experiences of those who identify as LGBTQ, has since been expanded to conceptualize the way in which a lifetime of discrimination, victimization, and harassment combine to impact the ability of individuals from minority groups to achieve and maintain mental and physical health. Maslow's Hierarchy of Needs codifies the ways in which higher-function needs (e.g., love and belonging) often necessarily take a back seat to more driving needs (e.g., food and shelter), thereby creating increased risk for behaviors that impact longer-term health (e.g., someone facing food insecurity is much less concerned over the nutritional value of their food than being able to secure it in the first place); as a result, impacting "health risk behaviors" may need to take an upstream approach to address the underlying factors limiting one's ability to meet basic needs. Finally, the Social Ecological Model provides a framework for understanding the ways in which an individual's beliefs and behaviors are influenced by their broader social, geographic, and cultural context across five intersecting layers (individual, interpersonal, community, organizational, and environment). Together, these theories and frameworks provide essential guidance in creating impactful health equity programs.

DISCUSSION QUESTIONS

- How can the Social Determinants of Health Framework help to explain the origins of disparities in lung cancer outcomes?

- Does Intersectionality Theory argue that the effects of being a member of multiple minority groups is additive, multiplicative, or varies depending upon the person? Why is that the case?

- What types of intervention targets would be most consistent with a health equity issue that has been conceptualized from the Minority Stress Theory perspective?

- Utilizing Maslow's Hierarchy of Needs as a backdrop, how might factors such as food insecurity and neighborhood crime ultimately decrease an individual's available social support?

- Describe a potential comprehensive intervention for asthma in Hispanic youth that targets each level of the Social Ecological Model.

REFERENCES

Bronfenbrenner, U. (1989). Ecological systems theory. In R. Vasta (Ed.), *Annals of child development* (Vol. 6, pp. 187–249). London, UK: Jessica Kingsley.

Chow, E. A., Foster, H., Gonzalez, V., & McIver, L. (2012). The disparate impact of diabetes on racial/ethnic minority populations. *Clinical Diabetes*, *30*(3), 130–133. doi:10.2337/diaclin.30.3.130

College Board. (2019). *Unemployment rates by education level and race/ethnicity, 2009.* Retrieved from https://trends.collegeboard.org/education-pays/figures-tables/unemployment-rates-education -level-and-race-ethnicity-2009

Crenshaw, K. (1989). Demarginalizing the intersection of race and sex: A Black feminist critique of antidiscrimination doctrine, feminist theory, and antiracist politics. *The University of Chicago Legal Forum, 1989*(1), 139–167. Retrieved from https://chicagounbound.uchicago.edu/cgi/viewcontent.cgi?article=1052&context=uclf

Dentato, M. P. (2012, Spring). The minority stress perspective. *Psychology and AIDS Exchange, 37*, 12–15. doi:10.1037/e565372012-003

Hendricks, M. L., & Testa, R. J. (2012). A conceptual framework for clinical work with transgender and gender nonconforming clients: An adaptation of the Minority Stress Model. *Professional Psychology: Research and Practice, 43*, 460–487. doi:10.1037/a0029597

Maslow, A. H. (1943). A theory of human motivation. *Psychological Review, 50*(4), 370–396. doi:10.1037/h0054346

Maslow, A. H. (1954). *Motivation and personality*. New York, NY: Harper.

Meyer, I. H. (1995). Minority stress and mental health in gay men. *Journal of Health and Social Behavior, 36*, 38–56. doi:10.2307/2137286

Meyer, I. H. (2003). Prejudice, social stress, and mental health in lesbian, gay, and bisexual populations: Conceptual issues and research evidence. *Psychological Bulletin, 129*(5), 674–697. doi:10.1037/0033-2909.129.5.674

Meyer, I. H. (2013). Prejudice, social stress, and mental health in lesbian, gay, and bisexual populations: Conceptual issues and research evidence. *Psychology of Sexual Orientation and Gender Diversity, 1*(Suppl.), 3–26. doi:10.1037/2329-0382.1.S.3

Office of Disease Prevention and Health Promotion. (n.d.). *Social determinants of health*. Retrieved from https://www.healthypeople.gov/2020/topics-objectives/topic/social-determinants-of-health

World Health Organization. (2019). *About social determinants of health*. Retrieved from https://www.who.int/social_determinants/sdh_definition/en

HEALTH EQUITY RESEARCH AND COLLABORATION APPROACHES: CBPR, MIXED METHODOLOGIES, AND COLLECTIVE IMPACT

JACOB C. WARREN ■ K. BRYANT SMALLEY

LEARNING OBJECTIVES

- Discuss the role of action, participation, and partnership in research
- Describe the core phases of community-based participatory research
- Define and discuss the importance of mixed methodology for health equity research
- Describe the five key principles of collective impact

INTRODUCTION

While the overall field of health equity research is relatively new, there are a number of robust methodologies that have been developed specifically for health equity work or adapted from existing methodologies. Some are designed specifically for accomplishing health equity research (e.g., community-based participatory research [CBPR] and mixed-methods research) and some are designed to provide a framework for conducting health equity promotion work (e.g., collective impact and multilevel interventions). While there are certainly other methods employed in researching and community organizing around health equity, these methods have particular promise that merit discussion. This chapter is not intended to serve as a roadmap for implementing the methodologies discussed; such detail is beyond the scope of this chapter. Our goal is to introduce them conceptually to serve as a springboard for additional study in the area.

COMMUNITY-BASED PARTICIPATORY RESEARCH

The methodology that is perhaps most directly tied to the field of health equity is that of CBPR, widely considered the gold standard in engaging communities impacted by health disparities in impactful research (Berge, Mendenhall, & Doherty, 2009; Israel, Schulz, Parker, & Becker, 1998; Wallerstein & Duran, 2006, 2010). The unique feature of CBPR is the dedication to not just representing or listening to, but being driven by the voice of the community as research projects are designed, implemented, analyzed, and interpreted.

To understand the concept of CBPR, it is important to first understand the role of action, participation, and partnership in the biomedical research enterprise. Traditional research has been investigator driven—typically a university-based faculty member draws upon her own experiences and knowledge to develop a research hypothesis, which she then systematically tests, analyzes, and interprets from a standpoint of scientific detachment (e.g., What is the gene responsible for this type of breast cancer?). Such an approach is devoid of all three concepts integral to CBPR: action, participation, and partnership.

Action research, in contrast to traditional research, is focused on both answering a question and upon changing the status quo. In essence, it is focused on developing a specific solution to the problem at hand (e.g., What are the removable barriers to mammography in African American communities, and what happens when they are removed?). While it is still scientific in nature, it is directly connected to changing the concept under investigation. Participatory research is research in which the individuals impacted by the research topic are a part of the research "process"—not just subjects in a study, but actively shaping the project itself (e.g., What do African American breast cancer survivors identify as ways to decrease depression in women post-mastectomy, and how would they design an intervention to do so?). This level of participation is foreign to many "classically-trained" researchers, as it shatters the wall many have been taught to place between research participants and the research itself. Research that combines both components is referred to as "participatory action research (PAR)," which is driven by those impacted to in turn impact the outcome under investigation (e.g., How can we establish an African American breast cancer survivor research network to develop and implement prevention strategies?).

Layered on top of levels of action and participation is levels of involvement of communities in research. Traditional research does not truly engage communities in the research process. Even if members of the community are participants in the research project, they are not a part of the process itself (e.g., How can we develop a new substance abuse prevention program by interviewing rural substance users?). Research that is community-placed takes a first step in the direction of community engagement by physically locating the research within the affected community—that is, rather than asking community members to come to you to participate in the study, you locate the study in the community itself (e.g., How can we place a substance abuse intervention delivery site directly within a remote Appalachian community?). The next step is community-based research, which actively engages the community in the design, conduct, interpretation, or dissemination of findings of research (e.g., How can we test a program that matches recovering substance abusers with peer support specialists?). In this example, the peer support specialists—who themselves are in recovery—become agents of change within the research process by serving as interventionists.

Bringing together all these concepts—action, participation, and community partnership—yields community-based participatory (action) research, or CBPR. CBPR takes community-based research to the next level by actively partnering with the community being affected by the outcome of interest in the design, conduct, interpretation, *and* dissemination of the findings of research. In its purest form, the investigator does not even select the research focus—it is selected collaboratively by the community itself (e.g., How can we, along with community leaders, collaboratively plan, execute, and interpret a study of the link between low self-esteem and substance use in rural children?).

While the individual methods used to accomplish each step vary widely from initiative to initiative, Israel, Eng, Schulz, and Parker (2005) delineate a six-step process for engaging in CBPR, with recommendations for each step provided by Kendall, Nguyen, Glick, and Seal (2017) summarized in Table 4.1. Step 1 involves forming the partnerships themselves. Step 2 focuses on assessing the community's strengths and dynamics to inform subsequent work. Step 3 builds from the assessment to identify priority health concerns and associated research questions. Step 4 focuses on designing and conducting epidemiologic, intervention, and/or policy-related research. Step 5 involves feeding results back to all partners and collaboratively interpreting research findings. Finally, Step 6 focuses on disseminating and translating the research findings to a broader

TABLE 4.1 Recommendations for Conducting Community-Based Participatory Research by Phase

PHASE	RECOMMENDATIONS
Partnership formation	▪ Establish a clear understanding of the strengths and limitations of each organization ▪ Build a strong belief in and commitment to compromise and equality ▪ Establish clear guidelines or a memorandum of understanding to guide partnership activities
Community assessment	▪ Establish shared leadership and power within the operating structure ▪ Have a co-facilitator structure between community and academic partners ▪ Have more community than non-community representatives on the board ▪ Create an environment where experience is as equally valued as academic knowledge
Prioritization of concerns	▪ Establish specific, long-term goals of the project ▪ Develop a detailed implementation plan ▪ Form a steering committee to provide leadership and oversight of project activities
Conducting study	▪ Consider establishment of a subcommittee or new board to guide study execution ▪ Engage more community members than academics on leadership of study execution ▪ Develop measurable outcomes for all partners ▪ Consider having an external evaluation team for the project
Feedback and interpretation	▪ Ensure community partners are engaged in this step of the research process ▪ Utilize member-checking with community members ▪ Be transparent and let results speak
Dissemination and translation	▪ Avoid jargon and fancy conceptual models ▪ Focus on key findings and do not overwhelm with statistics ▪ Focus on interpretation of findings and application to other projects and/or outcomes ▪ Include community partners as co-presenters

audience. Throughout the process, an intentional focus on maintaining, sustaining, and evaluating the CBPR partnership itself helps to promote long-term functioning of the group. This becomes particularly important because of the time- and labor-intensive nature of CBPR.

CBPR represents a significant departure for most university-based researchers, who largely were trained to feel that their education and experience were gained in order to develop their "own" research questions and who are often uncomfortable with the loss of "control" that CBPR partnerships entail. Their ability, however, to build extremely successful and sustainable partnerships that develop impactful initiatives is unquestioned (Coughlin, Smith, & Fernández, 2017).

MIXED-METHODS

Mixed methodology has existed for decades, and is closely tied to the field of behavioral intervention development. Because of its ability to diversify the type of data received in a study and triangulate multiple sources of data, it is particularly well-suited for health equity studies. While there are many variations of—and ongoing debate regarding—definitions for mixed-methods studies, the inaugural issue of the *Journal of Mixed Methods Research* defined the approach as "research in which the investigator collects and analyzes data, integrates the findings, and draws inferences using both qualitative and quantitative approaches or methods in a single study or a program of inquiry" (Tashakkori & Creswell, 2007, p. 4). They go on to specifically mention that mixed methods provides the opportunity to simultaneously examine research questions that are both participatory and preplanned, and to draw both emic and etic conclusions (i.e., "insider" vs. "outsider" perspective).

This ability to integrate insider and outsider perspectives while combining participatory and preplanned research questions is the core of mixed methodology's power in health equity research. Inherently, even if part of the community under investigation, researchers typically do not fully represent the community being investigated. For most communities impacted by health disparities, issues of socioeconomic security, educational levels, and health literacy are major concerns, and almost by default health equity researchers have an elevated level of each of these factors. Further, unless the researcher was a member of the specific geographic community under investigation, differences are inherent and methodologies that rely solely on investigator-driven data (e.g., quantitative) do not even leave the door open for exploring additional concepts and factors that may be just as, if not more, important than those developed by the investigator. Including a qualitative component allows for the voices of individuals affected by the outcome of interest to be heard, and provides the opportunity to be more inclusive of this diversity of thought. For communities historically disenfranchised and silenced, ensuring the ability to have their voice represented can make all the difference in the success of a study.

COLLECTIVE IMPACT

While CBPR provides an excellent framework for developing partnerships to collectively research health equity issues, it is not designed to support the implementation of large, social change initiatives often necessary to achieve health equity. In their seminal article on the topic, Kania and Kramer (2011) made the argument that "large-scale social change requires broad cross-sector coordination, yet the social sector remains focused on the isolated intervention of individual organizations." Their premise was that to truly see social change, such as the kind necessary to achieve

TABLE 4.2 Key Principles of Collective Impact

PRINCIPLE	DESCRIPTION
Common agenda	The group establishes a shared vision and conducts collaborative strategic planning to develop a common definition, joint approach, and mutually-endorsed action plans
Shared measurement	Common ground is reached on how success will be measured, all organizations measure common indicators, and outcomes are measured against predefined accountability goals
Mutually reinforcing activities	Rather than engaging in a single collaborative activity, each agency engages in their own, but built around a cohesive plan that builds intersections and synergy across agencies
Continuous communication	Partners are dedicated to full transparency and openness, trust and buy-in are continually reinforced, a common vocabulary is established, and common motivation is sustained
Backbone support	An identified agency with dedicated staff coordinates collective efforts with a specific focus on planning, managing, supporting, and convening

SOURCE: Adapted from Hanleybrown, F., Kania, J., & Kramer, M. (2012). Channeling change: Making collective impact work. *Stanford Social Innovation Review.* Retrieved from https://ssir.org/articles/entry/channeling_change_making_collective_impact_work

health equity, organizations must learn how to cooperate not in the execution of individual tasks and activities, but rather in coordinating the overall impact of what they are all seeking to accomplish. In this way, multiple organizations can coordinate their efforts such that each agency works within its own area of maximum impact, but is able to simultaneously extend upon or enhance the work of its collaborators. Defined as "the commitment of a group of important actors from different sectors to a common agenda for solving a specific social problem" (Kania & Kramer, 2011, para. 5), the use of the collective impact framework has exploded in the past decade.

Collective impact is guided by five key principles: common agenda, shared measurement, mutually reinforcing activities, continuous communication, and backbone support. These are described in Table 4.2. The overall collective impact process follows three phases: initiate action, organize for impact, and sustain action and impact (Hanleybrown, Kania, & Kramer, 2012).

Collective impact has been implemented by hundreds of coalitions and task forces spanning the public sector to industry, and will continue to be an important approach for community-driven initiatives to consider.

CONCLUSION

The field of health equity—both practice and research—draws upon several disciplines. Four approaches in particular have been effective in understanding and achieving health equity. CBPR focuses on the tenet of "nothing about us, without us" by partnering with communities affected by disparities in the design, implementation, evaluation, and dissemination of research projects through action, participation, and partnership. Mixed methodologies focus on integrating the strengths of both quantitative and qualitative research when designing new interventions and programs—by taking both an etic and an emic approach, richer information can be obtained. Finally, collective impact focuses on specific community engagement strategies designed to orient community coalitions to achieve shared goals through strategic and deliberate collaboration. These approaches are not designed to solve a specific issue—rather, they provide tools for health equity practitioners and researchers to develop and implement strategies to achieve equity.

DISCUSSION QUESTIONS

- How could the action and participation components of CBPR place the approach at odds with the tenets of scientific detachment and neutrality?

- How do CBPR approaches help to reveal the power of communities impacted by health disparities in ways that encourage their participation in research?

- How does a mixed-methods approach help to balance the emic and etic aspects of research? What are the advantages of having both perspectives in a single study?

- What are some of the barriers that agencies looking to implement collective impact might face, particularly with respect to establishing a common agenda?

REFERENCES

Berge, J., Mendenhall, T. J., & Doherty, W. J. (2009). Using community-based participatory research (CBPR) to target health disparities in families. *Family Relations, 58*(4), 475–488. doi:10.1111/j.1741-3729.2009.00567.x

Coughlin, S. S., Smith, S. A., & Fernández, M. E. (Eds.). (2017). *Handbook of community-based participatory research*. Oxford, UK: Oxford University Press.

Hanleybrown, F., Kania, J., & Kramer, M. (2012). Channeling change: Making collective impact work. *Stanford Social Innovation Review*. Retrieved from https://ssir.org/articles/entry/channeling_change_making_collective_impact_work

Israel, B. A., Eng, E., Schulz, A. J., & Parker, E. A. (Eds.). (2005). *Methods in community-based participatory research for health*. New York, NY: Wiley.

Israel, B. A., Schulz, A. J., Parker, E. A., & Becker, A. B. (1998). Review of community-based research: Assessing partnership approaches to improve public health. *Annual Review of Public Health, 19*, 173–202. doi:10.1146/annurev.publhealth.19.1.173

Kania, J., & Kramer, M. (2011). Collective impact. *Stanford Social Innovation Review*. Retrieved from https://ssir.org/articles/entry/collective_impact

Kendall, C., Nguyen, A. L., Glick, J., & Seal, D. (2017). Research methods and community-based participatory research. In S. S. Coughlin, S. A. Smith, & M. E. Fernández (Eds.), *Handbook of community-based participatory research* (pp. 21–38). Oxford, UK: Oxford University Press.

Tashakkori, A., & Creswell, J. W. (2007). The new era of mixed methods. *Journal of Mixed Methods Research, 1*(1), 3–7. doi:10.1177/2345678906293042

Wallerstein, N. B., & Duran, B. (2006). Using community-based participatory research to address health disparities. *Health Promotion Practice, 7*(3), 312–323. doi:10.1177/1524839906289376

Wallerstein, N. B., & Duran, B. (2010). Community-based participatory research contributions to intervention research: The intersection of science and practice to improve health equity. *American Journal of Public Health, 100*(Suppl. 1), S40–S46. doi:10.2105/AJPH.2009.184036

II

POPULATION PERSPECTIVES ON HEALTH EQUITY

AFRICAN AMERICAN HEALTH EQUITY

FAYE Z. BELGRAVE ▪ JASMINE A. ABRAMS ▪ K. BRYANT SMALLEY ▪ JACOB C. WARREN

LEARNING OBJECTIVES

- Describe the ways in which social determinants of health play a role in the existence and persistence of African American health disparities
- Describe the extent to which biology and genetics influence disparities and how both are influenced by broader social determinants of health
- Discuss the magnitude, source, and prevention of health disparities for African Americans in diabetes, cardiovascular disease, HIV, and cancer
- Discuss factors related to differences in mortality for health disparity outcomes among African Americans
- Describe approaches for achieving health equity for African Americans

INTRODUCTION

The field of health disparities and subsequently health equity has origins in the study of differences in health status and outcomes between African American and White populations. As a result, the literature surrounding health disparities and health equity among African Americans is arguably the most robust of any population-specific health disparity group. The U.S. Census (2018) defines "Black" or "African American" as "A person having origins in any of the Black racial groups of Africa." It includes people who indicate their race as "Black, African American, or Negro," or who provide written entries such as Afro American, Kenyan, Nigerian, or Haitian. Unfortunately, the depth of health disparities research among African Americans has not yet translated into systemic improvements in health outcomes across the United States and calls-to-action are still regularly made with regard to African American health (Negbenebor & Garza, 2018).

African American populations remain severely impacted by macrolevel structural issues that lead to many health disparities. Thus, the disparities remain, continuing a near 400-year trend starting with the arrival of African people in the "New World" (Hammonds & Reverby, 2019). In this chapter, we summarize the multi-level factors influencing the presence of health disparities for African Americans to provide context for subsequent discussion. We then summarize several of the most studied disparities, examining the cause-specific health determinants, outcome disparities, and cause-specific recommendations for intervention and prevention work. We conclude with a discussion of specific approaches to advance health equity among African Americans.

OUTCOMES OF FOCUS

Cardiovascular Disease

Cardiovascular disease (CVD), conditions that affect the heart and involve restricted or blocked blood vessels, is a $200 billion epidemic impacting the lives of an estimated 80 million people living in the United States. Among the most common forms of CVD are hypertension, coronary heart disease, and stroke. Killing one to two people each minute, CVD results in one of every four deaths among Americans annually. Compared to other racial/ethnic groups, African Americans experience a disproportionate CVD burden as they are more likely to have some form of CVD and experience increased CVD risk factors (Centers for Disease Control and Prevention [CDC], n.d.-a).

Given the disparities in prevalence, it is not surprising that African Americans, and African American women especially, are less likely to receive appropriate disease management treatments for CVD (Canto et al., 2000; Cook, Ayanian, Orav, & Hicks, 2009; G. Howard, Labarthe, Hu, Yoon, & Howard, 2007; Smedley, Stith, & Nelson, 2003; Vaccarino et al., 2005). In addition, African Americans are more likely to receive insufficient preventive care, which is essential to abating the personal, societal, and economic burden of CVD (Jha et al., 2003).

There are also strong mortality disparities related to CVD tied to higher prevalence, incidence, morbidity, and mortality (R. A. Williams, 2009). As shown in Figure 5.1, men have a 30% higher mortality rate, and women have a 37% higher mortality rate when compared with their White

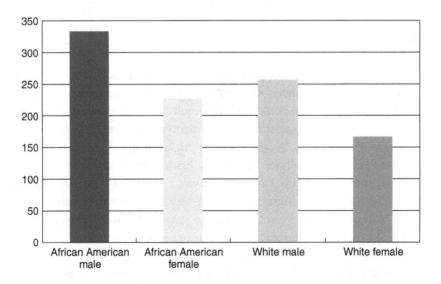

FIGURE 5.1 Age-adjusted heart disease mortality rates by race and gender.

NOTE: 1999 to 2016 age-adjusted cause-specific mortality rate per 100,000.

SOURCE: CDC WONDER Compressed Mortality Files. Retrieved from https://wonder.cdc.gov/cmf-icd10.html.

counterparts for heart disease. Because of the overall burden, however, this represents a massive absolute difference—the excess in heart disease mortality rate among African American men, for example, is more than the overall diabetes and stroke mortality rates in White men *combined*.

Biological and social factors have been identified as driving the disparities, with initial elevations in risk identified even in early childhood (Sowers, Ferdinand, Bakris, & Douglas, 2015). While a great deal of attention has focused on the potential role of genetics, the literature largely agrees that the role of genetics is minor (if present at all; Jamerson, 2004). Because of its clear relation to physiological factors such as allostatic load, experiences of racism and discrimination have been repeatedly associated with CVD risk in the literature, although debates regarding the strength of the association remain largely due to the methodological complexity of measuring discrimination experiences (Calvin et al., 2003; Dolezsar, McGrath, Herzig, & Miller, 2014; Sims et al., 2012). Other risk factors include lower awareness of heart disease symptoms, level of trust and confidence in providers, and social/neighborhood contexts that enhance risk factors (Cuffee et al., 2013; Lutfiyya, Cumba, McCullough, Barlow, & Lipsky, 2008; Morenoff et al., 2007; Thorpe, Brandon, & LaVeist, 2008). Specific targets in prevention have included hypertension control, lipid management, tobacco use cessation, promotion of physical activity, and prevention of heart failure, but relatively little focus has been placed on post-heart attack care (A. M. Davis, Vinci, Okwuosa, Chase, & Huang, 2007).

Recommendations to curb disparities include intentional focus on early detection and treatment, improving disease management self-efficacy, using multidisciplinary teams, implementing community outreach and community-level interventions (particularly involving community health workers), improving care transitions, promoting access and adherence to prescriptions, focusing on the cultural nature of many hypertension-related behavior changes (such as diet), and incorporating the importance of mental health into intervention modalities (Brownstein et al., 2005; A. M. Davis et al., 2007; Finkelstein, Khavjou, Mobley, Haney, & Will, 2004; Jamerson, 2004; Peters, Aroian, & Flack, 2006; Schoenthaler, Ogedegbe, & Allegrante, 2009; Williams, 2009). Unfortunately, advances that are made are not equally applied to African American and White populations. For instance, while the awareness of CVD has increased substantially over the past several decades for all women, the gap in awareness between African American and White women has not closed, which has helped to maintain disparities (A. H. Christian, Rosamond, White, & Mosca, 2007).

Stroke

Another form of CVD, stroke, is the leading cause of long-term disability in the United States (Gutierrez & Williams, 2014). As with diabetes and hypertension (two of the outcome's major risk factors), African Americans experience a highly disparate rate of stroke incidence and mortality that has been described as a "national crisis" (G. Howard & Howard, 2001). Particularly impacting African Americans in the South, the disparity is tied both to differences in the underlying burden of risk factors and to significant disparities in stroke care and stroke prevention (Cruz-Flores et al., 2011; G. Howard et al., 2007). As shown in Figure 5.2, the cause-specific mortality rate for African American men is 57% higher than among White men, and for women it is 34% higher.

Although there is no gender disparity for White men and women, who have virtually identical mortality rates, African American men have a stroke mortality rate 17% higher than African American women. The disparity in stroke widens in direct relation to underlying hypertension—for

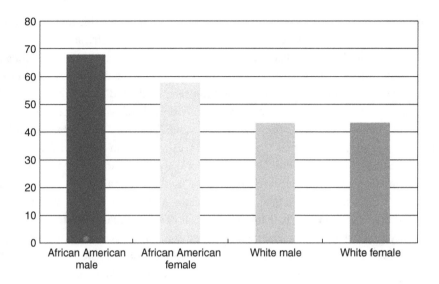

FIGURE 5.2 Age-adjusted stroke mortality rates by race and gender.
NOTE: 1999 to 2016 age-adjusted cause-specific mortality rate per 100,000.
SOURCE: CDC WONDER Compressed Mortality Files. Retrieved from https://wonder.cdc.gov/cmf-icd10.html.

every 10 mmHg increase in systolic blood pressure, African Americans experience an additional threefold risk of stroke in comparison to their White counterparts (Gutierrez & Williams, 2014). Disturbingly, while the incidence rate of stroke is higher in African Americans, the magnitude of difference is not as large as the difference seen in mortality—this suggests that there are systemic issues in the receipt of quality poststroke care that lead African Americans to be more likely to die after having a stroke (V. J. Howard et al., 2011). In addition, African Americans have greater neurologic impairment, increased risk of dysphagia, and poorer overall outcomes poststroke (Bussell & González-Fernández, 2011; Shen, Washington, & Aponte-Soto, 2004).

Numerous differences have been identified that contribute to this disparity beyond the frequently-cited differences in obesity and physical inactivity (McGruder, Malarcher, Antoine, Greenlund, & Croft, 2004). African Americans have been shown to be less aware of stroke symptoms, the need for seeking treatment urgently, and the causal connection between risk factors and stroke (Alkadry, Bhandari, Wilson, & Blessett, 2011; Cruz-Flores et al., 2011; Lutfiyya, Cumba, et al., 2008; Lutfiyya, Lipsky, et al., 2008). African Americans also utilize emergency medical services less, and even when they do seek services, they are less likely to receive life- and function-saving treatments, less likely to receive a CT within 25 minutes, less likely to receive cardiac monitoring and dysphagia screening, and less likely to be placed on secondary stroke prevention agents (J. B. Christian, Lapane, & Toppa, 2003; Cruz-Flores et al., 2011; Glasser et al., 2008; Jacobs et al., 2006). Factors contributing to this lack of awareness and associated action are related to insurance coverage, mistrust of the healthcare system, low representation of African American physicians, childhood and adult socioeconomic status, and institutional racism (Bravata et al., 2005; Cruz-Flores et al., 2011; Glymour, Avendaño, Haas, & Berkman, 2008). Strategies to decrease stroke incidence and mortality include focusing on family and community strengths, improving overall psychological health, utilizing community health worker–focused approaches, and using collaborative care teams focused on long-term management of symptoms and risk factors (Blixen et al., 2014; Glymour et al., 2012; Kuhajda et al., 2006).

HYPERTENSION

Often referred to as a "silent killer," hypertension almost always precedes CVD and African Americans experience disparities in diagnosis, morbidity, and mortality associated with hypertension and subsequent forms of CVD. Among African Americans over the age of 20, 42% of men and 44% of women have hypertension, compared to 30% for White men and approximately 29% for White women (National Center for Health Statistics, 2015). Although research demonstrates that control of hypertension can result in decreased risk for more advanced CVD, rates of hypertension control are lower for African Americans compared to other racial/ethnic groups (Ferdinand et al., 2017).

Corresponding hospitalization rates for hypertension are also disparate with African Americans up to eight times more likely to be hospitalized as a result of hypertension in comparison to Whites. However, African Americans are also less likely to receive cutting-edge diagnostic procedures, interventions, and treatments (Carlisle, Leake, & Shapiro, 1997; S. K. Davis, Liu, & Gibbons, 2003). The effect of hypertension on other health conditions (e.g., diabetes, cancer) outcomes is also significant—for instance, it has been estimated that 30% of the disparity in breast cancer survival between African American and White women is due to hypertension (Braithwaite et al., 2009).

Diabetes

African Americans are twice as likely to be diagnosed with diabetes, which is the seventh leading cause of death in the United States (Office of Minority Health, 2019). The disparity in diabetes mortality affecting African Americans is striking and is related to differences in biological, behavioral, social, environmental, and health system factors leading to higher prevalence, decreased diabetic control, and higher rates of complications such as renal failure and blindness (Horowitz, Colson, Hebert, & Lancaster, 2004; Peek, Cargill, & Huang, 2007; Spanakis & Golden, 2013). As shown in Figure 5.3, there exists stark racial and gender disparities in age-adjusted mortality related to diabetes. Specifically, the diabetes death rate is 96% and 140% higher for Black men and women, respectively, when compared to their White counterparts.

Many factors explain this disparity, including higher HbA1c levels, lower access to healthy foods, lower levels of health literacy, financial and cultural barriers to medication adherence, barriers to receiving timely and adequate medical care, lower levels of engagement with patient empowerment tools such as patient portals, and concerns over daily hassles, physician support, and perceived seriousness of diabetes (Black, 2002; Horowitz et al., 2004; Kirk et al., 2006; Osborn et al., 2011; Sarkar et al., 2011; Spencer et al., 2006). Specific recommendations for improving diabetes outcomes in African American populations include taking a multilevel approach (e.g., implementing interventions with individuals, providers, and systems), utilizing cultural tailoring techniques for intervention programs, conducting provider trainings that promote team-based care, utilizing community health worker models, fostering the creation of a diabetes support system, partnering with faith-based organizations to increase awareness and support, and implementing culturally-sensitive screening initiatives for providers (Austin & Claiborne, 2011; Black, 2002; Marshall, 2005; Peek et al., 2007; Spencer et al., 2011; Tang, Brown, Funnell, & Anderson, 2008).

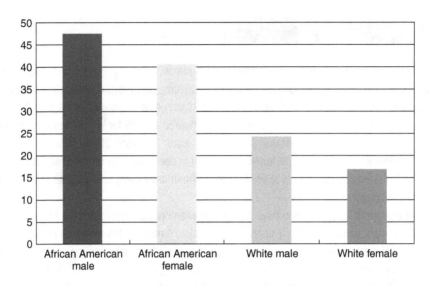

FIGURE 5.3 Age-adjusted diabetes mortality rates by race and gender.
NOTE: 1999 to 2016 age-adjusted cause-specific mortality rate per 100,000.
SOURCE: CDC WONDER Compressed Mortality Files. Retrieved from https://wonder.cdc.gov/cmf-icd10.html.

Cancer

Prominent disparities exist for many different cancer types (see Figure 5.4). While these disparities have been recognized for some time, survival rates remain lower for African Americans for
"most cancers at each stage of diagnosis" (DeSantis et al., 2016). African American men are 47%
more likely to die from colorectal cancer than White men, 130% more likely to die from prostate
cancer, and 67% more likely to die from breast cancer. African American women are 40% more
likely to die from colorectal cancer than White women, 37% more likely to die from breast cancer,
and 105% more likely to die from cervical cancer. For some cancers, disparities are much higher
for African American men than women. For example, while African American men are 22%
more likely to die from lung cancer than White men, African American women are 10% less likely
to die from lung cancer. Some of the largest cancer disparities are related to screening and early
detection (Ghafoor et al., 2002).

As with other disparities discussed throughout this chapter, differences in mortality are not
always associated with differences in incidence. For prostate cancer as an example, while African
American men are 40% more likely to be diagnosed with prostate cancer, they are over twice as
likely to die from it (Chornokur, Dalton, Borysova, & Kumar, 2011). This relates to established
differences in stage of presentation, diagnosis, treatment approaches utilized, survival rates, and
quality of life for African Americans with prostate cancer (Chornokur et al., 2011). For breast cancer, the disparity is more substantial—despite having a lower incidence rate, African American
women have a 50% higher breast cancer mortality rate (American Cancer Society, 2017; Newman,
2005). These disparities persist even when controlling for socioeconomic status, stage at diagnosis, and comorbidities (Alexander et al., 2007; Ward et al., 2004).

The literature on potential causal factors is large and often contradictory, with many researchers focusing on genetic and biological risk and others focusing on larger social determinants.

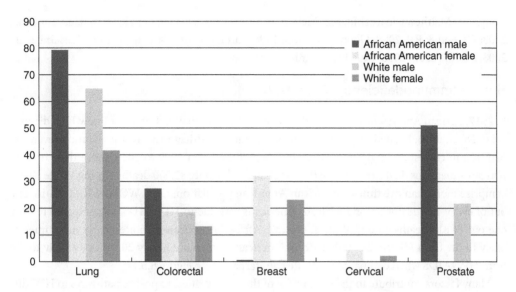

FIGURE 5.4 Age-adjusted cancer mortality rates by race and gender, various sites.

NOTE: 1999 to 2016 age-adjusted cause-specific mortality rate per 100,000.

SOURCE: CDC WONDER Compressed Mortality Files. Retrieved from https://wonder.cdc.gov/cmf-icd10.html.

While there is some evidence that biological factors and genetics play a minor role in the presence of cancer disparities, the overall scientific consensus is that these factors explain only a small portion of the disparities. This finding is supported by the fact that within-stage comparisons find disparities in mortality. For example, for most cancers 5-year survival rates are lower for African Americans at each stage of diagnosis (DeSantis, Naishadham, & Jemal, 2013). In addition, even some genetic predispositions are still subject to a broader source of disparities (e.g., social determinants): African American women are more likely to be diagnosed with triple-negative breast cancer (TNBC), which is particularly aggressive, but African American women with TNBC have even higher mortality rates than White women with TNBC (Dietze, Sistrunk, Miranda-Carboni, O'Regan, & Seewaldt, 2015).

Other contributing factors identified in the literature include mistrust of the medical system, lower levels of health literacy, higher levels of poverty, lower likelihood of having a primary care physician, lower likelihood of receiving recommended cancer screenings (e.g., colonoscopy), underinsurance, lack of insurance, cultural factors such as dietary risk, differences in receipt of appropriate pain management, and even differences in use of evidence-based treatments such as chemotherapy and radiation (Allen, Kennedy, Wilson-Glover, & Gilligan, 2007; Dimou, Syrigos, & Wasif Saif, 2009; Freeman, 2004; James, Greiner, Ellerbeck, Feng, & Ahluwalia, 2006; Payne, Medina, & Hampton, 2003). Recommendations for eliminating cancer disparities include use of culturally tailored programming and educational materials, use of community outreach through community health workers, providing support for patients (including through faith-based institutions), and increasing access to prevention. Other recommendations include utilizing patient navigation programs, promoting early detection, utilizing transdisciplinary research and clinical teams, increasing representation of African Americans in cancer clinical trials, and ensuring equal access to high-quality and newly developed treatments (Chornokur et al., 2011;

Coughlin, Matthews-Juarez, Juarez, Melton, & King, 2014; DeSantis et al., 2016; Gabram et al., 2008; Gerend & Pai, 2008; Gotay & Wilson, 1998; Guidry, Fagan, & Walker, 1998; Husaini et al., 2008; Molina et al., 2008; Murthy, Krumholz, & Gross, 2004).

Human Immunodeficiency Virus (HIV)

In 2017, African Americans represented 13% of the U.S. population but 43% of new HIV diagnoses (CDC, n.d.-b). Related disparities in diagnosis rates, postdiagnosis treatment, and prevention manifest in correspondingly stark mortality disparities. From 1999 to 2016, more than 104,000 African Americans died from HIV/AIDS, as compared to only 82,000 deaths among Whites (who comprise more than five times the African American population; CDC WONDER). In 2016, one out of every 104 deaths among African Americans was due to HIV/AIDS, as compared to only one out of 817 deaths among Whites. Overall, African American men are nearly nine times as likely to die from HIV/AIDS and African American women are nearly 20 times as likely to die from HIV/AIDS when compared to White counterparts (see Figure 5.5.).

Many factors contribute to the magnitude of these disparities. Exposure pathways to HIV differ markedly by gender: approximately 80% of new HIV cases in African American men occur through same-sex sexual activity, whereas approximately 90% of new HIV cases in African American women occur through opposite-sex sexual activity (HIV among sexual minority men of color is discussed in more detail in Chapter 12, LGBTQ Health Equity). Sexual transmission is therefore the largest source of HIV acquisition in African Americans. Further, because of elevated rates of stigma (both surrounding HIV and sexual minority status), African American men have been found to be less likely to disclose their HIV status to sexual partners of either gender (Bird, Fingerhut, & McKirnan, 2011). Earlier research found that beginning in adolescence, African Americans exhibited less knowledge of HIV risk factors and prevention practices, indicating

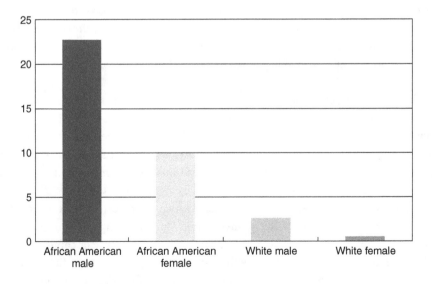

FIGURE 5.5 Age-adjusted AIDS mortality rates by race and gender.
NOTE: 1999 to 2016 age-adjusted cause-specific mortality rate per 100,000.
SOURCE: CDC WONDER Compressed Mortality Files. Retrieved from https://wonder.cdc.gov/cmf-icd10.html.

sexual health prevention efforts not adequately reaching the population (Swenson et al., 2010). However, recent research demonstrates that African American young adults engage in more preventive behaviors, as indicated by greater rates of testing and condom use, compared to White young adults. These findings highlight that HIV acquisition and associated disparities are not simply a function of individual behaviors (Moore, Javier, Abrams, McGann, & Belgrave, 2017).

Beyond disparities in prevalence, in terms of postdiagnosis care, only 46% of African Americans living with HIV had achieved viral suppression compared to 56.3% of Whites (Crepaz, Dong, Wang, Hernandez, & Hall, 2018). Viral suppression is critical to the prevention of HIV transmission and lower rates of viral control directly contribute to the ongoing disparities in new diagnoses. Further, despite representing 44% of individuals who meet indications for taking HIV pre-exposure prophylaxis medication (PrEP), only 11.2% of PrEP users are African American (Kuehn, 2018). Prevention is further complicated by lower access to medical and screening services; one out of every seven African Americans living with HIV do not know they have it (CDC, n.d.-b).

Avoidance of screening, disruptions in the continuum of HIV care, and lower adherence rates to HIV medication have been tied to factors ranging from lower access to medical services overall to HIV-specific mistrust of the medical community (Bogart, Wagner, Galvan, & Banks, 2010). High rates of stigma within the general population, within the African American community, and specifically within the African American faith community, have also been identified as key barriers to disclosure of HIV status, receipt of medical care, and engagement in preventive services/ programs (Muturi & An, 2010; Radcliffe et al., 2010; Vyavaharkar et al., 2010).

Because of the long-recognized racial disparity in HIV/AIDS outcomes, there is a robust body of literature in the prevention and treatment of HIV/AIDS among African American populations that is beyond the scope of this chapter; however, common intervention themes for both men and women include a focus on ethnic and gender pride, social skills development, sexual assertiveness and communication, condom use skills, disclosure, stress reduction, and substance abuse prevention (DiClemente & Wingood, 1995; Wohl et al., 2011). For women in particular, faith-based interventions (such as the P4 for Women modification of the well-known Sisters Informing Sisters about Topics on AIDS [SISTA] intervention) have been found to be particularly impactful (Wingood et al., 2013).

In summary, there are varied social determinants that create health disparities for African Americans across a number of outcomes. It is important to note that while magnitude differs across causes, to a large extent the underlying factors (e.g., access to quality care, availability of preventive screenings) repeat across outcomes. While these factors tend to require multi-level, large-scale initiatives to achieve health equity, these commonalities provide a unique opportunity to impact multiple health disparities through focused equity efforts.

DISPARITY-DRIVING FACTORS AMONG AFRICAN AMERICANS

When attempting to explain the health inequities experienced by African Americans, scholars often cite culture, historical discrimination, broad structural inequalities, and the intersection of these factors as central causes. Through the identification of causal, risk, and protective factors, scholars and practitioners have also identified many promising practices and recommendations for practitioners that are helping to shape programs across the country.

The discussion of the root of health disparities generally focuses on two broad categories: social determinants of health and a legacy of oppression and discrimination that began with the forced arrival of Blacks to the United States. More recently, genetics and biological factors have been implicated as causes of health disparities. Given that social determinants are discussed in depth elsewhere in this text (see Chapter 3, Health Equity Frameworks and Theories), we will not go into detail here defining the construct. However, factors such as income levels, educational attainment, neighborhood characteristics, individual and institutional discrimination, and even fundamental access to care are much more likely than biological factors to serve as barriers to achieving and maintaining health for African Americans. There is a clear and consistent relationship between income/educational level and health status, with a marked gradient among African Americans (Cutler & Lleras-Muney, 2006; Rivero-Becerra & Rodriguez, 2004; D. R. Williams, 2002). Unfortunately, among African American women in particular, employment does not translate to increased wealth—despite having higher employment rates than other races/ethnicities, African American women do not have correspondingly higher levels of income (United States Bureau of Labor Statistics, 2016).

As with many populations discussed in this book, the cumulative effects of marginalization, discrimination, and racism are profound. Racism and discrimination create barriers to health equity through several processes. Racial discrimination adversely impacts the quality and quantity of medical care. For example, perceived discrimination is linked to poor medication adherence (Forsyth, Schoenthaler, Chaplin, Ogedegbe, & Ravenell, 2014). Other research shows implicit bias held against African Americans by healthcare providers leads to biased treatment recommendations (Moskowitz, Stone, & Childs, 2012; D. R. Williams & Wyatt, 2015). In addition, the experiences of racial discrimination adversely affect health by creating psychological distress and other physiological changes (Brody et al., 2014) such as changes in heart rate variability (Hill et al., 2017).

Moreover, at a systems level, racism operates through many institutional structures such as residential segregation to impact the health of African Americans. Many African Americans live in communities where there are a high number of health-compromising conditions (e.g., environmental pollutants, high availability of tobacco and alcohol products, unhealthy food sources) and a lack of health-promoting resources (e.g., fresh farmers markets, full service grocery stores, and parks and recreation facilities; Corral et al., 2012; Smedley, 2012). See Chapter 2, Prejudice, Discrimination, and Health, for further discussion of racism and discrimination and health disparities.

As discussed in Chapter 3, Health Equity Frameworks and Theories, racism and discrimination also lead to "minority stress," which represents the lifetime of accumulated stress response and its related health risk behaviors and consequences. Beyond the cumulative effects of discrimination on health outcomes, direct barriers to accessibility and acceptability of care trace their roots to historic mistrust of the medical community. Mistrust of the medical community may account for some of the underutilization of healthcare by African Americans (Tucker, Moradi, Wall, & Nghiem, 2014) as distrust created by unethical medical experimentation (e.g., Tuskegee Syphilis Study) still manifests today. When combined with the high rates of reported discrimination within the healthcare setting (Corbie-Smith, Thomas, & St. George, 2002; Panza et al., 2019; Washington, 2006), it is easy to see how medical mistrust continues and may contribute to avoidance of care.

While the literature on potential genetic predispositions for health outcomes is broad, its findings are largely inconsistent and have failed to identify genetic sources that sufficiently account for a meaningful portion of documented health disparities. Recent work, however, has begun to focus more on the epigenetics of health disparities—that is, the ways in which genetic predispositions (be they related to race or not) are disproportionately activated in the high-stress environment that African Americans are more likely to experience. For instance, chronic stress has been related to outcomes and risk factors ranging from preterm birth to telomere length (Chue et al., 2014; Entringer, Buss, & Wadhwa, 2015). The emerging field of social epigenomics will provide important new insights into the role that genetics and biology play in health disparities; however, the general consensus is that differences that relate to these factors are almost always associated with an underlying trigger rooted in social determinants of health.

APPROACHES TO ACHIEVE EQUITY

While cause-specific approaches were discussed within each outcome, there are a number of general recommendations that can apply across many outcomes of interest. These include interventions and programs focused on stress reduction, social support, and empowerment delivered via approaches that include faith-based/community-based, online, community partnering, multilevel approaches, and socioenvironmental approaches (Belgrave & Abrams, 2016). Examples of outcomes investigated across these approaches, as summarized by Belgrave and Abrams (2016), are presented in Table 5.1. Stress reduction programs acknowledge the chronic and pervasive stress African Americans face every day due to structural discrimination and other social determinants of health. A variety of stress-reducing strategies have been found to be effective at reducing adverse health outcomes among African Americans (see Table 5.1). Mindfulness mediation and guided mediation have been found to be effective (Cox et al., 2013), as well as movement/rhythm and dance (Vinesett et al., 2017).

TABLE 5.1 Culturally-Sensitive Approaches to Achieve Health Equity for African Americans

APPROACH	EVIDENCE
Stress reduction	▪ Breast cancer (Monti et al., 2013) ▪ HIV (Jones et al., 2010) ▪ Weight loss (Cox et al., 2013) ▪ Intimate partner violence and post-traumatic stress disorder (PTSD; Dutton, Bermudez, Matas, Majid, & Myers, 2013) ▪ Quality of life and reduction of psychological distress (Vinesett et al., 2017)
Social support	▪ Intimate partner violence (Nicolaidis et al., 2013) ▪ Binge eating (Mason & Lewis, 2017) ▪ Pregnancy weight gain (Herring et al., 2016) ▪ Improved maternal and infant outcomes (Gabbe et al., 2017) ▪ Diabetes (Murrock, Higgins, & Killion, 2009) ▪ HIV medication adherence (Simoni, Pantalone, Plummer, & Huang, 2007) ▪ Sexual risk-taking (Belgrave, Corneille, Hood, Foster-Woodson, & Fitzgerald, 2010)

(continued)

TABLE 5.1 Culturally Sensitive Approaches to Achieve Health Equity for African Americans (*continued*)

APPROACH	EVIDENCE
Empowerment	▪ Depression and distress (Kaslow et al., 2010) ▪ HIV prevention (Wingood & DiClemente, 2006) ▪ Sexual risk (Akintobi et al., 2016)
Faith/community-based	▪ Breast cancer (Boyd & Wilmoth, 2006) ▪ Cardiovascular health (Tettey, Duran, Andersen, & Boutin-Foster, 2017) ▪ HIV prevention (Wingood et al., 2013) ▪ Weight loss (Timmons, 2015) ▪ Cancer screening (Haynes et al., 2014) ▪ Physical activity/hypertension (Duru, Sarkisian, Leng, & Mangione, 2010) ▪ Breast cancer screening, hypertensive control, nutrition, stroke knowledge, cancer knowledge (Linnan et al., 2014) ▪ Cancer prevention (Sadler et al., 2011)
Community partnering	▪ Cardiovascular risk reduction (Villablanca et al., 2016) ▪ Nutrition (Barnidge et al., 2015) ▪ Cancer screening (Fouad, Wynn, Martin, & Partridge, 2010) ▪ Multifocal initiatives (Ferré, Jones, Norris, & Rowley, 2010)
Online	▪ HIV prevention (Wingood et al., 2011) ▪ Support and well-being in cancer survivors (Johnson-Turbes et al., 2015) ▪ Weight control during pregnancy (Herring et al., 2016)

Social support draws upon culturally relevant communal values of interdependence and communalism (Belgrave & Allison, 2018). Social support can be emotional, cognitive, and tangible, structured or unstructured, and can come from either professionals (e.g., therapists, healthcare workers) or family and friends. An example of the effectiveness of social support is described in a study that found a community-based pregnancy support program (Moms2B) resulted in several improvements in maternal and infant health in the targeted community (Gabbe et al., 2017).

Within the social determinants of health, it is important to note the highly protective effect that a "strong ethnic identity for African Americans" has on health outcomes (Belgrave & Abrams, 2016). These protections affect outcomes ranging from eating disorders to risky sexual behaviors to CVD (Beadnell et al., 2003; Dagadu & Christie-Mizell, 2014; Rogers Wood & Petrie, 2010).

Empowerment programs focus on increasing knowledge and appreciation for Black culture by promoting ethnic pride and framing program activities using cultural values and behaviors of African Americans. These programs may use the Principles of Kwanza, African proverbs, and attend to and integrate other values and symbols of African and African American culture in activities (Akintobi et al. 2016, Belgrave & Allison, 2018). For example, Akintobi et al. implemented a culturally tailored HIV prevention program that utilized culturally relevant materials (i.e., hip hop, Ma'at Principles African American History, and Urban Cinema Clips) with young African American adults and saw reductions in HIV risk behaviors.

Faith-based institutions provide a culturally familiar context in which to implement health screenings, prevention, and treatment activities. A large majority of African Americans (83%) report they believe in God with absolute certainty and 75% report that religion is very important (Masci, 2018). Therefore, many health programs are implemented within faith-based institutions and other programs may rely on spiritual beliefs to frame implementation activities

(Tettley, Duran, Andersen, & Boutin-Foster, 2017; Whitney et al., 2017). An example of a program implemented in faith-based organizations targeted at weight loss is the "Witness Project" in which African American breast cancer survivors tell their stories through witnessing to others the importance of mammograms (Bailey, Erwin, & Belin, 2000). Whitney et al. (2017) translated a clinic-based diabetes education program into a faith-based education curriculum by incorporating biblical scripture (e.g., "Therefore encourage one another and build one another up, just as you are doing" [1 Thessalonians 5:11 English Standard Version [ESV]]). Personal stories and testimonials, traditions in the African American church, were also used in this program. See Table 5.1. for other faith-based programs that have proven effective in ameliorating negative health outcomes.

Culturally familiar organizations and businesses frequented by African Americans are also good venues in which to implement health screenings and prevention. For example, several effective health programs have been implemented in beauty salons and barber shops. Linnan, D'Angelo, and Harrington (2014) summarized findings on the effectiveness of barber shops and beauty salons for recruiting and implementing health-related interventions to racial/ethnic minority participants. Close to 75% of the interventions showed a statistically significant improvement for a variety of health outcomes. As an example, Sadler et al. (2011) trained Black cosmetologists in how to discuss the importance of early breast cancer detection with their clients and found that women in the intervention group reported significantly higher rates of mammography than women in the control group.

Community partnerships draw upon the expertise of varied and diverse perspectives and substantially and meaningfully engage multiple entities such as community stakeholders, community coalitions, academic researchers, healthcare providers, and residents, among others. Community partnerships have been successful in reducing cardiometabolic risk (Villablanca, Warford, & Wheeler, 2016), increasing recommended vegetable and fruit intake (Barnidge et al., 2015), and reducing multiple health problems in the community (Ferré, Jones, Norris, & Rowley, 2010). An example of a community partnership is a coalition developed in rural counties in Alabama that increased targeted cancer screening for African American women (Fouad, Wynn, Martin, & Partridge, 2010). Activities of the coalition included the development of work groups and training these groups to promote cancer screening. Central to the success of this partnership was the recruitment and utilization of volunteers from local communities who served as health advisors and who encouraged women to get regular mammograms.

Along with faith-based institutions and culturally familiar community ventures, another mechanism for delivering effective health programs includes e-health or Internet-based programs. E-health programs have shown effectiveness across a variety of health outcomes for African Americans including reductions in weight gain, improvements in psychological well-being, and prevention of HIV (Herring et al., 2016; Johnson-Turbes, Schlueter, Moore, Buchanan, & Fairley, 2015; Wingood et al., 2011). E-health programs may be particularly useful for scalable programming as they are low-cost, accessible, and feasible (Chisolm & Sarkar, 2015).

Finally, programs that address socio-environmental determinants of health implement systematic change—essential for reducing health disparities. These programs are discussed in much detail in Chapter 3, Health Equity Frameworks and Theories, and Chapter 4, Health Equity Research and Collaboration Approaches.

INTERSECTIONALITY SPOTLIGHT

As discussed in Chapter 3, Health Equity Frameworks and Theories, the concept of intersectionality is rooted in Black feminist thought and was developed to describe the layered experiences of oppression experienced by African American women. The experiences of African Americans who live in rural areas merits specific discussion. One out of 12 rural residents is African American (Housing Assistance Council, 2012), with the greatest representation in the Southern states. Overall health disparities faced by rural residents are discussed in detail in Chapter 13, Rural, Frontier, and Appalachian Health Equity, but there are clearly exacerbated disparities found for rural African Americans, who are more likely to be obese, less likely to exercise, less likely to be insured, have fewer physician encounters, and are less likely to have an identified "personal" physician (Housing Assistance Council, 2012; Hueston & Hubbard, 2000; Lemacks, Wells, Ilich, & Ralston, 2013; Scott & Wilson, 2011).

As a result of these and other barriers to health, rural African Americans are 20% more likely to have diabetes, have poorer diabetic control, and increased rates of diabetes complications than their urban African American peers (Connolly, Unwin, Sherriff, Belous, & Kelly, 2000; Saydan & Lochner, 2010; Bennett, Olatosi, & Probst, 2008). They are also less likely to have adequate hypertension control (Mainous, King, Garr, & Pearson, 2004) and rural African American women have the highest breast cancer mortality rate in the U.S. (Wilson-Anderson, Williams, Beacham, & McDonald, 2013). Overall, the health equity issues faced by rural African Americans compound and are much more than additive, indicating that the effects of intersectional oppression are strongly felt in rural communities (Warren et al., 2014).

Specific recommendations for achieving health equity for rural African Americans includes the creation of rural-specific culturally tailored intervention and prevention programs, focusing initiatives on nutrition and physical activity which have widespread effects on multiple outcomes, involvement of local churches, utilization of peer educators, and involvement of rural African Americans in the design and implementation of health promotion initiatives (e.g., through community-based participatory research principles; Frank & Grubbs, 2008; Lemacks et al., 2013; Warren & Smalley, 2014; Warren et al., 2014; Wilson-Anderson et al., 2013).

CASE STUDY   BLACK AIDS INSTITUTE AND BLACK TREATMENT ADVOCACY NETWORK (BTAN)

African American men who have sex with men make up the largest group of new HIV cases (Centers for Disease Control and Prevention [CDC], 2018) and half of African American gay men are projected to be diagnosed with HIV within their lifetime (CDC, 2016). African American heterosexual women comprise the fourth largest group for new HIV infections. However, a diagnosis of HIV is not a foregone conclusion for all African Americans. There are several efforts by the CDC and other federal, state, and local initiatives that target HIV prevention and treatment.

African Americans infected and affected by HIV are aggressively addressing HIV prevention and treatment through non-profit organizations and community organizing. One such

(continued)

organization is the Black AIDS Institute (BAI; https://blackaids.org). The stated mission of the BAI is "to stop the AIDS pandemic in Black communities by engaging and mobilizing Black institutions and individuals in unapologetically Black efforts to confront HIV." BAI has several programs and activities throughout the United States focused on ending HIV. One such program is the Black Treatment Advocates Network (https://blackaids.org/black-treatment-advocates-network-btan). BTAN addresses systematic barriers that maintain HIV disparities by ensuring that there are adequate numbers of Black-serving institutions and leaders who have the skills, capacity, and connections to ensure equitable access and utilization of current HIV prevention and treatment strategies. Thus, a large part of BTAN's efforts are directed at training and developing capacity within local communities to address HIV prevention and treatment.

Through a national network of chapters, individuals, and groups throughout the United States are provided with the trainings, workshops, networking opportunities, and other support to mobilize in the fight against HIV/AIDS. BTAN chapters are in cities and locales that are most affected by HIV and include persons living with HIV/AIDS, activists, students, and members of community-based and faith-based organizations. Each chapter is encouraged to develop and engage in community-based and policy-related activities guided by BTAN's overarching mission and four areas of focus reflected by the names of chapter committees: (a) Voluntary Disclosure, (b) Treatment Education, (c) Patient Navigation, and (d) Advocacy.

Voluntary Disclosure committee members work to identify and reduce barriers to status disclosure for individuals living with HIV. Efforts of this committee are generally focused on reducing stigma and discrimination. Example activities include developing a supporting group for people living with HIV/AIDS, engaging in role-playing exercises to simulate disclosure, hosting ethics trainings, and developing materials that address the intersectionality of disclosure (e.g., being transgender and HIV positive). Treatment Education committee members focus on promotion of health literacy and raising awareness of the epidemic as well as important new developments in prevention and treatment (e.g., PrEP, the once-daily pill that can prevent HIV). The goal of the Patient Navigation committee is to assist HIV-positive individuals with connecting to and retention in treatment and care via activities such as peer mentoring, encouragement of service utilization, and networking events for patients and providers. The goal of the Advocacy committee is to generate activism in policy via community meetings, representation at city, regional, and national HIV-planning meetings, and informing elected officials of policies that can help end HIV/AIDS in Black communities. Collectively, the efforts of BTAN's chapters have resulted in the launching of national awareness campaigns, a host of events and community forums that provide resources for screening, prevention, and treatment in African American communities, and collective action to support policies and healthcare institutions that advance HIV research, prevention, and treatment for African Americans.

DISCUSSION QUESTIONS

- What is the mission of the Black AIDS Institute and the Black Treatment Advocacy Network?
- Why do you think it is important that African Americans be aggressively involved in addressing HIV in their communities?

CURRENT EVENT

DO HAIR CARE PRODUCTS CONTRIBUTE TO HEALTH DISPARITIES FOR AFRICAN AMERICAN WOMEN?

Recent research suggests that chemicals in hair care products frequently used by African American women (e.g., relaxers) may contribute to health disparities. Although more African American women are choosing not to use hair relaxers but rather to wear their hair in its "natural" state, hair relaxers continue to be used by many African American women. A growing number of studies have implicated hair relaxers and other hair care products as an adverse health risk for African American women. Endocrine-disrupting chemicals (EDCs) found in hair care products include, but are not limited to, estrogens, which are used to promote hair growth; phthalates, which provide fragrance; and parabens, which act as preservatives (Wright, Gathers, Kapke, Johnson, & Joseph, 2010). African American women are more likely than any other ethnic group to use hair care products containing EDCs (e.g., relaxers, dyes, activators, oils; James-Todd, Senie, & Terry, 2011). EDC exposure has been associated with uterine fibroids and several forms of cancer, including breast, ovarian, and cervical cancer (Giulivo, Lopez de Alda, Capri, & Barceló, 2016; Katz, Yang, Treviño, Walker, & Al-Hendy, 2016; Stiel, Adkins-Jackson, Clark, Mitchell, & Montgomery, 2016). Other studies have shown that EDCs can affect women's reproductive health (Tiwary, 1998; Wise, Palmer, Reich, Cozier, & Rosenberg, 2012) and how the body processes lipids, suggesting a link between EDC exposure and obesity and diabetes (Giulivo et al., 2016). While research into cause and effect is still preliminary, the abundant amount of correlational evidence suggests that Black women should be cautious when using EDC products.

DISCUSSION QUESTIONS

- What are some culturally congruent programs and interventions for increasing health equities and reducing health disparities among African Americans?

- What is the role of racism and discrimination in health disparities for African Americans?

- Based upon the known factors influencing disparities in diabetes, CVD, HIV, and cancer, what types of programs may be particularly effective in achieving equity across all of these outcomes?

- Why are faith-based and community-based approaches to achieving health equity particularly powerful for African American communities?

- What types of prevention efforts are necessary to close the mortality gap that is seen beyond disparities in incidence and prevalence? How can these be achieved in a culturally informed way?

REFERENCES

Akintobi, T. H., Trotter, J., Zellner, T., Lenoir, S., Evans, D., Rollins, L., & Miller, A. (2016). Outcomes of a behavioral intervention to increase condom use and reduce HIV risk among urban African American young adults. *Health Promotion Practice*, 17(5), 751–759. doi:10.1177/1524839916649367

Alexander, D., Waterbor, J., Hughes, T., Funkhouser, E., Grizzle, W., & Manne, U. (2007). African-American and Caucasian disparities in colorectal cancer mortality and survival by data source: An epidemiologic review. *Cancer Biomarkers*, 3(6), 301–313. doi:10.3233/CBM-2007-3604

Alkadry, M. G., Bhandari, R., Wilson, C. S., & Blessett, B. (2011). Racial disparities in stroke awareness: African Americans and Caucasians. *Journal of Health and Human Services Administration*, *33*(4), 462–490. Retrieved from https://www.jstor.org/stable/41288105

Allen, J. D., Kennedy, M., Wilson-Glover, A., & Gilligan, T. D. (2007). African-American men's perceptions about prostate cancer: Implications for designing educational interventions. *Social Science & Medicine*, *64*(11), 2189–2200. doi:10.1016/j.socscimed.2007.01.007

American Cancer Society. (2017). *Breast cancer facts and figures*. Atlanta, GA: Author.

Austin, S. A., & Claiborne, N. (2011). Faith wellness collaboration: A community-based approach to address type II diabetes disparities in an African-American community. *Social Work in Health Care*, *50*(5), 360–375. doi:10.1080/00981389.2011.567128

Bailey, E. J., Erwin, D. O., & Belin, P. (2000). Using cultural beliefs and patterns to improve mammography utilization among African-American women: The Witness Project. *Journal of the National Medical Association*, *93*(3), 136–142.

Barnidge, E. K., Baker, E. A., Schootman, M., Motton, F., Sawicki, M., & Rose, F. (2015). The effect of education plus access on perceived fruit and vegetable consumption in a rural African American community intervention. *Health Education Research*, *30*, 773–785. doi:10.1093/her/cyv041

Beadnell, B., Stielstra, S., Baker, S., Morrison, D. M., Knox, K., Gutierrez, L., & Doyle, A. (2003). Ethnic identity and sexual risk-taking among African-American women enrolled in an HIV/STD prevention intervention. *Psychology, Health & Medicine*, *8*, 187–198. doi:10.1080/1354850031000087564

Belgrave, F. Z., & Abrams, J. A. (2016). Reducing disparities and achieving equity in African American women's health. *American Psychologist*, *71*(8), 723–733. doi:10.1037/amp0000081

Belgrave, F. Z., & Allison, K. W. (2018). *African American psychology: From Africa to America*. Thousand Oaks, CA: Sage.

Belgrave, F. Z., Corneille, M., Hood, K., Foster-Woodson, J., & Fitzgerald, A. (2010). The impact of perceived group support on the effectiveness of an HIV prevention intervention for African American women. *Journal of Black Psychology*, *36*, 127–143. doi:10.1177/0095798409356686

Bennett, K. J., Olatosi, B., & Probst, J. C. (2008). *Health disparities: A rural-urban chartbook*. Retrieved from https://sc.edu/study/colleges_schools/public_health/research/research_centers/sc_rural_health_research_center/documents/73healthdisparitiesaruralurbanchartbook2008.pdf

Bird, J. D. P., Fingerhut, D. D., & McKirnan, D. J. (2011). Ethnic differences in HIV-disclosure and sexual risk. *AIDS Care*, *23*(4), 444–448. doi:10.1080/09540121.2010.507757

Black, S. A. (2002). Diabetes, diversity, and disparity: What do we do with the evidence? *American Journal of Public Health*, *92*(4), 543–548. doi:10.2105/AJPH.92.4.543

Blixen, C., Perzynski, A., Cage, J., Smyth, K., Moore, S., Sila, C.,… Sajatovic, M. (2014). Stroke recovery and prevention barriers among young African-American men: Potential avenues to reduce health disparities. *Topics in Stroke Rehabilitation*, *21*(5), 432–442. doi:10.1310/tsr2105-432

Bogart, L. M., Wagner, G., Galvan, F. H., & Banks, D. (2010). Conspiracy beliefs about HIV are related to antiretroviral treatment nonadherence among African American men with HIV. *Journal of Acquired Immune Deficiency Syndrome*, *53*(5), 648–655. doi:10.1097/QAI.0b013e3181c57dbc

Boyd, A. S., & Wilmoth, M. C. (2006). An innovative community-based intervention for African American women with breast cancer: The Witness Project. *Health & Social Work*, *31*, 77–80. doi:10.1093/hsw/31.1.77

Braithwaite, D., Tammemagi, C. M., Moore, D. H., Ozanne, E. M., Hiatt, R. A., Belkora, J., … Esserman, L. (2009). Hypertension is an independent predictor of survival disparity between African-American and White breast cancer patients. *International Journal of Cancer*, *124*(5), 1213–1219. doi:10.1002/ijc.24054

Bravata, D. M., Wells, C. K., Gulanski, B., Kernan, W. N., Brass, L. M., Long, J., & Concato, J. (2005). Racial disparities in stroke risk factors: The impact of socioeconomic status. *Stroke*, *36*(7), 1507–1511. doi:10.1161/01.STR.0000170991.63594.b6

Brody, G. H., Lei, M. K., Chae, D. H., Yu, T., Kogan, S. M., & Beach, S. R. (2014). Perceived discrimination among African American adolescents and allostatic load: A longitudinal analysis with buffering effects. *Child Development*, *85*(3), 989–1002. doi:10.1111/cdev.12213

Brownstein, J. N., Bone, L. R., Dennison, C. R., Hill, M. N., Kim, M. T., & Levine, D. M. (2005). Community health workers as interventionists in the prevention and control of heart disease and stroke. *American Journal of Preventive Medicine, 29*(5), 128–133. doi:10.1016/j.amepre.2005.07.024

Bussell, S. A., & González-Fernández, M. (2011). Racial disparities in the development of dysphagia after stroke: Further evidence from the Medicare database. *Archives of Physical Medicine and Rehabilitation, 92*(5), 737–742. doi:10.1016/j.apmr.2010.12.005

Calvin, R., Winters, K., Wyatt, S. B., Williams, D. R., Henderson, F. C., & Walker, E. R. (2003). Racism and cardiovascular disease in African Americans. *The American Journal of the Medical Sciences, 325*(6), 315–331. doi:10.1097/00000441-200306000-00003

Canto, J. G., Shlipak, M. G., Roger, W. J., Malmgren, J. A., Frederick, P. D., Labmrew, C. T., . . . Kiefe, C. I. (2000). Prevalence, clinical characteristics, and mortality among patients with myocardial infarction presenting without chest pain. *Journal of the American Medical Association, 283*(24), 3223–3229. doi:10.1001/jama.283.24.3223

Carlisle, D. M., Leake, B. D., & Shapiro, M. F. (1997). Racial and ethnic disparities in the use of cardiovascular procedures: Associations with type of health insurance. *American Journal of Public Health, 87*(2), 263–267. doi:10.2105/AJPH.87.2.263

Centers for Disease Control and Prevention. (n.d.-a). *Heart disease fact sheet*. Retrieved from https://www.cdc.gov/dhdsp/data_statistics/fact_sheets/fs_heart_disease.htm

Centers for Disease Control and Prevention. (n.d.-b). *HIV and African Americans*. Retrieved from https://www.cdc.gov/hiv/group/racialethnic/africanamericans/index.html

Centers for Disease Control and Prevention. (2016). *Lifetime risk of HIV diagnosis*. Retrieved from https://www.cdc.gov/nchhstp/newsroom/2016/croi-press-release-risk.html

Centers for Disease Control and Prevention. (2018). HIV surveillance report, 2017. Retrieved from http://www.cdc.gov/hiv/library/reports/hiv-surveillance.html

Chisolm, D. J., & Sarkar, M. (2015). E-health use in African American internet users: Can new tools address old disparities? *Telemedicine and e-Health, 21*, 163–169. doi:10.1089/tmj.2014.0107

Chornokur, G., Dalton, K., Borysova, M. E., & Kumar, N. B. (2011). Disparities at presentation, diagnosis, treatment, and survival in African American men affected by prostate cancer. *The Prostate, 71*(9), 985–997. doi:10.1002/pros.21314

Christian, A. H., Rosamond, W., White, A. R., & Mosca, L. (2007). Nine-year trends and racial and ethnic disparities in women's awareness of heart disease and stroke: An American Heart Association national study. *Journal of Women's Health, 16*(1), 68–81. doi:10.1089/jwh.2006.M072

Christian, J. B., Lapane, K. L., & Toppa, R. S. (2003). Racial disparities in receipt of secondary stroke prevention agents among US nursing home residents. *Stroke, 34*(11), 2693–2697. doi:10.1161/01.STR.0000096993.90248.27

Chue, D. H., Nuru-Jeter, A. M., Adler, N. E., Brody, G. H., Lin, J., Blackburn, E. H., & Epel, E. S. (2014). Discrimination, racial bias, and telomere length in African-American men. *American Journal of Preventive Medicine, 46*(2), 103–111. doi:10.1016/j.amepre.2013.10.020

Connolly, V., Unwin, N., Sherriff, P., Belous, R., & Kelly, W. (2000). Diabetes prevalence and socioeconomic status: A population based study showing increased prevalence of type 2 diabetes mellitus in deprived areas. *Journal of Epidemiological Community Health, 54*, 173–177. doi:10.1136/jech.54.3.173

Cook, N. L., Avanian, J. Z., Orav, E. J., & Hicks, L. S. (2009). Differences in specialist consultations for cardiovascular disease by race, ethnicity, gender, insurance status, and site of primary care. *Circulation, 119*(18), 2463–2470. doi:10.1161/CIRCULATIONAHA.108.825133

Corbie-Smith, G., Thomas, S. B., & St. George, D. M. M. (2002). Distrust, race, and research. *Archives of Internal Medicine, 162*, 2458–2463. doi:10.1001/archinte.162.21.2458

Corral, I., Landrine, H., Hao, Y., Zhao, L., Mellerson, J. L., & Cooper, D. L. (2012). Residential segregation, health behavior and overweight/obesity among a national sample of African American adults. *Journal of Health Psychology, 17*(3), 371–378. doi:10.1177/1359105311417191

Coughlin, S. S., Matthews-Juarez, P., Juarez, P. D., Melton, C. E., & King, M. (2014). Opportunities to address lung cancer disparities among African Americans. *Cancer Medicine, 3*(6), 1467–1476. doi:10.1002/cam4.348

Cox, T. L., Krukowski, R., Love, S. J., Eddings, K., DiCarlo, M., Chang, J. Y., ... West, D. S. (2013). Stress management–augmented behavioral weight loss intervention for African American women: A pilot, randomized controlled trial. *Health Education & Behavior, 40*, 78–87. doi:10.1177/1090198112439411

Crepaz, N., Dong, X., Wang, X., Hernandez, A. L., & Hall, H. I. (2018). Racial and ethnic disparities in sustained viral suppression and transmission risk potential among persons receiving HIV care—United States, 2014. *Morbidity and Mortality Weekly Report, 67*(4), 113–118. doi:10.15585/mmwr.mm6704a2

Cruz-Flores, S., Rabinstein, A., Biller, J., Elkind, M. S. V., Griffith, P., Gorelick, P. B., ... Valderrama, A. L. (2011). Racial-ethnic disparities in stroke care: The American experience. *Stroke, 42*(7), 2091–2116. doi:10.1161/STR.0b013e3182213e24

Cuffee, Y. L., Hargraves, J. L., Rosal, M., Briesacher, B. A., Schoenthaler, A., Person, S., ... Allison, J. (2013). Reported racial discrimination, trust in physicians, and medication adherence among inner-city African Americans with hypertension. *American Journal of Public Health, 103*(11), e55–e62. doi:10.2105/AJPH.2013.301554

Cutler, D. M., & Lleras-Muney, A. (2006). *Education and health: Evaluating theories and evidence* (NBER Working Paper No. 12352). Cambridge, MA: National Bureau of Economic Research.

Dagadu, H. E., & Christie-Mizell, C. A. (2014). Heart trouble and racial group identity: Exploring ethnic heterogeneity among Black Americans. *Race and Social Problems, 6*(2), 143–160. doi:10.1007/s12552-013-9109-7

Davis, A. M., Vinci, L. M., Okwuosa, T. M., Chase, A. R., & Huang, E. S. (2007). Cardiovascular health disparities. *Medical Care Research and Review, 64*(5 Suppl.), 29S–100S. doi:10.1177/1077558707305416

Davis, S. K., Liu, Y., & Gibbons, G. H. (2003). Disparities in trends of hospitalization for potentially preventable chronic conditions among African Americans during the 1990s: Implications and benchmarks. *American Journal of Public Health, 93*(3), 447–455. doi:10.2105/AJPH.93.3.447

DeSantis, C. E., Naishadham, D., & Jemal, A. (2013). Cancer statistics for African Americans, 2013. *CA: A Cancer Journal for Clinicians, 63*(3), 151–166. doi:10.3322/caac.21173

DeSantis, C. E., Siegel, R. L., Golding Sauer, A., Miller, K. D., Fedewa, S. A., Alcaraz, K. I., & Jemal, A. (2016). Cancer statistics for African Americans, 2016: Progress and opportunities in reducing racial disparities. *CA: A Cancer Journal for Clinicians, 66*(4), 290–308. doi:10.3322/caac.21340

DiClemente, R. J., & Wingood, G. M. (1995). A randomized controlled trial of an HIV sexual risk-reduction intervention for young African-American women. *Journal of the American Medical Association, 274*(16), 1271–1276. doi:10.1001/jama.1995.03530160023028

Dietze, E. C., Sistrunk, C., Miranda-Carboni, G., O'Regan, R., & Seewaldt, V. L. (2015). Triple-negative breast cancer in African-American women: Disparities versus biology. *Nature Reviews Cancer, 15*, 248–254. doi:10.1038/nrc3896

Dimou, A., Syrigos, K. N., & Wasif Saif, M. (2009). Disparities in colorectal cancer in African-Americans vs Whites: Before and after diagnosis. *World Journal of Gastroenterology, 15*(30), 3734–3743. doi:10.3748/wjg.15.3734

Dolezsar, C. M., McGrath, J. J., Herzig, A. J. M., & Miller, S. B. (2014). Perceived racial discrimination and hypertension: A comprehensive systematic review. *Health Psychology, 33*(1), 20–34. doi:10.1037/a0033718

Duru, O. K., Sarkisian, C. A., Leng, M., & Mangione, C. M. (2010). Sisters in motion: A randomized controlled trial of a faith-based physical activity intervention. *Journal of the American Geriatrics Society, 58*, 1863–1869. doi:10.1111/j.1532-5415.2010.03082.x

Dutton, M. A., Bermudez, D., Matas, A., Majid, H., & Myers, N. L. (2013). Mindfulness-based stress reduction for low-income, predominantly African American women with PTSD and a history of intimate partner violence. *Cognitive and Behavioral Practice, 20*, 23–32. doi:10.1016/j.cbpra.2011.08.003

Entringer, S., Buss, C., & Wadhwa, P. D. (2015). Prenatal stress, development, health and disease risk: A psychobiological perspective—2015 Curt Richter Award paper. *Psychoneuroendocrinology, 62*, 366–375. doi:10.1016/j.psyneuen.2015.08.019

Ferdinand, K. C., Yadav, K., Nasser, S. A., Clayton-Jeter, H. D., Lewin, J., Cryer, D. R., & Senatore, F. F. (2017). Disparities in hypertension and cardiovascular disease in Blacks: The critical role of medication adherence. *Journal of Clinical Hypertension, 19*(10), 1015–1024. doi:10.1111/jch.13089

Ferré, C. D., Jones, L., Norris, K. C., & Rowley, D. L. (2010). The Healthy African American Families (HAAF) project: From community-based participatory research to community-partnered participatory research. *Ethnicity & Disease, 20*(1 Suppl. 2), 1–8. Retrieved from https://www.ncbi.nlm.nih.gov/pmc/articles/PMC3791221

Finkelstein, E. A., Khavjou, O. A., Mobley, L. R., Haney, D. M., & Will, J. C. (2004). Racial/ethnic disparities in coronary heart disease risk factors among WISEWOMAN enrollees. *Journal of Women's Health, 13*(5), 503–518. doi:10.1089/1540999041280963

Forsyth, J., Schoenthaler, A., Chaplin, W. F., Ogedegbe, G., & Ravenell, J. (2014). Perceived discrimination and medication adherence in Black hypertensive patients: The role of stress and depression. *Psychosomatic Medicine, 76*(3), 229–236. doi:10.1097/PSY.0000000000000043

Fouad, M., Wynn, T., Martin, M., & Partridge, E. (2010). Patient navigation pilot project: Results from the Community Health Advisors in Action Program (CHAAP). *Ethnicity & Disease, 20*, 155–161. Retrieved from https://www.ethndis.org/priorarchives/ethn-20-02-155.pdf

Frank, D., & Grubbs, L. (2008). A faith-based screening and education program for diabetes, CVD, and stroke in rural African Americans. *The Association of Black Nursing Faculty Journal, 19*, 96–101.

Freeman, H. P. (2004). Poverty, culture, and social injustice: Determinants of cancer disparities. *CA: A Cancer Journal for Clinicians, 54*(2), 72–77. doi:10.3322/canjclin.54.2.72

Gabbe, P. T., Reno, R., Clutter, C., Schottke, T. F., Price, T., Calhoun, K., … Lynch, C. D. (2017). Improving maternal and infant child health outcomes with community-based pregnancy support groups: Outcomes from Moms2B Ohio. *Maternal and Child Health Journal, 21*(5), 1130–1138. doi:10.1007/s10995-016-2211-x

Gabram, S. G. A., Lund, M. J. B., Gardner, J., Hatchett, N., Bumpers, H. L., Okoli, J.,… Brawley, O. W. (2008). Effects of an outreach and internal navigation program on breast cancer diagnosis in an urban cancer center with a large African-American population. *Cancer, 113*(3), 602–607. doi:10.1002/cncr.23568

Gerend, M. A., & Pai, M. (2008). Social determinants of Black-White disparities in breast cancer mortality: A review. *Cancer Epidemiology, Biomarkers, and Prevention, 17*(11), 2913–2923. doi:10.1158/1055-9965.EPI-07-0633

Ghafoor, A., Jemal, A., Cokkinides, V., Cardinez, C., Murray, T., Samuels, A., & Thun, M. J. (2002). Cancer statistics for African Americans. *CA: A Cancer Journal for Clinicians, 52*(6), 326–341. doi:10.3322/canjclin.52.6.326

Giulivo, M., Lopez de Alda, M., Capri, E., & Barceló, D. (2016). Human exposure to endocrine disrupting compounds: Their rold in reproductive systems, metabolic syndrome and breast cancer. A review. *Environmental Research, 151*, 251–264. doi:10.1016/j.envres.2016.07.011

Glasser, S. P., Cushman, M., Prineas, R., Kleindorfer, D., Prince, V., You, Z., … Howard, G. (2008). Does differential prophylactic aspirin use contribute to racial and geographic disparities in stroke and coronary heart disease? *Preventive Medicine, 47*(2), 161–166. doi:10.1016/j.ypmed.2008.05.009

Glymour, M. M., Avendaño, M., Haas, S., & Berkman, L. F. (2008). Lifecourse social conditions and racial disparities in incidence of first stroke. *Annals of Epidemiology, 18*(12), 904–912. doi:10.1016/j.annepidem.2008.09.010

Glymour, M. M., Yen, J. J., Kosheleva, A., Moon, J. R., Capistrant, B. D., & Patton, K. K. (2012). Elevated depressive symptoms and incident stroke in Hispanic, African-American, and White older Americans. *Journal of Behavioral Medicine, 35*(2), 211–220. doi:10.1007/s10865-011-9356-2

Gotay, C. C., & Wilson, M. E. (1998). Social support and cancer screening in African American, Hispanic, and Native American women. *Cancer Practice, 6*, 31–37. doi:10.1046/j.1523-5394.1998.1998006031.x

Guidry, J. J., Fagan, P., & Walker, V. (1998). Cultural sensitivity and readability of breast and prostate printed cancer education materials targeting African Americans. *Journal of the National Medical Association, 90*(3), 165–169. Retrieved from https://www.ncbi.nlm.nih.gov/pmc/articles/PMC2608327

Gutierrez, J., & Williams, O. A. (2014). A decade of racial and ethnic stroke disparities in the United States. *Neurology, 82*(12), 1080–1082. doi:10.1212/WNL.0000000000000237

Hammonds, E. M., & Reverby, S. M. (2019). Toward a historically informed analysis of racial health disparities since 1619. *American Journal of Public Health, 109*(10), 1348–1349. doi:10.2105/AJPH.2019.305262

Haynes, V., Escoffery, C., Wilkerson, C., Bell, R., & Flowers, L. (2014). Adaptation of a cervical cancer education program for African Americans in the faith-based community, Atlanta, Georgia, 2012. *Preventing Chronic Disease*, *11*, E67. doi:10.5888/pcd11.130271

Herring, S. J., Cruice, J. F., Bennett, G. G., Rose, M. Z., Davey, A., & Foster, G. D. (2016). Preventing excessive gestational weight gain among African American women: A randomized clinical trial. *Obesity*, *24*, 30–36. doi:10.1002/oby.21240

Hill, L. K., Hoggard, L. S., Richmond, A. S., Gray, D. L., Williams, D. P., & Thayer, J. F. (2017). Examining the association between perceived discrimination and heart rate variability in African Americans. *Cultural Diversity and Ethnic Minority Psychology*, *23*(1), 5–14. doi:10.1037/cdp0000076

Horowitz, C. R., Colson, K. A., Hebert, P. L., & Lancaster, K. (2004). Barriers to buying healthy foods for people with diabetes: Evidence of environmental disparities. *American Journal of Public Health*, *94*(9), 1549–1554. doi:10.2105/AJPH.94.9.1549

Housing Assistance Council. (2012). *HAC rural research brief: Race and ethnicity in rural America* (HAC tabulations of 2010 Census of Population and housing, Summary File 1). Retrieved from http://www.ruralhome.org/storage/research_notes/rrn-race-and-ethnicity-web.pdf

Howard, G., & Howard, V. J. (2001). Ethnic disparities in stroke: The scope of the problem. *Ethnicity & Disease*, *11*(4), 761–768.

Howard, G., Labarthe, D. R., Hu, J., Yoon, S., & Howard, V. J. (2007). Regional differences in African Americans' high risk for stroke: The remarkable burden of stroke for Southern African Americans. *Annals of Epidemiology*, *17*(9), 689–696. doi:10.1016/j.annepidem.2007.03.019

Howard, V. J., Kleindorfer, D. W., Judd, S. E., McClure, L. A., Safford, M. M., Rhodes, J. D., … Howard, G. (2011). Disparities in stroke incidence contributing to disparities in stroke mortality. *Annals of Neurology*, *69*(4), 619–627. doi:10.1002/ana.22385

Hueston, W., & Hubbard, E. (2000). Preventive services for rural and urban African American adults. *Archives of Family Medicine*, *9*, 262–266. doi:10.1001/archfami.9.3.263

Husaini, B. A., Reece, M. C., Emerson, J. S., Scales, S., Hull, P. C., & Levine, R. S. (2008). A church-based program on prostate cancer screening for African American men: Reducing health disparities. *Ethnicity and Disease*, *18*, 179–184. Retrieved from https://www.ethndis.org/priorsuparchives/ethn-18-02s2-179.pdf

Jacobs, B. S., Birbeck, G., Mullard, A. J., Hickenbottom, S., Kothari, R., Roberts, S., & Reeves, M. J. (2006). Quality of hospital care in African American and White patients with ischemic stroke and TIA. *Neurology*, *66*(6), 809–814. doi:10.1212/01.wnl.0000203335.45804.72

Jamerson, K. A. (2004). The disproportionate impact of hypertensive cardiovascular disease in African Americans: Getting to the heart of the issue. *The Journal of Clinical Hypertension*, *6*(s4), 4–10. doi:10.1111/j.1524-6175.2004.03563.x

James, T. M., Greiner, K. A., Ellerbeck, E. F., Feng, C., & Ahluwalia, J. S. (2006). Disparities in colorectal cancer screening: A guideline-based analysis of adherence. *Ethnicity and Disease*, *16*, 228–233. Retrieved from https://www.ethndis.org/priorarchives/ethn-16-01-228.pdf

James-Todd, T., Senie, R., & Terry, M. B. (2011). Racial/ethnic differences in hormonally-active hair product use: A plausible risk factor for health disparities. *Journal of Immigrant and Minority Health*, *14*, 506–511. doi:10.1007/s10903-011-9482-5

Jha, A. K., Varosy, P. D., Kanaya, A. M., Hunninghake, D. B., Hlatky, M. A., . . . Shlipak, M. G. (2003). Differences in medical care and disease outcomes among Black and White women with heart disease. *Circulation*, *108*, 1089–1094. doi:10.1161/01.CIR.0000085994.38132.E5

Johnson-Turbes, A., Schlueter, D., Moore, A. R., Buchanan, N. D., & Fairley, T. L. (2015). Evaluation of a web-based program for African American young breast cancer survivors. *American Journal of Preventive Medicine*, *49*(6, Suppl. 5), S543–S549. doi:10.1016/j.amepre.2015.09.003

Jones, D. L., Ishii Owens, M., Lydston, D., Tobin, J. N., Brondolo, E., & Weiss, S. M. (2010). Self-efficacy and distress in women with AIDS: The SMART/EST women's project. *AIDS Care*, *22*, 1499–1508. doi:10.1080/09540121.2010.484454

Kaslow, N. J., Leiner, A. S., Reviere, S., Jackson, E., Bethea, K., Bhaju, J., … Thompson, M. P. (2010). Suicidal, abused African American women's response to a culturally informed intervention. *Journal of Consulting and Clinical Psychology, 78*, 449–458. doi:10.1037/a0019692

Katz, T. A., Yang, Q., Treviño, L. S., Walker, C. L., & Al-Hendy, A. (2016). Endocrine disrupting chemicals and uterine fibroids. *Fertility and Sterility, 106*(4), 967–977. doi:10.1016/j.fertnstert.2016.08.023

Kirk, J. K., D'Agostino, R. B., Bell, R. A., Passmore, L. V., Bonds, D. E., Karter, A. J., & Narayan, K. M. V. (2006). Disparities in HbA1c levels between African-American and non-Hispanic White adults with diabetes. *Diabetes Care, 29*(9), 2130–2136. doi:10.2337/dc05-1973

Kuehn, B. (2018). PrEP disparities. *Journal of the American Medical Association, 320*(22), 2304. doi:10.1001/jama.2018.18947

Kuhajda, M. C., Cornell, C. E., Brownstein, J. N., Littleton, M. A., Stalker, V., Bittner, V. A., … Raczynski, J. M. (2006). Training community health workers to reduce health disparities in Alabama's Black belt: The Pine Apple Heart Disease and Stroke Project. *Family and Community Health, 29*(2), 89–102. doi:10.1097/00003727-200604000-00005

Lemacks, J., Wells, B., Ilich, J., & Ralston, P. (2013). Interventions for improving nutrition and physical activity behaviors in African American populations: A systematic review, January 2000 through December 2011. *Preventing Chronic Disease, 10*, 120256. doi:10.5888/pcd10.120256

Linnan, L. A., D'Angelo, H., & Harrington, C. B. (2014). A literature synthesis of health promotion research in salons and barbershops. *American Journal of Preventive Medicine, 47*, 77–85. doi:10.1016/j.amepre.2014.02.007

Lutfiyya, M. N., Cumba, M. T., McCullough, J. E., Barlow, E. L., & Lipsky, M. S. (2008). Disparities in adult African American women's knowledge of heart attack and stroke, symptomatology: An analysis of 2003-2005 behavioral risk factor surveillance survey data. *Journal of Women's Health, 17*(5), 805–813. doi:10.1089/jwh.2007.0599

Lutfiyya, M. N., Lipsky, M. S., Bales, R. W., Cha, I., & McGrath, C. (2008). Disparities in knowledge of heart attack and stroke symptoms among adult men: An analysis of behavioral risk factor surveillance survey data. *Journal of the National Medical Association, 100*(1), 1116–1124. doi:10.1016/S0027-9684(15)31483-8

Mainous, A., King, D., Garr, D., & Pearson, W. (2004). Race, rural residence, and control of diabetes and hypertension. *Annals of Family Medicine, 2*(6), 563–568. doi:10.1370/afm.119

Marshall, M. C. (2005). Diabetes in African Americans. *Postgraduate Medical Journals, 81*, 734–740. doi:10.1136/pgmj.2004.028274

Masci, D. (2018). *5 facts about the religious lives of African Americans*. Retrieved from https://www.pewresearch.org/fact-tank/2018/02/07/5-facts-about-the-religious-lives-of-african-americans

Mason, T. B., & Lewis, R. J. (2017). Examining social support, rumination, and optimism in relation to binge eating among Caucasian and African-American college women. *Eating and Weight Disorders, 22*(4), 693–698. doi:10.1007/s40519-016-0300-x

McGruder, H. F., Malarcher, A. M., Antoine, T. L., Greenlund, K. J., & Croft, J. B. (2004). Racial and ethnic disparities in cardiovascular risk factors among stroke survivors: United States 1999 to 2001. *Stroke, 35*(7), 1557–1561. doi:10.1161/01.STR.0000130427.84114.50

Molina, M. A., Cheung, M. C., Perez, E. A., Byrne, M. M., Franceschi, D., Moffat, F. L., … Koniaris, L. G. (2008). African American and poor patients have a dramatically worse prognosis for head and neck cancer. *Cancer, 113*(10), 2797–2806. doi:10.1002/cncr.23889

Monti, D. A., Kash, K. M., Kunkel, E. J., Moss, A., Mathews, M., Brainard, G., … Newberg, A. B. (2013). Psychosocial benefits of a novel mindfulness intervention versus standard support in distressed women with breast cancer. *Psycho-Oncology, 22*, 2565–2575. doi:10.1002/pon.3320

Moore, M. P., Javier, S. J., Abrams, J. A., McGann, A. W., & Belgrave, F. Z. (2017). Ethnic comparisons in HIV testing attitudes, HIV testing, and predictors of HIV testing among Black and White college students. *Journal of Racial and Ethnic Health Disparities, 4*(4), 571–579. doi:10.1007/s40615-016-0259-3

Morenoff, J. D., House, J. S., Hansen, B. B., Williams, D. R., Kaplan, G. A., & Hunte, H. E. (2007). Understanding social disparities in hypertension prevalence, awareness, treatment, and control: The role of neighborhood context. *Social Science & Medicine, 65*(9), 1853–1866. doi:10.1016/j.socscimed.2007.05.038

Moskowitz, G. B., Stone, J., & Childs, A. (2012). Implicit stereotyping and medical decisions: Unconscious stereotype activation in practitioners' thoughts about African Americans. *American Journal of Public Health, 102*(5), 996–1001. doi:10.2105/AJPH.2011.300591

Murrock, C. J., Higgins, P. A., & Killion, C. (2009). Dance and peer support to improve diabetes outcomes in African American women. *The Diabetes Educator, 35,* 995–1003. doi:10.1177/0145721709343322

Murthy, V. H., Krumholz, H. M., & Gross, C. P. (2004). Participation in clinical trials: Race-, sex-, and age-based disparities. *Journal of the American Medical Association, 291*(22), 2720–2726. doi:10.1001/jama.291.22.2720

Muturi, N., & An, S. (2010). HIV/AIDS stigma and religiosity among African American women. *Journal of Health Communication, 15*(4), 388–401. doi:10.1080/10810731003753125

National Center for Health Statistics. (2015). *Health, United States, 2015: With special feature on racial and ethnic health disparities.* Hyattsville, MD: Author. Retrieved from https://www.ncbi.nlm.nih.gov/books/NBK367640

Negbenebor, N. A., & Garza, E. W. (2018). Black lives matter, but what about our health? *Journal of the National Medical Association, 110*(1), 16–17. doi:10.1016/j.jnma.2017.06.006

Newman, L. A. (2005). Breast cancer in African-American women. *The Oncologist, 10*(1), 1–14. doi:10.1634/theoncologist.10-1-1

Nicolaidis, C., Wahab, S., Trimble, J., Mejia, A., Mitchell, S. R., Raymaker, D., ... Waters, A. S. (2013). The interconnections project: Development and evaluation of a community-based depression program for African American violence survivors. *Journal of General Internal Medicine, 28,* 530–538. doi:10.1007/s11606-012-2270-7

Office of Minority Health. (2019). *Diabetes and African Americans.* Retrieved from https://minorityhealth.hhs.gov/omh/browse.aspx?lvl=4&lvlid=18

Osborn, C. Y., Cavanaugh, K., Wallston, K. A., Kripalani, S., Elasy, T. A., Rothman, R. L., & White, R. O. (2011). Health literacy explains racial disparities in diabetes medication adherence. *Journal of Health Communication, 16*(Suppl. 3), 268–278. doi:10.1080/10810730.2011.604388

Panza, G. A., Puhl, R. M., Taylor, B. A., Zaleski, A. L., Livingston, J., & Pescatello, L. S. (2019). Links between discrimination and cardiovascular health among socially stigmatized groups: A systematic review. *PLoS One, 14*(6), e0217623. doi:10.1371/journal.pone.0217623

Payne, R., Medina, E., & Hampton, J. W. (2003). Quality of life concerns in patients with breast cancer. *Cancer, 91*(S1), 311–317. doi:10.1002/cncr.11017

Peek, M. E., Cargill, A., & Huang, E. S. (2007). Diabetes health disparities: A systematic review of health care interventions. *Medical Care Research and Review, 64*(5 Suppl.), 101S–156S. doi:10.1177/1077558707305409

Peters, R. M., Aroian, K. J., & Flack, J. M. (2006). African American culture and hypertension prevention. *Western Journal of Nursing Research, 28*(7), 831–854. doi:10.1177/0193945906289332

Radcliffe, J., Doty, N., Hawkins, L. A., Gaskins, C. S., Beidas, R., & Rudy, B. J. (2010). Stigma and sexual health risk in HIV-positive African American young men who have sex with men. *AIDS Patient Care and STDs, 24*(8), 493–499. doi:10.1089/apc.2010.0020

Rivero-Becerra, J., & Rodriguez, C. J. (2004). Effects of race and socioeconomic status in the incidence of hypertension and increased left ventricular mass: A review. *Brazilian Journal of Hypertension, 11,* 147–150.

Rogers-Wood, N. A., & Petrie, T. A. (2010). Body dissatisfaction, ethnic identity, and disordered eating among African American women. *Journal of Counseling Psychology, 57,* 141–153. doi:10.1037/a0018922

Sadler, G. R., Ko, C. M., Wu, P., Alisangco, J., Castañeda, S. F., & Kelly, C. (2011). A cluster randomized controlled trial to increase breast cancer screening among African American women: The Black Cosmetologists Promoting Health Program. *Journal of the National Medical Association, 103*(8), 735–745. doi:10.1016/S0027-9684(15)30413-2

Sarkar, U., Karter, A. J., Liu, J. Y., Adler, N. E., Nguyen, R., López, A., & Schillinger, D. (2011). Social disparities in internet patient portal use in diabetes: Evidence that the digital divide extends beyond access. *Journal of the American Medical Informatics Association, 18*(3), 318–321. doi:10.1136/jamia.2010.006015

Saydan, S., & Lochner, K. (2010). Socioeconomic status and risk of diabetes-related mortality in the United States. *Public Health Reports, 125*, 377–388. doi:10.1177/003335491012500306

Schoenthaler, A., Ogedegbe, G., & Allegrante, J. P. (2009). Self-efficacy mediates the relationship between depressive symptoms and medication adherence among hypertensive African Americans. *Health Education & Behavior, 36*(1), 127–137. doi:10.1177/1090198107309459

Scott, A., & Wilson, R. (2011). Social determinants of health among African Americans in a rural community in the Deep South: An ecological exploration. *Rural and Remote Health, 11*, 1634. Retrieved from https://www.rrh.org.au/journal/article/1634

Shen, J. J., Washington, E. L., & Aponte-Soto, L. (2004). Racial disparities in the pathogenesis and outcomes for patients with ischemic stroke. *Managed Care Interface, 17*(3), 28–34.

Simoni, J. M., Pantalone, D. W., Plummer, M. D., & Huang, B. (2007). A randomized controlled trial of a peer support intervention targeting antiretroviral medication adherence and depressive symptomatology in HIV-positive men and women. *Health Psychology, 26*, 488–495. doi:10.1037/0278-6133.26.4.488

Sims, M., Diez-Roux, A. V., Dudley, A., Gebreab, S., Wyatt, S. B., Bruce, M. A., … Taylor, H. A. (2012). Perceived discrimination and hypertension among African Americans in the Jackson heart study. *American Journal of Public Health, 102*(S2), S258–S265. doi:10.2105/AJPH.2011.300523

Smedley, B. D. (2012). The lived experience of race and its health consequences. *American Journal of Public Health, 102*(5), 933–935. doi:10.2105/AJPH.2011.300643

Smedley, B. D., Stith, A. Y., & Nelson, A. R. (Eds.). (2003). *Unequal treatment: Confronting racial and ethnic disparities in health care*. Washington, DC: National Academies Press.

Sowers, J. R., Ferdinand, K. C., Bakris, G. L., & Douglas, J. G. (2015). Hypertension-related disease in African Americans: Factors underlying disparities in illness and its outcome. *Postgraduate Medicine, 112*(4), 24–48. doi:10.3810/pgm.2002.10.1331

Spanakis, E., & Golden, S. H. (2013). Race/ethnic difference in diabetes and diabetic complications. *Current Diabetes Reports, 13*(6), 814–823. doi:10.1007/s11892-013-0421-9

Spencer, M. S., Kieffer, E. C., Sinco, B. R., Palmisano, G., Guzman, J. R., James, S. A., … Heisler, M. (2006). Diabetes-specific emotional distress among African Americans and Hispanics with type 2 diabetes. *Journal of Health Care for the Poor and Underserved, 17*(2), 88–105. doi:10.1353/hpu.2006.0082

Spencer, M. S., Rosland, A., Kieffer, E. C., Sinco, B. R., Valerio, M., Palmisano, G., … Heisler, M. (2011). Effectiveness of a community health worker intervention among African American and Latino adults with type 2 diabetes: A randomized controlled trial. *American Journal of Public Health, 101*(12), 2253–2260. doi:10.2105/AJPH.2010.300106

Stiel, L., Adkins-Jackson, P. B., Clark, P., Mitchell, E., & Montgomery, S. (2016). A review of hair product use on breast cancer risk in African American women. *Cancer Medicine, 5*(3), 597–604. doi:10.1002/cam4.613

Swenson, R. R., Rizzo, C. J., Brown, L. K., Vanable, P. A., Carey, M. P., Valois, R. F.,… Romer, D. (2010). HIV knowledge and its contribution to sexual health behaviors of low-income African American adolescents. *Journal of the National Medical Association, 102*(12), 1173–1182. doi:10.1016/S0027-9684(15)30772-0

Tang, T. S., Brown, M. B., Funnell, M. M., & Anderson, R. M. (2008). Social support, quality of life, and self-care behaviors among African Americans with type 2 diabetes. *The Diabetes Educator, 34*(2), 266–276. doi:10.1177/0145721708315680

Tettey, N. S., Duran, P. A., Andersen, H. S., Boutin-Foster, C. (2017). Evaluation of HeartSmarts, a faith-based cardiovascular health education program. *Journal of Religion and Health, 56*(1), 320–328. doi:10.1007/s10943-016-0309-5

Thorpe, R. J., Brandon, D. T., & LaVeist, T. A. (2008). Social context as an explanation for race disparities in hypertension: Findings from the Exploring Health Disparities in Integrated Communities (EHDIC) study. *Social Science & Medicine, 67*(10), 1604–1611. doi:10.1016/j.socscimed.2008.07.002

Timmons, S. M. (2015). Review and evaluation of faith-based weight management interventions that target African American women. *Journal of Religion and Health, 54*, 798–809. doi:10.1007/s10943-014-9912-5

Tiwary, C. M. (1998). Premature sexual development in children following the use of estrogen-or placenta-containing hair products. *Clinical Pediatrics, 37*(12), 733–739. doi:10.1177/000992289803701204

Tucker, C. M., Moradi, B., Wall, W., & Nghiem, K. (2014). Roles of perceived provider cultural sensitivity and health care justice in African American/Black patients' satisfaction with provider. *Journal of Clinical Psychology in Medical Settings, 21*(3), 282–290. doi:10.1007/s10880-014-9397-0

U.S. Bureau of Labor Statistics. (2016). *Black women in the labor force*. Retrieved from https://www.dol .gov/wb/media/Printer_Friendly_Black_Women_in_the_Labor_Force.pdf

U.S. Census Bureau. (2018). *About race*. Retrieved from https://www.census.gov/topics/population/race/ about.html

Vaccarino, V., Rathore, S. S., Wenger, N. K., Frederick, P. D., Abramson, J. L., Barron, H. V., . . . Krumholz, H. M. (2005). Sex and racial differences in the management of acute myocardial infarction, 1994 through 2002. *New England Journal of Medicine, 353*(7), 671–682. doi: 10.1056/NEJMsa032214

Villablanca, A. C., Warford, C., & Wheeler, K. (2016). Inflammation and cardiometabolic risk in African American women is reduced by a pilot community-based educational intervention. *Journal of Women's Health, 25,* 188–199. doi:10.1089/jwh.2014.5109

Vinesett, A. L., Whaley, R. R., Woods-Giscombe, C., Dennis, P., Johnson, M., Li, Y., ... & Wilson, K. H. (2017). Modified African Ngoma healing ceremony for stress reduction: A pilot study. *The Journal of Alternative and Complementary Medicine, 23*(10), 800–804. doi:10.1089/acm.2016.0410

Vyavaharkar, M., Moneyham, L., Corwin, S., Saunders, R., Annang, L., & Tavakoli, A. (2010). Relationships between stigma, social support, and depression in HIV-infected African American women living in the rural Southeastern United States. *Journal of the Association of Nurses in AIDS Care, 21*(2), 144–152. doi:10.1016/j.jana.2009.07.008

Ward, E. W., Jemal, A., Cokkinides, V., Singh, G. K., Cardinez, C., Ghafoor, A., & Thun, M. (2004). Cancer disparities by race/ethnicity and socioeconomic status. *CA: A Cancer Journal for Clinicians, 54*(2), 78–93. doi:10.3322/canjclin.54.2.78

Warren, J. C., & Smalley, K. B. (Eds.). (2014). *Rural public health: Best practices and preventive models*. New York, NY: Springer Publishing Company.

Warren, J. C., Smalley, K. B., Rimando, M., Barefoot, K. N., Hatton, A., & LeLeux-Labarge, K. (2014). Rural minority health: Race, ethnicity, and sexual orientation. In J. C. Warren & K. B. Smalley (Eds.), *Rural public health* (pp. 203–226). New York, NY: Springer Publishing Company.

Washington, H. A. (2006). *Medical apartheid: The dark history of medical experimentation on Black Americans from colonial times to the present*. New York, NY: Doubleday Books.

Whitney, E., Kindred, E., Pratt, A., O'Neal, Y., Harrison, R. C. P., & Peek, M. E. (2017). Culturally tailoring a patient empowerment and diabetes education curriculum for the African American church. *Diabetes Education, 43*(5), 441–448. doi:10.1177/0145721717725280

Williams, D. R. (2002). Racial/ethnic variations in women's health: The social embeddedness of health. *American Journal of Public Health, 92,* 588–597. doi:10.2105/AJPH.92.4.588

Williams, D. R., & Wyatt, R. (2015). Racial bias in health care and health: Challenges and opportunities. *Journal of the American Medical Association, 314*(6), 555–556. doi:10.1001/jama.2015.9260

Williams, R. A. (2009). Cardiovascular disease in African American women: A health care disparities issue. *Journal of the National Medical Association, 101*(6), 536–540. doi:10.1016/S0027-9684(15)30938-X

Wilson-Anderson, K., Williams, P., Beacham, T., & McDonald, N. (2013). Breast health teaching in predominantly African American rural Mississippi Delta. *The Association of Black Nurse Faculty Journal, 24,* 28–33.

Wingood, G. M., Card, J. J., Er, D., Solomon, J., Braxton, N., Lang, D., ... Diclemente, R. J. (2011). Preliminary efficacy of a computer-based HIV intervention for African-American women. *Psychology & Health, 26,* 223–234. doi:10.1080/08870446.2011.531576

Wingood, G. M., & DiClemente, R. J. (2006). Enhancing adoption of evidence-based HIV interventions: Promotion of a suite of HIV prevention interventions for African American women. *AIDS Education and Prevention, 18*(Suppl. A), 161–170. doi:10.1521/aeap.2006.18.supp.161

Wingood, G. M., Robinson, L. R., Braxton, N. D., Er, D. L., Conner, A. C., Renfro, T. L., ... DiClemente, R. J. (2013). Comparative effectiveness of a faith-based HIV intervention for African American women:

Importance of enhancing religious social capital. *American Journal of Public Health, 103*(12), 2226–2233. doi:10.2105/AJPH.2013.301386

Wise, L. A., Palmer, J. R., Reich, D., Cozier, Y. C., & Rosenberg, L. (2012). Hair relaxer use and risk of uterine leiomyomata in African-American women. *American Journal of Epidemiology, 175*(5), 432–440. doi:10.1093/aje/kwr351

Wohl, A. R., Galvan, F. H., Myers, H. F., Garland, W., George, S., Witt, M., … Lee, M. L. (2011). Do social support, stress, disclosure, and stigma influence retention in HIV care for Latino and African American men who have sex with men and women? *AIDS and Behavior, 15*(6), 1098–1110. doi:10.1007/s10461-010-9833-6

Wright, D. R., Gathers, R., Kapke, A., Johnson, D., & Joseph, C. L. M. (2010). Hair care practices and their association with scalp and hair disorders in African American girls. *Journal of the American Academy of Dermatology, 64*, 253–262. doi:10.1016/j.jaad.2010.05.037

HEALTH EQUITY IN U.S. LATINX POPULATIONS

CARMEN R. VALDEZ ■ MIGUEL PINEDO ■ LIANA PETRUZZI ■
MONIQUE VASQUEZ ■ DELIANA GARCIA

LEARNING OBJECTIVES

- Discuss the origins of the terms "Hispanic," "Latino," and "Latinx" and the implications of the usage of each of these terms
- Summarize the demographic profile of Latinx populations within the United States and how these factors influence health disparities
- Describe the health disparities that Latinx populations face
- Explain models for achieving health equity specific to Latinx populations and how these models can be applied to developing Latinx health equity initiatives
- Describe how intersectionality affects Latinx health equity

INTRODUCTION

Disproportionate health burden and inequitable opportunities for health and access to healthcare are barriers encountered by many U.S. Latinx populations. First, the chapter orients the reader to the terminology used to refer to members of Latin American descent in the United States and describes key demographics of the U.S. Latinx population. Then, the chapter reviews the literature on health status and the social and structural determinants of burden, healthcare access, and quality for U.S. Latinx populations; presents Latinx-specific models of health disparities/health equity; describes emerging interventions, programs, and policies for achieving health equity in this population; and offers best practice recommendations in designing such efforts. The chapter then illustrates select best practices with a case study.

TERMINOLOGY

The Federal Office of Management and Budget officially instituted the term "Hispanic" in 1978 to refer collectively to individuals, regardless of race, who came from a country that descended from Spain and, therefore, spoke Spanish (Alcoff, 2005). Although widely adopted in the Southwest, many groups rejected the term because of its colonial roots and a lack of connection with Spanish ancestry and language (e.g., Brazilians, indigenous communities; Alcoff, 2005; Comas-Díaz, 2000). The term "Latino" emerged in the 1980s as a form of political resistance (Hayes-Bautista & Chapa, 1987).

In recent years, "Latinx" has emerged as a more inclusive term that is gaining mobilization (Latinx Psychological Association, 2018). Adopting the term has important implications for health equity (Santos, 2017). First, by changing the Spanish language marker "o" (or its gender variant of "a/o") to "x," the term de-emphasizes male privilege and recognizes gender identity and expression as non-binary. Second, the term Latinx spotlights intersectionality, in that gender diversity is one of many interrelated factors, such as race, nationality, and language, affecting health among Latinx groups. Third, the term forces researchers, practitioners, and policy makers to reflect on the role of language in equity-promotion efforts, thus propelling authentic solidarity and social justice–driven practice with the Latinx community. As a result, we have elected to use the term Latinx throughout this chapter. We acknowledge that much of the literature we cite in this chapter used "Hispanic" or "Latino" to refer to U.S. Latinx populations.

KEY DEMOGRAPHICS

Population Growth

Consisting of 18% of the total U.S. population, Latinx individuals are a key demographic of the United States. In 2018, the U.S. Latinx population reached a record 59.9 million (Flores, Lopez, & Krogstad, 2019; U.S. Census Bureau, 2019a). Although Latinx population growth (2.0%) has decreased since 2011, it still accounted for 52% of U.S. growth and continued to outpace most racial/ethnic groups (Flores et al., 2019). Projections from 2017 by the U.S. Census Bureau estimate that the Latinx population will make up 27% of the total U.S. population by 2060 (Krogstad, 2019). The Latinx population is younger than the rest of the nation, with a median age of 28 years (Lopez, Krogstad, & Flores, 2018). In 2017, 31.5% of Latinx individuals were under the age of 18 in comparison to only 18.8% of non-Latinx Whites (U.S. Department of Health and Human Services [DHHS], 2019). The U.S. Latinx population is diverse based on ancestry, nativity, race, immigration status, and other important social indicators.

Nationality and Nativity

The U.S. Latinx population includes individuals whose ancestry derives from Mexico, the Caribbean (i.e., Puerto Rico, Cuba, and the Dominican Republic), South America, or Central America, regardless of race (DHHS, 2019). In 2018, Mexicans ranked as the largest subgroup at 62.4%, followed by Puerto Ricans (9.2%), Central Americans (8.8%), South Americans (6.7%), and Cubans (4.0%; U.S. Census Bureau, 2019b).

The U.S. Latinx population represents the largest foreign-born group in the United States. In 2018, 34.7% of Latinx individuals were foreign born (U.S. Census Bureau, 2019b), with the highest share migrating from Guatemala (61%), El Salvador (59%), Colombia (61%), Cuba (56%), and the Dominican Republic (55%; Flores, 2017). Within the context of language, 69% of Latinx individuals report speaking English only or being proficient in English (relative to 59% in 1980). Nevertheless, 73% of the U.S. mainland Latinx population in 2015 reported speaking a language other than English at home (DHHS, 2019).

Authorization Status

In 2017, an estimated 10.5 million people lacked authorization to live in the United States, including 8.1 million Latinx individuals (Passel & Cohn, 2019). Unauthorized or undocumented immigrants are those that entered the country unlawfully, or arrived lawfully with a visa but overstayed it. According to a Pew Research Center report, Mexicans constitute 47% of U.S. unauthorized immigrants in 2017, a rate that is declining due to more Mexicans leaving the United States than those arriving (Passel & Cohn, 2019). Similarly, crossings and apprehensions of Mexicans at the border have declined, while crossings and apprehensions of Guatemalans, Hondurans, and Salvadorians have increased over the past decade and especially since 2016 (Passel & Cohn, 2019).

Mobility

A large number of Latinx persons engage in seasonal farmwork. A migrant farmworker is an individual who is absent from their permanent place of residence within or outside the United States for the purpose of temporary or seasonal employment in agriculture. Many migrant farmworkers have their permanent U.S. residency, others lack authorization, and others yet have a temporary foreign certification (H2A workers) that allows them to enter the United States for the purpose of seasonal farmwork (Migrant Clinicians Network, n.d.). Farmworkers are typically from Mexico (68%) and they typically identify as male (78%) and married (59%; Velasco-Mondragon, Jimenez, Palladino-Davis, Davis, & Escamilla-Cejudo, 2016).

Education

In terms of education, 66% of Latinx have a high school diploma and 15% of Latinx have a bachelor's degree or higher, in comparison to 92% and 34.2% of non-Latinx Whites (DHHS, 2019). When examined by nationality, approximately half of foreign-born Salvadorians, Guatemalans, and Hondurans lack a high school diploma (Zong & Batalova, 2019).

Economic Stability and Poverty

The U.S. Latinx population is disproportionately affected by economic disadvantage. The Latinx real median household income grew for 3 consecutive years to $50,486 in 2017, above the income of non-Latinx Blacks ($40,258), but well below that of non-Latinx Asians ($81,331) and Whites ($68,145; Fontenot, Semega, & Kollar, 2018). Latinx earnings and purchasing power tend to be lower than for non-Latinx Whites, even after controlling for level of education (Williams, 2012). In 2017, data from the U.S. Census Bureau reported that 18.3% of Latinx persons in comparison to 8.7% of non-Latinx Whites were living below poverty thresholds, which is defined as $12,488 for single individuals under 65 or $25,094 for a family of four (Fontenot et al., 2018). Between 2007 and 2011, poverty rates were highest for Dominicans, Mexicans, and Puerto Ricans and lowest for Cubans and Salvadorians (Rabbitt, Smith, & Coleman-Jensen, 2016). More recently, Hondurans, Guatemalans, and Venezuelans share the highest poverty rates among immigrants of new-origin countries (Zong & Batalova, 2019). U.S. Latinx and other racial/ethnic minority populations are more likely than Whites to have experienced early economic and psychosocial adversity that can affect health (Williams, 2012). Although not entirely linked to economic stability, according to a report from the U.S. Department of Agriculture (Rabbitt et al., 2016), in 2011 to 2014, U.S. Latinx adults having Cuban origin were least food insecure, while those identifying themselves as having Puerto Rican origin were most food insecure. During that time frame, food insecurity was more prevalent among U.S. Latinx adults who were noncitizens (24.4%) than among those who were U.S. born (18.9%).

Environmental Exposures

U.S. Latinx populations are vulnerable to environmental exposures, such as lead poisoning, pesticides, and particulate matter (American Medical Association, 2015). These exposures are higher for those living in dense urban environments with heavy traffic or working in farming, most of whom are Mexican immigrants (Grineski, Collins, & Chakraborty, 2013). Mexican immigrants, who often reside in unsafe, inexpensive housing in high-income regions, are also exposed to high pollution levels (Bakhtsiyarava & Nawrotzki, 2017).

Racism and Discrimination

Finally, racism and perceived discrimination play a significant role in Latinx health. Increasing anti-immigrant climate amid ongoing political debate about migration has given rise to overt displays of racist and anti-immigrant images on social media as well as racist public acts (Lewis, Cogburn, & Williams, 2015). Heightened racism and discrimination against Latinx populations are in response to the criminalization of Latinx immigrants and the U.S. Latinx population overall (Chavez, 2013). In a recent example of hostility, a White gunman targeting what he called "Mexicans invading Texas" killed 22 people of predominant Mexican descent at an El Paso Walmart (Romo, 2019).

Compounding personal acts of racism and discrimination are systematic policy efforts to persecute and intimidate the Latinx population (Ayón & Becerra, 2013). Under the Trump administration, there have been family separations at the border (Jordan, 2019), increased raids and deportations, elimination of President Obama's Deferred Action for Childhood Arrivals (DACA; Pierce & Selee, 2017), and limitations on eligibility and legal residency for individuals using social services. Not surprisingly, recent polls indicate that the majority of Latinx individuals feel that racism is a problem in the United States and that their situation has worsened since the election of President Trump in 2016 (Latino Decisions, 2019; Lopez, Gonzalez-Barrera, & Krogstad, 2018). According to a Pew Research Center report, 4 in 10 Latinx individuals say they have experienced at least one form of harassment in the past 12 months because of their ethnic heritage (Lopez et al., 2018).

HEALTH OF LATINX POPULATIONS

Longevity and Mortality

Life expectancy is often considered the ultimate marker of the overall health of a population (Velasco-Mondragon et al., 2016). According to the National Center for Health Statistics (2018), life expectancy at birth in 2016 was longer for Latinx men (79.1 years) and women (84.2 years) than for non-Latinx White men (76.1 years) and women (81.1 years) or Black men (71.5 years) and women (77.9 years). Furthermore, although life expectancy for non-Latinx White and Black men decreased from 2016 to 2017, life expectancy for Latinx men remained unchanged. The age-adjusted death rate among non-Latinx Whites is 1.4 times that of Latinx in 2017, the former group having higher death rates for 11 of the 15 leading causes of death (Kochanek, Murphy, Xu, & Arias, 2019).

In addition, U.S. Latinx populations have the best birth outcomes (i.e., live births, fetal demise, and birth weight) among racial/ethnic minority groups despite their low socioeconomic profile. According to a report by the National Center for Health Statistics (2018), in 2016, low birth weight was found in only 7.32% of Latinx infants, a rate similar to non-Latinx Whites (7.07%), and almost half that of non-Latinx Blacks (13.3%). The prevalence of low birth weight ranges from a low of 6.90% (Mexican) to a high of 9.59% (Puerto Rican; National Center for Health Statistics, 2018).

Latinx Health Paradox

Although differences in longevity and birth outcomes in the general population have been attributed to socioeconomic factors that influence access to resources and medical care, the Latinx population has exhibited a phenomenon known as the Hispanic Health Paradox and the Immigrant Health Paradox (Velasco-Mondragon et al., 2016). The paradox applies to longevity, mortality, and a variety of physical and mental health outcomes and posits that Latinx immigrants enjoy superior health, compared with non-Latinx populations and U.S.-born Latinx individuals (Hall & Cuellar, 2016). The paradox is in the fact that immigrants are generally healthy upon entering the United States, which is counterintuitive because they disproportionately live in poverty and have limited access to economic resources, educational opportunities, and access to healthcare (Hall & Cuellar, 2016; Velasco-Mondragon et al., 2016). Many also flee violence and extreme economic insecurity prior to migration, while facing increasingly hostile contexts of reception in the United States (Schwartz et al., 2014).

One explanation for the health advantage is that Latinx individuals who are healthy are more likely than those experiencing poor health to migrate to the United States (Riosmena, Kuhn, & Jochem, 2017). Moreover, Latinx immigrants typically return to their country of origin when they are older, experience a chronic health concern or stress, or have more limited access to healthcare (Diaz, Koning, & Martinez-Donate, 2016). Latinx populations with low levels of acculturation to U.S. norms value close-knit family and social networks, which support health through sharing and exchanges of material and interpersonal supports (Heron, 2019).

The health paradox has a second component in that gains in health initially experienced by immigrants upon U.S. arrival decline over time with increasing length of stay and from one generation to another (Hall & Cuellar, 2016; Williams, 2012). In one study, recent Mexican immigrants with lower socioeconomic status (SES) resources and access to healthcare fared better in health outcomes than higher SES middle-aged U.S.-born Mexican Americans and foreign-born Mexican immigrants with long-term residence (see Williams, 2012). Loss of familial support, changes in dietary practices, downward social mobility, and chronic exposure to environmental hazards and threats may explain this part of the paradox (Galvez, 2013). Racism and restrictive immigration policy may intersect with these inequalities to undermine immigrants' sense of belonging, family preservation, and opportunities for advancement (Schwartz et al., 2014; Vesely, Bravo, & Guzzardo, 2019; Viruell-Fuentes, Miranda, & Abdulrahim, 2012).

Moreover, the paradox may obscure inequalities that exist among Latinx subgroups. For example, individual-level analysis from 1999 to 2015 of the National Health Interview Survey indicates that U.S.-born Puerto Rican men were disadvantaged in the number of years lived with morbidity. This discrepancy may reflect higher smoking rates among Puerto Rican men (28.5%) than the general Latinx population (10.1%; Centers for Disease Control and Prevention [CDC], n.d.-a; Riosmena et al., 2017). Foreign-born Cubans of all genders exhibited the healthiest outcomes of all groups. These findings highlight that benefits of increased longevity for older Latinx populations may be undermined if the additional years of life are characterized by chronic disease.

Major Health Burdens

Cancer

Unlike the non-Latinx population, for whom heart disease is the number one killer, cancer is the leading cause of death among Latinx populations. The illness accounts for similar death rates between Latinx individuals (20.6%) and non-Latinx Blacks (20.8%), but well below the rates of non-Latinx Whites (21.4%) and Asian and Pacific Islanders (25.1%; Heron, 2019). According to the Division of Vital Statistics, the cancer death rate for the U.S. Latinx population in 2017 decreased for men but remained stable for women (Heron, 2019). Subgroup statistics indicate 12% lower death rates among Puerto Ricans than non-Latinx White men, but 20% higher rates than for Mexican men (Velasco-Mondragon et al., 2016).

According to the National Center for Health Statistics (2017), the U.S. Latinx population is more likely to be diagnosed with infection-related cancers such as gastric, hepatic, and cervical, but are less likely to be diagnosed with prostate, breast, lung, and colorectal cancer, in comparison to non-Latinx Whites. Although Latinx women are less likely to be diagnosed with breast cancer, aggressive breast tumors affecting younger women are more common among Latinx and non-Latinx Black women living in poverty, and these tumors are less responsive to standard treatments and have a resulting poorer prognosis. Moreover, Latinx women are almost twice as likely to have liver cancer, stomach cancer, and cervical cancer and 1.4 times more likely to die from cervical cancer as compared to non-Latinx White women.

Lower rates of screening and higher prevalence of infection with human papillomavirus, hepatitis B virus, and the bacterium *Helicobacter pylori* in Latin America contributes to disparities in cervical, liver, and stomach cancer (National Cancer Institute, n.d.). There are also differences by nativity in that US-born Latinx men are twice as likely to develop hepatocellular carcinoma as foreign-born Latinx men (Velasco-Mondragon et al., 2016). Despite Latinx populations having lower rates of mortality and morbidity than non-Latinx Whites, they are more likely to be diagnosed with advanced-stage cancer (National Cancer Institute, n.d.), often attributed to lower access to preventive and diagnostic health services (Velasco-Mondragon et al., 2016).

Cardiovascular Disease

Although heart disease is the leading cause of death in the United States, it is the second leading cause of death in U.S. Latinx populations. Moreover, National Health Interview Survey data show that heart disease in 2017 was lower among Latinx populations (7.4%) in comparison to non-Latinx Blacks (9.5%) and Whites (11.5%). There is variation based on gender and ancestry, with Cuban, Puerto Rican, and Dominican men as well as Puerto Rican women showing the highest rates of coronary heart disease (see Balfour, Ruiz, Talavera, Allison, & Rodriguez, 2016). Latinx populations are less likely (14%) to be aware of the warning signs of a heart attack, compared to non-Latinx Whites (30%) and Blacks (16%; Balfour et al., 2016).

In the context of stroke, studies show lower prevalence rates of self-reported stroke in the U.S. Latinx population (2.3%) than non-Latinx Whites (2.6%; American Heart Association, 2018). Data from the Hispanic Community Health Study/Study of Latinos (NCHS/SOL) reveal that self-reported stroke is highest in Dominican men and Puerto Rican women (see Balfour et al., 2016). In contrast, studies using objective measures show an increased 3-year incidence of stroke among Mexican Americans compared to non-Latinx Whites, with a higher risk at younger versus older ages (Morgenstern et al., 2004).

Risk factors for heart disease include elevated rates of diabetes, obesity, hypertension, and cholesterol (CDC, 2019). A study using NCHS/SOL data showed that chronic stress burden was related to a higher prevalence of Latinx coronary heart disease and stroke, even after adjusting for sociodemographic, behavioral, and biological risk factors. Chronic stress also increased risk for diabetes and hypertension in the sample (Gallo et al., 2014). Another data set showed that among Latinx adults with hypertension, 45% report having their symptoms under control. In contrast, 50.8% of hypertensive non-Latinx White adults report control of their symptoms (Fryar, Ostchega, Hales, Zhang, & Kruszon-Moran, 2017).

Diabetes

Diabetes is the fifth leading cause of death among Latinx populations, outpacing Whites, for whom this disease is the seventh leading cause of death (CDC, 2015). In 2017, Latinx individuals were 60% more likely to die from diabetes than non-Latinx Whites (Health Resources and Services Administration, 2018). The prevalence of diabetes was 18.3% for Mexicans and 18% for both Puerto Ricans and Dominicans, and decreased to 10.2% for South Americans (Schneiderman et al., 2014). There is a clear link between diabetes and obesity, which is highest among Latinx children. Of children aged 2 to 19 years in 2015, 25.8% experienced obesity, relative to non-Latinx children who are Black (22%), White (14.1%), and Asian (11%; Hales, Carroll, Fryar, & Ogden, 2017).

Other risk factors for Latinx diabetes are smoking, obesity, and hypertension, which are influenced by low SES and other social determinants of health (SDOH; Health Resources and Services Administration, 2018). For example, the U.S. Latinx population with a high school education or lower are especially at risk of diabetes (Schneiderman et al., 2014). Compounding these risks is lack of insurance among Latinx immigrants, which is concerning because diabetes can be controlled with regular care (CDC, n.d.-b). Diabetes is associated with serious health complications, including chronic kidney disease, which can lead to kidney failure (CDC, n.d.-b). Latinx populations in the U.S. are about 1.5 times more likely to develop kidney failure and need regular dialysis or a kidney transplant to survive compared to non-Latinx populations (CDC, n.d.-b).

Mental Health

Overall, U.S. Latinx populations have lower rates of mental health problems than other racial/ethnic groups. A report by the Substance Abuse and Mental Health Service Administration (SAMHSA, 2018) shows the rate of mental illness among Latinx populations in 2017 to be 15.2%, only slightly higher than non-Latinx Asians (14.5%) and lower than White (20.4%) and Black (16.2%). This trend appears to apply to several mental health conditions. For example, data from the 2017 National Survey on Drug Use and Health (NSDUH; SAMHSA, 2018) indicated the past year prevalence of Major Depressive Disorder Episode (MDDE) was 5.4% for Latinx adults, a rate equal to non-Latinx Blacks and lower than Whites. Similarly, data from the National Asian and Latino Study (Alegría et al., 2008) show that U.S.-born Latinx populations have lower rates of depression and anxiety than non-Latinx Whites and that foreign-born Latinx have the lowest rates of depression and anxiety. Although these findings suggest protection for the foreign born, recent changes in immigration policy have heightened distress among those with undocumented status (Hilfinger Messias, McEwen, & Clark, 2015).

Age disparities in mental health status exist, in that Latinx seniors and adolescents have higher or equal rates of mental health problems than their non-Latinx White counterparts. The NSDUH 2017 data show a past year prevalence of MDDE for Latinx adolescents almost equal to that of non-Latinx Whites (14%) and greater to Blacks (9.5%; SAMHSA, 2018). In 2015, among Latinx students in grades 9 to 12, 18.9% had seriously considered attempting suicide, 15.7% had made a plan to attempt suicide, 11.3% had attempted suicide, and 4.1% had made a suicide attempt that resulted in an injury, poisoning, or overdose that required medical attention (American Psychiatric Association, 2017). These rates were consistently higher in Latinx students than in non-Latinx White and Black students, suggesting that Latinx youth may be exposed to immigration and acculturation stressors that make them particularly vulnerable to distress (American Psychiatric Association, 2017; Garcini et al., 2017). Among 16- to 25-year-old Latinx individuals, those with undocumented status are at risk for depression, anxiety, and substance abuse that is related to chronic immigration threats and minority stress (Garcini et al., 2017; Torres, Santiago, Walts, & Richards, 2018; Vargas, Juárez, Sanchez, & Livaudais, 2018).

Alcohol and Substance Use

Latinx populations are more likely to abstain from alcohol than other racial/ethnic groups. Approximately 32% of Latinx individuals have never had alcohol in their lifetime, while 16% of non-Latinx Whites report never drinking (National Institute on Alcohol Abuse and Alcoholism [NIAAA], 2019). Latinx groups are also less likely to be drinkers than other racial/ethnic groups; only about 54% of Latinx individuals report having at least one drink in the past year compared to 70% of non-Latinx Whites (NIAAA, 2019). However, despite a large proportion of Latinx persons being abstinent and nondrinkers, those who do drink are more likely to consume alcohol at higher volumes than Whites. National data suggest that U.S. Latinx populations consume more alcoholic drinks per occasion and report a higher frequency of heavy drinking days than other racial/ethnic groups (Chartier & Caetano, 2010; Kerr, Mulia, & Zemore, 2014). This level of drinking poses significantly great health and social risks for Latinx adults who do consume alcohol.

As a result, the U.S. Latinx population is impacted disproportionally by alcohol-related problems. Compared to non-Latinx Whites, Latinx individuals are more likely to experience negative social consequences (e.g., fights with friends or spouses), legal consequences (e.g., arrests for driving under the influence), alcohol-related injuries and accidents, and alcohol-related morbidity and mortality (e.g., liver disease). Latinx populations also tend to experience greater problem severity (i.e., a greater number of alcohol-dependence symptoms) and recurrent or persistent alcohol dependence than Whites (Chartier & Caetano, 2010; Mulia, Ye, Greenfield, & Zemore, 2009; Schmidt, Ye, Greenfield, & Bond, 2007; Witbrodt, Mulia, Zemore, & Kerr, 2014; Zemore et al., 2016). Even at comparable drinking levels, the U.S. Latinx population still experiences a greater burden of problems than non-Latinx

Whites (Witbrodt et al., 2014). Importantly, not all U.S. Latinx groups are equal when it comes to drinking and alcohol-related problems. Limited data suggest that those with Puerto Rican and Mexican origins tend to drink the most and are at greater risk for alcohol use disorders (AUDs) and alcohol-related problems than other Latinx subgroups (Caetano, Ramisetty-Mikler, & Rodriguez, 2009; Ramisetty-Mikler, Caetano, & Rodriguez, 2010; Vaeth, Caetano, Ramisetty-Mikler, & Rodriguez, 2009). Relatedly, individuals of Cuban origin are the least likely subgroup to engage in heavy drinking and experience alcohol-related problems (Vaeth et al., 2009).

Within the context of substance use, U.S. Latinx individuals commonly report lower use of illicit substances (9% past year; not including marijuana) than other racial/ethnic groups (NSDUH, 2017). However, despite a lower prevalence of illicit substance use, rates of abuse and dependence (i.e., substance use disorders) among Latinx persons tend to be comparable or slightly higher than non-Latinx Whites (Guerrero, Marsh, Khachikian, Amaro, & Vega, 2013). The most commonly used illicit substances among Latinx populations include marijuana, cocaine/crack, heroin, and hallucinogens (NSDUH, 2017). Some studies have found that certain substance-related consequences, such as mortality stemming from an overdose and transmission of blood-related infections (via injection), are more pronounced among Latinx persons than non-Latinx Whites (Alvarez, Jason, Olson, Ferrari, & Davis, 2007; Galea et al., 2003). Other studies have also found an increasing trend of overdose among the Latinx population (Bebinger, 2018).

Numerous factors have been documented to increase susceptibility to alcohol and substance use, including abuse and dependence, among the U.S. Latinx population. Substance use risk factors that tend to be salient among Latinx individuals include greater economic and social disadvantage, earlier age of onset use, laxer social norms regarding drinking and substance use, nativity, age of migration to the United States, and acculturation (Borges et al., 2011; Chartier & Caetano, 2010; Cherpitel, Li, Borges, & Zemore, 2017; Guerrero et al., 2013; Mulia, Ye, Zemore, & Greenfield, 2008; Pinedo, Zemore, Cherpitel, & Caetano, 2017).

Within the context of immigration, U.S.-born Latinx populations consistently report more alcohol and substance use and related problems than their foreign-born counterparts (Borges et al., 2011). Studies have also documented a protective effect among Latinx persons who migrate to the United States after the age of 12. Migrants who arrive before the age of 12 tend to report higher rates of substance use than Latinx migrants who arrived at older ages (Borges et al., 2011; Cherpitel et al., 2017). Finally, although greater acculturation to the United States has been associated with alcohol and substance use, it should be noted that acculturation has more consistently predicted substance use and associated problems among women than men (Pinedo et al., 2017). This may have to do with the adoption of more liberal norms surrounding women's substance use in the United States than in Latin America.

Healthcare Utilization and Access

Utilization and Access to Services

Data from the Medical Expenditure Panel Survey show that the U.S. Latinx population experienced worse access to care compared to non-Latinx Whites for a shocking 70% of care quality measures for 2015 to 2016 (Agency for Healthcare Research and Quality, 2019). At elevated risk for low access to care are Latinx immigrants, especially the undocumented, and those with substance use and mental health problems. Limitations to accessing care among immigrant Latinx populations include limited English proficiency, availability of and access to transportation, high cost, lack of knowledge of and familiarity with services, racism and discrimination, and stigma, among others (Warrier & Rose, 2016).

Latinx-undocumented immigrants are more likely to report lacking a usual source of care, are less likely to have a physician monitoring a health condition, and are less likely to experience excellent/good care in the past year, in comparison to the U.S.-born Latinx population (Rodríguez, Bustamante, & Ang, 2009). Reasons for low utilization of health services among this group include narrow eligibility criteria among social service agencies, mistrust and fear that healthcare providers will require proof of residency or report them to immigration authorities, and fear of public exposure (Hilfinger Messias et al., 2015). Undocumented women who experience gender-based violence by a partner who is a U.S. citizen are at the highest disadvantage, because seeking care and other protections might jeopardize their partner's sponsorship for their legal status (Warrier & Rose, 2016).

Regarding substance use and mental health problems, only 3% to 7% of Latinx persons with an alcohol or substance problem ever seek help, and those with lifetime substance use disorders are approximately 1.42 to 2.33 times less likely than non-Latinx Whites to have ever obtained help from a specialty substance abuse treatment program (Guerrero et al., 2013; Lê Cook & Alegría, 2011; Mulia, Tam, & Schmidt, 2014; Schmidt, Greenfield, & Mulia, 2006; Wells, Klap, Koike, & Sherbourne, 2001; Witbrodt et al., 2014). Perceptions that treatment is not culturally responsive and culturally related stigma may especially discourage Latinx persons from seeking substance use and mental health treatment (Pinedo, Zemore, & Rogers, 2018).

Health Insurance Coverage

Rates of health insurance coverage increased from 74% in 2013 to 83% in 2016 for nonelderly Latinx populations, in part due to the Affordable Care Act (ACA), but projected increases in insurance premiums signal a potential decline in insurance coverage among this population (Pagan & Howell, 2018). Latinx women have the least access to health coverage of any group of women, with 37% being uninsured compared to 14% of non-Latinx White women (Pagan & Howell, 2018). Health insurance coverage is particularly low among the noncitizen, nonelderly population, with data from the American Community Survey showing that 24% of lawfully permanent and 47% of undocumented adults were uninsured in 2017, compared to 10% of citizens (Kaiser Family Foundation, 2019). The report also found that 31% of undocumented children and 7% of U.S.-born children with at least one noncitizen parent were uninsured, relative to 4% of U.S.-born children with citizen parents. High uninsurance rates are the result of (a) undocumented immigrants not being eligible to enroll in Medicaid, Children's Health Insurance Program, or to purchase coverage through the ACA, and (b) full-time working adults within immigrant families often being employed in low-wage jobs and/or in industries that are less likely to offer employer-sponsored insurance (Kaiser Family Foundation, 2019).

LATINX HEALTH AND HEALTH EQUITY MODELS

Few health equity models exist in the literature that address Latinx health specifically. Creating these models is essential to better understand and address disparities among Latinx populations. Any health equity model applied to Latinx populations must account for the complex presentation of health burdens, distal social determinants and proximal risk factors, and healthcare quality and access. Moreover, such a model needs to acknowledge the diversity among Latinx subgroups based on ancestry, nativity, gender, immigration status, socioeconomic stability, and other intersecting identities (e.g., age, gender expression, sexual orientation, and skin color). The Pan American Health Organization (PAHO, 2018) Commission on Equity and Health Inequalities has adapted general models of health equity to Latinx populations. For example, PAHO adapted the Commission on Social Determinants model (Commission on Social Determinants of Health, 2008) to create a framework for the Latinx population that emphasizes colonialism, structural racism, and people's relationship to land. PAHO also added an overarching focus on intersectionality, which addresses multiple components of Latinx identity. Similar models are emerging, and this chapter describes two geared toward clinical practice before presenting a comprehensive model of Latinx health, SDOH, healthcare utilization, and access.

Latinx-Specific Models for Clinical Practice

The multidimensional ecosystemic comparative approach (MECA; Falicov, 2014) is a model for mental health practitioners that considers culture and the role of oppression in Latinx families, similarities and differences between and within families, and similarities and differences between families and practitioners. As shown in Figure 6.1, MECA identifies four key domains of the

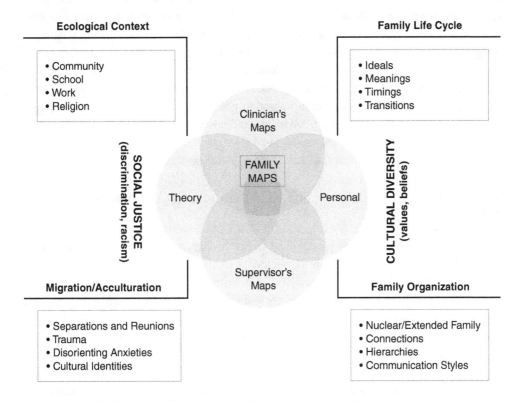

FIGURE 6.1 Multidimensional ecosystemic comparative approach.

SOURCE: From Falicov, C. J. (2014). *Latino families in therapy* (2nd ed.). New York, NY: Guilford Publications. Copyright 2013 by Guilford. Reprinted with permission of Guilford Press.

Latinx experience: ecological contexts, migration-acculturation, family life cycle, and family organization (Falicov, 2014). The first two domains pertain to sociopolitical factors and hence social justice, while the third and fourth domains reflect cultural diversity.

Assuming that the therapeutic space involves a cultural and sociopolitical encounter between two or more individuals, MECA incorporates the practitioner's intersecting identities, racial/ethnic experiences, privilege and bias, and cultural awareness and humility into the model. At the center, family and practitioner maps allow for the visualization of points of connection and potential bias that can affect the therapeutic encounter. The model promotes cultural humility on behalf of the practitioner, as well as interventions that address cultural diversity and social justice to break down power differentials and oppression (Falicov, 2014).

A second model for practice draws on global factors affecting Latinx immigrant populations. The Ulysses syndrome, proposed by Achotegui in 2002, borrows from the Greek literary hero Ulysses to explain how levels of stress experienced during migration impact mental and physical illness. Achotegui (2019) argues that "emigration presents stress levels of such intensity that they exceed the human capacity of adaptation" (p. 264). The result is not a discrete illness or symptom, but a complex dysregulation of stress response, which can, in turn, affect lifestyle and health behaviors and exacerbate illness expression.

Once immigrants arrive in the new country, they often face family separation, acculturative stressors, isolation, diminished social status, and fear of family separation and deportation. Achotegui describes seven forms of migratory mourning that affect those who emigrate, subsequent generations, and those who stayed behind. Forms of mourning include the loss of (a) family and loved ones, (b) language, (c) culture, (d) homeland, (e) social status, (f) belonging, and (g) the presence of physical risks. In light of these experiences of mourning, immigrant health can manifest in symptoms of migraines, nervousness, irritability, stomach pains, physical pain, and insomnia (Achotegui, 2019; Bianucci, Charlier, Perciaccante, Lippi, & Appenzeller, 2017). Achotegui calls for the recognition of immigration policy as mental health policy. The Ulysses syndrome model is important to practitioners to avoid misdiagnosing health problems or pathologizing the migrant experience. The model provides strategies for helping migrants to navigate phases of grief: negation, resistance, and acceptance (Achotegui, 2019).

A Comprehensive Model of Latinx Health and Social Determinants of Health

Velasco-Mondragon et al. (2016) proposed a comprehensive conceptual model of Latinx health in the United States. Developed from the socioecological framework and the life-span biopsychosocial model, the authors incorporate SDOH, proximal risk factors, and health care services and quality as factors that influence morbidity and mortality for Latinx populations. Figure 6.2 highlights the following SDOH: (A) environment, occupation and SES; (B) determinants such as poverty that can make individuals particularly vulnerable to health inequalities; and (C) behavioral and biological risk factors such as exercise, nutrition, and biological metabolic symptoms that affect health. These SDOH influence (D) morbidity and (E) mortality (Velasco-Mondragon et al., 2016). The model also demonstrates an interconnectedness with (F) policy, access, utilization, and quality of health services. For instance, high mortality from noninfectious chronic disease can influence policies to provide greater occupational or economic support.

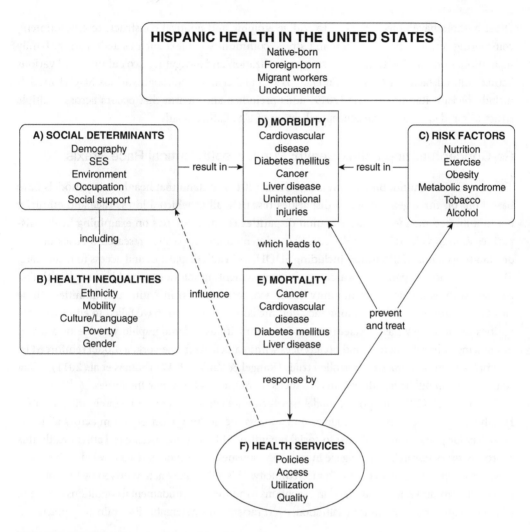

FIGURE 6.2 U.S. Latinx health and health services.

SES, socioeconomic status.
SOURCE: From Velasco-Mondragon, E., Jimenez, A., Palladino-Davis, A. G., Davis, D., & Escamilla-Cejudo, J. A. (2016). Hispanic health in the USA: A scoping review of the literature. *Public Health Reviews, 37*, 31. doi:10.1186/s40985-016-0043-2

A strength of this model is that it draws attention to health disparities and inequities among U.S. Latinx individuals who are native born, foreign born, migrant workers, and undocumented, all of whom are too often lumped together into one category. The flexibility in this approach allows policy makers and other stakeholders to design programs to increase access to safe, outside spaces, and healthy nutrition for foreign born-Latinx at risk for diabetes, while addressing acculturative and immigration stress that would hamper participation in such programs. A critique of this model is that social determinants (A and B) and behavioral and biological risk factors (C) are not displayed as interrelated constructs. A person's occupation or environment may affect risk factors such as exercise and nutrition because occupation, SES, and environmental factors affect where a person lives and whether they have the time and ability to exercise and purchase, easily access, or prepare nutritious food.

Other authors have noted the need to add geographic and political constructs to environment, considering residential segregation and stress, community context such as assimilation, family separation, immigration trauma/stress, marginalization and navigating two cultures, and various Latinx cultural factors (Ramirez García, 2019). Furthermore, although various SDOH models include racism, Ramirez García (2019) adds prejudice and racism that occurs across multiple structures and systems to the conceptualization of U.S. Latinx health.

Re-Conceptualizing Latinx Health: Public Health Critical Race Praxis

Thomas, Crouse Quinn, Butler, Fryer, and Garza (2011) contend that health equity models have been built on three generations of disparities research, all of which address race and ethnicity but in a limited manner. First-generation disparities research focuses on examining health disparities among vulnerable populations. Second-generation disparities research focuses on understanding causal relationships, including SDOH, of health disparities and access to healthcare. Third-generation disparities research involves implementing solutions for addressing health disparities, such as the use of community health workers (CHWs) in Latinx communities. These efforts have improved health among racial/ethnic communities, but have failed to eliminate disparities because they have treated race and/or ethnicity as a demographic variable or a factor influencing cultural practices and preferences within a deficits framework, a model reinforced by an emphasis on randomized controlled trials (Rangel & Valdez, 2017; Thomas et al., 2011). What is missing from public health systems is a focus on racism and systemic inequities.

Thomas et al. (2011) propose a model in which a fourth generation of research utilizes Public Health Critical Race Praxis to recognize and address the health impact of racism across all levels of society for populations subjected to social prejudice. Although not specific to Latinx health, this approach forces researchers to engage in race consciousness, reflect on and acknowledge their own biases, privilege, and experiences with race/ethnicity. This will require action driven by the voices of the community and lead to multilevel interventions to address the fundamental conditions of health, which for Latinx populations is racialization, overt racism, and systematic discriminatory practices.

EQUITY-ORIENTED PROGRAMS FOR LATINX POPULATIONS

Interventions Tailored to Latinx Populations

Although defined widely, interventions are generally focused on improving the quality of care or health outcomes of individuals that have already been diagnosed with a chronic condition; therefore, many interventions attempt to improve health outcomes at the most proximate level. Some of the most promising interventions for Latinx populations in the literature involve trained CHWs, also known as "lay health advisors," "health advocates," "health educators," *promotores de salud,*" or "patient navigators" (Albright et al., 2009). Interventions implemented by community members are considered more culturally appropriate (Fisher, Burnet, Huang, Chin, & Cagney, 2007; Hurtado et al., 2014) because community members "serve as bridges between the ethnic, cultural or geographic communities and healthcare providers" (Albright et al., 2009, p. 1). Other research suggests that the Latinx population particularly benefits from CHW programs due to low literacy rates and strong communal ties (Ramar & Desai, 2010). Several qualitative studies have explored why CHWs are effective change agents for improving Latinx health, with findings that suggest *promotores* empower patients, motivate behavioral and environmental change, and serve as community advocates (Albarran, Heilemann, & Koniak-Griffin, 2014; McCloskey, 2009).

CHWs have been used for over 30 years within the Latinx community, and many studies have indicated their efficacy at treating chronic diseases such as diabetes, cardiovascular disease, and HIV (Balcazar, Alvarado, & Ortiz, 2011; Little, Wang, Castro, Jimenez, & Rosal, 2014; Pérez-Escamilla, Hromi-Fiedler, Vega-López, Bermúdez-Millán, & Segura-Pérez, 2008; Rhodes, Foley, Zometa, & Bloom, 2007; Shommu et al., 2016). However, the role of the CHW and the intervention used has varied widely across studies. For example, in one diabetes intervention, the CHW acted like a care coordinator, which included reminding patients of upcoming appointments, attending appointments, and being a liaison between the healthcare providers and the patient (Corkery et al., 1997). The CHW intervention significantly improved diabetes knowledge, self-care practice, and hemoglobin A1c levels compared to a control group. In another study, a CHW provided individualized support for Latinx patients receiving hemodialysis, which included advanced care planning, care coordination, and health counseling (Cervantes et al., 2019). The intervention retention rate was 100%, and 95% of patients reported an improvement in their quality of life postintervention. Other interventions provided health education for diabetes, cardiovascular disease, and dietary behaviors (Balcazar et al., 2011; Little et al., 2014; Pérez-Escamilla et al., 2008). These studies suggest that CHW interventions can improve clinical outcomes, disease knowledge, and self-management skills.

Programs Tailored to Latinx Populations

Programs are generally focused on prevention and target individuals and communities that may be at risk for disease in the future; therefore, they attempt to address fundamental social conditions, known as "upstream" factors, and improve health outcomes at the community level. For example, multiple programs have attempted to improve access to primary care or health insurance in order to address access barriers that directly impact health outcomes (Abreu & Hynes, 2009; Blewett, Casey, & Call, 2004). Other programs have tried to address food security by providing food prescriptions or creating a community garden for Latinx farmworkers (Carney et al., 2012; RCHN Community Health Foundation, 2019).

Health promotion is another approach that has been successful within the Latinx community, and it typically focuses on building a safe community and educating on culturally relevant healthy lifestyles in order to prevent disease (Kumar & Preetha, 2012). For example, New York-Presbyterian Regional Health Collaborative utilized a population health model to create a "medical village," which connects Latinx community members to health services across the care continuum as well as community resources (Carillo et al., 2011). Finally, there are programs focused on improving the identification or treatment of preventable diseases, such as colorectal cancer, hypertension, or depression, through educational materials and community screenings (Aragones, Schwartz, Shah, & Gany, 2010; Coffman et al., 2017).

Many studies of programs are grounded in community-based participatory research (CBPR), which is an approach that "encourages equity and shared decision making between researchers and community members" (Bastida, Tseng, McKeever, & Jack, 2010, p. 16). CBPR engages communities to identify upstream SDOH such as access to healthcare or food that will make a larger impact on health equity (Valenzuela, McDowell, Cencula, Hoyt, & Mitchell, 2013). CBPR also reduces "parachute research," where community-based studies are only for the benefit of the researcher's career, as opposed to the community being served, which can cause further harm or exploitation (Bastida et al., 2010).

CBPR may be particularly effective at improving health disparities because it includes a needs assessment of the Latinx community, which then shapes the programs, interventions, or policies created (Cristancho, Garces, Peters, & Mueller, 2008). For example, a mental health intervention targeting mothers with depression, other caregivers, and their children was developed and implemented in community settings only after researchers partnered with local mental health and primary care clinics to understand the mental health needs of Latinx immigrant families in the area (Valdez, Ramirez-Stege, Martinez, D'Costa, & Chavez, 2018). Focus groups with families also informed the content and modality of the intervention, and the type of surface and deep level adaptations necessary to maximize recruitment and engagement of families into the 12-week intervention, as well as its benefit to families (Valdez et al., 2018). Training videos featured and were developed with involvement from families graduated from the program. In another example, after a community-needs assessment and community forum, one program held five health fairs over a 6-month period that was multifaceted and included screenings for diabetes, hypertension, and depression; primary care provider visits; and information about local healthcare and community-based resources (Coffman et al., 2017). After 1 year, primary care services increased from 33.8% at baseline to 48%, and 62% reported use of social services.

Policies Tailored to Latinx Populations

Policies are less focused on individuals or specific communities and are more focused on improving health equity for large segments of the population; therefore, they attempt to improve health outcomes at the most distal level and also present the best way to make improvements for a large number of people. Further, community-based techniques such as CBPR can still be implemented within policy-level work. One example is procedural justice, which are "equitable processes through which low-income communities of color, rural residents, and other marginalized groups can gain a seat at the table—and stay at the table, having a real voice in decision making affecting their lives" (Minkler, 2010, p. S81).

Affecting many Latinx populations is immigration policy at the federal and state levels. Immigration policies vary by state and trickle down to impact the Latinx community by dictating access to healthcare, higher education, employment, and housing, which all impact health outcomes (Wallace, Young, Rodríguez, & Brindis, 2018). Although a Latinx resident in Texas cannot access Medicaid unless they are a permanent legal resident/citizen, a Latinx DACA recipient in California can enroll in Medicaid, regardless of immigration status (Lucia, 2019). Moreover, recent immigration policies passed by the Trump administration have direct impacts on the health of the U.S. Latinx population. Examples include (a) the rescission of DACA that affected 800,000 young adults; (b) the passage of a "zero tolerance" law that led to family separation at the U.S.-Mexico border of more than 3,000 families; and (c) recent public-charge policies that prohibited eligibility for citizenship for immigrants participating in social assistance programs, such as Temporary Assistance for Needy Families (Justice in Aging, 2018; Vesely et al., 2019).

According to Browne et al. (2018), equity-oriented healthcare specifically recognizes the effects of structural inequities, the inequitable distribution of SDOH, the impact of multiple and intersecting forms of racism, discrimination and stigma on people's access to services and their experiences of care. This model of healthcare also recognizes the frequent mismatches between dominant approaches to care and the needs of people who are most affected by health and social inequities (Browne et al., 2018). Equity-oriented healthcare is an extension of patient-centered care and requires an in-depth understanding of the community being served and their specific needs (Kim, Molina, & Saadi, 2019).

BEST PRACTICE RECOMMENDATIONS IN DESIGNING NEW EQUITY EFFORTS FOR LATINX POPULATIONS

Protecting the health of the U.S. Latinx population is critical to the public health of the nation. Latinx individuals make up the largest minority racial/ethnic group and are impacted disproportionately by multiple health disparities across diverse outcomes, including physical health, mental and behavioral health, and access to healthcare (Flores, 2017; Vega, Rodriguez, & Gruskin, 2009). Though considerable work has been done to improve the health of Latinx populations and to reduce and eliminate existing health disparities, much work and research is still needed. The following sections provide best practices and recommendations for designing new interventions, programs, and policies aimed at progressing toward achieving health equity among U.S. Latinx populations.

Interventions and programs that are designed specifically for Latinx populations are key. Significant evidence indicates that culturally appropriate and tailored interventions targeting Latinx persons are effective in reducing health-damaging behaviors, increasing the adoption of health-promoting behaviors, and reducing poor health outcomes (Pérez-Escamilla et al., 2008; Victorson et al., 2014; Woodruff, Talavera, & Elder, 2002). Culturally appropriate programs take into account important social and contextual factors that are salient among Latinx populations and their lived experiences in the U.S. Such factors include the context of immigration (e.g., reasons for migration, receptivity of the host community), language barriers, and experiences of acculturation, racism, and discrimination, among others. Incorporating such factors in the design of interventions and programs can lead to increased feelings of belonging and validation, resulting in better outcomes (Pérez-Escamilla et al., 2008).

Further, it is important to note that various evidence-based interventions, treatments, and programs that were not designed specifically for Latinx populations have also been found to be effective. However, evidence-based programs can be enhanced by culturally adapting them for Latinx persons (Domenech Rodríguez, Baumann, & Schwartz, 2011; Lee et al., 2013; Parra Cardona et al., 2012). Culturally adapting an evidence-based intervention or program entails incorporating important cultural, social, and contextual factors that are prominent among Latinx groups, while retaining the core components of the original intervention or program. Evidence suggests that culturally adapted evidence-based programs can produce better outcomes than their nonadapted versions among Latinx groups, including increased retention and feelings of satisfaction (Lee et al., 2013; Parra Cardona et al., 2012; Rathod et al., 2018).

Improved data collection and research efforts are urgently needed to identify factors driving health inequities among U.S. Latinx populations. National data sets, particularly epidemiological and surveillance studies conducted by government and academic agencies, commonly fail to collect data on important factors shown to influence the health behaviors of the U.S. Latinx population. Such data include information on Latinx subgroups (e.g., Mexican, Puerto Rican, Cuban), cultural factors (e.g., cultural perceptions regarding health outcomes), immigration status, generation status, the effects of immigration enforcement, deportation experiences and the deportation of family members, and acculturation (Alegría et al., 2008; Lara, Gamboa, Kahramanian, Morales, & Bautista, 2005; Vargas et al., 2018). The lack of these data hinders comparative analyses with other racial/ethnic groups, which is key to determining if these factors may explain existing health disparities among Latinx groups. Such knowledge can inform the development of novel efforts designed specifically to address the health needs of the U.S. Latinx population.

Lastly, interventions and programs targeting Latinx populations must consider the role of the current hostile environment toward immigrants and Latinx persons. Effects of immigration enforcement and anti-immigration policies (e.g., deportations, increased surveillance of immigrant communities) also have spillover effects on the health of Latinx U.S citizens (Philbin, Flake, Hatzenbuehler, & Hirsch, 2018; Szkupinski Quiroga, Medina, & Glick, 2014). For example, greater number of state-level punitive immigration policies, perceived anti-immigration sentiments, and having a family member deported have been linked to poor mental health and greater feelings of discrimination among Latinx U.S. citizens and noncitizens alike (Hatzenbuehler et al., 2017; Vargas, Sanchez, & Juarez, 2017; Vargas et al., 2018). Thus, this work underscores that migration-related factors must be considered when addressing health equity and in the design of novel programs targeting the U.S. Latinx population.

Although there is substantial evidence indicating the effectiveness of culturally appropriate and community-based interventions and programs geared toward Latinx communities, long-term interventions, multilevel programs, and policy-based initiatives have received less attention (Trickett et al., 2011). Improving health equity within an entire population will take considerable time and will require sustainable funding and investment from communities, cities, counties, and businesses (Weinstein, Geller, Negussie, & Baciu, 2017). Public–private partnerships or broad-based collaborations can be difficult to maintain due to a narrow understanding of the problem, competing strategies and approaches, difficulty measuring population-level change, and limited literature to guide community- or population-level programs (Fawcett, Shultz, Watson-Thompson, Fox, & Bremby, 2010). However, Fawcett et al. (2010) offer a 12-step framework for collaborative public health action that includes identifying a common purpose, establishing a vision, implementing targeted action, documenting progress, and sustaining the work through ongoing investments. CBPR has much to offer when it comes to designing, implementing, and assessing community-specific health equity programs (Cacari-Stone, Wallerstein, Garcia, & Minkler, 2014). CBPR should be implemented across interventions, programs, and policies to address Latinx health disparities at the individual, community, and societal levels (Freudenberg & Tsui, 2014).

INTERSECTIONALITY SPOTLIGHT

Intersectionality recognizes that individuals hold overlapping social identities, such as sex, race, and sexual orientation, that each contribute to privilege or disfranchisement (Bowleg, 2012). Many of these identities are associated with their own health disparities, which further interact with Latinx identity and can lead to differential health outcomes. This chapter has identified various identities that influence health outcomes, such as immigration status, nationality, and sex. These variations are important to identify and recognize, especially when it comes to implementing health equity interventions, programs, or policies. Therefore, intersectionality should be used as a lens to better understand health disparities within the Latinx community and identify those who are most at risk of preventable disease or adverse outcomes.

Inequities Based on Sex

Latinx women are less likely to be screened for cervical cancer or diagnosed with breast cancer and more likely to die from cervical cancer compared to White women (National Cancer Institute, n.d.; National Center for Health Statistics, 2017). Latinx women are also at higher risk for maternal mortality compared to White women (Howland et al., 2019). Factors such as race or nationality can influence maternal outcomes. For example, one study found that Black Latinx women and Puerto Rican Latinx women had higher rates of infant mortality compared to Cuban Latinx women (Henry-Sanchez & Geronimus, 2013). Disparities in Latinx women may be explained by psychosocial factors, such as (a) women's lower social status and Latinx cultural values of self-sacrifice (Villarreal, 2007); (b) faster acculturation to U.S. norms by Latinx women than their male counterparts (Grzywacz, Rao, Gentry, Marin, & Arcury, 2009); and (c) disproportionate experiences of discrimination in healthcare due to Latinx women's fertility (Galvez, 2013).

Inequities Based on Race

Latinx identity is considered an ethnicity by the U.S. Census and separate from race; therefore, Latinx identity can also intersect with race. Although more research is needed in this area, there have been studies that compare health outcomes among Latinx participants based on race. One review paper identified 13 studies that compared Black Latinx samples to White Latinx samples across a variety of outcomes, including the prevalence of hypertension, self-reported health status, mental health, psychological distress, and discrimination (Cuevas, Dawson, & Williams, 2016). Unsurprisingly, many of the studies found that Black or "dark-skinned" Latinx participants had higher rates of discrimination, mental health concerns like depressive symptoms, and poorer self-reported health (Borrell & Crawford, 2006; Garcia, Sanchez, Sanchez-Youngman, Vargas, & Ybarra, 2015; Ortiz & Telles, 2012; Ramos, Jaccard, & Guilamo-Ramos, 2003).

Inequities Based on Sexual Orientation and Gender Identity

Five percent of the U.S. Latinx population identifies as LGBTQ and 9.8% of same-sex couples are Latinx (Brown, 2017; Pew Research Center, 2013). Although this may be a small section of the larger community, Latinx LGBTQ people experience significant oppression and discrimination. This is particularly true for Latinx transgender women, who face high rates of extreme poverty (28% compared to 5% of the general Latinx population), violence, and discrimination (Harrison-Quintana, Perez, & Grant, 2010). Although there are no national estimates of violence against Latinx transgender women, two studies found that 55% and 60% had been harassed or assaulted (Galvan & Bazargan, 2012; Lombardi, Wilchins, Priesing, & Malouf, 2002). Additionally, health disparities exist for the Latinx LGBTQ population. Although 16% of those newly diagnosed with HIV/AIDS in 2016 were Latinx, 87% were Latinx men who have sex with men (MSM; CDC, 2017). Similarly, compared to 2.6% of transgender people that have HIV/AIDS, 8.4% of Latinx transgender people have HIV/AIDS (Harrison-Quintana et al., 2010). Finally, Latinx LGBTQ adults are less likely to have health insurance or a primary source of healthcare than non-Latinx LGBTQ adults (Krehely, 2009). Therefore, it is particularly important to consider both sexual orientation and gender identity when assessing HIV health disparities within the Latinx community.

CASE STUDY **MATERNAL AND INFANT HEALTH IN MIGRANT LATINX WOMEN**

"Marina" and her family are migrant seasonal agricultural workers who are originally from Mexico. She began treatment for gestational diabetes in Florida at the end of January 2014, during her first trimester of pregnancy. Marina also had a toddler who was found to be beyond the acceptable weight range for a child of her age. It was also determined that the child was experiencing significant dental caries. On evaluation, Marina indicated that she helped the child soothe herself nightly with diluted fruit juice in a bottle. Because of her pregnancy, Marina's treatment for gestational diabetes would require a strict monitoring of her diet and regular checking of her blood sugar levels. Her child's diet was also adjusted by the physician as part of the normal course of treatment.

When the health center learned in February that the family planned to move to New Jersey, the clinician called Health Network, an organization focused on the mobile poor. By enrolling Marina and her child in Health Network, the department could be sure that despite their move out of the county and out of the state, Health Network staff would ensure that the management of her pregnancy would not be interrupted and that her care would be monitored.

A Health Network case manager attempted to contact Marina twice at the end of March to introduce herself and to explain how Health Network functions. The second attempt to reach Marina was successful. The case manager, fully bilingual in Spanish and English, verified Marina's address, confirmed that the family planned to move, explained that Health Network would be there to help her with her care, and, in that call, established a relationship of trust.

Over the course of 8 months, Health Network staff maintained communication, making seven contacts with the patient and her husband to monitor the health and treatment of Marina and her child. Marina did not move to New Jersey until July. Once there, the Health Network case manager confirmed that Marina and her child were being seen by a health center in the county to which they had moved and that her medical records were transferred. In August, Marina and her child returned to their home in Florida. Health Network once again saw that medical records were transferred back to the Florida health center in her county. Marina's child showed a marked improvement in her weight and overall health. She received extensive dental care in New Jersey that was continued in Florida. Soon after returning to Florida in August, Marina gave birth to a healthy baby at the end of September and completed her 6-week postpartum visit at the end of October. Health Network stayed in communication with the health center until the postpartum visit was completed to close the loop on care.

Although language barriers are often an obstacle to care, Health Network's bilingual staff demonstrated not only cultural awareness, but cultural responsiveness and humility. The case manager developed a rapport that enabled regular communication with both Marina and her husband in an atmosphere where they felt comfortable to talk about health concerns and personal plans. When Health Network staff made calls and left messages, Marina and her husband returned those calls. Because of Health Network's professionalism, health centers in two states received case completion records enabling them to close cases for an at-risk pregnancy for a patient on the move.

CURRENT EVENTS

DEFERRED ACTION FOR CHILDHOOD ARRIVALS

DACA is an immigration policy implemented under the Obama administration in 2012 that provides renewable 2-year deferments of deportation for individuals who were brought into the United States without documentation as children. The program allows individuals without a criminal background to obtain a work permit and stay in the United States rather than face deportation to a country where they may not even speak the local language. The Trump administration has announced plans to dismantle DACA, which have subsequently been put on hold by the U.S. Supreme Court pending their hearing of the case in the 2019 session. If ended, an estimated 700,000 people would face potential deportation.

Discussion Question: Given the current sociopolitical environment surrounding immigration, how could action in either direction—either upholding DACA or allowing it to be ended—affect the determinants of health discussed throughout this chapter?

ACCESSIBILITY OF BILINGUAL MENTAL HEALTH SERVICES

With the demographic changes occurring throughout the United States, it is estimated that there will be a 30% increase in the need for full-time mental health therapists by the year 2030. However, only 5% of therapists report they are competent in providing services in Spanish. Even for individuals who speak both English and Spanish, the ability to access services in their language of preference, or even to have the opportunity to express a particular emotion or sentiment in whichever language is most precise for the given topic, this presents major barriers to receipt of culturally and linguistically appropriate services.

Discussion Question: What kinds of changes throughout the educational system would be necessary to meet the demand for bilingual mental health professionals?

DISCUSSION QUESTIONS

- What are three demographic characteristics that make the U.S. Latinx population heterogeneous with respect to health status?
- What are the two components of the Latinx health paradox?
- Which health burden affects Latinx youth more than adults? Why?
- What challenges do Latinx populations encounter in accessing healthcare services?
- What are two distal SDOH and two proximal risk factors in Latinx health?
- How can Public Health Critical Race Praxis improve efforts to achieve health equity among Latinx populations in the United States?
- What is the promise of CBPR in the design of interventions, programs, and policies for Latinx populations?
- How can practitioners engage Latinx populations based on the case study presented?
- What are two recommendations you would like to see to improve health equity among Latinx populations? Why?
- How does intersectionality influence Latinx health?

REFERENCES

Abreu, M., & Hynes, H. P. (2009). The Latino Health Insurance Program: A pilot intervention for enrolling Latino families in health insurance programs, East Boston, Massachusetts, 2006-2007. *Preventing Chronic Disease*, 6(4), A129. Retrieved from https://www.ncbi.nlm.nih.gov/pmc/articles/PMC2774643/

Achotegui, J. (2019). Migrants living in very hard situations: Extreme migratory mourning (the Ulysses syndrome). *Psychoanalytic Dialogues*, 29(3), 252–268. doi:10.1080/10481885.2019.1614826

Agency for Healthcare Research and Quality. (2019). *2017 national healthcare quality and disparities report*. Retrieved from https://www.ahrq.gov/research/findings/nhqrdr/nhqdr17/index.html

Albarran, C. R., Heilemann, M. V., & Koniak-Griffin, D. (2014). Promotoras as facilitators of change: Latinas' perspectives after participating in a lifestyle behaviour intervention program. *Journal of Advanced Nursing*, 70(10), 2303–2313. doi:10.1111/jan.12383

Albright, A., Araujo, R., Brownson, C., Heffernan, D., Shield, D. I., Maryniuk, M., ... Secraw, P. (2009). *AADE position statement: Community health workers in diabetes management and prevention*. Chicago, IL: American Association of Diabetes Educators. Retrieved from https://www.diabeteseducator.org/docs/default-source/legacy-docs/_resources/pdf/CommunityHealthWorkerPositionStatement2009.pdf

Alcoff, L. M. (2005). Latino vs. Hispanic: The politics of ethnic names. *Philosophy and Social Criticism*, 31(4), 395–407. doi:10.1177/0191453705052972

Alegría, M., Canino, G., Shrout, P. E., Woo, M., Duan, N., Vila, D., ... Meng, X. L. (2008). Prevalence of mental illness in immigrant and non-immigrant US Latino groups. *American Journal of Psychiatry*, 165(3), 359–369. doi:10.1176/appi.ajp.2007.07040704

Alvarez, J., Jason, L. A., Olson, B. D., Ferrari, J. R., & Davis, M. I. (2007). Substance abuse prevalence and treatment among Latinos and Latinas. *Journal of Ethnicity in Substance Abuse*, 6(2), 115–141. doi:10.1300/J233v06n02_08

American Heart Association. (2018). Heart disease and stroke statistics—2018 update. *Circulation*, 137, e67–e492. Retrieved from https://www.ahajournals.org/doi/pdf/10.1161/CIR.0000000000000558

American Medical Association. (2015). *3 environmental issues disproportionately affecting Hispanic patients*. Retrieved from https://www.ama-assn.org/delivering-care/population-care/3-environmental-issues-disproportionately-affecting-hispanic

American Psychiatric Association. (2017). *Mental health disparities: Hispanics and Latinos*. Retrieved from https://www.psychiatry.org/File%20Library/Psychiatrists/Cultural-Competency/Mental-Health-Disparities/Mental-Health-Facts-for-Hispanic-Latino.pdf

Aragones, A., Schwartz, M. D., Shah, N. R., & Gany, F. M. (2010). A randomized controlled trial of a multilevel intervention to increase colorectal cancer screening among Latino immigrants in a primary care facility. *Journal of General Internal Medicine*, 25(6), 564–567. doi:10.1007/s11606-010-1266-4

Ayón, C., & Becerra, D. (2013). Mexican immigrant families under siege: The impact of anti-immigrant policies, discrimination, and the economic crisis. *Advances in Social Work*, 14(1), 206–228. doi:10.18060/2692

Bakhtsiyarava, M., & Nawrotzki, R. J. (2017). Environmental inequality and pollution advantage among immigrants in the United States. *Applied Geography*, 81, 60–69. doi:10.1016/j.apgeog.2017.02.013

Balcazar, H., Alvarado, M., & Ortiz, G. (2011). Salud Para Su Corazon (health for your heart) community health worker model: Community and clinical approaches for addressing cardiovascular disease risk reduction in Hispanics/Latinos. *The Journal of Ambulatory Care Management*, 34(4), 362. doi:10.1097/JAC.0b013e31822cbd0b

Balfour, P. C., Ruiz, J. M., Talavera, G. A., Allison, M. A., & Rodriguez, C. J. (2016). Cardiovascular disease in Hispanics/Latinos in the United States. *Journal of Latina/o Psychology*, 4(2), 98–113. doi:10.1037/lat0000056

Bastida, E. M., Tseng, T.-S., McKeever, C., & Jack, L., Jr. (2010). Ethics and community-based participatory research: Perspective from the field. *Health Promotion Practice*, 11(1), 16–20. doi:10.1177/1524839909352841

Bebinger, M. (2018, May 17). What explains the rising overdose rate among Latinos? *Kaiser Health News*. Retrieved from https://khn.org/news/what-explains-the-rising-overdose-rate-among-latinos

Bianucci, R., Charlier, P., Perciaccante, A., Lippi, D., & Appenzeller, O. (2017). The "Ulysses syndrome": An eponym identifies a psychosomatic disorder in modern migrants. *European Journal of Internal Medicine*, *41*, 30–32. doi:10.1016/j.ejim.2017.03.020

Blewett, L. A., Casey, M., & Call, K. T. (2004). Improving access to primary care for a growing Latino population: The role of safety net providers in the rural Midwest. *The Journal of Rural Health*, *20*(3), 237–245. doi:10.1111/j.1748-0361.2004.tb00034.x

Borges, G., Breslau, J., Orozco, R., Tancredi, D. J., Anderson, H., Aguilar-Gaxiola, S., & Mora, M.-E. M. (2011). A cross-national study on Mexico-US migration, substance use and substance use disorders. *Drug and Alcohol Dependence*, *117*(1), 16–23. doi:10.1016/j.drugalcdep.2010.12.022

Borrell, L. N., & Crawford, N. D. (2006). Race, ethnicity, and self-rated health status in the behavioral risk factor surveillance system survey. *Hispanic Journal of Behavioral Sciences*, *28*(3), 387–403. doi:10.2105/AJPH.2004.058172

Bowleg, L. (2012). The problem with the phrase women and minorities: Intersectionality—An important theoretical framework for public health. *American Journal of Public Health*, *102*(7), 1267–1273. doi:10.2105/AJPH.2012.300750

Brown, A. (2017). 5 key findings about LGBT Americans. *Pew Research Center*. Retrieved from https://www.pewresearch.org/fact-tank/2017/06/13/5-key-findings-about-lgbt-americans

Browne, A. Varcoe, C., Ford-Gilboe, M., & Wathen, C. N., Smye, V., Jackson, B. E., ... Garneau, A. B. (2018). Disruption as opportunity: Impacts of an organizational health equity intervention in primary care clinics. *International Journal for Equity in Health*, *17*, 154. doi:10.1186/s12939-018-0820-2

Cacari-Stone, L., Wallerstein, N., Garcia, A. P., & Minkler, M. (2014). The promise of community-based participatory research for health equity: A conceptual model for bridging evidence with policy. *American Journal of Public Health*, *104*(9), 1615–1623. doi:10.2105/AJPH.2014.301961

Caetano, R., Ramisetty-Mikler, S., & Rodriguez, L. A. (2009). The Hispanic Americans Baseline Alcohol Survey (HABLAS): The association between birthplace, acculturation and alcohol abuse and dependence across Hispanic national groups. *Drug and Alcohol Dependence*, *99*(1–3), 215–221. doi:10.1016/j.drugalcdep.2008.08.011

Carney, P. A., Hamada, J. L., Rdesinski, R., Sprager, L., Nichols, K. R., Liu, B., ... Shannon, J. (2012). Impact of a community gardening project on vegetable intake, food security and family relationships: A community-based participatory research study. *Journal of Community Health*, *37*(4), 874–881. doi:10.1007/s10900-011-9522-z

Carrillo, J. E., Shekhani, N. S., Deland, E. L., Fleck, E. M., Mucaria, J., Guimento, R., ... Corwin, S. J. (2011). A regional health collaborative formed By New York-Presbyterian aims to improve the health of a largely Hispanic community. *Health Affairs*, *30*(10), 1955–1964. doi:10.1377/hlthaff.2011.0635

Centers for Disease Control and Prevention. (n.d.-a). *Hispanics/Latinos and tobacco use*. Retrieved from https://www.cdc.gov/tobacco/disparities/hispanics-latinos/index.htm

Centers for Disease Control and Prevention. (n.d.-b). *Hispanic health: Preventing type-2 diabetes*. Retrieved from https://www.cdc.gov/features/hispanichealth/index.html

Centers for Disease Control and Prevention. (2015). Hispanic health: ¡A la Buena salud!—To good Health! *CDC Vitalsigns*. Retrieved from https://www.cdc.gov/vitalsigns/pdf/2015-05-vitalsigns.pdf

Centers for Disease Control and Prevention. (2017). *Diagnoses of HIV infection in the United States and dependent areas, 2017* (HIV surveillance report, Volume 29). Retrieved from https://www.cdc.gov/hiv/pdf/library/reports/surveillance/cdc-hiv-surveillance-report-2017-vol-29.pdf

Centers for Disease Control and Prevention. (2019). *Health, United States spotlight: Racial and ethnic disparities in heart disease*. Retrieved from https://www.cdc.gov/nchs/hus/spotlight/HeartDiseaseSpotlight_2019_0404.pdf

Cervantes, L., Chonchol, M., Hasnain-Wynia, R., Steiner, J. F., Havranek, E., Hull, M., ... Fischer, S. (2019). Peer navigator intervention for Latinos on hemodialysis: A single-arm clinical trial. *Journal of Palliative Medicine*, *22*(7), 838–843. doi:10.1089/jpm.2018.0439

Chartier, K., & Caetano, R. (2010). Ethnicity and health disparities in alcohol research. *Alcohol Research & Health*, *33*(1/2), 152. Retrieved from https://www.ncbi.nlm.nih.gov/pmc/articles/PMC3887493

Chavez, L. R. (2013). *The Latino threat: Constructing immigrants, citizens and the nation*. Stanford, CA: Stanford University Press.

Cherpitel, C. J., Li, L., Borges, G., & Zemore, S. (2017). Age at immigration and substance use and problems among males and females at the US–Mexico border. *Journal of Studies on Alcohol and Drugs, 78*(6), 827–834. doi:10.15288/jsad.2017.78.827

Coffman, M. J., de Hernandez, B. U., Smith, H. A., McWilliams, A., Taylor, Y. J., Tapp, H., … Dulin, M. (2017). Using CBPR to decrease health disparities in a suburban Latino neighborhood. *Hispanic Health Care International, 15*(3), 121–129. doi:10.1177/1540415317727569

Comas-Díaz, L. (2000). An ethnopolitical approach to working with people of color. *American Psychologist, 55*(11), 1319–1325. doi:10.1037//0003-066X.55.11.1319

Commission on Social Determinants of Health. (2008). *Closing the gap in a generation: Health equity through action on the social determinants of health. Final Report of the Commission on Social Determinants of Health*. Geneva, Switzerland: World Health Organization. Retrieved from https://www.who.int/social_determinants/final_report/csdh_finalreport_2008.pdf

Corkery, E., Palmer, C., Foley, M. E., Schechter, C. B., Frisher, L., & Roman, S. H. (1997). Effect of a bicultural community health worker on completion of diabetes education in a Hispanic population. *Diabetes Care, 20*(3), 254–257. doi:10.2337/diacare.20.3.254

Cristancho, S., Garces, D. M., Peters, K. E., & Mueller, B. C. (2008). Listening to rural Hispanic immigrants in the Midwest: A community-based participatory assessment of major barriers to health care access and use. *Qualitative Health Research, 18*(5), 633–646. doi:10.1177/1049732308316669

Cuevas, A. G., Dawson, B. A., & Williams, D. R. (2016). Race and skin color in Latino health: An analytic review. *American Journal of Public Health, 106*(12), 2131–2136. doi:10.2105/AJPH.2016.303452

Diaz, C. J., Koning, S. M., & Martinez-Donate, A. P. (2016). Moving beyond Salmon Bias: Mexican return migration and health selection. *Demography, 53*(6), 2005–2030. doi:10.1007/s13524-016-0526-2

Domenech Rodríguez, M. M., Baumann, A. A., & Schwartz, A. L. (2011). Cultural adaptation of an evidence based intervention: From theory to practice in a Latino/a community context. *American Journal of Community Psychology, 47*(1-2), 170–186. doi:10.1007/s10464-010-9371-4

Falicov, C. J. (2014). *Latino families in therapy* (2nd ed.). New York, NY: Guilford Publications.

Fawcett, S. B., Schultz, J., Watson-Thompson, J., Fox, M., & Bremby, R. (2010). Building multisectoral partnerships for population health and health equity. *Preventing Chronic Disease, 7*(6), 1–7. Retrieved from https://www.ncbi.nlm.nih.gov/pmc/articles/PMC2995607

Fisher, T. L., Burnet, D. L., Huang, E. S., Chin, M. H., & Cagney, K. A. (2007). Cultural leverage. *Medical Care Research and Review, 64*(5 Suppl.), 243S–282S. doi:10.1177/1077558707305414

Flores, A. (2017). Facts on U.S. Latinos, 2015. *Pew Research Center (Hispanic Trends Series)*. Retrieved from https://www.pewresearch.org/hispanic/2017/09/18/facts-on-u-s-latinos

Flores, A., Lopez, M. H., & Krogstad, J. M. (2019). U.S. Hispanic population reached new high in 2018, but growth has slowed. *Pew Research Center (Fact Tank Series)*. Retrieved from https://www.pewresearch.org/fact-tank/2019/07/08/u-s-hispanic-population-reached-new-high-in-2018-but-growth-has-slowed

Fontenot, K., Semega, J., & Kollar, M. (2018). *Income and poverty in the United States: 2017* (Current Population Reports, P60-263). Suitland-Silver Hill, MD: U.S. Census Bureau. Retrieved from https://census.gov/library/publications/2018/demo/p60-263.html

Freudenberg, N., & Tsui, E. (2014). Evidence, power, and policy change in community-based participatory research. *American Journal of Public Health, 104*(1), 11–14. doi:10.2105/AJPH.2013.301471

Fryar, C. D., Ostchega, Y., Hales, C. M., Zhang, G., & Kruszon-Moran, D. (2017). *Hypertension prevalence and control among adults: United States, 2015-2016*. Hyattsville, MD: National Center for Health Statistics. Retrieved from https://www.cdc.gov/nchs/products/databriefs/db289.htm

Galea, S., Ahern, M. J., Tardiff, K., Leon, A., Coffin, M. P. O., Derr, M. K., & Vlahov, D. (2003). Racial/ethnic disparities in overdose mortality trends in New York City, 1990–1998. *Journal of Urban Health, 80*(2), 201–211. doi:10.1093/jurban/jtg023

Gallo, L. C., Roesch, S. C., Fortmann, A. L., Carnethon, M. R., Penedo, F. J., Perreira, K., ... Isasi, C. R. (2014). Associations of chronic stress burden, perceived stress, and traumatic stress with cardiovascular disease prevalence and risk factors in the Hispanic Community Health Study/Study of Latinos Sociocultural Ancillary Study. *Psychosomatic Medicine, 76*(6), 468–475. doi:10.1097/PSY.0000000000000069

Galvan, F. H., & Bazargan, M. (2012). *Interactions of transgender Latina women with law enforcement.* UCLA: The Williams Institute. Retrieved from https://escholarship.org/uc/item/62p795s3

Galvez, A. (2013). *Patient citizens, immigrant mothers. Mexican women, public prenatal care, and the birth weight paradox.* New Brunswick, NJ: Rutgers University Press.

Garcia, J. A., Sanchez, G. R., Sanchez-Youngman, S., Vargas, E. D., & Ybarra, V. D. (2015). Race as lived experience: The impact of multi-dimensional measures of race/ethnicity on the self-reported health status of Latinos. *Du Bois Review: Social Science Research on Race, 12*(2), 349–373. doi:10.1017/S1742058X15000120

Garcini, L. M., Peña, J. M., Galvan, T., Fagundes, C. P., Malcarne, V., & Klonoff, E. A. (2017). Mental disorders among undocumented Mexican immigrants in high-risk neighborhoods: Prevalence, comorbidity, and vulnerabilities. *Journal of Consulting and Clinical Psychology, 85*(10), 927–936. doi:10.1037/ccp0000237

Grineski, S. E., Collins, T. W., & Chakraborty, J. (2013). Hispanic heterogeneity and environmental injustice: Intra-ethnic patterns of exposure to cancer risks from traffic-related air pollution in Miami. *Population and Environment, 35*(1), 26–44. doi:10.1007/s11111-012-0184-2

Grzywacz, J. G., Rao, P., Gentry, A., Marin, A., & Arcury, T. A. (2009). Acculturation and conflict in Mexican immigrants' intimate partnerships: The role of women's labor force participation. *Violence Against Women, 15*, 1194–1212. doi:10.1177/1077801209345144

Guerrero, E. G., Marsh, J. C., Khachikian, T., Amaro, H., & Vega, W. A. (2013). Disparities in Latino substance use, service use, and treatment: Implications for culturally and evidence-based interventions under health care reform. *Drug and Alcohol Dependence, 133*(3), 805–813. doi:10.1016/j.drugalcdep.2013.07.027

Hales, C. M., Carroll, M. D., Fryar, C. D., & Ogden, C. L. (2017). *Prevalence of obesity among adults and youth: United States, 2015–2016.* Hyattsville, MD: National Center for Health Statistics. Retrieved from https://stacks.cdc.gov/view/cdc/49223

Hall, E., & Cuellar, N. G. (2016). Immigrant health in the United States: A trajectory toward change. *Journal of Transcultural Nursing, 27*(6), 611–626. doi:10.1177/1043659616672534

Harrison-Quintana, J., Perez, D., & Grant, J. (2010). *Injustice at every turn: A look at Latino/a respondents in the National Transgender Discrimination Survey.* Retrieved from http://transequality.org/sites/default/files/docs/resources/ntds_latino_english_2.pdf

Hatzenbuehler, M. L., Prins, S. J., Flake, M., Philbin, M., Frazer, M. S., Hagen, D., & Hirsch, J. (2017). Immigration policies and mental health morbidity among Latinos: A state-level analysis. *Social Science & Medicine, 174*, 169–178. doi: 10.1016/j.socscimed.2016.11.040

Hayes-Bautista, D. E., & Chapa, J. (1987). Latino terminology: Conceptual bases for standardized terminology. *American Journal of Public Health, 77*(1), 61–68. doi:10.2105/AJPH.77.1.61

Health Resources and Services Administration, Office of Health Equity. (2018). *Health equity report 2017.* Rockville, MD: U.S. Department of Health and Human Services. Retrieved from https://www.hrsa.gov/sites/default/files/hrsa/health-equity/2017-HRSA-health-equity-report.pdf

Henry-Sanchez, B. L., & Geronimus, A. T. (2013). Racial/ethnic disparities in infant mortality among US Latinos: A test of the segmented racialization hypothesis. *Du Bois Review: Social Science Research on Race, 10*(1), 205–231. doi:10.1017/S1742058X13000064

Heron, M. (2019). Deaths: Leading causes for 2017. *National Vital Statistics Reports* (Vol. 68, no. 6). Hyattsville, MD: National Center for Health Statistics. Retrieved from https://www.cdc.gov/nchs/data/nvsr/nvsr68/nvsr68_06-508.pdf

Hilfinger Messias, D. K., McEwen, M. M., & Clark, L. (2015). The impact and implications of undocumented immigration on individual and collective health in the United States. *Nursing Outlook, 63*, 86–94. doi:10.1016/j.outlook.2014.11.004

Howland, R. E., Angley, M., Won, S. H., Wilcox, W., Searing, H., Liu, S. Y., & Johansson, E. W. (2019). Determinants of severe maternal morbidity and its racial/ethnic disparities in New York City, 2008–2012. *Maternal and Child Health Journal, 23*(3), 346–355. doi:10.1007/s10995-018-2682-z

Hurtado, M., Spinner, J. R., Yang, M., Evensen, C., Windham, A., Ortiz, G., … Ivy, E. D. (2014). Peer reviewed: Knowledge and behavioral effects in cardiovascular health: Community health worker health disparities initiative, 2007–2010. *Preventing Chronic Disease*, *11*, E22. doi:10.5888/pcd11.130250

Jordan, M. (2019, January 17). Family separations may have hit thousands more migrant children than reported. *The New York Times*. Retrieved from https://www.nytimes.com/2019/01/17/us/family-separation-trump-administration-migrants.html

Justice in Aging. (2018). *Public charge: A threat to the health & well-being of older adults in immigrant families*. Retrieved from https://www.justiceinaging.org/wp-content/uploads/2018/09/Public-Charge_A-Threat-to-the-Health-Wellbeing-of-Older-Adults-in-Immigrant-Families.pdf

Kaiser Family Foundation. (2019). *Health coverage of immigrants* (Fact Sheet). San Francisco, CA: Author. Retrieved from http://files.kff.org/attachment/Fact-Sheet-Health-Coverage-for-Immigrants

Kerr, W. C., Mulia, N., & Zemore, S. E. (2014). US trends in light, moderate, and heavy drinking episodes from 2000 to 2010. *Alcoholism: Clinical and Experimental Research*, *38*(9), 2496–2501. doi:10.1111/acer.12521

Kim, G., Molina, U. S., & Saadi, A. (2019). Should immigration status be included in a patient's health record? *American Medical Association Journal of Ethics*, *21*, E8–E16. doi:10.1001/amajethics.2019.8

Kochanek, K. D., Murphy, S. L., Xu, J. Q., & Arias, E. (2019). Deaths: Final data for 2017. *National Vital Statistics Reports 68*(9). Hyattsville, MD: National Center for Health Statistics. Retrieved from https://www.cdc.gov/nchs/data/nvsr/nvsr68/nvsr68_09-508.pdf

Krehely, J. (2009). *How to close the LGBT health disparities gap: Disparities by race and ethnicity*. Washington, DC: Center for American Progress. Retrieved from https://cdn.americanprogress.org/wp-content/uploads/issues/2009/12/pdf/lgbt_health_disparities_race.pdf

Krogstad, J. M. (2019). A view of the nation's future through kindergarten demographics. *Pew Research Center (FactTank Series)*. Retrieved from https://www.pewresearch.org/fact-tank/2019/07/31/kindergarten-demographics-in-us

Kumar, S., & Preetha, G. S. (2012). Health promotion: An effective tool for global health. *Indian Journal of Community Medicine*, *37*(1), 5–12. doi:10.4103/0970-0218.94009

Lara, M., Gamboa, C., Kahramanian, M. I., Morales, L. S., & Bautista, D. E. (2005). Acultruation and Latino health in the United States: A review of the literature and its sociopolitical context. *Annual Review of Public Health*, *26*, 367–397. doi:10.1146/annurev.publhealth.26.021304.144615

Latino Decisions. (2019, July 17). *In lead up to 2020, Latinos strongly reject racist attitudes and language*. Retrieved from https://latinodecisions.com/blog/in-2020-latinos-reject-racism/

Latinx Psychological Association. (2018). *NLPA renamed the National Latinx Psychological Association*. Retrieved from https://www.nlpa.ws/assets/docs/NLPA%20Name%20Change%20Press%20Release%20.pdf

Lê Cook, B., & Alegría, M. (2011). Racial-ethnic disparities in substance abuse treatment: The role of criminal history and socioeconomic status. *Psychiatric Services*, *62*(11), 1273–1281. doi:10.1176/ps.62.11.pss6211_1273

Lee, C. S., López, S. R., Colby, S. M., Rohsenow, D., Hernández, L., Borrelli, B., & Caetano, R. (2013). Culturally adapted motivational interviewing for Latino heavy drinkers: Results from a randomized clinical trial. *Journal of Ethnicity in Substance Abuse, 12*(4) 356–373.

Lewis, T. T., Cogburn, C. D., & Williams, D. R. (2015). Self-reported experiences of discrimination and health: Scientific advances, ongoing controversies, and emerging issues. *Annual Review in Clinical Psychology*, *11*, 10.1–10.34. doi:10.1146/annurev-clinpsy-032814-112728

Little, T. V., Wang, M. L., Castro, E. M., Jiménez, J., & Rosal, M. C. (2014). Community health worker interventions for Latinos with type 2 diabetes: A systematic review of randomized controlled trials. *Current Diabetes Reports*, *14*(12), 558. doi:10.1007/s11892-014-0558-1

Lombardi, E. L., Wilchins, R. A., Priesing, D., & Malouf, D. (2002). Gender violence: Transgender experiences with violence and discrimination. *Journal of Homosexuality*, *42*(1), 89–101. doi:10.1300/j082v42n01_05

Lopez, M. H., Gonzalez-Barrera, A., & Krogstad, J. M. (2018). More Latinos have serious concerns about their place in America under Trump. *Pew Research Center (Hispanic Trends)*. Retrieved from https://www.pewresearch.org/hispanic/2018/10/25/more-latinos-have-serious-concerns-about-their-place-in-america-under-trump

Lopez, M. H., Krogstad, J. M., & Flores, A. (2018). Key facts about young Latinos, one of the nation's fastest-growing populations. *Pew Research Center (FactTank)*. Retrieved from https://www.pewresearch.org/fact-tank/2018/09/13/key-facts-about-young-latinos

Lucia, L. (2019). *Towards universal health coverage: Expanding medical to low-income undocumented adults*. UC Berkeley Center for Labor Research and Education. Retrieved from http://laborcenter.berkeley.edu/medi-calundocumentedadults

McCloskey, J. (2009). Promotores as partners in a community-based diabetes intervention program targeting Hispanics. *Family & Community Health, 32*(1), 48–57. doi:10.1097/01.FCH.0000342816.87767.e6

Migrant Clinicians Network. (n.d.). *The migrant/seasonal farmworker*. Retrieved from https://www.migrantclinician.org/issues/migrant-info/migrant.html

Minkler, M. (2010). Linking science and policy through community-based participatory research to study and address health disparities. *American Journal of Public Health, 100*(S1), S81–S87. doi:10.2105/AJPH.2009.165720

Morgenstern, L. B., Smith, M. A., Lisabeth, L. D., Risser, J. M. H., Uchino, K., Garcia, N., ... Moyé, L. A. (2004). Excess stroke in Mexican Americans compared with non-Hispanic Whites: The Brain Attack Surveillance in Corpus Christi Project. *American Journal of Epidemiology, 160*, 376–383. doi:10.1093/aje/kwh225

Mulia, N., Tam, T. W., & Schmidt, L. A. (2014). Disparities in the use and quality of alcohol treatment services and some proposed solutions to narrow the gap. *Psychiatric Services, 65*(5), 626–633. doi:10.1176/appi.ps.201300188

Mulia, N., Ye, Y., Greenfield, T. K., & Zemore, S. E. (2009). Disparities in alcohol-related problems among White, Black, and Hispanic Americans. *Alcoholism: Clinical and Experimental Research, 33*(4), 654–662. doi:10.1111/j.1530-0277.2008.00880.x

Mulia, N., Ye, Y., Zemore, S. E., & Greenfield, T. K. (2008). Social disadvantage, stress, and alcohol use among Black, Hispanic, and White Americans: Findings from the 2005 US National Alcohol Survey. *Journal of Studies on Alcohol and Drugs, 69*(6), 824–833. Retrieved from https://www.ncbi.nlm.nih.gov/pmc/articles/PMC2583375/pdf/jsad824.pdf

National Cancer Institute. (n.d.). *Examples of cancer health disparities*. Retrieved from https://www.cancer.gov/about-nci/organization/crchd/about-health-disparities/examples#racial

National Center for Health Statistics. (2017). *Health, United States, 2015: With special feature on racial and ethnic health disparities*. Hyattsville, MD: Author. Retrieved from https://www.cdc.gov/nchs/data/hus/hus15.pdf

National Center for Health Statistics. (2018). *Health, United States, 2017: With special feature on mortality*. Hyattsville, MD: Author. Retrieved from https://www.cdc.gov/nchs/data/hus/hus17.pdf

National Institute on Alcohol Abuse and Alcoholism. (2019). *Alcohol and the Hispanic community*. Retrieved from https://www.niaaa.nih.gov/sites/default/files/hispanicFact.pdf

Ortiz, V., & Telles, E. (2012). Racial identity and racial treatment of Mexican Americans. *Race and Social Problems, 4*(1), 41–56. doi:10.1007/s12552-012-9064-8

Pagan, J. A., & Howell, E. (2018). Access to maternal and health care services for Latinas. In M. Valerio, D. N., Derige, & N. Hojvat-Gallin (Eds.), *2018 Latina maternal & child health report.* (pp. 11–12). Toronto, ON, Canada: Urban Strategies. Retrieved from https://www.urbanstrategies.us/2018lmchreview

Pan American Health Organization. (2018). *Just societies: Health equity and dignified lives. Executive summary of the Report of the Commission of the Pan American Health Organization on Equity and Health Inequalities in the Americas.* Washington, DC: Author. Retrieved from http://www.instituteofhealthequity.org/resources-reports/commission-of-the-pan-american-health-organisation-on-equity-and-health-inequalities-in-the-americas

Parra Cardona, J. R., Domenech Rodríguez, M., Forgatch, M., Sullivan, C., Bybee, D., Holtrop, K., ... Bernal, G. (2012). Culturally adapting an evidence-based parenting intervention for Latino immigrants: the need to integrate fidelity and cultural relevance. *Family Process, 51*(1), 56–72. doi:10.1111/j.1545-5300.2012.01386.x

Passel, J. S., & Cohn, D. (2019). Mexicans decline to less than half the U.S. unauthorized immigrant population for the first time. *Pew Research Center (FactTank Series)*. Retrieved from https://www.pewresearch.org/fact-tank/2019/06/12/us-unauthorized-immigrant-population-2017

Pérez-Escamilla, R., Hromi-Fiedler, A., Vega-López, S., Bermúdez-Millán, A., & Segura-Pérez, S. (2008). Impact of peer nutrition education on dietary behaviors and health outcomes among Latinos: A systematic literature review. *Journal of Nutrition Education and Behavior*, *40*(4), 208–225. doi:10.1016/j .jneb.2008.03.011

Pew Research Center. (2013). *A survey of LGBT Americans: Attitudes, experiences, and values in changing times*. Retrieved from https://www.pewsocialtrends.org/wp-content/uploads/sites/3/2013/06/SDT _LGBT-Americans_06-2013.pdf

Philbin, M. M., Flake, M., Hatzenbuehler, M. L., & Hirsch, J. S. (2018). State-level immigration and immigrant-focused policies as drivers of Latino health disparities in the United States. *Social Science & Medicine*, *199*, 29–38. doi:10.1016/j.socscimed.2017.04.007

Pierce, S., & Selee, A. (2017). Immigration under Trump: A review of policy shifts in the year since the election. *Migration Policy Institute*. Retrieved from https://www.migrationpolicy.org/research/ immigration-under-trump-review-policy-shifts

Pinedo, M., Zemore, S., Cherpitel, C., & Caetano, R. (2017). Acculturation and alcohol use: The role of environmental contexts. In S. J. Schwartz & J. Unger (Eds.), *The Oxford handbook of acculturation and health*. Oxford, UK: Oxford University Press.

Pinedo, M., Zemore, S., & Rogers, S. (2018). Understanding barriers to specialty substance abuse treatment among Latinos. *Journal of Substance Abuse Treatment*, *94*, 1–8. doi:10.1016/j.jsat.2018.08.004

Rabbitt, M. P., Smith, M. D., & Coleman-Jensen, A. (2016). *Food security among Hispanic adults in the United States, 2011-2014*. Washington, DC: United States Department of Agriculture (Economic Research Service). Retrieved from https://www.ers.usda.gov/publications/pub-details/?pubid=44083

Ramar, C. N., & Desai, G. J. (2010). Hispanic Americans face diabetes challenges and complications. *American Osteopathic Association Health Watch*. Retrieved from https://www.cecity.com/aoa/healthwatch/aug_10/ print5.pdf

Ramírez García, J. I. (2019). Integrating Latina/o ethnic determinants of health in research to promote population health and reduce health disparities. *Cultural Diversity and Ethnic Minority Psychology*, *25*(1), 21–31. doi:10.1037/cdp0000265

Ramisetty-Mikler, S., Caetano, R., & Rodriguez, L. A. (2010). The Hispanic Americans Baseline Alcohol Survey (HABLAS): Alcohol consumption and sociodemographic predictors across Hispanic national groups. *Journal of Substance Use*, *15*(6), 402–416. doi:10.3109/14659891003706357

Ramos, B., Jaccard, J., & Guilamo-Ramos, V. (2003). Dual ethnicity and depressive symptoms: Implications of being Black and Latino in the United States. *Hispanic Journal of Behavioral Sciences*, *25*(2), 147–173. doi:10.1177/0739986303025002002

Rangel, D. E., & Valdez, C. R. (2017). A culturally sensitive approach to large-scale prevention studies: A case study of randomized controlled trial with low-income Latino communities. *Journal of Primary Prevention*, *38*(6), 627–645. doi:10.1007/s10935-017-0487-2

Rathod, S., Gega, L., Degnan, A., Pikard, J., Khan, T., Husain, N., . . . Naeem, F. (2018). The current status of culturally adapted mental health interventions: a practice-focused review of meta-analyses. *Neuropsychiatric Disease and Treatment*, *14*, 165–178. doi:10.2147/NDT.S138430

RCHN Community Health Foundation. (2019). *Improving population health, advancing health equity*. Retrieved from https://www.rchnfoundation.org/wp-content/uploads/2019/03/Improving-Population-Health-Advancing-Health-Equity-RCHN-CHF-2019.pdf

Rhodes, S. D., Foley, K. L., Zometa, C. S., & Bloom, F. R. (2007). Lay health advisor interventions among Hispanics/Latinos: A qualitative systematic review. *American Journal of Preventive Medicine*, *33*(5), 418–427. doi:10.1016/j.amepre.2007.07.023

Riosmena, F., Kuhn, R., & Jochem, W. C. (2017). Explaining the immigrant health advantage: Self-selection and protection in health-related factors among five major national-origin immigrant groups in the United States. *Demography*, *54*(1), 175–200. doi:10.1007/s13524-016-0542-2

Rodríguez, M. A., Bustamante, A. V., & Ang, A. (2009). Perceived quality of care, receipt of preventive care, and usual source of health care among undocumented and other Latinos. *Journal of General Internal Medicine*, *24*, 508. doi:10.1007/s11606-009-1098-2

Romo, V. (2019). 'I'm the shooter,' El Paso suspect allegedly told police. National Public Radio. Retrieved from https://www.npr.org/2019/08/09/749954115/el-paso-alleged-gunman-admitted-i-m-the-shooter-police-say

Santos, C. (2017). The history, struggles, and potential of the term Latinx. Latina/o Psychology Today, 4(2), 7–14. Retrieved from https://www.researchgate.net/publication/322075861_The_history_struggles_and_potential_of_the_term_Latinx

Schmidt, L., Greenfield, T., & Mulia, N. (2006). Unequal treatment: Racial and ethnic disparities in alcoholism treatment services. Alcohol Research and Health, 29(1), 49. Retrieved from https://europepmc.org/articles/pmc6470902

Schmidt, L. A., Ye, Y., Greenfield, T. K., & Bond, J. (2007). Ethnic disparities in clinical severity and services for alcohol problems: Results from the National Alcohol Survey. Alcoholism: Clinical and Experimental Research, 31(1), 48–56. doi:10.1111/j.1530-0277.2006.00263.x

Schneiderman, N., Llabre, M., Cowie, C. C., Barnhart, J., Carnethon, M., Gallo, L. C., … Avilés-Santa, S. (2014). Prevalence of diabetes among Hispanics/Latinos from diverse backgrounds: The Hispanic community health study/study of Latinos (HCHS/SOL). Diabetes Care, 37(8), 2233–2239. doi:10.2337/dc13-2939

Schwartz, S. J., Unger, J. B., Lorenzo-Blanco, E. I., Des Rosiers, S. E., Villamar, J. A., Soto, D. W., … Szapocznik, J. (2014). Perceived context of reception among recent Hispanic immigrants: Conceptualization, instrument development, and preliminary validation. Cultural Diversity and Ethnic Minority Psychology, 20(1), 1–15. doi:10.1037/a0033391

Shommu, N. S., Ahmed, S., Rumana, N., Barron, G. R., McBrien, K. A., & Turin, T. C. (2016). What is the scope of improving immigrant and ethnic minority healthcare using community navigators: A systematic scoping review. International Journal for Equity in Health, 15(1), 6. doi:10.1186/s12939-016-0298-8

Substance Abuse and Mental Health Services Administration. (2018). Key substance use and mental health indicators in the United States: Results from the 2017 National Survey on Drug Use and Health (HHS Publication No. SMA 18-5068, NSDUH Series H-53). Rockville, MD: Center for Behavioral Health Statistics and Quality, Substance Abuse and Mental Health Services Administration. Retrieved from https://www. samhsa.gov/data/

Szkupinski Quiroga, S., Medina, D. M., & Glick, J. (2014). In the belly of the beast: Effects of anti-immigration policy on Latino community members. American Behavioral Scientist, 58(13), 1723–1742. doi:10.1177/0002764214537270

Thomas, S. B., Crouse-Quinn, S., Butler, J., Fryer, C. S., & Garza, M. A. (2011). Toward a fourth generation of disparities research to achieve health equity. Annual Review of Public Health, 32, 399–416. doi:10.1146/annurev-publhealth-031210-101136

Torres, S. A., Santiago, C. D., Walts, K. K., & Richards, M. H. (2018). Immigration policy, practices, and procedures: The impact on the mental health of Mexican and Central American youth and families. American Psychologist, 73(7), 843–854. doi:10.1037/amp0000184843

Trickett, E. J., Beehler, S., Deutsch, C., Green, L. W., Hawe, P., McLeroy, K., … Trimble, J. E. (2011). Advancing the science of community-level interventions. American Journal of Public Health, 101(8), 1410–1419.

U.S. Census Bureau. (2019a). Population estimates show aging across race groups differs. Retrieved from https://www.census.gov/newsroom/press-releases/2019/estimates-characteristics.html

U.S. Census Bureau. (2019b). The Hispanic population in the United States: 2018 [Data file Table 7: Nativity and citizenship status by sex, Hispanic origin, and race: 2018]. Retrieved from https://www.census.gov/data/tables/2018/demo/hispanic-origin/2018-cps.html

U.S. Department of Health and Human Services. (2019). Profile: Hispanic/Latino Americans. Washington, DC: Author. Retrieved from https://minorityhealth.hhs.gov/omh/browse.aspx?lvl=3&lvlid=64

Vaeth, P. A., Caetano, R., Ramisetty-Mikler, S., & Rodriguez, L. A. (2009). Hispanic Americans Baseline Alcohol Survey (HABLAS): Alcohol-related problems across Hispanic national groups. Journal of Studies on Alcohol and Drugs, 70(6), 991–999. doi:10.15288/jsad.2009.70.991

Valdez, C. R., Ramirez-Stege, A., Martinez, E., D'Costa, S., & Chavez, T. (2018). A community-responsive adaptation to reach and engage Latino families affected by maternal depression. Family Process, 57, 539–556. doi:10.1111/famp.1231

Valenzuela, J. M., McDowell, T., Cencula, L., Hoyt, L., & Mitchell, M. J. (2013). ¡ Hazlo Bien! A participatory needs assessment and recommendations for health promotion in growing Latino communities. *American Journal of Health Promotion, 27*(5), 339–346. doi:10.4278/ajhp.101110-QUAL-366

Vargas, E. D., Juárez, M., Sanchez, G. R., & Livaudais, M. (2018). Latinos' connections to immigrants: How knowing a deportee impacts Latino health. *Journal of Ethnic and Migration Studies, 49*, 2971–2988. doi:10.1080/1369183X.2018.1447365

Vargas, E. D., Sanchez, G. R., & Juarez, M. (2017). Fear by association: Perceptions of anti-immigrant policy and health outcomes. *Journal of Health Politics, Policy and Law, 42*(3), 459–483. doi:10.1215/03616878-3802940

Vega, W. A., Rodríguez, M. A., & Gruskin, E. (2009). Health disparities in the Latino population. *Epidemiologic Reviews, 31*, 99–112. doi:10.1093/epirev/mxp008

Velasco-Mondragon, E., Jimenez, A., Palladino-Davis, A. G., Davis, D., & Escamilla-Cejudo, J. A. (2016). Hispanic health in the USA: A scoping review of the literature. *Public Health Reviews, 37*, 31. doi:10.1186/s40985-016-0043-2

Vesely, C. K., Bravo, D. Y., & Guzzardo, M. T. (2019). *Immigrant families across the life course: Policy impacts on physical and mental health*. St. Paul, MN: National Council on Family Relations. Retrieved from https://www.ncfr.org/sites/default/files/2019-07/Immigrant_Families_Policy_Brief_July_23_2019.pdf

Victorson, D., Banas, J., Smith, J., Languido, L., Shen, E., Gutierrez, S., . . . Flores L. (2014). eSalud: Designing and implementing culturally competent eHealth research with Latino patient populations. *American Journal of Public Health, 104*(12), 2259–2265. doi:10.2105/AJPH.2014.302187

Villarreal, M. I. (2007). Women and health disparities: Implications for treating Hispanic women in rural and urban communities. *Alcoholism Treatment Quarterly, 25*(4), 91–110. doi:10.1300/J020v25n04_07

Viruell-Fuentes, E. A., Miranda, P. Y., & Abdulrahim, S. (2012). More than culture: Structural racisms, intersectionality theory, and immigrant health. *Social Science and Medicine, 75*, 2099–2106. doi:10.1016/j.socscimed.2011.12.037

Wallace, S. P., Young, M.-E. D. T., Rodríguez, M. A., & Brindis, C. D. (2018). A social determinants framework identifying state-level immigrant policies and their influence on health. *SSM-Population Health, 7*, 100316. doi:10.1016/j.ssmph.2018.10.016

Warrier, S., & Rose, J. (2016). Women, gender-based violence, and immigration. In F. Chang-Muy & E. P. Congress (Eds.), *Social work with immigrants and refugees: Legal issues, clinical skills, and advocacy* (2nd ed., pp. 237–256). New York, NY: Springer Publishing Company.

Weinstein, J. N., Geller, A., Negussie, Y., & Baciu, A. (Eds.). (2017). *Communities in action: Pathways to health equity*. Washington, DC: National Academies Press. Retrieved from https://www.ncbi.nlm.nih.gov/books/NBK425848

Wells, K., Klap, R., Koike, A., & Sherbourne, C. (2001). Ethnic disparities in unmet need for alcoholism, drug abuse, and mental health care. *American Journal of Psychiatry, 158*(12), 2027–2032. doi:10.1176/appi.ajp.158.12.2027

Williams, D. R. (2012). Miles to go before we sleep: Racial inequities in health. *Journal of Health and Social Behavior, 53*(3), 279–295. doi:10.1177/0022146512455804

Witbrodt, J., Mulia, N., Zemore, S. E., & Kerr, W. C. (2014). Racial/ethnic disparities in alcohol-related problems: Differences by gender and level of heavy drinking. *Alcoholism: Clinical and Experimental Research, 38*(6), 1662–1670. doi:10.1111/acer.12398

Woodruff, S. I., Talavera, G. A., & Elder, J. P. (2002). Evaluation of a culturally appropriate smoking cessation intervention for Latinos. *Tobacco Control, 11*(4), 361–367.

Zemore, S. E., Ye, Y., Mulia, N., Martinez, P., Jones-Webb, R., & Karriker-Jaffe, K. (2016). Poor, persecuted, young, and alone: Toward explaining the elevated risk of alcohol problems among Black and Latino men who drink. *Drug and Alcohol Dependence, 163*, 31–39. doi:10.1016/j.drugalcdep.2016.03.008

Zong, J., & Batalova, J. (2019). Immigrants from new origin countries in the United States. *Migration Policy Institute*. Retrieved from https://www.migrationpolicy.org/article/immigrants-new-origin-countries-united-states

ASIAN AMERICAN HEALTH EQUITY

SAHNAH LIM ▪ SHILPA PATEL ▪ SIMONA C. KWON ▪ EDWARD TEPPORN

LEARNING OBJECTIVES

- Describe the ways in which immigration policies have shaped the demographic profile of Asian Americans
- Discuss ways in which social determinants of health (e.g., English proficiency) relate to Asian health disparities
- Summarize the disparities in morbidity and mortality faced by Asian populations in the United States
- Articulate how community-based participatory research is a particularly effective approach in working with Asian populations
- Name and describe organizations working to achieve health equity for Asian groups

INTRODUCTION

In 1882, Congress passed the Chinese Exclusion Act, which was one of the first laws to restrict immigration for a particular ethnic group. Asian immigration to the U.S. continued to be severely restricted until the 1960s, primarily characterized by temporary immigration of laborers who often returned to their native countries after a short period of time (Tseng, 2009). This anti-immigrant legislation continued until the passage of the Immigration and Naturalization Act of 1965, which permitted a new wave of immigrants based on occupational skills, family reunification, and refugee status. Although originally envisioned as creating greater diversity of European immigrants, this Act unintentionally opened the doors for large waves of Asian and other non-Western European immigration into the U.S. Accordingly, between 1960 and 1980, Asian immigration steadily increased from 9% to 44% (U.S. Immigration and Naturalization Service, 1960–1978, 1979–1992) and included mostly Japanese, Chinese, and Filipinos (Barringer, Gardner, & Levin, 1993).

Asian Americans (AAs) are now the fastest growing minority group in the U.S. By 2060, it is projected that the AA population will increase to about 30 million people and represent approximately 9.3% of the U.S. population (Colby & Ortman, 2015). Chinese Americans comprise the largest subgroup, followed by Asian Indian, Filipino, Vietnamese, and Korean Americans

(Hoeffel, Rastogi, Kim, & Shahid, 2012). AAs are an incredibly diverse group in terms of country of origin, religion, socioeconomic status, and language. Yet, the model minority myth depicts AAs as homogenous and socioeconomically successful (Crystal, 1989). The model minority myth was an idea advanced by sociologist William Peterson in 1966 and has been used as a justification to continue to exclude AAs from resources, research, and political participation.

Supporting this erroneous view of AAs as uniformly well-off and successful is the lack of disaggregated data by AA subgroups (Trinh-Shevrin, Kwon, Park, Nadkarni, & Islam, 2015). There have been minimal efforts to oversample or collect subgroup ethnicity data, although recent advocacy efforts have made strides toward more granular data collection efforts (Islam, Trinh-Shevrin, & Rey, 2009). Even when aggregated, analysis of national data sets with AAs is challenging due to statistical unreliability since they are geographically concentrated in certain cities, resulting in small cell sizes in other geographic areas (Ghosh, 2009).

The data that are available demonstrate substantial variations in socioeconomic status by ethnic subgroup. While the median household income among AAs is higher than the national average ($73,060 among AAs vs. $53,600 among all U.S. households; López, Ruiz, & Patten, 2017), more AAs remain in poverty (Mayor's Office of Operations, 2016). Data on income show a istinct bimodal distribution in which AAs occupy very low and high ends of the spectrum. The Immigration and Naturalization Act of 1965, in part, contributed to this bimodal distribution, with occupation-based immigration often occurring among the more socioeconomically privileged and with refugee-based immigration occurring among the less privileged. Median annual household income is highest among Asian Indians ($100,000), while Nepalese and Burmese households report less than half of that income ($43,500 and $36,000, respectively; López et al., 2017). Even in the aggregate, social disadvantages persist, with approximately one in four AAs not graduating from high school (U.S. Census Bureau, 2015) and with more than 30% of AAs having limited English proficiency (LEP; U.S. Census Bureau, 2015).

HEALTH DISPARITIES AMONG ASIAN AMERICANS

The model minority myth also extends to the health domain; AAs are portrayed as a healthy minority group that does not deserve or require additional research or resources. However, there is substantial evidence that AAs are disproportionately impacted by chronic diseases (Deurenberg, Deurenberg-Yap, & Guricci, 2002; Gupta, Wu, Young, & Perlman, 2011; Yi, Kwon, Wyatt, Islam, & Trinh-Shevrin, 2015) as well as other communicable diseases such as chronic hepatitis B and tuberculosis (Centers for Disease Control and Prevention [CDC], n.d.-a; El-Serag, 2012; Pollack et al., 2014). Although cancer risk among AAs is lower compared to their White counterparts, cancer (not heart disease) is the leading cause of death among AAs (Torre et al., 2016), and some AAs have a higher risk for certain infection-related cancers. For example, risk of stomach and liver cancer among AAs is twice as high when compared to non-Hispanic Whites (Torre et al., 2016). When stratified by ethnic subgroup, Cambodians and Vietnamese have significantly higher human papillomavirus–related cervical cancer incidence (13% and 10%, respectively) compared to their non-Hispanic White counterparts (7%; Torre et al., 2016). Gender and other sociodemographic disparities (e.g., nativity) in cancer risk factors must also be taken into account. Alcohol consumption is a known risk factor for several cancers (International Agency for Research and Cancer, 2012); while fewer AAs (49%) consume alcohol than non-Hispanic Whites (72%), the prevalence is substantially higher in AA men (60%) compared to AA women (39%; Torre et al., 2016).

In addition to cancer disparities, AAs have higher rates of both depression and anxiety compared to non-Hispanic Whites and face greater difficulty in accessing mental health services (Brown, Meadows, & Elder, 2007; Okazaki, 1997). Similar to other diseases, these disparities are heightened among specific AA subgroups. For example, national suicide rates among Korean Americans nearly doubled between the years of 2003 and 2012 and are the highest compared to all other subgroups (Kung et al., 2016). Diabetes is another noteworthy example as diabetes rates are elevated among AAs as a whole, and in particular among South Asians and Filipinos with nearly one in three at risk (King et al., 2012). National data indicate lower diabetes screening among AAs (Tung, Baig, Huang, Laiteerapong, & Chua, 2017) and poorer management of diabetes among certain subgroups such as South Asians (Community Prevention Services Task Force, 2016).

MULTILEVEL FACTORS INFLUENCING HEALTH DISPARITIES AMONG ASIAN AMERICANS

Using an ecological perspective, Ma and Daus (2009) developed a comprehensive framework to guide health intervention and programming among AAs. This multilevel framework is useful for understanding health disparities among AAs and includes the following levels: individual, family, community, organization, government, and society. In this current chapter, we focus on the individual, organization, and government levels.

At the individual level, factors such as degree of acculturation, nativity (i.e., foreign vs. native born), income, educational attainment, health literacy, English proficiency, and immigration status influence health outcomes. There has been a growing recognition that public health research on immigration has not adequately integrated the concept of immigration into the social determinants of health (SDOH) framework (National Academies of Sciences, Engineering, and Medicine [NASEM], 2018). SDOH are upstream factors that determine health risk and outcomes; applying an SDOH framework is a key strategy to advance health equity, especially among AAs (Trinh-Shevrin, Kwon, et al., 2015). Proceedings from a recent workshop in 2018 hosted by the NASEM called for increased recognition of immigration as a consequence of SDOH, an SDOH in its own right (NASEM, 2018). Despite the misconception that most immigrants in the U.S. are Latinos, AAs are the only major racial/ethnic group in the U.S. for whom immigrants comprise a majority of the population (NASEM, 2018). Further, of the 11 million undocumented immigrants in the United States, about one in seven (1.8 million) are Asian immigrants (Migration Policy Institute, n.d.). Immigration, whether documented or undocumented, is an important individual-level SDOH that has major consequences for health and access to care (NASEM, 2018).

Another individual-level factor is health insurance coverage, which is related to both employment status and immigration status. National trends indicate that uninsurance rates for all groups have declined in recent years, with AAs having the second lowest rates compared to other racial/ethnic categories (Barnett & Marina, 2016). When looking across different national data sets and by AA subgroup, however, Korean Americans rank the worst in coverage; this is likely due to high rates of self-employment (Ponce, 2009). Currently available data may mask the disparities among AA subgroups since few studies have been conducted in cities with larger numbers of recently arrived and underserved immigrant populations (Ponce, 2009).

At the organization level, Ma and Daus (2009) challenge the assumption driving common behavior theories that are based on individual autonomy, particularly in light of the often collectivistic nature of Asian cultures. Instead, a more culturally appropriate health service or program might consider the importance of family identity among AAs as well as the different decision-making structures (e.g., matriarchal vs. patriarchal patterns of decision-making) embedded within those families. Healthcare services or programs that are not culturally tailored to incorporate cultural values and decision-making structures are perceived as less relevant and ultimately may affect healthcare use and outcomes.

Language access is another critical issue in quality of care among AAs. As mentioned previously, a significant amount of AAs are LEP, which, in turn, can seriously impact the quality of communication with a medical provider, a decision to seek care in the first place, and ultimately health outcomes such as mortality (Ro, Park, & Jang, 2009). On December 22, 2000, the Office of Minority Health of the U.S. Department of Health and Human Services [DHHS] released its National Standards on Culturally and Linguistically Appropriate Services in Health Care (65 Fed. Reg. 80865-79, 2000). These standards included various mandates related to language access for LEP patients, including the requirement that language assistance should be provided at no cost (Ro et al., 2009). As mentioned previously, however, the perception that immigrant populations are predominantly Hispanic may lead providers to not be adequately prepared to meet the linguistic needs of Asian populations.

These and other federal and state policies, however, are not regulatory, and implementation can widely vary across institutions. Issues of enforcement and additional mechanisms to ensure successful implementation (e.g., increased supply of bilingual providers and trained interpreters) must be addressed in order to address language access disparities among AAs (Ro et al., 2009). Limited language access in research and data collection is another important issue. Most national health surveys do not collect data with LEP AAs (i.e., surveys are often administered only in English and non-Asian languages), which likely biases the results by excluding the more underserved segment within the AA population.

At the government level, federal policies and funding directly influence access to public benefits such as Medicaid, food stamps, and welfare. Driven by anti-immigrant sentiments and colored by notions of the model minority myth, government (and nongovernment) funding and support for health research targeting AAs have been sparse (Ghosh, 2009). Most notably, federal guidelines that determine funding, such as the DHHS Healthy People 2020, are based on aggregated data and exclude diseases highly prevalent among AAs, such as liver cancer (Ghosh, 2009). While funding for research comes from both public and private sources, federal government funding is the largest and most influential. Other sources of funding for health research and programs come from foundations, yet only 0.3% of foundation funding was targeted to AA, Native Hawaiian (NH), and Pacific Islander (PI) communities combined (Asian Americans/Pacific Islanders in Philanthropy, 2015). A partial consequence of insufficient funding for AA health research has been a lack of data specific to AAs. For example, Ghosh (2003) found through a review of peer-reviewed health research that only 0.01% of articles between 1966 and 2000 involved AA and PI populations (Ghosh, 2003). Lack of data, in turn, influences policy makers' allocation of resources to social and health programs that ultimately affect the well-being of AA populations.

One critical factor influencing AA health disparities and one that straddles all different levels of influence (e.g., individual, government, society) is racial discrimination. Calling attention to discrimination is important because doing so provides a longitudinal, historical perspective to the health disparities currently experienced by AAs. The model minority myth has racist origins and intentions and is a form of ongoing racial discrimination. While the model minority myth portrays AAs as examples of success, it also positions AAs as perpetual foreigners; that is, no matter how long an individual, family, or community has resided in the U.S., they will always be seen as the "other" by the majority society of the U.S. (Devos & Banaji, 2005).

A notable example is the Immigration Act of 1882 and the Chinese Exclusion Act of 1882, which prohibited the entry of Chinese laborers and denied permanent legal status to Chinese already in the U.S. (Tseng, 2009). The Japanese American internment in labor camps during World War II is another example and one that has led to elevated levels of anxiety, trauma, and other health issues across generations of Japanese Americans (Janson & Hazel, 2004; Nagata & Takeshita, 2002). More recently after the September 11, 2001, attacks, many South Asian and other Muslim populations reported increased discrimination that adversely affected their employment, housing, and educational opportunities (New York City Commission on Human Rights, 2003) and increased hate violence (South Asian Americans Leading Together, 2014). Discrimination and prejudice, in turn, have been linked to numerous and adverse health outcomes, such as increased stress, increased substance use, and decreased satisfaction with care (Gee & Ro, 2009; Yi, Kwon, Sacks, & Trinh-Shevrin, 2016; Yi et al., 2015). Similar to recognizing immigration as a social determinant of health, Gee and Ro (2009) underscore the importance of racial discrimination as an SDOH and call for more refined measures, theories, and methodologies to further advance the paucity of research on the mechanisms by which racism impacts the health of AAs.

A COMMUNITY-BASED PARTICIPATORY RESEARCH APPROACH TO ADVANCE HEALTH EQUITY IN ASIAN AMERICANS

As discussed in Chapter 4, Health Equity Research and Collaboration Approaches, community-based participatory research (CBPR) is a collaborative approach that necessitates equitable community partner involvement throughout all stages of the research process. There are eight key principles of CBPR as first set forth by Israel, Schulz, Parker, and Becker (1998):

1. Recognizes community as a unit of identity

2. Builds on strengths and resources within the community

3. Facilitates collaborative partnerships in all phases of the research

4. Integrates knowledge and action for mutual benefit of all partners

5. Promotes a co-learning and empowering process that attends to social inequalities

6. Involves a cyclical and iterative process

7. Addresses health from both positive and ecological perspectives

8. Disseminates findings and knowledge gained to all partners

There is a significant amount of evidence demonstrating CBPR's ability to reduce health inequities in underserved and minority communities, which has been similarly mirrored by funding agencies' enthusiasm and more explicit requirement for funding recipients to apply CBPR approaches in their work and the call by many Asian health researchers for its incorporation specifically into approaches to reduce Asian health disparities (Tandon & Kwon, 2009). CBPR principles are not only salient in the case of health equities but are also congruent with social determinants of health frameworks (Trinh-Shevrin, Kwon, et al., 2015). Specifically, because CBPR focuses on garnering context from community partners to inform research studies, it necessarily guides researchers to incorporate and address SDOH of communities in their planning, development, implementation, and dissemination. Equally important, CBPR is particularly well suited for populations that are heterogeneous like AA communities since they require a tailoring of approaches via local expertise that can be elicited only through participation from trusted community partners (Tandon & Kwon, 2009). As such, CBPR approaches can be applied not only to inform research studies but can also be incorporated into program implementation and policy/advocacy efforts.

ORGANIZATIONS AND PROGRAMS WORKING TOWARD HEALTH EQUITY AMONG ASIAN AMERICANS

There are a number of programs across the U.S. that incorporate principles of CBPR to advance health equity among AA communities. New York University (NYU) Center for the Study of Asian American Health (NYU CSAAH) uses CBPR principles to guide multiple initiatives and activities, including the identification of health priority conditions and issues, and to inform the implementation of programs and projects. Established in 2003 through a National Institutes of Health (NIH) National Center for Minority Health Disparities Project EXPORT (Excellence in Partnership, Outreach, Research and Training) Center grant, the NYU CSAAH is the only center of its kind focused on AA health and health disparities. Guided by a population health equity framework and CBPR (Trinh-Shevrin, Islam, Nadkarni, Park, & Kwon, 2015; Trinh-Shevrin, Kwon, et al., 2015), the mission of CSAAH is to identify health priorities and reduce health disparities in the AA community through research, training, and partnership. CSAAH has identified and established seven key strategies for advancing a transdisciplinary population health equity agenda:

- Using a SDOH approach by performing ongoing descriptive and longitudinal research for monitoring quantitative changes in social factors and population health outcomes

- Performing disaggregated data collection in order to fill information gaps and promote equitable collection, reporting, and analysis of data for informing areas of health equity research and identifying the needs of underserved populations

- Advancing sustainable development of internal structures by strengthening infrastructures of organizations and communities

- Building human and social capital by integrating community leaders and community health workers (CHWs) in design and implementation of healthcare programs

- Conducting research that is directed by multisectoral coalitions for recognizing the role of SDOH equity and incorporating health considerations into decision-making across sectors and policy areas

▨   Engaging community-based ethnic coalitions, pan-ethnic advisory groups, and diverse stakeholders

▨   Fostering connections and access to care by working with healthcare systems and disseminating information through social service agencies and community-based organizations (NYU CSAAH, n.d.)

NYU CSAAH is one of the few academic medical centers in the United States to hold both the NIH and the CDC designations as Centers of Excellence, as well as the CDC designation as a Prevention Research Center. Informed by its community partnership and population health equity approach, CSAAH has identified the following priority research areas for achieving health equity in Asian populations: (a) cardiovascular disease (CVD) and diabetes disparities, (b) infection-related cancers and cancer prevention disparities, (c) mental health disparities, (d) ealthy aging, and (e) sexual and reproductive health. Other organizations and programs that incorporate principles of CBPR to advance health equity for AA communities are highlighted as follows:

1. **Asian American Network for Cancer Awareness, Research and Training**
    Housed at the University of California (UC) Davis Comprehensive Cancer Center and established in 2000, the mission of Asian American Network for Cancer Awareness, Research and Training (AANCART) is to reduce cancer health disparities by conducting community-based participatory education, training, and research by, for, and with AAs. AANCART is the only National Cancer Institute–designated Nation Center Reducing Asian-American Cancer Health Disparities. AANCART focuses especially on the cancer risk profile of individuals with Chinese, Filipino, Hmong, Korean, and Vietnamese ancestry (UC Davis Health). Examples of AANCART research studies and programs include a culturally competent peer education program targeted to among women in California to educate and improve cervical cancer screening, and the Sacramento Collaborative to Advance Testing and Care for Hepatitis B (SCrATCH B) program that seeks to increase hepatitis B virus testing among AAs at risk for chronic hepatitis B in the area (UC Davis Health).

2. **Asian & Pacific Islander American Health Forum**
    Established in 1986, Asian & Pacific Islander American Health Forum (APIAHF) is the oldest and largest health advocacy organization focused on AA, NH, and PI communities in the U.S. and its affiliated territories. The mission of APIAHF is to influence policy, mobilize communities, and strengthen programs and organizations to improve the health of their target communities (APIAHF, n.d.). The organization supports local AA, NH, and PI communities and organizations that serve these communities by providing services such as grants, training, technical assistance, and consulting, especially in the areas of healthcare access, healthcare quality, and health equity. One of the major initiatives from APIAHF was the Health Through Action (HTA) program, which was a $16.5 million, 5-year partnership between APIAHF and the W.K. Kellogg Foundation. At the time, it was the largest private foundation investment ever in the AA and NHPI community. HTA sought to improve health and reduce healthcare disparities for AA, NH, and PI communities across the country. As part of this program, APIAHF partnered with 17 AA and NHPI coalitions and organizations in 14 states through

subgrants, technical assistance, and convenings. A few of these organizations are high-lighted as follows:

a. *Center for Pan Asian Community Services*—For the HTA program, the Atlanta-based Center for Pan Asian Community Services served as the lead agency in a coalition to improve the overall health of AA and NHPIs in Georgia.

b. *Asian American Coalition for Children and Families*—This organization in New York City led the Project CHARGE (Coalition for Health Access to Reach Greater Equity) coalition to increase access to health insurance for AAs. Activities that Project CHARGE focused on during this program included culturally competent and language-accessible enrollment initiatives and expansion of enabling services.

c. *Asian Services in Action*—The goal of this Ohio-based coalition for HTA was to create a statewide coalition to advocate for resources and actions related to hepatitis B for AAs, including funding and systems and policy change.

d. *National Tongan American Society*—The goal of National Tongan American Society (NTAS) for this program was to develop and implement a program to reduce obesity and the prevalence of diabetes among PIs.

3. **Association of Asian Pacific Community Health Organizations**
   The Association of Asian Pacific Community Health Organizations (AAPCHO) is an association created in 1987 by a collective of community health centers for medically underserved AAs and NHPIs and their providers. The mission of AAPCHO is to promote advocacy, collaboration, and leadership within the AA and NHPI community in the United States to improve their health, especially in terms of increasing health access (AAPCHO, n.d.). The organization focuses on five specific areas to serve their mission: (a) health disparities, (b) technical assistance and training, (c) research capacity training, (d) patient-centered health outcomes, and (e) health information technology.

4. **Center for Asian Health**
   Established in 2000 and part of Temple University Katz School of Medicine, the mission of the Center for Asian Health (CAH) is to reduce health disparities and improve health equity among underserved AAs through activities such as research, community outreach and engagement, as well as patient navigation and support for clinical providers and organizations to enhance culturally and linguistically appropriate healthcare (CAH, n.d.-a). Working with a network of community, institutional, and clinical partners, the CAH focuses on four areas in their research program—cancer, tobacco, CVD, and global health (CAH, n.d.-b).

BEST-PRACTICE RECOMMENDATIONS IN DESIGNING NEW PROGRAMS

Using CBPR as a framework, there are a number of best-practice recommendations for designing new programs to reduce health disparities among AA communities in the United States (Trinh-Shevrin, Kwon, et al., 2015):

(continued)

1. *Leverage trusted partnerships and community assets*—A history of collaboration with community-based organizations increases the likelihood that communities will engage in health prevention and promotion activities. Further, leveraging community assets builds on existing community resources and increases capacity for health promotion and prevention activities.

2. *Focus on SDOH*—In order to achieve health equity, programs should focus on SDOH that reflect factors or conditions where communities live, work, and play, such as socioeconomic status, housing, racism, and cultural beliefs (Marmot, Friel, Bell, Houweling, & Taylor, 2008). In order to positively affect health, programs should address not only the immediate health concern but also the contextual and upstream factors that may affect health outcomes.

3. *Utilize a multisectoral coalition to develop and implement programs*—In addition to health partners and community-based organizations, programs should incorporate the perspectives of sectors such as non–health government agencies (e.g., education, criminal justice), business and commerce, faith-based organizations, and policy makers.

4. *Create flexible programs that can be adapted at multiple levels*—Evidence-based programs and policies are often not demonstrated and/or validated in AA communities. To increase relevance and success of programs, communities must be allowed to adapt them to address not only the cultural considerations but also the geographic and site-specific context of the community.

5. *Sustainability should be addressed from the outset*—Programs should utilize the principles of CBPR to create programs that can increase the capacity of communities and organizations that serve them so they can be sustained after funding ends.

INTERSECTIONALITY SPOTLIGHT

Unfortunately, research on intersectionality among AA populations is very limited and has focused largely on differences by gender. Data on the health status of AA women are still scarce, including those that are disaggregated by AA subgroup. Nonetheless, sexual and reproductive health and violence against women are issues through which to examine the multiple disadvantages that AA women may face compared to their male counterparts.

Park-Tanjasiri and Nguyen (2009) define sexual and reproductive rights for AA women as "the ability to access a broad range of services, including … birth control, emergency contraception, abortion, family planning, counseling, nutrition, prenatal care, sexual freedom, culturally appropriate services, bilingual and interpreter services, health insurance, and preventive care" (pp. 151–152). However, barriers related to being AA such as discrimination, linguistic and cultural limitations, and geographic isolation impede AA women from the realization of their sexual and reproductive rights. For example, Laotian American women are at elevated risk of delivering low-birth infants and maternal mortality, in part due to low rates of uptake in prenatal

(*continued*)

care (National Asian Women's Health Organization, 1997). In addition, cultural taboos against issues regarding sex (e.g., sexually transmitted infections, abortion) in many AA communities impede women from seeking treatment for important sexual and reproductive health issues. For example, studies have shown that AA women are least likely among all racial/ethnic groups to discuss sexually transmitted infections with their doctors (Park Tanjasiri & Nguyen, 2009).

AA women's health is also significantly impacted by gender-based violence. The Asian Pacific Institute on Gender-Based Violence compiled results from various community-based studies and reported that approximately 25% to 55% of AA women experience some type of violence during their lifetime (Yoshihama & Dabby, 2015). There is a lack of national studies on the prevalence of gender-based violence among AAs, particularly by Asian ethnic subgroups, which complicates the ability to gain a full picture of the issue. The Bureau of Justice Statistics conducts its National Crime Victimization Survey but does not publish data on victimization rates for AAs, including disaggregated data by gender. While one national study conducted in 2010 reported that AA women were the least likely to experience gender-based violence (20%) compared to other race/ethnic groups (Black et al., 2010), advocates and scholars have argued that smaller victimization rates likely reflect underreporting due to cultural values that emphasize family honor and harmony that discourage Asian women from reporting (Tjaden & Thoennes, 2000). Further, national data are collected from English-speaking women who have documented immigration status and likely exclude those that are LEP and have undocumented immigration status; this is particularly impactful, given the fact that (as presented earlier) the majority of AAs are immigrants. In addition to lack of reporting, it has been suggested that oppressive cultural values (e.g., value of endurance, conflict avoidance) and patriarchal systems influence both the occurrence and help-seeking behaviors of AA women (Wong et al., 2003).

There is a need for additional research, programming, and policies for AAs as a broad community but also for particular demographic groups (e.g., immigrant, women, LGBTQ, smaller ethnic groups, multiracial individuals). Equally important, research, programming, and policies are needed for those who live in the intersection of these identities. This section specifically draws attention to the multiplicative effects—of being a woman, an undocumented immigrant, and being AA—on the sexual and reproductive health of AA women. Disaggregated data among AA subgroups are also needed in order to explore culturally specific differences across subgroups on this topic; thoughtful dissemination must be accompanied with such sensitive data so that certain communities are not inadvertently shamed.

CASE STUDY   RACIAL AND ETHNIC APPROACHES TO COMMUNITY HEALTH FOR ASIAN AMERICANS PROGRAM

Rates of hypertension (HTN) and CVD are disproportionately high among certain racial and ethnic communities, especially among AAs (Klatsky, Tekawa, & Armstrong, 1996; Mohanty, Woolhandler, Himmelstein, & Bor, 2005). Research has shown that population- and evidence-based CVD prevention and HTN management strategies and programs that promote healthy lifestyle changes

(continued)

and enhance linkage to healthcare can reduce the risk of these chronic diseases (Appel et al., 2006; Boeing et al., 2012; Brownson, Haire-Joshu, & Luke, 2006; Burke, Dunbar-Jacob, & Hill, 1997; Kamphuis et al., 2006). However, these programs are often limited in their effectiveness for racial and ethnic communities such as AAs (George, Duran, & Norris, 2014; Merzel & D'Afflitti, 2003) due to a lack of cultural adaptation and relevance for these communities (Chen, Reid, Parker, & Pillemer, 2013; Lew & Chen, 2013). Thus, in order to achieve a positive impact in the AA community, these population- and evidence-based strategies and programs must be translated to community settings in a culturally sensitive and sustainable manner (Brownson et al., 2006; George et al., 2014; Han, Kim, & Kim, 2007; Merzel & D'Afflitti, 2003; Nierkens et al., 2013).

In 2014, with support from a 3-year grant of $1,000,000 by CDC (n.d.-b), the Center for the Study of Asian American Health at NYU Langone Health launched the Racial and Ethnic Approaches to Community Health for Asian Americans (REACH FAR) program to prevent CVD disease in AAs in the New York/New Jersey (NY/NJ) metropolitan area (Kum et al., 2018). Guided by a socioecological framework, social marketing principles, and principles of CBPR, the REACH FAR program increases access to healthy foods and culturally tailored health-coaching programs to improve high blood pressure (HBP) management in targeted AA communities—Bangladeshi, Filipino, Korean, and Asian Indian. The REACH FAR program worked with a multisectoral coalition comprised of a lead academic agency, four organizations and coalitions serving the target communities (Kalusugan Coalition, Korean Community Services of Metropolitan New York, NYU Center for the Study of Asian American Health, and UNITED SIKHS), community-based organizations, faith-based organizations (FBOs), local businesses, healthcare professionals, healthcare institutions, and local and state governmental agencies to implement multilevel, evidence-based strategies to fight HBP and CVD in a variety of community-based venues. These strategies include (a) increasing access to healthy foods and drinks in FBOs, (b) increasing access to healthy foods and drinks in restaurants and grocery stores, (c) increasing access to blood pressure screenings and coaching efforts in faith-based and community settings by offering the New York City Department of Health and Mental Hygiene's (NYC DOHMH) Keep on Track (KOT) blood pressure monitoring program, and (d) increasing access to translated, culturally tailored health information from the Million Hearts initiative (millionhearts.hhs.gov) disseminated through pharmacists and healthcare providers (Center for Asian Health, n.d.-b).

A significant priority for the REACH FAR program is to ensure HTN and CVD strategies, educational materials, and resources are culturally congruent and accessible to the diverse AA communities in the NY/NJ metropolitan area. Strategy development, implementation, and sustainability are adapted at various levels to ensure relevance to AA communities. For example, to increase access to healthy foods and drinks in FBOs, the REACH FAR program worked with mosques, churches, and gurudwaras (Sikh houses of worship) to implement nutrition policies to increase access to healthy food and drink during their communal meals. This list was based on the New York City Food Standards created by the NYC DOHMH (2011), but culturally adapted to increase relevance across all denominations and target communities. For instance, FBOs could implement a nutrition policy that ensured a whole-grain option was available to the

(continued)

congregation during the communal meal. This whole-grain option could include not only brown rice but also whole-grain naan, which is found in many South Asian FBOs. To complement strategy implementation, the REACH FAR coalition partnered with APartnership (http://apartnership.com/), an award winning AA media company to create a health campaign with HTN and healthy living messages that were culturally and linguistically appropriate to the target communities. Materials for the health campaign included posters, adapted plate planners, restaurant tent cards, and decals to support healthy eating as well as pharmacy postcards, magnets, and adapted NYC DOHMH and Million Hearts materials to support HTN prevention and management. In addition to being distributed at participating REACH FAR sites, messages and materials were also disseminated through multiple media outlets, including social, ethnic, and mainstream media (CDC's Division of Nutrition, Physical Activity, and Obesity, 2018). See Figure 7.1 for an example of an adapted plate planner in Bengali language.

The REACH FAR program found that significant modifications and adaptations needed to be made across all evidence-based strategies to ensure they were relevant to the diverse communities. Additionally, incorporating a CBPR approach in the REACH FAR program increased the effectiveness of strategy implementation and sustainability as it ensured meaningful participation from all coalition partners and that cultural adaptations were appropriate for the target communities (Kwon et al., 2017).

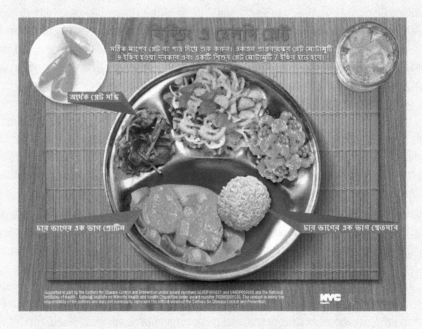

FIGURE 7.1 Adapted plate planner in Bengali.

SOURCE: Racial and Ethnic Approaches to Community Health for Asian Americans. (2016). *Nutrition plate planner–Bangla*. Retrieved from https://med.nyu.edu/asian-health/sites/default/files/asian-health2/plate-planner-preview-bangladeshi.pdf

CURRENT EVENT

THE HEALTH CARE RIGHTS LAW

At the time of publication of this text, there is ongoing activity within the federal government to amend the Health Care Rights Law to remove a large portion of the protections it provided to individuals with LEP. Under current law and regulations, antidiscrimination statutes based on national origin have been extended to cover LEP, given the clear and close correlation between the two. The federal government is now arguing that extending protections to ensure language access to all individuals receiving HHS funds is overly onerous and that the guidelines should be changed to allow more flexibility. As mentioned previously, more than 30% of AAs have LEP (U.S. Census Bureau, 2015), so any changes in regulations that affect the ability of LEP individuals to access care will have a substantial impact on AAs.

Discussion Question: What Asian subpopulations would be especially vulnerable to the effects of no longer being able to access healthcare in their own language? What kinds of Asian health disparities could be particularly affected as a result?

DISCUSSION QUESTIONS

- How did legal policies (including those related to immigration) shape the demographic profile of Asians in the U.S.? How do they contribute to the racism and stereotyping of Asian Americans that persist today?

- Asian Americans are considered to be a low English-proficient community. How does this impact healthcare practices and access and exacerbate health disparities for this population?

- What are some of the major institutional-, community-, and individual-level challenges to collecting data in the Asian American community? What are some effective strategies that can be implemented to address these challenges?

- How do cultural and structural factors impact the occurrence of and help-seeking related to gender-based violence against Asian American women? Identify some strategies to address these barriers in developing programs and outreach to address these factors.

- How could you apply an ecological model to developing a health intervention for an Asian American subgroup? How does this differ from approaches that focus primarily on individual behaviors?

- Identify a chronic disease and discuss potential community partners and strategies to integrate community participation and engagement in developing and implementing a health promotion intervention.

REFERENCES

Appel, L. J., Brands, M. W., Daniels, S. R., Karanja, N., Elmer, P. J., & Sacks, F. M. (2006). Dietary approaches to prevent and treat hypertension: A scientific statement from the American Heart Association. *Hypertension, 47*(2), 296–308. doi:10.1161/01.HYP.0000202568.01167.B6

Asian & Pacific Islander American Health Forum. (n.d.). *About.* Retrieved from https://www.apiahf.org/about

Asian Americans/Pacific Islanders in Philanthropy. (2015). *A call to action: Aligning public and private investments in Asian American, Native Hawaiian and Pacific Islander communities.* Oakland, CA: Author. Retrieved from https://aapip.org/sites/default/files/publication/files/ppp_call_to_action.6.pdf

Association of Asian Pacific Community Health Organizations. (n.d.). *About AAPCHO.* Retrieved from http://www.aapcho.org/wp/wp-content/uploads/2016/05/ABOUT-AAPCHO-info-sheet_052417.pdf

Barnett, J. C., & Marina, S. V. (2016). Health insurance coverage in the United States: 2015. *Current Population Reports.* Retrieved from https://www.census.gov/content/dam/Census/library/publications/2016/demo/p60-257.pdf

Barringer, H., Gardner, R. W., & Levin, M. J. (1993). *Asians and Pacific Islanders in the United States.* New York, NY: Russell Sage Foundation.

Black, M., Basille, K., Breiding, M., Smith, S., Walters, M., Merick, M., … Stevens, M. (2010). *National intimate partner and sexual violence survey: 2010 summary report.* Atlanta, GA: National Center for Injury Prevention and Control, Centers for Disease Control and Prevention. Retrieved from https://www.cdc.gov/violenceprevention/pdf/nisvs_report2010-a.pdf

Boeing, H., Bechthold, A., Bub, A., Ellinger, S., Haller, D., Kroke, A., … Watzl, B. (2012). Critical review: Vegetables and fruit in the prevention of chronic diseases. *Europe Journal of Nutrition,51*(6), 637–663. doi:10.1007/s00394-012-0380-y

Brown, J. S., Meadows, S. O., & Elder, G. H., Jr. (2007). Race-ethnic inequality and psychological distress: Depressive symptoms from adolescence to young adulthood. *Developmental Psychology, 43*(6), 1295–1311. doi:10.1037/0012-1649.43.6.1295

Brownson, R. C., Haire-Joshu, D., & Luke, D. A. (2006). Shaping the context of health: A review of environmental and policy approaches in the prevention of chronic diseases. *Annual Review of Public Health, 27,* 341–370. doi:10.1146/annurev.publhealth.27.021405.102137

Burke, L. E., Dunbar-Jacob, J. M., & Hill, M. N. (1997). Compliance with cardiovascular disease prevention strategies: A review of the research. *Annals of Behavioral Medicine, 19*(3), 239–263. doi:10.1007/BF02892289

Center for Asian Health. (n.d.-a). *About.* Retrieved from https://medicine.temple.edu/departments-centers/research-centers/center-asian-health/about

Center for Asian Health. (n.d.-b). *Research programs.* Retrieved from https://medicine.temple.edu/departments-centers/research-centers/center-asian-health/research-programs

Centers for Disease Control and Prevention. (n.d.-a). Health disparities in HIV/AIDS, viral hepatitis, STDs, and TB. Retrieved from https://www.cdc.gov/nchhstp/healthdisparities/asians.html

Centers for Disease Control and Prevention. (n.d.-b). *REACH 2014.* Retrieved from https://www.cdc.gov/nccdphp/dnpao/state-local-programs/reach/2014/index.html

Centers for Disease Control and Prevention, Division of Nutrition, Physical Activity, and Obesity. (2018, October). *Implementation guide for the notice of funding opportunity—Racial and ethnic approaches to community health program.* Retrieved from https://www.cdc.gov/nccdphp/dnpao/state-local-programs/pdf/REACH-Implementation-Guide-508.pdf

Chen, E. K., Reid, M. C., Parker, S. J., & Pillemer, K. (2013). Tailoring evidence-based interventions for new populations: A method for program adaptation through community engagement. *Evaluation & the Health Professions, 36*(1), 73–92. doi:10.1177/0163278712442536

Colby, S. L., & Ortman, J. M. (2015). *Projections of the size and composition of the U.S. population: 2014 to 2060.* Retrieved from https://www.census.gov/content/dam/Census/library/publications/2015/demo/p25-1143.pdf

Community Prevention Services Task Force. (2016). *Diabetes prevention and control: Intensive lifestyle interventions for patients with type 2 diabetes.*

Crystal, D. (1989). Asian Americans and the myth of the model minority. *Social Casework, 70,* 405–413. doi:10.1177/104438948907000702

Deurenberg, P., Deurenberg-Yap, M., & Guricci, S. (2002). Asians are different from Caucasians and from each other in their body mass index/body fat per cent relationship. *Obesity Reviews, 3*(3), 141–146. doi:10.1046/j.1467-789X.2002.00065.x

Devos, T., & Banaji, M. R. (2005). American = White? *Journal of Personality and Social Psychology, 88,* 447–466. doi:10.1037/0022-3514.88.3.447

El-Serag, H. B. (2012). Epidemiology of viral hepatitis and hepatocellular carcinoma. *Gastroenterology, 142*(6), 1264–1273.e1. doi:10.1053/j.gastro.2011.12.061

Gee, G. C., & Ro, A. (2009). Racism and discrimination. In C. Trinh-Shevrin, N. S. Islam, & M. J. Rey (Eds.), *Asian American communities and health* (pp. 364–402). San Francisco, CA: Jossey-Bass.

George, S., Duran, N., & Norris, K. (2014). A systematic review of barriers and facilitators to minority research participation among African Americans, Latinos, Asian Americans, and Pacific Islanders. *American Journal of Public Health, 104*(2), e16–e31. doi:10.2105/AJPH.2013.301706

Ghosh, C. (2003). Healthy People 2010 and Asian Americans/Pacific Islanders: Defining a baseline of information. *American Journal of Public Health, 93*(12), 2093–2098. doi:10.2105/AJPH.93.12.2093

Ghosh, C. (2009). Asian American health research. In C. Trinh-Shevrin, N. S. Islam, & M. J. Rey (Eds.), *Asian American communities and health* (pp. 73–104). San Francisco, CA: Jossey-Bass.

Gupta, L. S., Wu, C. C., Young, S., & Perlman, S. E. (2011). Prevalence of diabetes in New York City, 2002–2008: Comparing foreign-born South Asians and other Asians with U.S.-born Whites, Blacks, and Hispanics. *Diabetes Care, 34*(8), 1791–1793. doi:10.2337/dc11-0088

Han, H. R., Kim, K. B., & Kim, M. T. (2007). Evaluation of the training of Korean community health workers for chronic disease management. *Health Education Research, 22*(4), 513–521. doi:10.1093/her/cyl112

Hoeffel, E. M., Rastogi, S., Kim, M. O., & Shahid, H. (2012). *The Asian population: 2010.* 2010 Census Briefs. Retrieved from https://www.census.gov/prod/cen2010/briefs/c2010br-11.pdf

International Agency for Research on Cancer. (2012). *Personal habits and indoor combustions* (IARC monographics on the evaluation of carcinogenic risks to humans, *Vol. 100*(Pt. E), pp. 1–538). Lyon, France: Author. Retrieved from https://www.ncbi.nlm.nih.gov/books/NBK304391

Islam, N. S., Trinh-Shevrin, C., & Rey, M. J. (2009). Toward a contextual understanding of Asian American Health. In C. Trinh-Shevrin, N. S. Islam, & M. J. Rey (Eds.), *Asian American communities and health* (pp. 3–22). San Francisco, CA: Jossey-Bass.

Israel, B. A., Schulz, A. J., Parker, E. A., & Becker, A. B. (1998). Review of community-based research: Assessing partnership approaches to improve public health. *Annual Review of Public Health,19,* 173–202. doi:10.1146/annurev.publhealth.19.1.173

Janson, G., & Hazel, R. J. (2004). Trauma reactions of bystanders and victims to repetitive abuse experiences. *Violence and Victims, 19,* 239–255. doi:10.1891/vivi.19.2.239.64102

Kamphuis, C. B., Giskes, K., de Bruijn, G. J., Wendel-Vos, W., Brug, J., & van Lenthe, F. J. (2006). Environmental determinants of fruit and vegetable consumption among adults: A systematic review. *British Journal of Nutrition, 96*(4), 620–635. doi:10.1079/BJN20061896

King, G. L., McNeely, M. J., Thorpe, L. E., Mau, M. L., Ko, J., Liu, L. L., … Chow, E. A. (2012). Understanding and addressing unique needs of diabetes in Asian Americans, Native Hawaiians, and Pacific Islanders. *Diabetes Care,35*(5), 1181–1188. doi:10.2337/dc12-0210

Klatsky, A. L., Tekawa, I. S., & Armstrong, M. A. (1996). Cardiovascular risk factors among Asian Americans. *Public Health Reports, 111*(Suppl. 2), 62–64. doi:10.2105/ajph.81.11.1423

Kum, S. S., Patel, S., Garcia, M. J., Kim, S. S., Kavathe, R., Choy, C., … Kwon, S. C. (2018). Visualizing reach of racial and ethnic approaches to community health for Asian Americans: The REACH FAR project in New York and New Jersey. *Preventing Chronic Disease, 15,* E112. doi:10.5888/pcd15.180026

Kung, A., Hastings, K. G., Kapphahn, K. I., Wang, E. J., Cullen, M. R., Ivey, S. L., … Chung, S. (2016). Cross-national comparisons of increasing suicidal mortality rates for Koreans in the Republic of Korea and

Korean Americans in the USA, 2003–2012. *Epidemiology and Psychiatric Sciences, 27*, 62–73. doi:10.1017/S2045796016000792

Kwon, S. C., Patel, S., Choy, C., Zanowiak, J., Rideout, C., Yi, S., … Islam, N. S. (2017). Implementing health promotion activities using community-engaged approaches in Asian American faith-based organizations in New York City and New Jersey. *Translational Behavioral Medicine, 7*(3), 444–466. doi:10.1007/s13142-017-0506-0

Lew, R., & Chen, W. W. (2013). Promising practices to eliminate tobacco disparities among Asian American, Native Hawaiian and Pacific Islander communities. *Health Promotion Practice, 14*(5 Suppl.), 6S–9S. doi:10.1177/1524839913497717

López, G., Ruiz, N. G., & Patten, E. (2017). *Key facts about Asian Americans, a diverse and growing population.* Retrieved from http://www.pewresearch.org/fact-tank/2017/09/08/key-facts-about-asian-americans

Ma, G. X., & Daus, G. P. (2009). Health interventions. In C. Trinh-Shevrin, N. S. Islam, & J. R. Mariano (Eds.), *Asian American communities and health* (pp. 443–463). San Francisco, CA: Jossey-Bass.

Marmot, M., Friel, S., Bell, R., Houweling, T. A., & Taylor, S. (2008). Closing the gap in a generation: Health equity through action on the social determinants of health. *Lancet, 372*(9650), 1661–1669. doi:10.1016/S0140-6736(08)61690-6

Mayor's Office of Operations. (2016). *CEO poverty measure 2005-2014.* Retrieved from https://www1.nyc.gov/assets/opportunity/pdf/16_poverty_measure_report.pdf

Merzel, C., & D'Afflitti, J. (2003). Reconsidering community-based health promotion: Promise, performance, and potential. *American Journal of Public Health, 93*(4), 557–574. doi:10.2105/AJPH.93.4.557

Migration Policy Institute. (n.d.). *Unauthorized immigrant populations by country and region, top states and counties of residence, 2012–16.* Retrieved from https://www.migrationpolicy.org/programs/data-hub/charts/unauthorized-immigrant-populations-country-and-region-top-state-and-county

Mohanty, S. A., Woolhandler, S., Himmelstein, D. U., & Bor, D. H. (2005). Diabetes and cardiovascular disease among Asian Indians in the United States. *Journal of General Internal Medicine, 20*(5), 474–478. doi:10.1111/j.1525-1497.2005.40294.x

Nagata, D. K., & Takeshita, Y. J. (2002). Psychological reactions to redress: Diversity among Japanese Americans interned during World War II. *Cultural Diversity and Ethnic Minority Psychology, 8*(1), 41–59. doi:10.1037/1099-9809.8.1.41

National Academies of Sciences, Engineering, and Medicine. (2018). *Immigration as a social determinant of health: Proceedings of a workshop.* Washington, DC: Author.

National Asian Women's Health Organization. (1997). *Expanding options: A reproductive and sexual health survey of Asian American women.* Washington, DC: National Academies Press.

New York City Commission on Human Rights. (2003). *Discrimination against Muslims, Arabs, and South Asians in New York City since 9/11.* Retrieved from http://chhayacdc.org/wp-content/uploads/2014/09/Discrimination-Against-Muslims-Arabs-and-South-Asian-in-New-York-City-Since-9-11.pdf

New York City Department of Health & Mental Hygiene. (2011). *New York City food standards.* Retrieved from http://www.nyc.gov/html/dycd/downloads/pdf/2012/City_Agency_Food_Standards.pdf

New York University Center for the Study of Asian American Health. (n.d.). *Approach.* Retrieved from https://med.nyu.edu/asian-health/about-us/approach

Nierkens, V., Hartman, M. A., Nicolaou, M., Vissenberg, C., Beune, E. J., Hosper, K., … Stronks, K. (2013). Effectiveness of cultural adaptations of interventions aimed at smoking cessation, diet, and/or physical activity in ethnic minorities. A systematic review. *PLoS One, 8*(10), e73373. doi:10.1371/journal.pone.0073373

Okazaki, S. (1997). Sources of ethnic differences between Asian American and White American college students on measures of depression and social anxiety. *Journal of Abnormal Psychology, 106*(1), 52–60. doi:10.1037/0021-843X.106.1.52

Park-Tanjasiri, S., & Nguyen, T. (2009). The health of women. In C. Trinh-Shevrin, N. S. Islam, & M. J. Rey (Eds.), *Asian American communities and health* (pp. 132–161). San Francisco, CA: Jossey-Bass.

Pollack, H. J., Kwon, S. C., Wang, S. H., Wyatt, L. C., Trinh-Shevrin, C., & AAHBP Coalition. (2014). Chronic hepatitis B and liver cancer risks among Asian immigrants in New York City: Results from a large, community-based screening, evaluation, and treatment program. *Cancer Epidemiology Biomarkers & Prevention, 23*(11), 2229–2239. doi:10.1158/1055-9965.EPI-14-0491

Ponce, N. A. (2009). Health insurance. In C. Trinh-Shevrin, N. S. Islam, & M. J. Rey (Eds.), *Asian American communities and health* (pp. 344–361). San Francisco, CA: Jossey-Bass.

Racial and Ethnic Approaches to Community Health for Asian Americans. (2016). *Nutrition plate planner-- Bangla*. Retrieved from https://med.nyu.edu/asian-health/sites/default/files/asian-health2/plate-planner-preview-bangladeshi.pdf

Ro, M., Park, J. J., & Jang, D. (2009). Language access. In C. Trinh-Shevrin, N. S. Islam, & M. J. Rey (Eds.), *Asian American communities and health* (pp. 323–343). San Francisco, CA: Jossey-Bass.

South Asian Americans Leading Together. (2014). *Under suspicion, under attack: Xenophobic political rhetoric and hate violence against South Asian, Muslim, Sikh, Hindu, Middle Eastern, and Arab communities in the United States*. Takoma Park, MD: Author. Retrieved from http://saalt.org/wp-content/uploads/2013/06/SAALT_report_execsum.pdf

Tandon, S. D., & Kwon, S. C. (2009). Community-based participatory research. In C. Trinh-Shevrin, N. S. Islam, & M. J. Rey (Eds.), *Asian American communities and health* (pp. 464–503). San Francisco, CA: Jossey-Bass.

Tjaden, P., & Thoennes, N. (2000). *Full report of the prevalence, incidence, and consequences of violence against women*. Washington, DC: U.S. Department of Justice. Retrieved from https://www.ncjrs.gov/pdffiles1/nij/183781.pdf

Torre, L. A., Sauer, A. M., Chen, M. S., Jr., Kagawa-Singer, M., Jemal, A., & Siegel, R. L. (2016). Cancer statistics for Asian Americans, Native Hawaiians, and Pacific Islanders, 2016: Converging incidence in males and females. *CA: A Cancer Journal for Clinicians, 66*(3), 182–202. doi:10.3322/caac.21335

Trinh-Shevrin, C., Islam, N. S., Nadkarni, S., Park, R., & Kwon, S. C. (2015). Defining an integrative approach for health promotion and disease prevention: A population health equity framework. *Journal of Health Care for the Poor and Underserved, 26*(2 Suppl.), 146–163. doi:10.1353/hpu.2015.0067

Trinh-Shevrin, C., Kwon, S. C., Park, R., Nadkarni, S. K., & Islam, N. S. (2015). Moving the dial to advance population health equity in New York City Asian American populations. *American Journal of Public Health, 105*(Suppl. 3), e16–e25. doi:10.2105/AJPH.2015.302626

Tseng, W. (2009). Social, demographic, and cultural characteristics of Asian Americans. In C. Trinh-Shevrin, N. S. Islam, & M. J. Rey (Eds.), *Asian American communities and health*. San Francisco, CA: Jossey-Bass.

Tung, E. L, Baig, A. A., Huang, E. S., Laiteerapong, N., & Chua, K.-P. (2017). Racial and ethnic disparities in diabetes screening between Asian Americans and other adults: BRFSS 2012–2014. *Journal of General Internal Medicine, 32*, 423–429. doi:10.1007/s11606-016-3913-x

U.S. Census Bureau. (2015). *American Fact Finder: 2015 American Community Survey 1 year estimates, selected population profile in the United States (S0201)*. Retrieved from https://factfinder.census.gov/faces/tableservices/jsf/pages/productview.xhtml?src=bkmk

U.S. Immigration and Naturalization Service. (1960–1978). *Annual reports*. Washington, DC: Author.

U.S. Immigration and Naturalization Service. (1979–1992). *Statistical yearbook*. Washington, DC: Author.

Wong, J., Huang, V., Chan, S., Park, S., Jung, D., & Lee, D. (2003). S.O.S.: Shame, obligation, and survival: Asian Americans and domestic violence. In L. Zhan (Ed.), *Asian Americans: Vulnerable populations, model interventions, and clarifying agendas* (pp. 135–169). Boston, MA: Jones & Bartlett.

Yi, S. S., Kwon, S. C., Sacks, R., & Trinh-Shevrin, C. (2016). Commentary: Persistence and health-related consequences of the model minority stereotype for Asian Americans. *Ethnicity & Disease, 26*(1), 133–138. doi:10.18865/ed.26.1.133

Yi, S. S., Kwon, S. C., Wyatt, L., Islam, N., & Trinh-Shevrin, C. (2015). Weighing in on the hidden Asian American obesity epidemic. *Preventive Medicine, 73*, 6–9. doi:10.1016/j.ypmed.2015.01.007

Yoshihama, M., & Dabby, C. (2015). *Domestic violence in Asian & Pacific Islander homes*. Facts & Stats Report. Retrieved from https://s3.amazonaws.com/gbv-wp-uploads/wp-content/uploads/2019/02/01204358/Facts-Stats-Report-DV-API-Communities-2015-formatted2019.pdf

AMERICAN INDIAN AND ALASKA NATIVE HEALTH EQUITY

ROYLEEN J. ROSS ▪ IVA GREYWOLF ▪ K. BRYANT SMALLEY ▪
JACOB C. WARREN

LEARNING OBJECTIVES

- Discuss the diversity of American Indian and Alaska Native populations
- Describe historical injustices against American Indian and Alaska Native populations and their relationship to health outcomes
- Define and describe how historical trauma impacts health equity for American Indian and Alaska Native populations
- Describe the presence, predictors, and protective factors for disparities in alcohol/substance use disorder, diabetes, and violence for American Indian and Alaska Native populations
- Identify best-practice approaches for achieving health equity among American Indian and Alaska Native populations

INTRODUCTION

Because the American Indian and Alaska Native (AIAN) population of the U.S. has a legal right to healthcare services based on a series of "treaties, court decisions, acts of Congress, Executive Orders, and other legal bases" resulting from the forced relocation of AIAN tribes throughout American history (Warne, Kaur, & Perdue, 2012, p. 18), people often incorrectly assume that this guarantees access to quality healthcare and that AIAN individuals have health status and outcomes comparable to other racial/ethnic groups. While AIAN populations exhibit remarkable resilience and fortitude in the face of systemic oppression, disparities in health status and outcomes still exist, and access to care remains a significant challenge for AIAN populations. The Indian Health Service (IHS, the branch of the federal government responsible for provision of healthcare to AIANs) has been identified as one of the most critically underfunded segments of government. Despite having the legal obligation to provide for the healthcare of AIAN individuals, the U.S. government provides less than 40% of the equivalent U.S. per capita healthcare expenditures to the IHS and the Service often runs out of funds prior to the end of their fiscal year (Warne et al., 2012). The failure of the IHS to meet the needs of AIAN people continues a centuries-long pattern of injustices against AIAN populations that have resulted in severe and systemic health disparities.

More than 4 million U.S. citizens identify their race as American Indian (AI) or Alaska Native (U.S. Census Bureau, 2019), making AIAN the third largest minority group in the United States. However, the health and well-being of AIAN populations is rarely discussed in broader health equity circles, and the literature surrounding AIAN health remains limited in comparison to the size of the AIAN population. This is partially driven by structural separations that exist between the IHS and other Department of Health and Human Services (DHHS) agencies; however, the broader historical context of the historical atrocities committed against AIAN people, and the resulting legacy of those atrocities, cannot be ignored when discussing AIAN health equity. Similarly, the remarkable ability of AIAN people to thrive in the midst of inequities and historical trauma serves as an example of how cultural resilience can play a major role in promoting health equity.

When considering healthcare for AIAN people, the IHS is fraught with betrayals that have led to historical mistrust in the agency as a whole. While a full history of the horrors inflicted upon AIAN people by the U.S. government is beyond the scope of this chapter, the mistreatment of AIAN populations has been severe and systemic, including massacres, theft of land, forced removal of children to boarding schools (see callout box), repeated breaking of forced treaties, and numerous medical injustices. While several of these injustices are discussed throughout this chapter, they are not simply historical—for example, in the 1970s, the U.S. government admitted to sterilizing thousands of AI women against their will, and studies have estimated that 25% to 40% of all AI women of childbearing age were sterilized by the IHS during the early 1970s (Lawrence, 2000). There have been a number of reported cases of IHS healthcare providers abusing patients, including a recent conviction on multiple counts of an IHS pediatrician who sexually abused Indian children and adolescents over a 40-year period (Rosenblaum, 2018). The passage of the Indian Self-Determination and Education Assistance Act (PL 93-638) placed control of health services back in the hands of tribes at their discretion (Warne et al., 2012). While these services are most frequently offered on reservations, Urban Indian Health Centers/Urban Indian Organizations are operated in 41 locations in 22 states (National Council of Urban Indian Health, n.d.).

A key factor that complicates AIAN health equity work is a prevailing misunderstanding of the composition of the AIAN population. While all AIAN groups share a common history of persecution, it is also very important to remember that the AIAN population is not a monolithic group—there are 574 federally-recognized tribes across 35 states, each with its own unique culture that intersects with underlying factors impacting health equity. It is critical to remember that findings in one sample may not translate to another sample not because of limitations in design, but due to fundamental differences between the groups being considered. Recognizing and taking into consideration the types of diversity *within* the AIAN population is critical to truly advancing the field of AIAN health equity. Unfortunately, in order to achieve adequate sample size for many studies, recruitment must occur across tribes and/or reservations within a tribe, which can complicate interpretation of negative findings and impacts the interpretation and external validity of studies (Greenfield & Venner, 2012; Whitbeck, Walls, & Welch, 2012). Another complicator in studying AIAN health equity is the separation between rural and urban AIAN groups. There is a widespread misperception that AIAN populations are rural-residing; while AIANs are the only racial/ethnic group in the United States that has a higher representation within rural areas than urban areas, nearly half of AIANs still live in an urban area (Dewees & Marks, 2017), and there is a lack of literature adequately describing, comparing, and meeting the health needs of reservation-residing, rural non-reservation residing, and urban-residing AIAN populations. Even within rural, there is often overlooked diversity—as an example, many AIAN individuals reside in remote/frontier locations that are very difficult to access, at times accessible only via plane or snow machine. Such locations are dramatically underrepresented in the research literature and present unique considerations for pursuing AIAN health equity work.

Despite the current limitations in the field, the consistency of the literature surrounding several key issues supports the presence of numerous health disparities that deserve a much higher level of attention within the field of health equity. AIAN populations share many types of risk, including sociodemographic and historical. At the sociodemographic level, AIAN populations as a whole are half as likely to obtain a college degree and have higher rates of unemployment than the general U.S. population (U.S. Census Bureau, 2007) and, as a result, face a markedly increased risk for poverty (up to four times the national average; Castor et al., 2006). This discrepancy is fueled by inadequate preparation for college and colleges most often being located great distances from their home communities. This social isolation is a factor of acculturation stress, which also includes factors such as racism, discrimination, stigma, social injustice, and suppression of Native values. The stress is magnified for AIAN students that hold traditional values as they carry their history and witness the ongoing taking of land and natural resources (Flynn, Olson, & Yellig, 2014). These sociodemographic factors are tied to a correspondingly high rate of morbidity and early mortality for AIAN people (Grandbois, 2009). Historical trauma also plays a substantial role in AIAN health disparities. Historical trauma is defined by Brave Heart (2003) as "cumulative emotional and psychological wounding over the lifespan and across generations emanating from massive group trauma experiences," such as the centuries-long history of violence, discrimination, and treachery experienced by AIAN people at the hands of not only other people but the U.S. government as well. Similar to minority stress theory (see Chapter 3, Health Equity Frameworks and Theories), the related concept of Historical Trauma Response posits that there is a constellation of disparities that result from this historical and ongoing oppression, including depression, self-injury, suicide, anxiety, and substance use disorder (Brave Heart, 2003; Wiechelt, Gryczynski, Johnson, & Caldwell, 2012).

THE NATIONAL ATROCITY OF BOARDING SCHOOLS

While the history of forced removal of AIAN populations and the theft of sovereign land is commonly known, there are other injustices that do not have the same level of cultural awareness. As part of the broader 19th- to 20th-centuries attack on AIAN culture and attempts at forced assimilation into "mainstream" U.S. culture to address the "Indian problem," the U.S. government enacted a policy of forced removal of AIAN children for the purpose of "civilizing" them in boarding schools to eradicate their "savagism" (Adams, 1995). While it is difficult to quantify the number of children subjected to forced removal, it is estimated that by 1930, nearly half of AIAN children were enrolled in boarding schools that were sometimes thousands of miles away from their family and culture. At these boarding schools, children were "forbidden to engage in cultural practices or speak their languages and suffered harsh punishment if they disobeyed"

(continued)

(Evans-Campbell, Walters, Pearson, & Campbell, 2012, p. 421). They had their clothes and hairstyles replaced with White American styles, were renamed with English names, and were subjected to high rates of child abuse (Adams, 1995). In 1928, a scathing federal report (the "Meriam report") "found that children at federal boarding schools were malnourished, overworked, harshly punished and poorly educated" in a system that had inadequate sanitation, violated federal child labor laws, and failed to meet basic physical needs such as food and shelter (Bear, 2008, "The Problem of Indian Administration"). Despite these findings, many boarding schools remained operational, and a 1969 follow-up report (the "Kennedy report") called the system in its very title "a national tragedy." Schools continued to close after the Kennedy report, and the landmark 1975 Indian Self-Determination and Education Assistance Act finally codified the ability of the federal government to make grants and contracts directly with tribes for the tribes themselves to operate their own educational systems. However, it was an additional 3 years later with the passage of the Indian Child Welfare Act (ICWA) that AIAN parents finally "gained the legal right to deny their children's placement in off-reservation schools" (Northern Plains Reservation Aid, 2019, para. 17). The historical trauma of these boarding schools cannot be overstated. A history of boarding school attendance has been tied not only to substance use and suicidality in those who attended but also to increased rates of anxiety, post-traumatic stress disorder (PTSD), and suicidality in the children of those who attended (Evans-Campbell et al., 2012). These outcomes have further impaired parenting skills and alienation from culture, impacting multiple generations of Native families, and will continue to influence future generations.

OUTCOMES OF FOCUS

Disparities in health status and health outcomes for AIAN populations have been recognized for nearly 500 years (Jones, 2006), and a full discussion of each recognized disparity is beyond the scope of this chapter. Instead, we will focus on three health inequities that considerably affect AIAN populations: alcohol and substance use disorders, diabetes, and violence. Other outcomes with demonstrated disparities include suicide, depression, dental caries, postneonatal death, obesity, cardiovascular disease, and metabolic syndrome (Baldwin et al., 2009; Barker, Goodman, & DeBeck, 2017; Hutchinson & Shin, 2014; Manson, 2001; Nash & Nagel, 2005; Phipps, Ricks, Manz, & Blahut, 2012; Wilson, Civic, & Glass, 1995).

Alcohol and Substance Use Disorders

Alcohol and substance use disorders are often recognized as one of the largest disparities faced by AIAN populations (Hawkins, Cummins, & Marlatt, 2004). There is disagreement in the literature, however, about not only the magnitude of the disparity, but also about its existence. Some national studies have shown higher rates of abstinence among AIAN populations in comparison to White Americans (Cunningham, Solomon, & Muramoto, 2016), as well as high levels of success in maintaining abstinence among individuals with alcohol use disorder (Bezdek & Spicer, 2006). There is also emerging evidence that the firewater myth, defined as "the notion that American Indians and Alaska Natives . . . are more susceptible to the effects of alcohol and vulnerable to alcohol problems," creates a self-fulfilling prophecy in which individuals who ascribe to the firewater myth are in turn more likely to have problems with alcohol (Gonzalez & Skewes, 2016, p. 838).

While the literature is conflicted regarding the level of alcohol use among AIAN populations, the effects of alcohol abuse on AIAN populations are profound—alcohol has been implicated in the deaths of more than 10% of all deaths among AIAN people, and in certain states AIAN people have double to triple the death rates seen in other racial/ethnic groups (Centers for Disease Control and Prevention, 2008; Gonzales, Roeber, et al., 2014). In addition, elevated rates of marijuana use and inhalants have been demonstrated in AIAN youth (Hawkins et al., 2004). Because of the remote nature of many AIAN communities, elevated rates of methamphetamine production/use and opioid abuse seen across rural populations are also common—estimates suggest that rates of methamphetamine use may be as high as four times all other racial/ethnic groups (Brown, 2010; Iritani, Hallfors, & Bauer, 2007). Interestingly, local studies have also found increasing rates of methamphetamine use among specific urban AIAN populations that suggest the methamphetamine epidemic may be impacting AIAN individuals nationwide particularly hard (Spear, Crevecoeur, Rawson, & Clark, 2007). Unfortunately, rural-residing AIAN have been shown to have lower access to facilities offering medication-assisted treatment than their urban counterparts, complicating receipt of evidence-based treatment (Hirchak & Murphy, 2016). Substantial variation has been demonstrated, however, between tribes and between reservation-dwelling and urban AIAN, and it is important to not draw conclusions about individual tribes and/or communities without first having learned of their own health status (O'Connell, Novins, Beals, & Spicer, 2005).

Alcohol abuse for AIAN women is particularly complex. While they do exhibit elevated rates of alcohol abuse, AIAN women are also more likely to abstain from alcohol (Duran et al., 2004)—this bimodal distribution underscores the importance of understanding the full context of alcohol use within AIAN communities when implementing intervention programs. As with women of all races and ethnicities, increases in alcohol abuse are also related to increases in other risks, such as fetal alcohol spectrum disorder (Russo, Purohit, Foudin, & Salin, 2004).

Overall risk factors for alcohol and substance use for AIAN people include poverty, life stress, social norms, cultural disruption, discrimination, a history of forced boarding school attendance, perceived lack of social activities, family history of substance use disorder, exposure to trauma, and genetic factors (Beauvais & LaBoueff, 1985; Edwards & Edwards, 1988; Evans-Campbell et al., 2012; LeMaster, Connell, Mitchell, & Manson, 2002; Mulligan et al., 2003; Novins et al., 2012; Oetting & Donnermeyer, 1998; Spindler & Spindler, 1978; Wall, Garcia-Andrade, Wong, Lau, & Ehlers, 2006; Whitbeck, Hoyt, McMorris, Chen, & Stubben, 2001). Protective factors include academic achievement, participation in traditional tribal activities and ceremonies, increased sense of cultural self-concept, and involvement with Native American churches or Christian churches (Kulis, Hodge, Ayers, Brown, & Marsiglia, 2012; Kulis, Napoli, & Marisglia, 2002; LeMaster et al., 2002; Thurman & Green, 1997).

When considering treatment, complicating care is the fact that AIAN individuals are at substantially increased risk for the multimorbidity of alcohol abuse, depression, and diabetes when compared to the non-Hispanic White population (Tann, Yabiku, Okamoto, & Yanow, 2007). Substance use disorder has also been tied to a strikingly high two-thirds to three-fourths of suicides and suicide attempts among AIAN youth (Barlow et al., 2012), indicating the substance use disorder disparity is complex and interwoven with many other AIAN health equity issues. These disparities are further exacerbated by acculturation stress, poverty, institutional racism, and ongoing colonization. For example, with the Alaska Native population, statehood is only at the 60-year mark.

Because of the complexity of substance use disorder and its connection to other outcomes, in recent decades, a movement summarized as "our culture is our treatment" has sought to radically change the model of substance use disorder treatment and prevention for AIAN populations. Referred to as "culture-as-treatment," the movement focuses on providing a cultural immersion "designed to approximate the day-to-day experiences of pre-reservation ancestors" (Gone & Calf Looking, 2011, p. 291). The premise is that the wounds of historical trauma are best healed through a focus on rebuilding what that history has damaged—cultural identity and self-realization. Empirical support for culture-as-treatment continues to grow in both rural and urban AIAN populations (Spicer, 2001) and has begun to show effects in other mental health areas as well (e.g., suicide prevention; Barker et al., 2017). Other techniques with demonstrated or emerging effectiveness include culturally-tailored parent–child interaction therapy, community-based systems of care, life skills interventions connected to traditional cultural practices such as canoe journeys, equine-assisted prevention programs, talking circles, traditional drumming, family-based interventions, Positive Indian Parenting, and traditional storytelling interventions (Bigfoot & Funderburk, 2011; Dickerson, Robichaud, Teruya, Nagaran, & Hser, 2012; Kumpfer, Alvarado, Smith, & Bellamy, 2002; Lowe, Liang, Riggs, & Henson, 2012; Mallory & Whitbeck, 2007 as cited in Whitbeck et al., 2012; Marlatt et al., 2003; Thomas, Donovan, Sigo, Austin, & Marlatt, 2009; Wexler, 2014).

SUICIDE AMONG AIAN POPULATIONS

The impact of suicide among AIAN populations has received increased attention in recent years. While some prior studies failed to demonstrate a markedly elevated suicide rate, recent studies have begun to recognize the diversity of the AIAN population and conduct more robust analyses that incorporate geographic region and age. A study of death certificate data combined with IHS patient data found that from 1999 to 2009, the adjusted death rate from suicide was 50% higher than among Whites, who have the next-highest suicide death rate (Herne, Bartholomew, & Weahkee, 2014). There are substantial variations, however, within the AIAN population that complicate both research and prevention efforts. Rates are highest among Alaska Natives and in the Northern Plains, who have up to three times the risk of their White, age- and gender-matched counterparts. In addition, Herne et al. (2014) found substantial variations by age, reporting decreasing risk and increasing protection across the life span, with AIAN individuals under the age of 25 years having more than three times the risk of suicide as their White counterparts, but AIAN individuals over the age of 85 years having less than half the risk of suicide. There is an urgent need for age- and culturally specific suicide prevention efforts designed specifically to reach younger AIAN individuals, Alaska Natives, and AIAN residents of the Northern Plains, and there have been calls for lawmakers and psychologists to come together to address the evident crisis (Dorgan, 2010). The National Action Alliance for Suicide Prevention's American Indian and Alaska Native Task Force assembled a list of recommendations in 2015 (Wexler et al., 2015) that included focusing on taking an expansive commitment to indigenous approaches to

(continued)

inquiry; taking a holistic perspective on suicide; incorporating the past, present, and future into understanding and preventing suicide; conceptualizing suicide as a social problem; examining suicide rates at the local level within the specific community context; developing community capacity and collaborating with communities on the creation of local programs; and emphasizing the importance of protective factors, resilience, and well-being.

Diabetes

Diabetes rates among AIAN populations are higher than any racial/ethnic group in the United States, estimated at four to eight times the general population (Lee et al., 1995; Sittner, Greenfield, & Walls, 2018), with certain tribes having the highest documented diabetes prevalence among all populations in the world (Knowler, Pettit, Saad, & Bennett, 1990). Increased risk for diabetes begins in youth and has increased across the life span—for example, AIAN youth aged 15 to 19 saw a 68% increase in diabetes prevalence from just 1994 to 2004 and Alaska Native adults saw a more than twofold increase from 1985 to 2006 (Narayanan et al., 2010; Nsiah-Kumi et al., 2013; Satterfield, DeBruyn, Santos, Alonso, & Frank, 2016). Disparities also exist in prognosis and sequelae of diabetes—AIAN adults with diabetes receiving care through the IHS have been shown to have higher rates of hypertension, stroke, kidney failure, amputations, and liver disease than commercially insured U.S. adults, with morbidity burden exceeding that of non-AIAN groups by 50% (O'Connell, Wilson, Manson, & Acton, 2010). In addition, AIAN women with diabetes who experience discrimination in the healthcare setting are less likely to receive clinically indicated breast examinations and Pap tests, impacting other health domains even beyond their diabetes (Gonzales, Harding, Lambert, Fu, & Henderson, 2013).

Risk factors for diabetes in AIAN groups include psychological distress, negative family support, vitamin D insufficiency, a history of trauma, racial microaggressions, and various genetic factors such as genetic markers and shortened telomeres (Dill et al., 2016; Goins, Noonan, Gonzales, Winchester, & Bradley, 2017; Hanson et al., 2014; Nsiah-Kumi et al., 2012; Sittner et al., 2018; Zhao et al., 2014). Medical discrimination plays a significant role in limiting access to supportive care—more than two-thirds of AI women with diabetes report having experienced medical discrimination, which is associated with lower rates of dental exams, blood pressure checks, and vaccinations, as well as inadequate glycemic control (Gonzales, Lambert, Fu, Jacob, & Hardin, 2014). Distinct structural barriers also exist—for example, nearly the entire state of Alaska and nearly all of the Navajo Nation is classified as a food desert (Pardilla, Prasad, Suratkar, & Gittelsohn, 2013; U.S. Department of Agriculture, 2019). There simply is not access to fresh fruits and vegetables in many of these isolated communities. Protective factors have not been as thoroughly studied, but include cultural spirituality, adherence to traditional diets, and general involvement with traditional tribal culture (Carlson et al., 2017; Dill et al., 2016; McLaughlin, 2010). The diabetes disparity has also been tied to the ways in which the U.S. government institutionalized systems of physical inactivity, high-calorie but poor-nutrition diets, and psychological distress in their management of reservation systems (Wiedman, 2012). The governmental commodity food program has been specifically tied to multigenerational diabetes risk and disparities through its direct tie to high-calorie, low-nutrition foods and through its disproportionate impact on AI people with food insecurity, thereby being linked with adverse childhood experiences

(Warne & Lajimodiere, 2015). While there is significant variation in the perception of diabetes across various tribes, many tribes attribute diabetes onset to a loss of traditional ways and the external influence of non-AIAN populations (McLaughlin, 2010). To counteract these effects, some prevention efforts have focused on restoring community capacity, including programs working on food environment through school-based, food-store, and social services programs (Gittelsohn & Rowan, 2011).

Facilitators to diabetic control identified by AIAN groups in qualitative studies include receipt of culturally-relevant diabetes education, social support from peers with diabetes, culture and spirituality, and self-efficacy (Shaw, Brown, Khan, Mau, & Dillard, 2013). Barriers include lack of knowledge of nutrition and diet, dietary restriction–related social difficulties, and the impact of comorbid conditions (Shaw et al., 2013). As mentioned previously, however, it is important to remember the immense diversity within the AIAN community and recognize that findings in a given study may not translate to all AIAN groups—as an example, a study within a single tribe revealed two divergent cultural models of diabetes care with different implications for treatment and prevention (Henderson, 2010). In another example, the well-established relationship between depression and poor glycemic control across AIAN populations was found to be completely mediated by low social support in the Eastern Band of Cherokee specifically (Goins et al., 2017). Researchers and practitioners are, therefore, strongly encouraged to actively validate programs and models within their own communities served prior to implementing prevention and/or intervention programs.

With respect to national movements in diabetes, the Diabetes Prevention Program (DPP) has become a leading evidence-based practice in diabetes intervention; however, it was developed using Western ideals and normed in non-AIAN populations. The IHS Division of Diabetes Treatment and Prevention adapted DPP into the Special Diabetes Program for Indians (SDPI) and has implemented it in more than 300 community-driven programs (McLaughlin, 2010). While the evidence is mixed regarding the impact of traditional DPP on outcomes for AIAN populations, cultural adaptations of DPP have shown impact on weight, blood pressure, and lipid levels (Jiang et al., 2013). Other programs that have been developed include the CBPR-driven Family Education Diabetes Series (Mendenhall et al., 2010), the Traditional Foods Project that combines cultural education with reclamation of traditional food systems (Satterfield et al., 2016), a Medicine Wheel Model of nutrition-based intervention (Kattelmann, Conti, & Ren, 2010), a home-visiting program for AIAN youth with diabetes (Chambers et al., 2015), and a comprehensive K–12 diabetes prevention curriculum that integrates diabetes science with cultural context (Francis & Chino, 2012).

Longitudinal studies have found general improvements in the health status of AIAN populations with diabetes over the past several decades, offering hope that a continued focus on achieving equity in diabetes diagnoses and outcomes can help to eliminate the effects of this striking disparity (Looker et al., 2010).

Domestic Violence and Sexual Assault

Domestic violence and sexual assault are disturbingly high among AIAN populations. Beginning in adolescence, AIAN populations are more likely than their non-AIAN peers to be victims of both serious violence and simple assault and are also more likely to witness violence inflicted upon others (Manson, Beals, Klein, & Croy, 2005; Rennison, 2001; Rosay, 2016). Violence impacts AIAN women particularly hard—nearly 90% of AIAN women report that they have been abused in their lifetime, up to half are estimated to experience sexual abuse (typically by a romantic partner), and nearly half experience domestic violence (Bohn, 2003; Chester, Robin, Koss, Lopez, & Goldman, 1994; Evans-Campbell, Lindhorst, Huang, & Walters, 2006). AIAN women also face staggeringly high risk for homicide—in Minnesota, for example, AI women are 10 times more likely to be murdered than White women (Smith, 2015). However, despite the known elevations in risk, fewer than 15% of AIAN women report ever having been screened for violence (Harwell, Moore, & Spence, 2003). The number of missing and murdered AIAN women in the United States has reached epidemic proportions. According to the Urban Indian Health Institute (UIHI), in 2016 there were 5,712 reports of missing American Indian and Alaska Native women and girls (UIHI, 2018).

Because of the ways in which historical denigration of AIAN women compounds experiences of violence, the trauma associated with experiencing physical and sexual violence is profound and often beyond that seen in other groups (Evans-Campbell et al., 2006; Smith, 2015). Recommendations for minimizing trauma's long-term effects and for preventing violence altogether include actively ensuring women feel validated in their experience and reactions, increasing compassion among caregivers, providing opportunities to seek help in both Western and traditional Native contexts, implementing community-level programs such as awareness campaigns and supportive shelters, and basing programs outside traditional "office" environments (Evans-Campbell et al., 2006; Norton & Manson, 1997; Oetzel & Duran, 2004). The need for tribal-associated shelters has been repeatedly highlighted as an essential method for ensuring women in need of services feel comfortable and supported in receiving those services (Tehee & Esqueda, 2008).

Complicating cross-cultural comparisons of violence, as well as the implementation of Western-developed intervention and prevention programs, is the fact that AIAN women and White women have been shown to have drastically different conceptualizations of domestic violence and the reasons behind it (Tehee & Esqueda, 2008). For example, AIAN women are more likely to view domestic violence as physical rather than emotional and are more likely to attribute the issue to broader social determinants of health (e.g., poverty, unemployment) than are White women (Tehee & Esqueda, 2008). AIAN women are also much more likely to state that the legal system does not work in handling domestic violence (Tehee & Esqueda, 2008).

It is upsetting, but unsurprising, that AIAN women express distrust of the legal system. Before the Violence Against Women Act (VAWA) of 1994, tribes were legally unable to bring criminal charges against non-AIAN people who perpetrated domestic violence against AIAN women (Ross, GreyWolf, Tehee, Henry, & Cheromiah et al., 2018). Even with the passage of VAWA, tribes remained unable to prosecute sexual assault, sex trafficking, and crimes against children if perpetrated by a non-AIAN assailant (Ross et al., 2018). VAWA expired in 2019, and while a reauthorization bill passed the House in April 2019 that includes an expansion of tribal jurisdiction to include sexual violence, sex trafficking, stalking, child abuse, and violence against tribal law enforcement, the Senate has refused to bring the bill forward for a vote (Onco, 2019).

The effects of violence are multigenerational, with AIAN children more likely to witness domestic violence than their non-AIAN counterparts (Costello et al., 1997). AIAN youth are also more likely to experience trauma and other adverse childhood events than their non-AIAN counterparts, although this association has been largely accounted for by associated socioeconomic differences between racial/ethnic groups (Kenney & Singh, 2016; Manson et al., 2005; Whitesell, Beals, Mitchell, Manson, & Turner, 2009). Experiences of childhood maltreatment among AIAN populations have been tied to later incidence of mental disorders and substance use disorder, suicidal behavior, and relationship problems (Sarche & Spicer, 2008). It is important to note, however, that while adverse childhood experiences (ACEs) may be more commonly experienced, AIAN communities are also "rich with protective factors that provide ... essential, positive experiences, including native traditions, language, spirituality, elders, and connectedness" that help to counteract the negative effects of ACEs (Association of American Indian Physicians, n.d.).

When discussing the origins of these disparities, it is essential to not reify stereotypes of AIAN populations as inherently violent. First, it is essential to note that nearly 100% of AIAN victims of violence report at least one episode of physical and/or sexual violence by a non-AIAN perpetrator (Rosay, 2016). In addition, even for AIAN perpetrators, historical studies have repeatedly shown that violence—particularly against women—has increased markedly since colonialization and does not in any way reflect a general manifestation of AIAN culture. The role of colonialization and government-sanctioned violence against AIAN of any gender cannot be ignored, but is often mentioned only as an afterthought due to the complexities in quantifying its impact—however, experts have made clear connections between the historical denigration of AIAN identities and physical bodies and the subsequent view of AIAN individuals, and in particular women, as something less than human and not worthy of bodily respect (e.g., Smith, 2015; Weaver, 2009). A full coverage of the depth of these associations is beyond the scope of this chapter, but readers are encouraged to read the work of Smith (2015) for a compelling history of colonialization's effect on modern violence against AIAN people.

AIAN-specific risk factors for violence identified within the literature include substance use, lack of screening in primary care, economic deprivation, ethnic heterogeneity, and family disruption (Hamby, 2000; Lanier & Huff-Corzine, 2006; Oetzel & Duran, 2004). AIAN women have been consistently shown to receive a lower intensity law enforcement response, with over 40% of AIAN women who were murdered being killed by someone who had previously violated a protective order against them (Bachman, Zaykowski, Kallmyer, Poteyeva, & Lanier, 2008; Oetzel & Duran, 2004). Law enforcement response is complicated by complex jurisdictional issues that can impede investigations and active distrust of external law enforcement (Hamby, 2008). Protective factors against violence include connectedness, family caring, parental monitoring, tribal cultural involvement, prosocial behaviors, self-image, positive affect, and community connectedness (Bearinger et al., 2005; Pu et al., 2013).

AIAN CHILDREN AND THE FOSTER CARE SYSTEM

The literature on AIAN children in the foster care system is still in its infancy. This line of work is complicated by centuries of atrocities committed against AIAN families ranging from the previously discussed history of forced boarding school removal to the theft of AIAN children into foster and adoptive homes at rates that reached 25% to 35% in the 1970s (Jacobs, 2013). While steps have been taken to protect AIAN children from being removed from tribal lands, concerns still remain—AIAN children not residing on reservations continue to be disproportionately removed

(continued)

from homes and placed in foster care (Carter, 2010), and AIAN children who enter nontribal foster care have been shown to have worse educational and employment outcomes than their non-AIAN counterparts in foster care (O'Brien et al., 2010). While other racial/ethnic groups are also overrepresented in the foster care system, there is emerging evidence that the factors influencing the removal of AIAN children remain driven by factors other than what influences the removal of African American and Hispanic children from their homes (Lawler, LaPlante, Giger, & Norris, 2012). Specific identified causes include institutional racism, institutional bias, and the legacy of colonialism (Crofoot & Harris, 2012).

In the case of children residing on reservations, it is essential to support additional expansion of tribal-run family services such as child protective services through local/state policy change and training of local tribal leaders and community members. Returning the power and funding to tribes to support their own children's needs helps to repair the historical trauma of forced removal of children, upholds the intent of ICWA, helps children remain in their communities when the intervention of social services is needed, and promotes more successful family reunification (Cross, Earle, & Simons, 2000; Landers & Danes, 2016).

METHODS TO ACHIEVE EQUITY

While there are barriers to achieving health equity for AIAN populations, there is also tremendous movement in developing culturally-driven methods to do so. Commonly cited barriers for work in the area of AIAN health disparities include mistrust of the research and medical communities, linguistic and cultural disconnects, a lack of culturally-grounded approaches, limited/selective access to members of AIAN communities, and a general lack of population-level data on AIAN health (Sarche & Spicer, 2008; Walters & Simoni, 2009). Discrimination within the healthcare setting remains, and experiences of discrimination have been associated with cardiac events, depression, and hospitalization (Walls, Gonzalez, Gladney, & Onello, 2015). Another barrier to advancing health equity for AIAN populations are the significant barriers in place for "traditional" educational attainment, including mistrust of educational systems (due to historical oppression, e.g., forced boarding schools), disparities in educational quality, role burdens, marginalization of lines of research inquiry related to AIAN health, and overt discrimination (Walters & Simoni, 2009).

However, researchers have identified numerous ways to counteract these barriers and ensure that culturally relevant and community-driven solutions are developed to achieve AIAN health equity. An important movement in recent decades has been toward an intentional focus on community-based participatory research (CBPR) and other community–academic partnership models (McOliver et al., 2015; Ross, 2018; Whitesell, Beals, Big Cros, Mitchell, & Novins, 2012). Such approaches naturally yield culturally-appropriate health education, educational opportunities in the health professions for AIAN learners, and create natural mentoring programs for AIAN professionals (Eschiti, 2004). Community-driven efforts also lead to integration of, and founding in, cultural practices (Hawkins et al., 2004; Legha & Novins, 2012). For non-AIAN researchers, and even for AIAN researchers working within a different tribe, it is important to learn about the culture and traditions specific to the tribal community with which partnerships are being built and to directly encourage support and involvement of the local community and tribal leaders (McLaughlin, 2010). AIAN health equity experts also recommend an intentional focus on community-level interventions that not only have broader impact but also help to connect to the broader cultural awareness of community and collaboration often found in AIAN cultures (Beauvais & LaBouef, 1985; Edwards & Edwards, 1988; Petoskey, Van Stelle, & De Jong, 1998).

Other recommendations for achieving AIAN health equity include use of peer-led programs (Mellanby, Rees, & Tripp, 2000), bicultural competence interventions (Schinke et al., 1988), and the specific inclusion of AIAN lay health educators/community health workers (McLaughlin, 2010) in delivering interventions and programs. Further, there is a strong call for the development of AIAN-specific therapeutic approaches. For example, CBT has been identified as having a particularly "Western" approach that is not as culturally relevant within AIAN communities (Boyd & Hunsaker, 2018). This is a common problem in health equity work, but becomes even more magnified with AIAN populations because of the strong distinction between mainstream culture and many AIAN cultures. This can lead "evidence-based practices" to be seen as "culturally insensitive and intrusive" (Whitbeck et al., 2012). To counteract this issue, there has been intense focus in recent years on formal cultural tailoring, wherein interventions proven effective in non-AIAN populations are methodically altered and tailored to the cultural realities of a specific tribe (ideally in direct collaboration with the tribe itself; Whitbeck et al., 2012). Finally, there is substantial need to support the development and mentoring of AIAN individuals as health equity researchers and practitioners—increasing the diversity of the health equity workforce will only help to create more diverse and inclusive solutions for AIAN health.

INTERSECTIONALITY SPOTLIGHT

Throughout this chapter, the intersectional nature of gender and rurality have been discussed; however, there is an intersectionality that is unique to AIAN populations. AIAN culture has long had a more expansive view of gender and sexual orientation than Western culture, with the concept of "two-spirit" individuals long preceding modern discussions of sexual orientation and transgender identities. In many tribes, including Crow, Lakota, Navajo, and Ojibwe, there are long-standing words and often ceremonial roles for individuals who identified outside of the gender binary, viewing them instead as a distinct, third gender. Some cultures even sanctioned same-sex spouses for two-spirit individuals. As cultural war was waged on AIAN tribes, this recognition of a third gender and support of same-sex relationships was often a primary target, and violence against two-spirit individuals became common during colonialization. "Two-spirit" is a modern term developed to represent the umbrella of third genders from throughout AIAN culture, and as a result, many AIAN individuals actually reject the term two-spirit, instead preferring to use the historical term from their traditional language. Interestingly, the concept of two-spirit has begun to be appropriated within the LGBTQ community, with some non-AIAN individuals identifying with the term. It is unclear how the usage of this term will continue to evolve and if AIAN populations will resist its appropriation by the broader community.

CASE STUDY	THE USE OF TRADITIONAL HEALING CEREMONIES

Traditional healing ceremonies are an integral part of Native spirituality. Health and spirituality cannot be separated for the traditional indigenous person. Until 1978, with the American Indian Religious Freedom Act (AIRFA), AI, Alaska Native, and Native Hawaiian people could not openly participate in traditional healing ceremonies. For almost 100 years before AIRFA, there was a concerted effort to eradicate Indian ceremonies and practices through harsh punishments. Ceremonies and ceremonial participation continued, but with great secrecy. Today, many tribal members residing in remote, rural, and urban settings continue to utilize Native healing ceremonies. These daily rituals are implemented by individuals, regardless of environment, setting, and circumstances. The use of tribal ceremonies as healing and wellness mechanisms are beginning to be acknowledged as having credibility in Western-integrated healthcare settings. Among the Navajo, use of Native healers for medical conditions is common, and this corroborates other research suggesting that alternative medicine is widely used by many cultural groups for common diseases (Kim & Kwok, 1998). Traditional treatment is often sought in lieu of Western medical and psychological interventions for serious medical conditions. Unfortunately, blatant cultural appropriation has resulted in healers directing patients not to reveal the methodologies, interventions, ceremony, or even their personal identity because there have been medical providers that badger traditional healers and seek to analyze every portion of the healing that has been successful. How does one analyze the spirit?

The use of tribal ceremonies to promote mental health is also common. We have many Native warriors returning home from military conflicts carrying psychological burdens. Native people have an extended history of enlisting in military service at greater rates than any other ethnic group even before they were officially recognized as American citizens. Native people have their own systems of protection and healing seldom recognized by dominant society. Upon return to their tribal homelands, some of these veterans have opted to go the traditional way and use traditional ceremony as their healing intervention of choice. In the Arizona desert, wounded warriors from the Hopi Nation can join in a ceremony called Wiping Away the Tears. The traditional cleansing ritual helps dispel a chronic "ghost sickness" that can haunt survivors of battle. These and other traditional healing therapies are the treatment of choice for many Native American veterans—half of whom say usual PTSD treatments don't work (Phillips, 2014; Urquhart, Hale, Shah, & Erdman, 2016). Villanueva (2003) conducted a study in a Southwestern tribe pertaining to the correlation between PTSD and alcohol. He found the lowest scores on PTSD instrumentation in those males that had been "initiated into the highest (traditional) religious societies" (p. 1375). In a study conducted by Ogle, Kyle, and West (2010), 35 Native American veterans were surveyed about their participation in Pow Wow gatherings and Sweat Lodge ceremonies and sobriety and PTSD symptoms. Of those that were surveyed with PTSD symptoms, 18 participated in Pow Wows with 89% indicating participation positively impacted their symptoms; of the 14 that participated in Sweat Lodge, 90% "agreed" or "strongly agreed" that participation positively impacted their PTSD symptoms. Gone (2019) has argued for a further expansion of traditional practices in mental health, stating it is essential to recover indigenous knowledge traditions in psychology to create an "AlterNative" to current psychology. In doing

(continued)

so, he argues that "ceremonial petition is therapeutically beneficial because in yielding a 'good, clean mind' it restores one's facility and potency for exercising thought-wish toward bringing one's desires into reality" (p. 11).

Therefore, based upon these examples, implementation of traditional knowledge, traditional ways of knowing, and ceremony continue to have beneficial healing qualities for Native people. Empirically, there also exists proof from a scientific standpoint that indigenous biopsychosocial methodological models are effective in disabling distress, increasing healing, and promoting wellness for Native peoples (Gone, 2019). From this perspective, mental health services, encased in aboriginal psychological interventions and ceremony, can work to remedy the most severe psychological concerns. These traditional forms of healing are egalitarian to Western ways of healing. When fully acknowledged and credentialed as such, the Native American model of health, incorporating a holistic worldview and collectivistic perspectives, will complement, or supersede, other forms of healing.

CURRENT EVENT

THE MASTER SETTLEMENT AGREEMENT

The Master Settlement Agreement, focusing on the health burden created by cigarette manufacturers knowingly distributing an addictive and carcinogenic product, has generated more than $100 billion in prevention funding across the United States. The Agreement, originally reached between 46 states and multiple territories, was designed to "repay" states for the cost of tobacco-related healthcare. However, as sovereign nations, tribes were not included in the Agreement and have not benefited proportional to need from the massive prevention campaigns the Agreement has supported (Warne et al., 2012). Many perceived the Agreement as a panacea for prevention, yet the population in most need of prevention work was excluded from the settlement. There have been decades of attempts to hold tobacco companies equally accountable to the impact on AIAN populations, but there has been little legal traction gained and federal courts have repeatedly dismissed cases tribes have brought related to their exclusion from the settlement agreement. It is currently up to individual states to determine the degree to which settlement funds will be used to address prevention directly within AIAN communities.

DISCUSSION QUESTIONS

- How does the diversity of AIAN populations affect the ways in which evidence-based practices should be implemented?

- In what ways could historical mistrust affect participation in health promotion programs, even those designed to be culturally affirming?

- How can community-based methods of health equity research help to counteract the effects of historical trauma for AIAN populations?

- What are some of the social determinants of health that impact pressing health disparities in AIAN populations, and how can they be addressed appropriately?

- What are some of the facets of AIAN culture that provide unique opportunities for the development of impactful, culturally driven interventions and programs?

REFERENCES

Adams, D. W. (1995). *Education for extinction: American Indians and the boarding school experience, 1875–1928*. Lawrence: University of Kansas Press.

American Indian Religious Freedom Act, Public Law No. 95-341, 92 Stat. 469 (Aug. 11, 1978).

Association of American Indian Physicians. (n.d.). *Strengthening our Native communities: How understanding adverse childhood experiences can help*. Retrieved from https://www.aaip.org/programs/aces-toolkit/

Bachman, R., Zaykowski, H., Kallmyer, R., Poteyeva, M., & Lanier, C. (2008). *Violence against American Indian and Alaska Native women and the criminal justice response: What is known*. Washington, DC: Center for Victim Research. Retrieved from https://ncvc.dspacedirect.org/handle/20.500.11990/197

Baldwin, L., Grossman, D. C., Murowchick, E., Larson, E. H., Hollow, W. B., Sugarman, J. R., . . . Hart, L. G. (2009). Trends in perinatal and infant health disparities between rural American Indians and Alaska Natives and rural Whites. *American Journal of Public Health, 99*(4), 638–646. doi:10.2105/AJPH.2007.119735

Barker, B., Goodman, M. A., & DeBeck, K. (2017). Reclaiming indigenous identities: Culture as strength against suicide among indigenous youth in Canada. *Canadian Journal of Public Health, 108*, e208–e210. doi:10.17269/CJPH.108.5754

Barlow, A., Tingey, L., Cwik, M., Goklish, N., Larzelere-Hinton, F., Lee, A., ... Walkup, J. T. (2012). Understanding the relationship between substance use and self-injury in American Indian youth. *The American Journal of Drug and Alcohol Abuse, 38*(5), 403–408. doi:10.3109/00952990.2012.696757

Bear, C. (2008). American Indian boarding schools haunt many. *National Public Radio Morning Edition*. Retrieved from https://www.npr.org/templates/story/story.php?storyId=16516865

Bearinger, L. H., Pettingell, S., Resnick, M. D., Skay, C. L., Potthoff, S. J., & Eichhorn, J. (2005). Violence perpetration among urban American Indian youth: Can protection offset risk? *Archives of Pediatric Adolescent Medicine, 159*(3), 270–277. doi:10.1001/archpedi.159.3.270

Beauvais, F., & LaBoueff, S. (1985). Drug and alcohol abuse intervention in American Indian communities. *International Journal of the Addictions, 20*, 139–171. doi:10.3109/10826088509074831

Bezdek, M., & Spicer, P. (2006). Maintaining abstinence in a Northern Plains tribe. *Medical Anthropology Quarterly, 20*(2), 160–181. doi:10.1525/maq.2006.20.2.160

Bigfoot, D., & Funderburk, B. (2011). Honoring children, making relatives: The cultural translation of parent-child interaction therapy for American Indian and Alaska Native families. *Journal of Psychoactive Drugs, 43*, 309–318. doi:10.1080/02791072.2011.628924

Bohn, D. K. (2003). Lifetime physical and sexual abuse, substance abuse, depression, and suicide attempts among Native American women. *Issues in Mental Health Nursing, 24*(3), 333–352. doi:10.1080/01612840305277

Boyd, B., & Hunsaker, R. (2018). Cognitive behavioral models, measures, and treatments for stress disorders in American Indians and Alaska Natives. In E. C. Chang, C. A. Downey, J. K. Hirsch, & E. A. Yu (Eds.), *Cultural, racial, and ethnic psychology book series. Treating depression, anxiety, and stress in ethnic and racial groups: Cognitive behavioral approaches* (pp. 313–336). Washington, DC: American Psychological Association.

Brave Heart, M. Y. H. (2003). The historical trauma response among Natives and its relationship with substance abuse: A Lakota illustration. *Journal of Psychoactive Drugs, 35*(1), 7–13. doi:10.1080/02791072.2003.10399988

Brown, R. A. (2010). Crystal methamphetamine use among American Indian and White youth in Appalachia: Social context, masculinity, and desistance. *Addiction Research & Theory, 18*(3), 250–269. doi:10.3109/16066350902802319

Carlson, A. E., Aronson, B. D., Unzen, M., Lewis, M., Benjamin, G. J., & Walls, M. L. (2017). Apathy and type 2 diabetes among American Indians: Exploring the protective effects of traditional cultural involvement. *Journal of Health Care for the Poor and Underserved, 28*(2), 770–783. doi:10.1353/hpu.2017.0073

Carter, V. B. (2010). Factors predicting placement of urban American Indian/Alaska Natives into out-of-home care. *Children and Youth Services Review, 32*(5), 657–663. doi:10.1016/j.childyouth.2009.12.013

Castor, M. L., Smyser, M. S., Taualii, M. M., Park, A. N., Lawson, S. A., & Forguera, R. A. (2006). A nationwide population-based study identifying health disparities between American Indians/Alaska Natives and the general populations living in select urban counties. *American Journal of Public Health, 96*(8), 1478–1484. doi:10.2105/AJPH.2004.053942

Centers for Disease Control and Prevention. (2008). Alcohol-attributable deaths and years of potential life lost among American Indians and Alaska Natives: United States, 2001–2005. *Morbidity and Mortality Weekly Report, 57*(34), 938–941. Retrieved from https://www.cdc.gov/mmwr/preview/mmwrhtml/mm5734a3.htm

Chambers, R. A., Rosenstock, S., Neault, N., Kenney, A., Richards, J., Begay, K., ... Barlow, A. (2015). A home-visiting diabetes prevention and management program for American Indian youth: The Together on Diabetes trial. *The Diabetes Educator, 41*(6), 729–747. doi:10.1177/0145721715608953

Chester, B., Robin, R. W., Koss, M. P., Lopez, J., & Goldman, D. (1994). Grandmother dishonored: Violence against women by male partners in American Indian communities. *Violence and Victims, 9*(3), 249–258. doi:10.1891/0886-6708.9.3.249

Costello, E. J., Farmer, E. M., Angold, A., Burns, B. J., & Erkanli, A. (1997). Psychiatric disorders among American Indian and white youth in Appalachia: The Great Smoky Mountains Study. *American Journal of Public Health, 87*(5), 827–832. doi:10.2105/AJPH.87.5.827

Crofoot, T. L., & Harris, M. S. (2012). An Indian Child Welfare perspective on disproportionality in child welfare. *Children and Youth Services Review, 34*(9), 1667–1674. doi:10.1016/j.childyouth.2012.04.028

Cross, T. A., Earle, K. A., & Simmons, D. (2000). Child abuse and neglect in Indian country: Policy issues. *Families in Society, 81*(1), 49–58. doi:10.1606/1044-3894.1092

Cunningham, J. K., Solomon, T. A., & Muramoto, M. L. (2016). Alcohol use among Native Americans compared to whites: Examining the veracity of the "Native American elevated alcohol consumption" belief. *Drug and Alcohol Dependence, 160*, 65–75. doi:10.1016/j.drugalcdep.2015.12.015

Dewees, S., & Marks, B. (2017). *Twice invisible: Understanding rural Native America (Research Note #2)*. Longmont, CO: First Nations Development Institute. Retrieved from https://www.usetinc.org/wp-content/uploads/bvenuti/WWS/2017/May%202017/May%208/Twice%20Invisible%20-%20Research%20Note.pdf

Dickerson, D., Robichaud, F., Teruya, C., Nagaran, K., & Hser, Y. (2012). Utilizing drumming for American Indians/Alaska Natives with substance use disorders: A focus group study. *The American Journal of Drug and Alcohol Abuse, 38*(5), 505–510. doi:10.3109/00952990.2012.699565

Dill, E. J., Manson, S. M., Jiang, L., Pratte, K. A., Gutilla, M. J., Knepper, S. L., ... Roubideaux, Y. (2016). Psychosocial predictors of weight loss among American Indian and Alaska Native participants in a diabetes prevention translational project. *Journal of Diabetes Research, 2016*, 1546939. doi:10.1155/2016/1546939

Dorgan, B. L. (2010). The tragedy of Native American youth suicide. *Psychological Services, 7*(3), 213–218. doi:/10.1037/a0020461

Duran, B., Sanders, M., Skipper, B., Waitzkin, H., Malcoh, L. H., Paine, S., & Yager, J. (2004). Prevalence and correlates of mental disorders among Native American women in primary care. *American Journal of Public Health, 94*(1), 71–77. doi:10.2105/AJPH.94.1.71

Edwards, E. D., & Edwards, M. E. (1988). Alcoholism prevention treatment and Native American youth: A community approach. *Journal of Drug Issues, 18*, 103–115. doi:10.1177/002204268801800110

Eschiti, V. S. (2004). Holistic approach to resolving American Indian/Alaska Native health care disparities. *Journal of Holistic Nursing, 22*(3), 200–208. doi:10.1177/0898010104266713

Evans-Campbell, T., Lindhorst, T., Huang, B., & Walters, K. L. (2006). Interpersonal violence in the lives of urban American Indian and Alaska Native women: Implications for health, mental health, and help-seeking. *American Journal of Public Health, 96*(8), 1416–1422. doi:10.2105/AJPH.2004.054213

Evans-Campbell, T., Walters, K. L., Pearson, C. R., & Campbell, C. D. (2012). Indian boarding school experience, substance use, and mental health among urban two-spirit American Indian/Alaska Natives. *The American Journal of Drug and Alcohol Abuse, 38*(5), 421–427. doi:10.3109/00952990.2012.701358

Flynn, S. V., Olson, S. D., & Yellig, A. D. (2014). American Indian acculturation: Tribal lands to predominately white postsecondary settings. *Journal of Counseling and Development, 92*, 280–293.

Francis, C. D., & Chino, M. (2012). Type 2 diabetes science and American Indian/Alaska Native culture: Creating a national K–12 curriculum prevention strategy for Native youth. *Diabetes Spectrum, 25*(1), 23–25. doi:10.2337/diaspect.25.1.23

Gittelsohn, J., & Rowan, M. (2011). Preventing diabetes and obesity in American Indian communities: The potential of environmental interventions. *The American Journal of Clinical Nutrition, 93*(5), 1179S–1183S. doi:10.3945/ajcn.110.003509

Goins, R. T., Noonan, C., Gonzales, K., Winchester, B., & Bradley, V. L. (2017). Association of depressive symptomology and psychological trauma with diabetes control among older American Indian women: Does social support matter? *Journal of Diabetes and Its Complications, 31*(4), 669–674. doi:10.1016/j.jdiacomp.2017.01.004

Gone, J. P. (2019). "The thing happened as he wished": Recovering an American Indian cultural psychology. *American Journal of Community Psychology, 64*(1/2), 172–184. doi:10.1002/ajcp.12353

Gone, J. P., & Calf Looking, P. E. (2011). American Indian culture as a substance abuse treatment: Pursuing evidence for a local intervention. *Journal of Psychoactive Drugs, 43*(4), 291–296. doi:10.1080/02791072.2011.628915

Gonzales, K., Roeber, J., Kanny, D., Tran, A., Saiki, C., ... Geiger, S. D. (2014). Alcohol-attributable deaths and years of potential life lost - 11 states, 2006-2010. *Morbidity and Mortality Weekly Report, 63*(1), 213–216. Retrieved from https://www.cdc.gov/mmwr/preview/mmwrhtml/mm6310a2.htm

Gonzales, K. L., Harding, A. K., Lambert, W. E., Fu, R., & Henderson, W. G. (2013). Perceived experiences of discrimination in health care: A barrier for cancer screening among American Indian women with type 2 diabetes. *Women's Health Issues, 23*(1), e61–e67. doi:10.1016/j.whi.2012.10.004

Gonzales, K. L., Lambert, W. E., Fu, W. E., Jacob, M., & Hardin, A. K. (2014). Perceived racial discrimination in health care, completion of standard diabetes services, and diabetes control among a sample of American Indian women. *The Diabetes Educator, 40*(6), 747–755. doi:10.1177/0145721714551422

Gonzalez, V. M., & Skewes, M. C. (2016). Association of the firewater myth with drinking behavior among American Indian and Alaska Native college students. *Psychology of Addictive Behaviors, 30*(8), 838–849. doi:10.1037/adb0000226

Grandbois, D. (2009). Stigma of mental illness among American Indian and Alaska Native nations: Historical and contemporary perspectives. *Issues in Mental Health Nursing, 26*(10), 1001–1024. doi:10.1080/01612840500280661

Greenfield, B. L., & Venner, K. L. (2012). Review of substance use disorder treatment research in Indian country: Future directions to strive toward health equity. *The American Journal of Drug and Alcohol Abuse, 38*(5), 483–492. doi:10.3109/00952990.2012.702170

Hamby, S. (2008). The path of helpseeking: Perceptions of law enforcement among American Indian victims of sexual assault. *Journal of Prevention and Intervention in the Community, 36*(1/2), 89–104. doi:10.1080/10852350802022340

Hamby, S. L. (2000). The importance of community in a feminist analysis of domestic violence among American Indians. *American Journal of Community Psychology, 28*(5), 649–669. doi:10.1023/A:1005145720371

Hanson, R. L., Muller, Y. L., Kobes, S., Guo, T., Bian, L., ... Baier, L. J. (2014). A genome-wide association study in American Indians implicates DNER as a susceptibility locus for type 2 diabetes. *Diabetes, 63*(1), 369–376. doi:10.2337/db13-0416

Harwell, T. S., Moore, K. R., & Spence, M. R. (2003). Physical violence, intimate partner violence, and emotional abuse among adult American Indian men and women in Montana. *Preventive Medicine, 37*(4), 297–303. doi:10.1016/S0091-7435(03)00136-1

Hawkins, E. H., Cummins, L. H., & Marlatt, G. A. (2004). Preventing substance abuse in American Indian and Alaska Native youth: Promising strategies for healthier communities. *Psychological Bulletin, 130*(2), 304–323. doi:10.1037/0033-2909.130.2.304

Henderson, L. C. (2010). Divergent models of diabetes among American Indian elders. *Journal of Cross-Cultural Gerontology*, *25*, 303–316. doi:10.1007/s10823-010-9128-4

Herne, M. A., Bartholomew, M. L., & Weahkee, R. L. (2014). Suicide mortality among American Indians and Alaska Natives, 1999–2009. *American Journal of Public Health*, *104*(S3), S336–S342. doi:10.2105/AJPH.2014.301929

Hirchak, K. A., & Murphy, S. M. (2016). Assessing differences in the availability of opioid addiction therapy options: Rural versus urban and American Indian reservation versus nonreservation. *Journal of Rural Health*, *33*(1), 102–109. doi:10.1111/jrh.12178

Hutchinson, R. N., & Shin, S. (2014). Systematic review of health disparities for cardiovascular diseases and associated factors among American Indian and Alaska Native populations. *PLoS One*, *9*(1), e80973. doi:10.1371/journal.pone.0080973

Iritani, B. J., Hallfors, D. D., & Bauer, D. J. (2007). Crystal methamphetamine use among young adults in the USA. *Addiction*, *102*(7), 1102–1113. doi:10.1111/j.1360-0443.2007.01847.x

Jacobs, M. D. (2013). Forgotten child: The American Indian child welfare crisis of the 1960s and 1970s. *American Indian Quarterly*, *37*(1/2), 136–159. doi:10.1353/aiq.2013.0014

Jiang, L., Manson, S. M., Beals, J., Henderson, W. G., Huang, H., Acton, K. J., … Roubideaux, Y. (2013). Translating the Diabetes Prevention Program into American Indian and Alaska Native communities. *Diabetes Care*, *36*(7), 2027–2034. doi:10.2337/dc12-1250

Jones, D. S. (2006). The persistence of American Indian health disparities. *American Journal of Public Health*, *96*(12), 2122–2134. doi:10.2105/AJPH.2004.054262

Kattelmann, K. K., Conti, K., & Ren, C. (2010). The medicine wheel nutrition intervention: A diabetes education study with the Cheyenne River Sioux tribe. *Journal of the American Dietetic Association*, *110*(5), S44–S51. doi:10.1016/j.jada.2010.03.003

Kenney, M. K., & Singh, G. K. (2016). Adverse childhood experiences among American Indian/Alaska Native children: The 2011-2012 National Survey of Children's Health. *Scientifica*, *2016*, 7424239. doi:10.1155/2016/7424239

Kim, C., & Kwok, Y. S. (1998). Navajo use of native healers. *Archives of Internal Medicine*, *158*(20), 2245–2249. doi:10.1001/archinte.158.20.2245

Knowler, W. C., Pettit, D. J., Saad, M. F., & Bennett, P. H. (1990). Diabetes mellitus in the Pima Indians: Incidence, risk, factors, and pathogenesis. *Diabetes Metabolism Research and Reviews*, *6*(1), 1–27. doi:10.1002/dmr.5610060101

Kulis, S., Hodge, D. R., Ayers, S. L., Brown, E. F., & Marsiglia, F. F. (2012). Spirituality and religion: Intertwined protective factors for substance use among urban American Indian youth. *The American Journal of Drug and Alcohol Abuse*, *38*(5), 444–449. doi:10.3109/00952990.2012.670338

Kulis, S., Napoli, M., & Marsiglia, F. F. (2002). Ethnic pride, biculturalism, and drug use norms of urban American Indian adolescents. *Social Work Research*, *26*(2), 101–112. doi:10.1093/swr/26.2.101

Kumpfer, K. L., Alvarado, R., Smith, P., & Bellamy, N. (2002). Cultural sensitivity in universal family-based prevention interventions. *Prevention Science*, *3*, 241–244. doi:10.1023/A:1019902902119

Landers, A. L., & Danes, S. M. (2016). Forgotten children: A critical review of the reunification of American Indian children in the child welfare system. *Children and Youth Services Review*, *71*, 137–147. doi:10.1016/j.childyouth.2016.10.043

Lanier, C., & Huff-Corzine, L. (2006). American Indian homicide: A county-level analysis utilizing social disorganization theory. *Homicide Studies*, *10*(3), 181–194. doi:10.1177/1088767906288573

Lawler, M. J., LaPlante, K. D., Giger, J. T., & Norris, D. S. (2012). Overrepresentation of Native American children in foster care: An independent construct? *Journal of Ethnic and Cultural Diversity in Social Work*, *21*(2), 95–110. doi:10.1080/15313204.2012.647344

Lawrence, J. (2000). The Indian Health Service and the sterilization of Native American women. *American Indian Quarterly*, *24*(3), 400–419. doi:10.1353/aiq.2000.0008

Lee, E. T., Howard, B. V., Savage, P. J., Cowan, L. D., Fabsitz, R. R., Oopik, A. J., … Welty, T. K. (1995). Diabetes and impaired glucose tolerance in three American Indian populations aged 45–74 years: The Strong Heart Study. *Diabetes Care*, *18*(5), 599–610. doi:10.2337/diacare.18.5.599

Legha, R. K., & Novins, D. (2012). The role of culture in substance abuse treatment programs for American Indian and Alaska Native communities. *Psychiatric Services*, *63*(7), 686–692. doi:10.1176/appi.ps.201100399

LeMaster, P. L., Connell, C. M., Mitchell, C. M., & Manson, S. M. (2002). Tobacco use among American Indian adolescents: Protective and risk factors. *Journal of Adolescent Health*, *30*, 426–432. doi:10.1016/S1054-139X(01)00411-6

Looker, H. C., Krakoff, J., Andre, V., Kobus, K., Nelson, R. G., Knowler, W. C., & Hanson, R. L. (2010). Secular trends in treatment and control of type 2 diabetes in an American Indian population: A 30-year longitudinal study. *Diabetes Care*, *33*(11), 2383–2389. doi:10.2337/dc10-0678

Lowe, J., Liang, H., Riggs, C., & Henson, J. (2012). Community partnership to affect substance abuse among Native American adolescents. *The American Journal of Drug and Alcohol Abuse*, *38*(5), 450–455. doi:10.3109/00952990.2012.694534

Mallory, A., & Whitbeck, L. (2007). *Shonga ska: Sacred horse society* (Final report to the Omaha Tribe). Unpublished tribal report, Lincoln, NE.

Manson, S. M., Beals, J., Klein, S. A., & Croy, C. D. (2005). Social epidemiology of trauma among 2 American Indian reservation populations. *American Journal of Public Health*, *95*(5), 851–859. doi:10.2105/AJPH.2004.054171

Manson, S. P. (2001). Behavioral health services for American Indians: Need, use, and barriers to effective care. In M. Dixon & Y Roubideaux (Eds.), *Promises to keep: Public health policy for American Indians and Alaska Natives in the 21st century* (pp. 167–192). Washington, DC: American Public Health Association.

Marlatt, G. A., Larimer, M. E., Mail, P. D., Hawkins, E. H., Cummins, L. H., Blume, A. W., ... Gallion, S. (2003). Journeys of the circle: A culturally congruent life skills intervention for adolescent Indian drinking. *Alcoholism: Clinical and Experimental Research*, *27*(8), 1327–1329. doi:10.1097/01.ALC.0000080345.04590.52

McLaughlin, S. (2010). Traditions and diabetes prevention: A healthy path for Native Americans. *Diabetes Spectrum*, *23*(4), 272–277. doi:10.2337/diaspect.23.4.272

McOliver, C. A., Campter, A. K., Doyle, J. T., Eggers, M. J., Ford, T. E., Lila, M. A., ... Donatuto, J. (2015). Community-based research as a mechanism to reduce environmental health disparities in American Indian and Alaska Native communities. *International Journal of Environmental Research in Public Health*, *12*, 4076–4100. doi:10.3390/ijerph120404076

Mellanby, A. R., Rees, J. B., & Tripp, J. H. (2000). Peer-led and adult-led school health education: A critical review of available comparative research. *Health Education Research*, *15*, 533–545. doi:10.1093/her/15.5.533

Mendenhall, T. J., Berge, J. M., Harper, P., GreenCrow, B., LittleWalker, N., WhiteEagle, S., & BrownOwl, S. (2010). The Family Education Diabetes Series (FEDS): Community-based participatory research with a Midwestern American Indian community. *Nursing Inquiry*, *17*(4), 359–372. doi:10.1111/j.1440-1800.2010.00508.x

Mulligan, C. J., Robin, R. W., Osier, M. V., Sambuughin, N., Goldfarb, L. G., Kittles, R. A., ... Long, J. C. (2003). Allelic variation at alcohol metabolism genes (ADH1B, ADH1C, ALDH2) and alcohol dependence in an American Indian population. *Human Genetics*, *113*(4), 325–336. doi:10.1007/s00439-003-0971-z

Narayanan, M. L., Schraer, C. D., Bulkow, L. R., Koller, K. R., Asay, E., Mayer, A. M., & Raymer, T. W. (2010). Diabetes prevalence, incidence, complications, and mortality among Alaska Native people 1985–2006. *International Journal of Circumpolar Health*, *69*(3), 236–252. doi:10.3402/ijch.v69i3.17618

Nash, D. A., & Nagel, R. J. (2005). Confronting oral health disparities among American Indian/Alaska Native children: The pediatric oral health therapist. *American Journal of Public Health*, *95*(8), 1325–1329. doi:10.2105/AJPH.2005.061796

National Council of Urban Indian Health. (n.d.). *NCUIH membership*. Retrieved from https://www.ncuih.org/UIHOs_locations

Northern Plains Reservation Aid. (2019). *History and culture: Boarding schools*. Retrieved from http://www.nativepartnership.org/site/PageServer?pagename=airc_hist_boardingschools

Norton, I. M., & Manson, S. M. (1997). Domestic violence intervention in an urban Indian Health Center. *Community Mental Health Journal*, *33*, 331–337. doi:10.1023/A:1025051325351

Novins, D. K., Boyd, M. L., Brotherton, D. T., Fickenscher, A., Moore, L., & Spicer, P. (2012). Walking on: Celebrating the journeys of traumatized Native American adolescents with substance use problems on the winding road to healing. *Journal of Psychoactive Drugs, 44*(2), 153–159. doi:10.1080/02791072.2012 .684628

Nsiah-Kumi, P. A., Erickson, J. M., Beals, J. L., Ogle, E. A., Whiting, M., Brushbreaker, C., … Larsen, J. L. (2012). Vitamin d insufficiency is associated with diabetes risk in Native American children. *Clinical Pediatrics, 51*(2), 146–153. doi:10.1177/0009922811417290

Nsiah-Kumi, P. A., Lasley, S., Whiting, M., Brushbreaker, C., Erickson, J. M., Qiu, F., … Larsen, J. L. (2013). Diabetes, pre-diabetes, and insulin resistance screening in Native American children and youth. *International Journal of Obesity, 37*, 540–545. doi:10.1038/ijo.2012.199

O'Brien, K., Pecora, P. J., Echohawk, L. A., Evans-Campbell, T., Palmanteer-Holder, N., & White, C. R. (2010). Educational and employment achievements of American Indian/Alaska Native alumni of foster care. *Families in Society, 91*(2), 149–157. doi:10.1606/1044.3894.3974

O'Connell, J., Yi, R., Wilson, C., Manson, S. M., & Acton, K. J. (2010). Racial disparities in health status: A comparison of the morbidity among American Indian and U.S. adults with diabetes. *Diabetes Care, 33*(7), 1463–1470. doi:10.2337/dc09-1652

O'Connell, J. M., Novins, D. K., Beals, J., & Spicer, P. (2005). Disparities in patterns of alcohol use among reservation-based and geographically dispersed American Indian populations. *Alcoholism: Clinical and Experimental Research, 29*(1), 107–116. doi:10.1097/01.ALC.0000153789.59228.FC

Oetting, E. R., & Donnermeyer, J. F. (1998). Primary socialization theory: The etiology of drug use and deviance. *Substance Use & Misuse, 33*, 995–1026. doi:10.3109/10826089809056252

Oetzel, J., & Duran, B. (2004). Intimate partner violence in American Indian and/or Alaska Native communities: A social ecological framework of determinants and interventions. *American Indian and Alaska Native Mental Health Research, 11*(3), 49–68. doi:10.5820/aian.1103.2004.49

Ogle, D. R., Kyle, P., & West, D. (2010). Efficacy of traditional Native American practices: *Powwow gatherings and sweat lodge ceremony on veteran populations.* Paper session presented at the meeting of 19th Annual Convention of the Western Psychological Association, Cancun, Mexico.

Onco, L. T. (2019). *Victory: The Violence Against Women Act passes House with Tribal provisions.* Retrieved from https://www.fcnl.org/updates/victory-the-violence-against-women-act-passes-house-with-tribal -provisions-2036

Pardilla, M., Prasad, D., Suratkar, S., & Gittelsohn, J. (2013). High levels of household food insecurity on the Navajo Nation. *Public Health Nutrition, 17*(1), 58–65. doi:10.1017/S1368980012005630

Petoskey, E. L., Van Stelle, K. R., & De Jong, J. A. (1998). Prevention through empowerment in a Native American community. *Drugs and Society, 12*, 147–162. doi:10.1300/J023v12n01_10

Phillips, R. E. (2014). Ceremonial PTSD therapies favored by Native American veterans. *Washington State University Insider.* Retrieved from https://news.wsu.edu/2014/06/17/ceremonial-ptsd-therapies-favored-by -native-american-veterans

Phipps, K. R., Ricks, T. L., Manz, M. C., & Blahut, P. (2012). Prevalence and severity of dental caries among American Indian and Alaska Native preschool children. *Journal of Public Health Dentistry, 72*(2), 208–215. doi:10.1111/j.1752-7325.2012.00331.x

Pu, J., Chewning, B., St. Clair, I. D., Kokotailo, P. K., Lacourt, J., & Wilson, D. (2013). Protective factors in American Indian communities and adolescent violence. *Maternal and Child Health Journal, 17*, 1199–1207. doi:10.1007/s10995-012-1111-y

Rennison, C. M. (2001). *Violent victimization and race, 1993-98.* Washington, DC: U.S. Department of Justice, Bureau of Justice Statistics. Retrieve from http://ncdsv.org/images/BJS_ViolentVictimization AndRace1993-1998_3-2001.pdf

Rosay, A. B. (2016). *Violence against American Indian and Alaska Native women and men: 2010 findings from The National Intimate Partner and Sexual Violence Survey.* Washington, DC: U.S. Department of Justice, National Institute of Justice. Retrieved from https://www.ncjrs.gov/pdffiles1/nij/249736.pdf

Rosenblaum, T. (2018). Sexual assault trial: Pediatrician's coworker had concerns after 2 months. *Great Falls Tribune.* Retrieved from https://www.greatfallstribune.com/story/news/2018/09/04/ browning-montana-blackfeet-indian-reservation-pediatrician-sexual-assault-trial/1198098002

Ross, R. J. (2018). *American Indian Biculturalism Inventory - Pueblo.* Proquest Theses and Dissertations. Retrieved from https://commons.und.edu/theses/2327

Ross, R. J., GreyWolf, I., Tehee, M., Henry, S. M., & Cheromiah, M. (2018). Missing and murdered indigenous women and girls. *Society of Indian Psychologists,* 1–6. doi:10.17605/OSF.IO/4KMNS

Russo, D., Purohit, V., Foudin, L., & Salin, M. (2004). Workshop on alcohol use and health disparities 2002: A call to arms. *Alcohol, 32*(1), 37–43. doi:10.1016/j.alcohol.2004.01.003

Sarche, M., & Spicer, P. (2008). Poverty and health disparities for American Indian and Alaska Native children: Current knowledge and future prospects. *Annals of the New York Academy of Science, 1136,* 126–136. doi:10.1196/annals.1425.017

Satterfield, D., DeBruyn, L., Santos, M., Alonso, L., & Frank, M. (2016). Health promotion and diabetes prevention in American Indian and Alaska Native communities: Traditional Foods Project, 2008-2014. *Morbidity and Mortality Weekly Report, 65*(1), 4–10. doi:10.15585/mmwr.su6501a3

Schinke, S. P., Botvin, G. J., Trimble, J. E., Orlandi, M. A., Gilchrist, L. D., & Locklear, V. S. (1988). Preventing substance abuse among American Indian adolescents: A bicultural competence skills approach. *Journal of Counseling Psychology, 35,* 87–90. doi:10.1037/0022-0167.35.1.87

Shaw, J. L., Brown, J., Khan, B., Mau, M. K., & Dillard, D. (2013). Resources, roadblocks, and turning points: A qualitative study of American Indian/Alaska Native adults with type 2 diabetes. *Journal of Community Health, 38*(1), 86–94. doi:10.1007/s10900-012-9585-5

Sittner, K. J., Greenfield, B. L., & Walls, M. L. (2018). Microaggressions, diabetes distress, and self-care behaviors in a sample of American Indian adults with type 2 diabetes. *Journal of Behavioral Medicine, 41,* 122–129. doi:10.1007/s10865-017-9898-z

Smith, A. (2015). *Conquest: Sexual violence and American Indian genocide.* Durham, NC: Duke University Press.

Spear, S., Crevecoeur, D. A., Rawson, R. A., & Clark, R. (2007). The rise in methamphetamine use among American Indians in Los Angeles county. *American Indian and Alaska Native Mental Health Research, 14*(2), 1–15. doi:10.5820/aian.1402.2007.1

Spicer, P. (2001). Culture and the restoration of self among former American Indian drinkers. *Social Science & Medicine, 53*(2), 227–240. doi:10.1016/S0277-9536(00)00333-6

Spindler, G. D., & Spindler, L. S. (1978). Identity, militancy, and cultural congruence: The Menomonee and Kainai. *Annals of the American Academy of Political and Social Science, 436,* 73–85. doi:10.1177/000271627843600108

Tann, S. S., Yabiku, S. T., Okamoto, S. K., & Yanow, J. (2007). triADD: The risk for alcohol abuse, depression, and diabetes multimorbidity in the American Indian and Alaska Native population. *American Indian and Alaska Native Mental Health Research, 14*(1), 1–23. doi:10.5820/aian.1401.2007.5

Tehee, M., & Esqueda, C. W. (2008). American Indian and European American women's perceptions of domestic violence. *Journal of Family Violence, 23*(1), 25–35. doi:10.1007/s10896-007-9126-7

Thomas, L. R., Donovan, D. M., Sigo, R. L. W., Austin, L., & Marlatt, G. A. (2009). The community pulling together: A tribal community–university partnership project to reduce substance abuse and promote good health in a reservation tribal community. *Journal of Ethnicity and Substance Abuse, 8,* 283–296. doi:10.1080/15332640903110476

Thurman, P. J., & Green, V. A. (1997). American Indian inhalant use. *American Indian and Alaska Native Mental Health Research, 8,* 24–40. doi:10.5820/aian.0801.1997.24

Urban Indian Health Institute. (2018). *Missing and Murdered Indigenous Women and Girls Report.* Retrieved from https://www.uihi.org/wp-content/uploads/2018/11/Missing-and-Murdered-Indigenous -Women-and-Girls-Report.pdf

Urquhart, G., Hale, M., Shah, N. A., & Erdman, P. (2016). *Native American veteran treatment preferences: Results from an ongoing survey.* Retrieved from https://openjournals.wsu.edu/index.php/mestizo/article/ view/1450/836

U.S. Census Bureau. (2007). *We the People: American Indians and Alaska Natives in the United States, 2007.* Retrieved from https://www.census.gov/prod/2006pubs/censr-28.pdf

U.S. Census Bureau. (2019). *QuickFacts: United States.* Retrieved from https://www.census.gov/quickfacts/ fact/table/US/PST045218

U.S. Department of Agriculture. (2019). *USDA food access research atlas*. Retrieved from https://www.ers.usda.gov/data-products/food-access-research-atlas/go-to-the-atlas

Villanueva, M. (2003). Posttraumatic stress disorder, alcohol, and tribes: Obstacles to research. *Alcoholism: Clinical and Experimental Research, 27*(8), 1374–1380. doi:10.1097/01.ALC.0000080163.54436.3F

Walters, K. L., & Simoni, J. M. (2009). Decolonizing strategies for mentoring American Indians and Alaska Natives in HIV and mental health research. *American Journal of Public Health, 99*(s1), s71–s76. doi:10.2105/AJPH.2008.136127

Wall, T. L., Garcia-Andrade, C., Wong, V., Lau, P., & Ehlers, C. L. (2006). Parental history of alcoholism and problem behaviors in Native-American children and adolescents. *Alcoholism: Clinical and Experimental Research, 24*(1), 30–34. doi:10.1111/j.1530-0277.2000.tb04549.x

Walls, M. L., Gonzalez, J., Gladney, T., & Onello, E. (2015). Unconscious bias: Racial microaggressions in American Indian health care. *Journal of the American Board of Family Medicine, 28*(2), 231–239. doi:10.3122/jabfm.2015.02.140194

Warne, D., Kaur, J., & Perdue, D. (2012). American Indian/Alaska Native cancer policy: Systemic approaches to reducing cancer disparities. *Journal of Cancer Education, 27*(s1), 18–23. doi:10.1007/s13187-012-0315-6

Warne, D., & Lajimodiere, D. (2015). American Indian health disparities: Psychosocial influences. *Social and Personality Psychology Compass, 9/10*, 567–579. doi:10.1111/spc3.12198

Weaver, H. N. (2009). The colonial context of violence: Reflections on violence in the lives of Native American women. *Journal of Interpersonal Violence, 24*(9), 1552–1563. doi:10.1177/0886260508323665

Wexler, L. (2014). Looking across three generations of Alaska Natives to explore how culture fosters indigenous resilience. *Transcultural Psychiatry, 51*(1), 73–92. doi:10.1177/1363461513497417

Wexler, L., Chandler, M., Gone, J. P., Cwik, M., Kirmayer, L. J., LaFromboise, T., . . . Allen, J. (2015). Advancing suicide prevention research with rural American Indian and Alaska Native populations. *American Journal of Public Health, 105*(5), 891–899. doi:10.2105/AJPH.2014.302517

Whitbeck, L. B., Hoyt, D. R., McMorris, B. J., Chen, A., & Stubben, J. D. (2001). Perceived discrimination and early substance abuse among American Indian children. *Journal of Health and Social Behavior, 42*, 405–424. doi:10.2307/3090187

Whitbeck, L. B., Wells, M. L., & Welch, M. L. (2012). Substance abuse prevention in American Indian and Alaska Native communities. *The American Journal of Drug and Alcohol Abuse, 38*(5), 428–435. doi:10.3109/00952990.2012.695416

Whitesell, N. R., Beals, J., Big Cros, C., Mitchell, C., & Novins, D. K. (2012). Epidemiology and etiology of substance use among American Indians and Alaska Natives: Risk, protection, and implications for prevention. *The American Journal of Drug and Alcohol Abuse, 38*(5), 376–382. doi:10.3109/00952990.2012.694527

Whitesell, N. R., Beals, J., Mitchell, C. M., Manson, S. M., & Turner, R. J. (2009). Childhood exposure to adversity and risk of substance-use disorder in two American Indian populations: The meditational role of early substance-use initiation. *Journal of Studies on Alcohol and Drugs, 70*(6), 971–981. doi:10.15288/jsad.2009.70.971

Wiechelt, S. A., Gryczynski, J., Johnson, J. L., & Caldwell, D. (2012). Historical trauma among urban American Indians: Impact on substance abuse and family cohesion. *Journal of Loss and Trauma, 17*(4), 319–336. doi:10.1080/15325024.2011.616837

Wiedman, D. (2012). Native American embodiment of the chronicities of modernity: Reservation food, diabetes, and the metabolic syndrome among the Kiowa, Comanche, and Apache. *Medical Anthropology Quarterly, 26*(4), 595–612. doi:10.1111/maq.12009

Wilson, C., Civic, D., & Glass, D. (1995). Prevalence and correlates of depressive syndromes among adults visiting an Indian Health Service primary care clinic. *American Indian and Alaska Native Mental Health Research, 6*(2), 1–12. doi:10.5820/aian.0602.1995.1

Zhao, J., Zhu, Y., Lin, J., Matsuguchi, T., Blackburn, E., Zhang, Y., . . . & Howard, B. V. (2014). Short leukocyte telomere length predicts risk of diabetes in American Indians: The Strong Heart Family Study. *Diabetes, 63*(1), 354–362. doi:10.2337/db13-0744

HEALTH EQUITY FOR KĀNAKA 'ŌIWI, THE INDIGENOUS PEOPLE OF HAWAI'I

SHELLEY SOONG ■ MELE A. LOOK ■ JOSEPH KEAWE'AIMOKU KAHOLOKULA ■ MOMI AKANA ■ EARL KAWA'A

LEARNING OBJECTIVES

- Describe the history of occupation and militarization of Hawai'i and the ways in which it influences Kānaka 'Ōiwi health

- Contrast culturally adapted programs, culturally grounded programs, and promising programs in achieving health equity

- Summarize key aspects of Kānaka 'Ōiwi culture that are important in developing health equity initiatives

- Describe key policy changes that could help to improve Kānaka 'Ōiwi health

- Discuss the need for additional work in intersectionality in Kānaka 'Ōiwi health

INTRODUCTION

There exists a well-recognized vitality, resilience, and strength among Kānaka 'Ōiwi (Native Hawaiians; Goodyear-Ka'opua, Hussey, & Wright, 2014). Despite having faced occupation, militarization, and social injustices by the United States, Kānaka 'Ōiwi continue to be an intelligent, strong, resilient, and united people (Chun, 2011; Goodyear-Ka'opua et al., 2014; Kawa'a, 2018). The U.S. Office of Management and Budget aggregates Kānaka 'Ōiwi and all other Pacific Islander groups in the U.S. into a single Native Hawaiian and Other Pacific Islander (NHOPI) racial/ethnic category. NHOPI represents a diverse set of Pacific Islander groups, and Kānaka 'Ōiwi make up the largest subpopulation at 43% (Hixson, Hepler, & Kim, 2012). NHOPI is one of the fastest growing racial/ethnic groups in the nation having grown by 40% from 874,000 in 2000 to 1.2 million in 2010 (Hixson et al., 2012). In 2018, 1.6 million individuals in the U.S. identified as NHOPI (U.S. Census Bureau, 2018), with the largest NHOPI populations residing in Hawai'i, California, Washington, Texas, and Florida (Hixson et al., 2012). In addition to Kānaka 'Ōiwi, other Pacific Islander groups in the U.S. include Samoans, Tongans, Guamanian/Chamorro, Micronesians (people of the Federated States of Micronesia,

Palau, Marshall Islands, and the Commonwealth of the Northern Mariana), and Fijians, each with different languages, customs, histories, acculturation statuses (e.g., indigenous, immigrant, and migrant), and aspirations (Look, Trask-Batti, Agres, Mau, & Kaholokula, 2013; Marck, 2000; Teaiwia, 1994). This chapter will focus on Kānaka ʻŌiwi, the indigenous people of Hawaiʻi.

Kānaka ʻŌiwi continue to experience a greater health burden compared to the overall U.S. racial and ethnic populations (Balabis, Pobutsky, Baker, Tottori, & Salvail, 2007). Compared to the total U.S. population, Kānaka ʻŌiwi not only have a disproportionately higher prevalence of chronic medical conditions, such as diabetes, obesity, and cardiovascular disease (CVD; Aluli, Reyes, & Tsark, 2007; Aluli et al., 2010; Mau, Sinclair, Saito, Baumhofer, & Kaholokula, 2009), but also have greater mortality rates for cancer, stroke, heart disease, and diabetes (Johnson, Oyama, LeMarchand, & Wilkens, 2004). Along with other underrepresented racial and ethnic groups in the U.S. (i.e., American Indians and Alaska Natives [AI/AN], Blacks or African Americans, and Hispanics or Latinos), Kānaka ʻŌiwi have continued to remain part of racial and ethnic health disparities that relentlessly continue to exist in the U.S., despite decades of federal initiatives to achieve health equity (Galinsky, Zelaya, Simile, & Barnes, 2017; Johnson et al., 2004).

As with other indigenous populations, Kānaka ʻŌiwi health disparities continue and can be attributed to a variety of complex and interconnected social determinants of health that include historical trauma, discrimination, and lifestyle changes (Blaisdell, 1995; Kaholokula, Iwane, & Nacapoy, 2010). Historical trauma can be described as a type of psychological wounding experienced by indigenous communities because of past and present transgressions (e.g., interpersonal violence, forced displacement from ancestral lands, cultural and language loss, compulsory acculturation strategies, and overt and covert discrimination); in addition, this trauma can be intergenerational (i.e., transmitted from one generation to the next) and relived by indigenous peoples through both narrative forms and their lived experiences of stigmatization (Kaholokula, Miyamoto, Hermosura, & Inada, 2020; Sotero, 2006). The complexity of the problem has been further heightened by an overlay of socioeconomic and sociocultural challenges (Kaholokula, Nacapoy, & Dang, 2009). In order to comprehensively understand Kānaka ʻŌiwi health disparities, it is important to understand the broader historical and sociopolitical framework that has led to their existence.

In this chapter, we first provide a post-Western contact, historical overview of Kānaka ʻŌiwi, because their history is often overlooked in U.S. history and thus unfamiliar to most people in the U.S., especially as it relates to the emphasis of this book—achieving health equity. We then describe emerging health disparities and inequities among Kānaka ʻŌiwi. We then discuss culturally responsive programs and case studies that have been successfully implemented in the efforts to achieve health equity for Kānaka ʻŌiwi. Finally, we conclude with recommendations and best practices for health equity work.

BEGINNINGS OF INEQUITY

Prior to and up until Western foreign intrusion in 1778 when British explorer Captain James Cook first arrived in Hawaiʻi, it is estimated Kānaka ʻŌiwi numbered 300,000 to 800,000 (Bushnell, 1993; Stannard, 1989). Historical accounts indicate his expedition, which began the sustained Western contact on Hawaiʻi, encountered a vibrant and robust people that were physically, emotionally, and spiritually healthy (Beaglehole, 1967). The healthy lifestyle practices of Kānaka ʻŌiwi were clearly evident in their well-ordered society in which a *kapu* (sacred) system dictated rules for land, hygiene, and relationships; this in turn allowed them the opportunity to follow a lifestyle that included a well-ordered communal society, and a well-balanced nutritious diet and active lifestyle that resulted in holistic wellness and disease prevention (Blaisdell, 2001; Hughes, 2001). The well-ordered society of Kānaka 'Ōiwi contributed to their overall health and well-being as a people. This all changed, however, once Westerner foreigners settled upon their land.

Over the decades that followed the initial arrival of Western Europeans, foreign sailors and merchants came to Hawai'i and brought a flood of diseases from Europe, the Americas, and Asia. These outsiders came with the plague, influenza, small pox, measles, and other diseases that killed up to a thousand people a day; this resulted in massive disease epidemics that crushed the Kānaka 'Ōiwi population such that by the mid-19th century, the Kānaka 'Ōiwi population plummeted to 30,000 (Bushnell, 1993; Pa Martin, 1991). Kānaka 'Ōiwi health was decimated.

As a result of foreign settlers, in addition to the tragic reduction of the overall Kānaka 'Ōiwi population, many Kānaka 'Ōiwi lost their land rights through the alien concept of land privatization known as the Great Māhele of 1848 (Blaisdell, 2001). Not surprisingly, this concept was at complete odds with the Hawaiian perspective on land, in which it was the proper use of the land, not its ownership, which was of importance (Handy, Handy, & Pukui, 1991). Kānaka 'Ōiwi were not only disenfranchised from their ancestral lands, but disconnected from their traditional food sources, and forced to abandon many of their cultural practices. The ability for Kānaka 'Ōiwi to practice their ancestral *kuleana* (responsibility) to honor their direct ancestral relationship to the land was severed. As Kānaka 'Ōiwi tragically suffered through devastating population decline, and loss of land, governance, and economy, foreign settlers momentously benefited as an increasing number of missionaries and whaling ships arrived to Hawai'i (Trask, 1984). They facilitated a system that enabled foreigners to acquire large tracts of land and thereby develop a profitable plantation system (Mokuau et al., 2016; Silva, 2004). As missionaries developed boarding schools, Kānaka 'Ōiwi children were removed and detached from their homes and families (McCubbin, Ishikawa, & McCubbin, 2008). The Western culture, along with Christianity, were strictly enforced as Hawaiian political and economic control was undermined; Hawaiian cultural practices and language were deemed to be primitive, and English replaced the Hawaiian language (Warner, 1999). During the mid-1800s and early 1900s as a result of not only the significant population decline, but also the disapproval of Kānaka 'Ōiwi to work on sugar plantations that were built on their sacred ancestral lands, foreign laborers from China, Japan, Korea, and the Philippines were hired to work in the plantation industries (Blaisdell, 2001). Sadly, these laborers, and the missionaries and businessmen that preceded their arrival, eventually outnumbered Kānaka 'Ōiwi (Blaisdell, 2001). These tragic events eventually led to the illegal overthrow of the Hawaiian Kingdom in 1893 through the forced removal of the Hawaiian reigning monarch, Queen Lili'uokalani, by a U.S. military-backed group of businessmen and missionary descendants (Kana'iaupuni & Malone, 2006). Wrongfully without a vote from the general citizenry, and with documented objection by Kānaka 'Ōiwi, in 1898, the U.S. illegally forced annexation of Hawai'i; made Hawai'i a territory of the U.S.; and took 1.8 million acres of the Hawaiian Kingdom's crown and government lands in the process (Blaisdell, 2001). By 1959, Hawai'i became the 50th state of the U.S. and has since become the most densely militarized state in the nation (e.g., on the island of O'ahu alone, the U.S. military controls 22.4% of its land; Niheu, Turbin, & Yamada, 2007).

Despite the disheartening history of oppression Kānaka 'Ōiwi had to withstand by the U.S., their resilience and strength as a people endured (Niheu, 2014; Osorio, 2006; Tengan, 2008). In the 1960s and 1970s, a vital chapter in modern Hawaiian history occurred through a cultural awakening and revitalization of Hawaiian identity often called the "Hawaiian Renaissance." This momentous period was distinct with a revival of traditional Hawaiian music, dance, language, voyaging, and also importantly through political activism that sought political sovereignty and policy to achieve equity (Kanahele, 1979). A landmark was grassroot activism that ended U.S. military bombing and control of Kaho`olawe, the eighth largest island of Hawai'i (Kanahele & Kanahele, 1992).

This vibrant period instigated important policy landmarks in the areas of health, education, and political self-determination. Towards the later years of this period, federal legislations were enacted to address clear inequities. The Native Hawaiian Health Care Improvement Act, 1988 (P.L.100-579) developed from nearly two decades of research documenting inequities, and formed the basis of the E Ola Mau: The Native Hawaiian Health Needs Study. The study identified four key findings for Hawaiians: (a) significant inequity in rates of chronic disease; (b) poor accessibility to health services; (c) shortages of Native Hawaiians in health services; and (d) preference of culturally-relevant services and programs. Under the Act, the Native Hawaiian Health Care Systems was established along with a health scholarship program for Native Hawaiians (Akau et al., 1998; Papa Ola Lokahi, 1998). Along the same timeline, inequities in Native Hawaiian education achievements were documented and federal legislation established the Native Hawaiian Education Council, which provided funding for various areas including Hawaiian language immersion schools, and culturally-relevant curriculum. A significant policy landmark was the passing by Congress in 1993 of a resolution apologizing for the illegal overthrow of the Kingdom of Hawai'i by the U.S. and the devastating effects that Hawai'i's historical experiences left on its people. As noted by Mokuau et al. (2016):

> Although the overthrow of the Kingdom of Hawai'i occurred more than a century ago, historical loss of population, land, culture, and self-identity have shaped the economic and psychosocial landscapes of Hawai'i's people, and limits their ability to actualize optimal health. (p. 2)

HEALTH INEQUITIES AND DISPARITIES

Similar to other indigenous populations in the U.S., Kānaka 'Ōiwi share a sociopolitical history of forced incorporation into the U.S. that has contributed to documented higher prevalence of a number of chronic diseases in comparison to majority populations in the U.S. The leading causes of death are generally consistent, but Kānaka 'Ōiwi consistently have higher disease prevalence, often with onset a decade earlier than other populations (Balabis et al., 2007; Mau et al., 2009). Racial and ethnic longevity disparities have also been clearly evident in past decades, and this trend continues to persist with Kānaka 'Ōiwi continuing to have the shortest life expectancy compared to the majority longest-living racial/ethnic groups (Johnson et al. 2004; Nakagawa, Koenig, Asai, Chang, & Seto, 2013; Nakagawa, MacDonald, & Asai, 2015; Wu et al., 2017).

Cardiovascular Disease

CVD is the leading cause of death for Kānaka 'Ōiwi (Aluli et al., 2007). The specific causes of CVD include coronary heart disease (CHD) and cerebrovascular accident (stroke), with stroke being the third leading cause of death in Kānaka 'Ōiwi (Aluli et al., 2010; Balabis et al., 2007; Johnson et al., 2004). In Hawai'i, CVD prevalence is 68% higher among Kānaka 'Ōiwi compared to other racial/ethnic groups (Johnson et al., 2004), and Kānaka ʻŌiwi have a 34% higher CVD mortality rate than that of the general Hawaiʻi population (Balabis et al., 2007). Kānaka ʻŌiwi also have a higher prevalence of stroke, being two times more likely to have a stroke, and be afflicted by stroke an average of 10 years younger, than other racial/ethnic groups in Hawaiʻi (Nakagawa et al., 2013). Prevalence of hypertension, a CHD and stroke risk factor, is also disproportionately higher among Kānaka ʻŌiwi (Nakagawa et al., 2013), and a higher prevalence of hypertension has been linked to perceptions of racism in Kānaka ʻŌiwi (Kaholokula et al., 2010).

Cancer

Cancer is the second leading cause of death for Kānaka ʻŌiwi, and overall cancer mortality rates are highest for both Kānaka ʻŌiwi men and women compared to other racial/ethnic groups (Johnson et al., 2004). Kānaka ʻŌiwi tend to not only be diagnosed with cancer at a younger age, but experience lower survival rates compared to other racial groups (Blaisdell, 1998; Terada, Carney, Kim, Ahn, & Miyamura, 2016). Cancer incidence rates are the highest for Kānaka ʻŌiwi women, as they continue to have the highest incidence and mortality rates for breast cancer (American Cancer Society, 2004). NHOPI patients have also been found to have significantly higher secondary admission rates following hysterectomy for endometrial cancer compared to non-NHOPI patients (Terada et al., 2016). From 1990 through 2008, lung cancer was among the top three cancer sites in NHOPI, and Kānaka ʻŌiwi and Samoan men consistently displayed higher incidence rates of lung cancer in comparison with non-Hispanic Whites (Liu et al., 2013). These disparities relate to a variety of factors and include the lack of culturally appropriate interventions, late detection, diagnoses at more advanced stages, genetic markers of tumor aggressiveness, and high prevalence of tobacco use (Tsark & Braun, 2009; Mokuau, Braun, & Daniggelis, 2012).

Diabetes

Diabetes is the fourth leading cause of death in Kānaka ʻŌiwi, and their mortality rate due to diabetes is twice that for the entire state of Hawaiʻi (Johnson et al., 2004). Kānaka ʻŌiwi have an age-adjusted death rate of 38.8 (per 100,000) due to diabetes compared to 12.5 in Whites and 16.3 in the general population of Hawaiʻi (Johnson et al., 2004). NHOPI overall have continued to have a higher prevalence of type 2 diabetes compared to other racial/ethnic groups (Hsu et al., 2012); for instance, diagnosis of diabetes among NHOPI is twice that of European Americans (11.6% vs. 5.1%; Nguyen & Salvail, 2013). NHOPI also have a higher prevalence not only of diabetes, but also of diabetes complications. NHOPI are most likely to have end-stage renal disease induced by diabetes compared with other causes of end-stage renal disease among other racial/ethnic groups (Mau et al., 2003). Studies also indicate Kānaka ʻŌiwi have the highest occurrence of chronic kidney disease compared to other racial/ethnic groups (Mau et al., 2007). In a 2007 study, Kānaka ʻŌiwi in Hawaiʻi that were discharged with a diagnosis of diabetes were found to have the second highest number of individuals with lower-extremity amputations, with amputations occurring at the youngest age compared to other racial/ethnic groups (Pobutsky, Balabis, Nguyen, & Tottori, 2010). Preventable hospitalization rates due to diabetes are also significantly higher for Kānaka ʻŌiwi males compared to Whites, even after adjusting for ethnic-specific prevalence of diabetes and demographic factors (Sentell et al., 2014).

Overweight/Obesity

Overweight and obesity are major risk factors for CVD, hypertension, diabetes, cancer, hyperlipidemia, and sleep apnea, diseases highly prevalent in Kānaka ʻŌiwi, and many of which are premature (before the age of 60 years; Mau et al., 2009; Wong & Kataoka-Yahiro, 2017; World Health Organization, 2013). NHOPI have the highest prevalence of overweight/obesity (BMI ≥25) in Hawaiʻi (76.3%) compared to 54.6% of Caucasians, 55.1% of Filipinos, and 46.2% of Japanese (Hawaiʻi Health Data Warehouse, 2017). Kānaka ʻŌiwi alone have been found to have the highest proportion of overweight and obese compared to other racial/ethnic groups (Maskarinec et al., 2016). In a study examining the prevalence and correlates of obesity among young adults (18–24 years) in rural Hawaiʻi, 30.7% of NHOPI overall were obese compared to 10.6% of Asian Americans and 9.2% of European Americans (Madan et al., 2012). NHOPI are also less likely to have a healthy weight (BMI <25 kg/m^2) at 16.9% compared to Asians, Whites, and Blacks (56%, 36.6% and 26.4%, respectively; Hawley & McGarvey, 2015).

Behavioral Health

Kānaka ʻŌiwi have among the highest prevalence of behavioral health problems compared to other racial/ethnic groups in the U.S. These behavioral health problems include depression (Office of Hawaiian Affairs, 2017); anxiety (Hishinuma, Miyamoto, Nishimura, & Nahulu, 2000); suicide (Else, Andrade, & Nahulu, 2007); substance use (Lowry, Eaton, Brener, & Kann, 2011); family adversity (e.g., family disruption, family criminality, and poor family health; Goebert et al., 2000); adverse childhood experiences (Ye & Reyes-Salvail, 2014); and serious psychological distress (Galinsky et al., 2017). Kānaka ʻŌiwi also report greater trauma (e.g., depression, anxiety, post-traumatic stress disorder, and sleep disturbances) related to accidents and abuse over the life course compared to other racial/ethnic groups in Hawaiʻi (Klest, Freyd, & Foynes, 2013). Kānaka ʻŌiwi living in Hawaiʻi have a higher prevalence of depression (13%) compared to the state's population (8%; Salvail & Smith, 2007), and depression in NHOPI is associated with aggression (Makini et al., 1996), substance use (Kaholokula, Grandinetti, Crabbe, Chang, & Kenui, 1999), and suicide (Yuen, Nahulu, Hishinuma, & Miyamoto, 2000). The overall suicide rate among Kānaka ʻŌiwi is among the highest in the U.S. (Else et al., 2007).

STRIVING FOR HEALTH EQUITY

Given the significant health disparities that Kānaka ʻŌiwi continue to experience, achieving health equity is imperative. It is important, however, to note that the term "health equity" is a Western concept; whereas health equity can be understood as the absence of systematic disparities in health between different racial/ethnic groups (Braveman & Gruskin, 2003), the Kānaka ʻŌiwi understanding of health equity is quite different. Fundamental to a Kānaka ʻŌiwi understanding of health is the concept of *lokahi* (harmony) and *pono* (equity) in the relationship between *kanaka* (mankind, both self and others), *ʻāina* (land), and *na akua* (gods, spirits; Blaisdell, 1991; Kamaka, Wong, Carpenter, Kaulukukui, & Maskarinec, 2017). Illness results when this harmonic relationship is altered or impaired. The psychological distress and interrelated health problems caused by Western oppression and cultural disruptions can be described as the *kaumaha* (heavy, sad, depressed) syndrome (Rezentes, 1996). Kānaka ʻŌiwi of modern times share a "collective sadness and moral outrage" (Rezentes, 1996) and *hōʻinoʻino* (abuse, inure) or broken-spirit (Crabbe, 1999), which is a result of centuries of oppression and cultural discord that has disrupted the harmonious relationship they once had. Wellness can be restored by correcting these impaired relationships (Blaisdell, 1991). Equity in health is essentially achieving this harmony through knowledge, specifically ancestral knowledge.

Ancestral knowledge is the essence of equity for Kānaka ʻŌiwi. In *kahiko* (ancient) time, spirituality was not a second thought; it was a way of life. This is consistent with research indicating that spiritual and social well-being are important to the overall well-being of Kānaka ʻŌiwi living with chronic disease, despite the physical limitations caused by the disease (Kaholokula et al., 2008; Kaʻopua, Mitschke, & Kloezeman, 2008). On the personal level, the Hawaiian worldview of health integrates harmony of mind and body through ancestral knowledge and spirituality (Blaisdell, 1991). The ability of Kānaka ʻŌiwi to adhere to the ancestral knowledge that is central to their identity and social relations is intimately tied to their physical and emotional well-being.

Establishing Culturally Relevant Evidence-Based Programs

The U.S. government has called for the implementation of evidence-based programs (EBP) for health promotion as part of a national movement to improve health disparities, and the overall quality and accountability of the delivery of healthcare services (Isaacs, Huang, Hernandez, & Echo-Hawk, 2005). The Institute of Medicine (2001) defines programs based on evidence-based practices as "an integration of the best research evidence with clinical expertise and patient values" (pp. 45–46). There are increasing demands from payers and policy makers for EBP in an effort to reliably produce practical and cost-effective interventions. Federal agencies consider the implementation of EBP as a means of reaching national objectives and ensuring funds are directed toward programs that improve population health. Failure to implement an EBP is often considered a lost opportunity to improve health outcomes (Brownson, Fielding, & Maylahn, 2009).

The increasing reliance on EBP, however, leaves indigenous communities at a disadvantage as there are limited evidence-based health promotion interventions designed by or for indigenous people (Echo-Hawk, 2011; Novins et al., 2011; Pyett, Waples-Crowe, & Van Der Sterren, 2008; Walters et al., 2018). Methodologies to establish evidence-based health intervention programs are from quantitative research and controlled clinical trials (Echo-Hawk, 2011; Ernst, 2012; Isaacs et al., 2005). Yet these procedures and designs often do not fit well with indigenous populations as they lack attention to the sociocultural factors that are significant to indigenous people (e.g., family structure, community roles, and regional differences; Echo-Hawk, 2011; Ernst, 2012). As funding sources often require the use of EBP, indigenous communities are challenged with having to select from the limited number of EBP designed by or for indigenous people, or from EBP that were created in social and cultural contexts with no known effectiveness to their indigenous community (Novins et al., 2011).

Community-based participatory research (CBPR) has been well-received by indigenous populations, including Kānaka ʻŌiwi, particularly in health promotion and disease prevention EBP (Townsend Ing, Delafield, & Soong, 2017). A set of CBPR guiding principles (Israel, Schulz, Parker, & Becker, 1998) that are cited by CBPR researchers with increasing frequency, have also been used in successful Kānaka ʻŌiwi health research studies (Kaholokula et al., 2014; Sinclair et al., 2013). As described in Chapter 4, Health Equity Research and Collaboration

Approaches, the promise of CBPR is to build trust that mutually benefits all stakeholders and lasts through and beyond the study (Schulz, Israel, Selig, Bayer, & Griffin, 1998). Developing culturally congruent interventions for health promotion in Kānaka ʻŌiwi communities through CBPR has become an acceptable strategy in NHOPI communities to tackle the daunting NHOPI health disparities that continue to exist (Kaholokula et al., 2012).

CBPR has been effective in building and strengthening the research capacity of Kānaka ʻŌiwi communities by involving community members at the onset of research planning, and continuing their active involvement in the study's design, implementation, evaluation, dissemination, and manuscript authorship (Kaholokula et al., 2014; Sinclair et al., 2013; Townsend et al., 2017). Through skillful implementation and acceptability by all parties, CBPR has enhanced sustainability in the research process for Kānaka ʻŌiwi communities by advocating for NHOPI community needs (e.g., collaborating on community projects that are instigated by the community); honoring and respecting all stakeholders while both supporting and protecting their interests (e.g., encouraging and supporting community investigators to obtain advanced graduate degrees); disseminating findings and creating awareness to other NHOPI communities (e.g., facilitating the collaboration of different NHOPI community organizations in various NHOPI communities); and recognizing needed and available resources in the community (Townsend et al., 2017).

The necessity of having partnerships in place between researchers and NHOPI communities to help ensure culture-centered interventions are developed and sustained in a culturally appropriate manner is integral to achieve health equity (Dickerson et al., 2020). The value of understanding the cultural context as the basis for creating an equitable partnering process has been suggested by CBPR researchers (Wallerstein, Duran, Oetzel, & Minkler, 2018), and this has been evident in research studies with Native Hawaiian communities (Kaholokula et al., 2017). Through effective community involvement, there exists the potential to promote culture-centered interventions and achieve intervention sustainability through the transferability of study findings (Belone et al., 2017). One such example is the Ulu Network, a community coalition committed to improving NHOPI cardiometabolic health and well-being (Chung-Do et al., 2016). The Ulu Network, facilitated by the University of Hawaiʻi at Mānoa's John A. Burns School of Medicine Department of Native Hawaiian Health (DNHH) and Center for Native and Pacific Health Disparities Research, is a coalition of 38 NHOPI-serving community organizations with more than 80 sites spanning across Hawaiʻi and reaching into California. Ulu Network organizations collaborate with DNHH researchers to develop, evaluate, implement, and disseminate culturally-relevant EBP for NHOPI using a CBPR approach. Through the Ulu Network, EBP that utilize Native Hawaiian and Pacific values, cultural practices, and beliefs as their foundation are accessible to NHOPI organizations that desire to implement and sustain EBPs in their communities.

Culturally Responsive Programs

Rather than present a single case study illustrating methods to improve Kānaka ʻŌiwi health, we instead present three that highlight the varied ways in which culturally responsive programs are conceptualized: culturally adapted, culturally-grounded, and promising programs. A description of each type of program is followed by an illustrative case study.

Culturally adapted programs. Researchers and community health educators have relied on culturally adapting EBP for Indigenous populations (Ernst, 2012; Kaholokula et al., 2014; Sinclair et al., 2013; Walters et al., 2018). Challenges are presented, however, in the development of culturally adapted interventions for indigenous populations when indigenous knowledge systems are used within Western-based intervention paradigms (Dickerson et al., 2020). Using a CBPR framework, and taking the time to build strong and enduring collaborative partnerships, has been a step to overcome this challenge and lead to successful program development and production of positive health outcomes (Kaholokula et al., 2014; Sinclair et al., 2013; Walters et al., 2018).

Cultural adaptation of EBP has been done through formative mixed qualitative and quantitative methods, with the rationale for cultural adaptation coming from initial formative work (Dickerson et al., 2020). Qualitative studies with Kānaka ʻŌiwi populations often identify the importance of extended family systems, values of cooperation and collectivism, pride in cultural heritage and traditions, and spirituality (Browne et al., 2014; Oneha, 2001; Oneha, Magnussen, & Shoultz, 2010). In adapting an EBP for Kānaka ʻŌiwi, it is important to consider these factors may be directly or indirectly associated with health-related behaviors and/or with acceptance and adoption of health promotion programs into communities.

A frequent complaint by NHOPI is the insensitivity to the nuances of different Pacific populations. For example, Micronesians, a fast growing Pacific Islander group, is made up of multiple island nations, each with its own distinct languages, family structures, and traditions. In order to have successful culturally appropriate programs and materials, program planners must be able to develop and plan health initiatives from a Hawaiian perspective. Thereby, in adapting an EBP using a CBPR approach, the recognition of community agency and local adaptation of health interventions based on populations they are targeting to serve can ultimately improve their efficacy and sustainability in achieving health outcomes (Dickerson et al., 2020; Kaholokula et al., 2014).

CASE STUDY   PILI ʻOHANA

The PILI ʻOhana Program (PILI) is a culturally adapted EBP built upon a long-standing community–academic partnership using a CBPR approach. PILI was adapted from the prominent evidence-based Diabetes Prevention Program (Hamman et al., 2006) to become a weight loss maintenance program for NHOPI. PILI was developed and tested by a partnership of seven community, academic, and state organizations. The aim of PILI was to integrate community wisdom and expertise with scientific methods to conduct research on NHOPI health disparities. Community members serve as coinvestigators with academic researchers and play an active role in the planning, decision-making, and carrying out of all research activities. PILI's culturally-adapted and community-placed program lessons are designed to improve diet, physical activity, and time and stress management for NHOPI; in addition, the program fosters a supportive environment and allows participants to actively engage in their health (Kaholokula et al., 2012). In addition to being efficacious in a randomized controlled trial, PILI's cultural-congruence and effectiveness has also been demonstrated as it was delivered and evaluated in real-world settings by community peer educators of partnering community-based organizations (Kaholokula et al., 2014).

PILI goes back to ancient Hawaiian wisdom on how health and well-being should be. Community members and leaders are researchers and key individuals in addressing their own health, as it starts in their own homes and community. By changing the way health is viewed, healthcare is no longer just between a patient and physician, but between an individual's family,

(continued)

neighbors, and community members. PILI is not just weight management, but making lifestyle changes such as spending more quality time with one's family and community. The goal of PILI, going beyond the health intervention, is building community capacity, specifically by empowering communities to engage with academic science researchers on issues that affect them in a meaningful way.

The group setting of PILI provides a safety net to allow participants to support one another, while at the same time being educated and informed on the benefits of making healthy lifestyle choices. As shared by one participant, "Losing weight together and participating in the Great Aloha Run [8-mile walk/run event] together were my most memorable memories with PILI." Throughout the program, participants naturally develop rapport with one another. As shared by one participant, "We looked forward to meeting each other, week after week. We couldn't get enough of each other." Participants not only build trust and accountability with each other, but are able to share personal accounts of their lifestyle habits with each other. Ultimately, participants realize they are not alone in changing their lifestyle. As shared by one participant, "Everyone ended the class with a great sense of camaraderie by helping and encouraging each another to lose weight." In respect to who is accountable to one's health, PILI returns to ancient wisdom and puts health back into the hands of the community by helping community members be accountable to each other.

RECOMMENDATIONS

Kānaka ʻŌiwi are a distinguished population with unique cultural traditions, practices, and beliefs that directly impact their health and well-being. Despite having faced historical trauma and grave injustices within the social, economic, and political realms, Kānaka ʻŌiwi remain a resilient and steadfast people. Health inequities, however, continue to be a barrier to Kānaka ʻŌiwi achieving optimal health. As culture is a significant part of what distinguishes a population, particularly at-risk indigenous peoples, it is vital that a group's culture is the cornerstone of disease prevention, treatment, and management programs. For Kānaka ʻŌiwi and other Pacific Islanders, establishing sustainable, culturally-responsive health intervention programs through cultural adaptation of existing EBP, development of culturally grounded EBP, and implementation of promising programs, will encourage effective health program development and revitalization of cultural practices. The case studies described in this chapter can serve as successful templates for programs and program development for Kānaka ʻŌiwi communities, and are clearly applicable to other Pacific Island peoples as well.

A community-driven CBPR approach is essential to effectively develop, implement, evaluate, and disseminate culturally adapted and culturally grounded EBPs. While obtaining and sustaining community partnership for EBP research can be laborious and a time-consuming requirement, it deeply enriches the process and the outcomes from design to dissemination. Close and trusting relationships with community partners naturally bring forth central core culture and community values. For Kānaka ʻŌiwi the values of *aloha*, *ʻohana*, and *ʻāina* are foundations in life (Rezentes, 1996). These values, however, are complex concepts. For example, the term "aloha" may be understood as merely a greeting to those external to the Hawaiian culture, when in actuality it refers to many aspects including love, affection, compassion, mercy, sympathy, pity, kindness, sentiment, grace, and charity (Pukui & Elbert, 1986). Kānaka ʻŌiwi will seek, evaluate, accept, and reject a program based on their assessment of the presence of "aloha," not only in program staff, but throughout all components of a given program. Thereby, intrinsic understanding of cultural values should be required and entrenched in the research team, which includes community partners as well.

In regard to formative research, qualitative approaches are an essential methodology to assist in building culturally responsive and grounded EBPs for Kānaka ʻŌiwi. Qualitative methods resonate with Pacific Islander communities, where face-to-face or direct presence is the preferred interaction. It is important that when information for intervention adaptation or development is gathered, this approach is used to ensure the data not only facilitates health promotion, but is grounded in cultural values and practices significant to the community. A conceptual model to guide culturally-responsive intervention development and evaluation can also be produced through formative research, particularly when there is limited relevant published literature to guide the intervention. Through this process, it is also important to assess factors important to the community and incorporate the measurement of these factors into the development of evaluation plans (Kaholokula, Ing, Look, Delafield, & Sinclair, 2018).

As demonstrated in the case studies described in this chapter, to successfully implement culturally responsive programs and achieve positive outcomes, it is integral to have families and communities participating together in a group setting. Empowering both family and community members to participate in a program, while recognizing each participating member as an important contributing member to the class, will increase the likelihood of program participant retention and achieving positive outcomes for program participants as a whole. The successful culturally responsive programs mentioned in this chapter occurred over the course of, at minimum, a 3-month period in which family and/or community members met weekly and built unity amongst each other. The network of interpersonal relationships of the family are a strong source of support and identity that shape the processes of self-determination and decision-making for Pacific Islander peoples (Ewalt & Mokuau, 1995). In implementing culturally-responsive programs based on family and community engagement to achieve health equity, it is important to recognize that the process of building family and community capacity to make lifestyle changes takes time.

In order to successfully implement culturally-responsive programs, effective organizational policies that support Kānaka ʻŌiwi and other Pacific Islander health initiatives in a culturally appropriate manner are needed. EBPs designed by and for Kānaka ʻŌiwi using a CBPR approach represent a unique opportunity for Kānaka ʻŌiwi to control the future of their health. Although organizations exist that are dedicated to providing education, research, and health services for Kānaka ʻŌiwi, continued efforts are needed. These efforts can be assisted by the establishment and accountability of culturally sensitive organizations, institutions, and systems that will affirmatively seek out Kānaka ʻŌiwi to conduct research.

There must also be an organizational commitment to recruit Kānaka ʻŌiwi to develop and implement culturally responsive EBPs to achieve health equity. This can be done, however, only if there are sufficient numbers of Kānaka ʻŌiwi in the health science workforce. Effective health science education and training programs are needed to recruit, train, and retain Kānaka ʻŌiwi and increase the pool of Kānaka ʻŌiwi health science researchers that will focus on culturally responsive EBPs. Through a dedicated appreciation and commitment to respect and honor the history and culture of Kānaka ʻŌiwi, the development and implementation of future successful culturally responsive programs can be implemented to achieve health equity for Kānaka ʻŌiwi.

INTERSECTIONALITY SPOTLIGHT

Unfortunately, because of the overall dearth of research investigating the health of Kānaka 'Ōiwi and other Pacific Islander populations, research into the effect of intersectionality on NHOPI is extremely limited. As community-driven solutions continue to be developed, it will be important to apply an intersectional lens where possible to help illuminate what differences might exist. Such knowledge will best be gained through partnerships within NHOPI states, territories, and countries and in other population centers worldwide, as the low levels of representation of NHOPI in most research studies lead to methodologically-flawed collapsing of the diversity within NHOPI groups into a single analytic group—even in intersectionality research.

Culturally Grounded Evidence-Based Programs

CASE STUDY   OLA HOU I KA HULA (RESTORE HEALTH THROUGH HULA)

The design, development, and implementation of culturally grounded health research has fairly recently emerged as a necessary approach to disease prevention in indigenous communities (Walters et al., 2018). Researchers have compared and contrasted the cultural adaptation approach to the cultural grounded approach and found that studies using cultural adaptation approaches have yielded mixed results (Okamoto et al., 2014). Although limited, evidence of successful culturally grounded evidence-based health promotion interventions that restore traditional practices has been found to be impactful in reducing risks of chronic medical conditions in NHOPI (Kaholokula et al., 2017). Cultural grounding and culture-centeredness strives to draw from the strengths of a culture through the agency, power, and language of a people to direct health changes in their communities (Dutta, 2007). As noted by Dickerson et al. (2020), "harnessing community-based knowledge in the development of culturally centered interventions has the potential to help indigenous communities both decolonize and reclaim their cultural beliefs, practices, and aspirations that promote health and well-being."

For Kānaka 'Ōiwi, an individual's health and well-being are interrelated in the health of their family, community, and environment (Goodyear-Ka'ōpua et al., 2014); given this notion, to improve Native Hawaiian health, the design of health promotion interventions must promote loyalty, unity, and reciprocity within Hawaiian communities, and uphold family supports as critical assets (Kaholokula et al., 2012). Obtaining cultural knowledge and perspectives from NHOPI to aid in intervention development is critical in designing sustainable health promotion programs for NHOPI communities. Cultural grounding deeply ingrains community involvement and power to directly influence specific interventions that incorporate essential knowledge systems that are based on ancestral knowledge, history, languages, values, and healing traditions (Dickerson et al., 2020; Dutta, 2007).

(continued)

The cultural dance of hula is popular across Hawaiʻi and is performed by both genders and at all ages. While often mistaken as presented mostly for tourists, in actuality it is the indigenous dance form of Kānaka ʻŌiwi and is a deep part of the community fabric in Hawaiʻi, with diverse ethnicities participating in school performances, family gatherings, and formal theater presentations. Over the past decade a formidable CBPR collaboration developed between biomedical researchers at the University of Hawaiʻi medical school, *kumu hula* (hula experts and educators), and NHOPI community leaders to leverage this cultural strength to address CVD in NHOPI communities. The collaboration successfully developed and implemented the *Ola Hou i ka Hula* (Ola Hou) program as a form of cardiac rehabilitation for individuals recovering from heart bypass surgery (Look, Kaholokula, Carvahlo, Seto, & de Silva, 2012; Maskarinec et al., 2015). Then, in response to the collaboration's NHOPI community leaders' commitment to CVD prevention, the group moved forward to develop and test a hypertension management program based on 3 months of hula training and a modest 3 hours of culturally-relevant heart health education in a rigorous randomized clinical trial (Kaholokula et al., 2017). The evidence proved that poorly managed hypertension would significantly improve through participation in the Ola Hou program (Kaholokula et al., 2017). The approach resonates strongly amongst NHOPI. As one NHOPI participant from a rural community described:

> *I have hypertension and type 2 diabetes, and have been having the worst time trying to incorporate physical activity into my lifestyle. I have always told my family that I would like to go back to dancing hula, as that was a passion of mine when I was growing up, and later had to stop. Having the chance to dance hula again has been so awesome. I look forward to the hula class where I am surrounded by other women who want to learn hula, learn how to take care of their hypertension, have fitness, but most of all fellowship with each other.*

Traditional hula training incorporates many NHOPI values, including familial relationships, cooperation, and *aloha*—ongoing kindness and acceptance of others. Hula experts explain that this cultural dance incorporates the integrated Hawaiian view of health where aspects of physical, mental, and spiritual development are involved (de Silva, Look, Tolentino, & Maskarinec, 2017; Look et al., 2014).

The program's community collaboration also made a commitment to build community capacity and enable widespread implementation. Throughout its 10 years of research studies, they conducted annual community trainings for kumu hula and for interested health organizations. Over this period, 31 kumu hula were trained and over 16 sites including five community health clinics have been offering the Ola Hou program specifically for hypertension management or for general heart health and disease prevention. As a health clinic program facilitator explained:

> *Our patients love it, it has become a "super-support group," they not only help each other, they want to share the hula at our clinic community events, at family celebrations, and holiday gatherings. Our doctors even are writing in-house prescriptions that say the patient should join the Ola Hou hula class.*

Promising Programs

CASE STUDY   KEIKI O KA ʻĀINA BOARD AND STONE

The restoration of traditional cultural practices in everyday life has emerged as much-needed and necessary steps to address the daunting health inequities Kānaka ʻŌiwi are faced with (Ho-Lastimosa et al., 2019). Cultural knowledge and practice is distinctly important when describing Kānaka ʻŌiwi health, and the interest and need for place-based and culturally relevant strategies rooted in Hawaiian epistemology is widely apparent in Native Hawaiian communities (Ho-Lastimosa et al., 2019; Meyer, 2001; Mokuau, 2011; Mokuau et al., 2016; Niheu et al., 2007). Although not yet tested as an EBP like the adapted EBP and culturally grounded EBP mentioned previously, promising health promotion intervention programs have been developed through grassroots community efforts. These distinct programs address the health inequities and sociocultural needs of Kānaka ʻŌiwi; restore cultural practices; and have the potential of reducing risks of chronic medical conditions.

Kānaka ʻŌiwi believe that a balanced system integrates not only all aspects of the self, which includes the biological, psychological, social, cognitive, and spiritual, but also with the world, which includes the individual, family, community, and environment; it is the balance of all these facets that brings about optimal health (McMullin, 2005; Mokuau, 2011). Among these programs that consistently draw support of NHOPI communities are those that encourage the revitalization of *kalo* (taro) farming, the restoration of ancient *loko iʻa* (fish ponds), traditional open ocean canoe voyaging, and the practice of *poi* pounding (Goodyear-Kaʻōpua et al., 2014; Ho-Lastimosa, Hwang, & Lastimosa, 2014; Kawaʻa, 2018).

The *Keiki O Ka ʻĀina* (Children of the Land) Board and Stone Program (Board and Stone) is a place-based, family-centered cultural practice class. Striving to eventually be an EBP, Board and Stone is a promising program to achieve health equity as participants not only learn how to make *poi*, the primary food staple for Kānaka ʻŌiwi, but also make the traditional hand-carved Hawaiian implements, *pa wili ʻai* (board) and *pohaku* (stone) pounder, which are traditionally used to make *poi* from cooked taro root, called *kalo* in the Hawaiian language. *Kalo* has a spiritual significance to Kānaka ʻŌiwi for in origin stories, the first *kalo* plant was the elder sibling to man. In Hawaiian genealogical traditions, there is a reciprocal relationship where older siblings care for those younger and in turn, the younger must honor, care for, respect, and abide their elders. Imbedded in this cultural belief and practice is the understanding Kānaka ʻŌiwi follow that by caring for *kalo* and the *ʻāina* (land), it will in turn provide food, shelter, and all necessary things needed to sustain their health and well-being (Handy et al., 1991).

Since Board and Stone first began 10 years ago, over 9,000 family members have participated in the program, and enrollment continues to increase. The popularity of the program is a phenomenon, with extensive wait-lists and primarily word-of-mouth program promotion. What started in a class at a single site in Kalihi Valley on the island of Oahu, the program has since grown to multiple sites on different islands, and particularly in rural communities where Kānaka ʻŌiwi often reside. The Board and Stone movement has emerged in these Hawaiian communities and created an increased desire to have kalo and poi as a regular food in their diet. Board and Stone began monthly poi pounding events, and initially brought in 200 lbs of kalo monthly;

(continued)

the demand for kalo has since increased, and Board and Stone now brings in a monthly 800 to 1,000 lbs of kalo. Along with the increase in access to this traditional practice and food, there has also been an increase in Board and Stone *alaka'i* (teachers) with the knowledge, skills, and passion to lead and train others. Board and Stone gives individuals and families the opportunity to learn the ways of their ancestors; connect them to their roots and heritage; find and redefine themselves; and strengthen their families. The classes have been described by participants as both rewarding and life changing. As shared by one participant:

> It brought us together as a family. We took turns. Where she [my wife] struggled, she left it for me; and if I struggled, I left it more to my son. We all shared and took turns. It was a family project. Even carving the pohaku, it was wonderful. It really brought us closer as a family.

Participation involves significantly more than simply making a board and stone to pound poi; the classes provide a safe environment for family strengthening, teaching and empowering families to perpetuate and connect with their culture, and improving their overall health and well-being. As shared by another participant, fathers have also learned to become better parents and husbands through program participation:

> In the past, my husband would go to the beach or forest alone every chance he had. After taking the board and stone class, he took [lead instructor] Kawa'a's teaching to heart willingly, and the light within him began to turn on. My husband began taking our three girls and me to the mountains and beach, and now we go all the time. I fell in love with him all over again.

Through Board and Stone, the cultural practice of poi pounding is no longer just a practice done by ancestors of the past, but a practice done regularly by individuals and families as they invest in the health of themselves, their family, and their future by gaining the skills and knowledge of their ancestors. As shared by one participant:

> The class helped me to come to a realization that I gotta do something now to help myself to live longer. Even just the kalo, it tells me that we have good things coming from our culture that was helpful to our ancestors, and if I can change to be more healthy for my family, then I can help them. We can do something now by taking care of our health now.

CURRENT EVENTS

THE IMPORTANCE OF THE CENSUS

Hawai'i has historically had a low response rate to the U.S. Census due to a combination of language barriers, logistical challenges, and a historically-justified mistrust of the U.S. government. However, each person who is not counted leads to more than $2,000 in lost federal funding to the state. As a result, many Kānaka 'Ōiwi community groups are working to increase participation in the Census to ensure their

(continued)

representation is accurately counted, even while other groups feel that participation in the Census is a tacit acceptance of the still-disputed relationship between Hawai'i and the U.S. government. Groups in favor of increased Census response rates argue that not only will accurate counting increase the overall flow of money to the state, but it will also help to more accurately establish the number of Kānaka 'Ōiwi within Hawai'i that can open doors to additional funds specifically for health equity.

Discussion Question: What are the implications of under-estimating the size of the Kānaka 'Ōiwi population in Hawai'i as compared to other states, and how could this affect response to Kānaka 'Ōiwi health disparities?

PROTECTING NATURAL RESOURCES IN HAWAI'I

Recently, a group of taro farmers in East Maui launched an appeal to the Hawai'i Supreme Court to block a ruling that allows use of public water sources by private users without having to conduct an environmental review and implement an associated impact mitigation plan. Farmers argue that over the past 30 years, billions of gallons of public water have been diverted to plantations that have caused unknown damage to the overall ecosystem and impacted their ability to maintain their own farming endeavors.

Discussion Question: How do decisions regarding environmental regulations have a particular impact on the development and implementation of Kānaka 'Ōiwi health equity initiatives?

DISCUSSION QUESTIONS

- How has post-Western contact Hawaiian history influenced Kānaka 'Ōiwi health disparities?
- What is the difference between culturally adapted, culturally grounded, and promising programs to achieve health equity?
- How can promising programs described in this chapter become EBP?
- How can the Western concept of health equity be achieved through the Kānaka 'Ōiwi perspective of health?
- What policy changes can be made to achieve health equity for Kānaka 'Ōiwi?

REFERENCES

Akau, M., Akutagawa, W., Birnie, K., Chang, M., Kinney, E., Nissanka, S., … Spoehr, H. (1998). Ke ala ola pono: The Native Hawaiian community's effort to heal itself. *Pacific Health Dialog, 5*(2), 232–238. Retrieved from http://pacifichealthdialog.org.fj/

Aluli, N., Reyes, P., & Tsark, J. (2007). Cardiovascular disease disparities in Native Hawaiians. *Journal of the Cardiometabolic Syndrome, 2,* 250–253. doi:10.1111/j.1559-4564.2007.07560.x

Aluli, N. E., Reyes, P. W., Brady, S. K., Tsark, J. U., Jones, K. L., Mau, M., … Howard, B. V. (2010). All-cause and CVD mortality in Native Hawaiians. *Diabetes Research and Clinical Practice, 89*(1), 65–71. doi:10.1016/j.diabres.2010.03.003

Balabis, J., Pobutsky, A., Baker, K. K., Tottori, C., & Salvail, F. (2007). *The burden of cardiovascular disease in Hawaii 2007.* Honolulu, Hawai'i: Hawaii State Department Health. Retrieved from http://hawaii.gov/health/statistics/brfss/reports/CVDBurden_Rpt2007.pdf

Beaglehole, J. C. (Ed.). (1967). *The journals of Captain James Cook on his voyages of discovery: Volume III, Part I: The voyage of the resolution and discovery 1776–1780.* Cambridge, MA: Hakluyt Society at the University Press.

Belone, L., Orosco, A., Damon, E., Smith-McNeal, W., Rae, R., Sherpa, M. L., … Wallerstein, N. (2017). The piloting of a culturally centered American Indian family prevention program: A CBPR partnership between Mescalero Apache and the University of New Mexico. *Public Health Reviews, 38,* 30. doi:10.1186/s40985-017-0076-1

Blaisdell, R. K. (1991, August). *Historical and philosophical aspects of lapaʻau traditional Kānaka Maoli healing practices.* Paper presented at the Puʻuhonua in Hawaiian Culture, Kahua Naʻauao, Honolulu, Hawaiʻi. Retrieved from http://www.inmotionmagazine.com/kekuni.html

Blaisdell, R. K. (1995, June). *Update on Kanaka Maoli (indigenous Hawaiian) health.* Paper presented at the Asian American and Pacific Islander Health Summit, San Francisco, CA. Retrieved from http://www.inmotionmagazine.com/kekuni3.html

Blaisdell, R. K. (1998). Culture and cancer in Kanaka Maoli (Native Hawaiians) abstract. *Asian American and Pacific Islander Journal of Health, 6*(2), 400.

Blaisdell, R. K. (2001). The impact of disease on Hawaiʻi's history. *Hawaii Medical Journal, 60,* 295–296.

Braveman, P., & Gruskin, S. (2003). Defining equity in health. *Journal of Epidemiology and Community Health, 57,* 254–258. doi:10.1136/jech.57.4.254

Browne, C. V., Mokuau, N., Kaʻopua, L. S., Kim, B. J., Higuchi, P., & Braun, K. L. (2014). Listening to the voices of native Hawaiian elders and ʻohana caregivers: Discussions on aging, health, and care preferences. *Journal of Cross-Cultural Gerontology, 29*(2), 131–151. doi:10.1007/s10823-014-9227-8

Brownson, R. C., Fielding, J. E., & Maylahn, C. M. (2009). Evidence-based public health: A fundamental concept for public health practice. *Annual Review of Public Health, 30*(1), 175–201. doi:10.1146/annurev.publhealth.031308.100134

Bushnell, O. A. (1993). *The gifts of civilization: Germs and genocide in Hawaiʻi.* Honolulu: University of Hawaiʻi Press.

Chung-Do, J. J., Look, M. A., Mabellos, T., Trask-Batti, M., Burke, K., & Mau, M. K. (2016). Engaging Pacific Islanders in research: Community recommendations. *Progress in Community Health Partnerships: Research, Education, and Action, 10*(1), 63–71. doi:10.1353/cpr.2016.0002

Crabbe, K. (1999). Conceptions of depression: A Hawaiian perspective. *Pacific Health Dialog, 61*(1), 122–126. Retrieved from http://pacifichealthdialog.org.fj/

De Silva, M., Look, M. A., Tolentino, K., & Maskarinec, G. G. (2017). Research, hula, and health. In W. L. Lee & M. A. Look (Eds.), *Hoʻi Hou ka Mauli Ola* (pp. 136–144). Honolulu: University of Hawaiʻi Press.

Dickerson, D., Baldwin, J. A., Belcourt, A., Belone, L., Gittelsohn, J., Kaholokula, J. K., … Wallerstein, N. (2020). Encompassing cultural contexts within scientific research methodologies in the development of health promotion interventions. *Prevention Science, 21*(Suppl. 1), 33–42. doi:10.1007/s11121-018-0926-1

Dutta, M. J. (2007). Communicating about culture and health: Theorizing culture-centered and cultural sensitivity approaches. *Communication Theory, 17,* 304–328. doi:10.1111/j.1468-2885.2007.00297.x

Echo-Hawk, H. (2011). Indigenous communities and evidence building. *Journal of Psychoactive Drugs, 43*(4), 260–275. doi:10.1080/02791072.2011.628920

Else, I. R. N., Andrade, N. N., & Nahulu, L. B. (2007). Suicide and suicidal-related behaviors among Indigenous Pacific Islanders in the United States. *Death Studies, 31*(5), 479–501. doi:10.1080/07481180701244595

Ernst, A. J. (2012, September). *Evidence-based practices in tribal communities: Challenges and solutions* [Abstract]. Webinar presentation held by the Council of State Governments Justice Center, New York, NY. Retrieved from http://www.corrections.com/news/article/31557-evidence-based-practices-in-tribal-communities-challenges-and-solutions

Ewalt, P. L., & Mokuau, N. (1995). Self-determination from a Pacific perspective. *Social Work, 40*(2), 168–175. doi:10.1093/sw/40.2.168

Galinsky, A. M., Zelaya, C. E., Barnes, P. M., & Simile, C. (2017). Selected health conditions among Native Hawaiian and Pacific Islander adults: United States, 2014. *NCHS Data Brief, No 277.* Hyattsville, MD: National Center for Health Statistics.

Goebert, D., Nahulu, L., Hishinuma, E., Bell, C., Yuen, N., Carlton, B., ... Johnson, R. (2000). Cumulative effect of family environment on psychiatric symptomatology among multiethnic adolescents. *Journal of Adolescent Health, 27*(1), 34–42. doi:10.1016/S1054-139X(00)00108-7

Hamman, R. F., Wing, R. R., Edelstein, S. L., Lachin, J. M., Bray, G. A., Delahanty, L., ... Wylie-Rosett, J. (2006). Effect of weight loss with lifestyle intervention on risk of diabetes. *Diabetes Care, 29*(9), 2102–2107. doi:10.2337/dc06-0560

Handy, E. S. C., Handy, E. G., & Pukui, M. K. (1991). *Native planters in old Hawaii: Their life, lore, and environment.* Honolulu, Hawai'i: Bishop Museum Press.

Hawai'i Health Data Warehouse. (2017). *Hawaii State Department of Health, Behavioral Risk Factor Surveillance System. Adults who are obese by race/ethnicity, 2015–2017.* Retrieved from http://ibis.hhdw.org/ibisph-view

Hawley, N. L. & McGarvey, S. T. (2015). Obesity and diabetes in Pacific Islanders: The current burden and the need for urgent action. *Current Diabetes Reports, 15,* 29. doi:10.1007/s11892-015-0594-5

Hishinuma, E. S., Miyamoto, R. H., Nishimura, S. T., & Nahulu, L. B. (2000). Differences in state-trait anxiety inventory scores for ethnically diverse adolescents in Hawaii. *Cultural Diversity and Ethnic Minority Psychology, 6*(1), 73–83. doi:10.1037/1099-9809.6.1.73

Hixson, L., Hepler, B. B., & Kim, M. O. (2012). *The Native Hawaiian and other Pacific Islander population: 2010.* Suitland-Silver Hill, MD: U.S. Census Bureau. Retrieved from http://www.census.gov/prod/cen2010/briefs/c2010br-12.pdf

Ho-Lastimosa, I., Chung-Do, J. J., Hwang, P. W., Radovich, T. R., Rogerson, I., Ho, K., ... Spencer, M. S. (2019). Integrating Native Hawaiian tradition with the modern technology of aquaponics. *Global Health Promotion, 26*(3), 87–92. doi:10.1177/1757975919831241

Ho-Lastimosa, I., Hwang, P. W., & Lastimosa, B. (2014). Insights in public health: Community strengthening through canoe culture: Ho'omana'o Mau as method and metaphor. *Hawai'i Journal of Medicine & Public Health, 73*(12), 397–399.

Hsu, W. C., Boyko, E. J., Fujimoto, W. Y., Kanaya, A., Karmally, W., Karter, A., ... Arakaki, R. (2012). Pathophysiologic differences among Asians, Native Hawaiians, and other Pacific Islanders and treatment implications. *Diabetes Care, 35*(5), 1189–1198. doi:10.2337/dc12-0212

Hughes, C. K. (2001). Uli'eo Koa—Warrior preparedness. *Pacific Health Dialog, 8*(2), 393–400. Retrieved from http://pacifichealthdialog.org.fj/

Institute of Medicine. (2001). *Committee on quality of health care in America. Crossing the quality chasm: A new health system for the 21st century.* Washington, DC: National Academies Press. Retrieved from https://www.ncbi.nlm.nih.gov/books/NBK222272/

Isaacs, M. R., Huang, L. N., Hernandez, M., & Echo-Hawk, H. (2005). *The road to evidence: The intersection of evidence-based practices and cultural competence in children's mental health.* Washington, DC: National Alliance of Multi-Ethnic Behavioral Health Associations.

Israel, B. A., Schulz, A. J., Parker, E. A., & Becker, A. B. (1998). Review of community-based research: Assessing partnership approaches to improve public health. *Annual Review of Public Health, 19*(1), 173–202. doi:10.1146/annurev.publhealth.19.1.173

Johnson, D. B., Oyama, N., LeMarchand, L., & Wilkens, L. (2004). Native Hawaiians mortality, morbidity, and lifestyle: Comparing data from 1982, 1990, and 2000. *Pacific Health Dialog, 11,* 120–130. Retrieved from https://www.ncbi.nlm.nih.gov/pubmed/16281689

Kaholokula, J. K., Grandinetti, A., Crabbe, K. M., Chang, H. K., & Kenui, C. K. (1999). Depressive symptoms and cigarette smoking among Native Hawaiians. *Asia-Pacific Journal of Public Health, 11*(2), 60–64. doi:10.1177/101053959901100202

Kaholokula, J. K., Ing, C. T., Look, M. A., Delafield, R., & Sinclair, K. (2018). Culturally responsive approaches to health promotion for Native Hawaiians and Pacific Islanders. *Annals of Human Biology, 45*(3), 249–263. doi:10.1080/03014460.2018.1465593

Kaholokula, J. K., Iwane, M. K., & Nacapoy, A. H. (2010). Effects of perceived racism and acculturation on hypertension in Native Hawaiians. *Hawaii Medical Journal, 69*(Suppl. 2), 11–15. Retrieved from https://www.ncbi.nlm.nih.gov/pmc/articles/PMC3158444/

Kaholokula, J. K., Look, M. A., Mabellos, T., Zhang, G., de Silva, M., Yoshimura, S., ... Sinclair, K. A. (2017). Cultural dance program improves hypertension management in Native Hawaiians and Pacific Islanders: A pilot randomized trial. *Journal of Racial and Ethnic Health Disparities, 4,* 35–46. doi:10.1007/s40615-015-0198-4

Kaholokula, J. K., Mau, M. K., Efird, J. T., Leake, A., West, M., Palakiko, D. M., ... Gomes, H. (2012). A family and community focused lifestyle program prevents weight regain in Pacific Islanders: A pilot randomized controlled trial. *Health Education & Behavior, 39*(4), 386–395. doi:10.1177/1090198110394174

Kaholokula, J. K., Miyamoto, R. E. S., Hermosura, A. H., & Inada, M. (2020). Prejudice, stigma, and oppression on the behavioral health of Native Hawaiians and Pacific Islanders. In L. Benuto, M. Duckworth, A. Masuda, & W. O'Donohue (Eds.), *Prejudice, stigma, privilege, and oppression: A behavioral health handbook.* New York, NY: Springer.

Kaholokula, J. K., Nacapoy, A. H., & Dang, K. L. (2009). Social justice as a public health imperative for Kānaka Maoli. *AlterNative: An International Journal of Indigenous Peoples, 5*(2), 117–137. doi:10.1177/117718010900500207

Kaholokula, J. K., Wilson, R. E., Townsend, C. K., Zhang, G. X., Chen, J., Yoshimura, S. R., ... Mau, M. K. (2014). Translating the Diabetes Prevention Program in Native Hawaiian and Pacific Islander communities: The PILI ʻOhana project. *Translational Behavioral Medicine, 4*(2), 149–159. doi:10.1007/s13142-013-0244-x

Kanahele, G. H., & Kanahele, G. S. (1992). *Ku kanaka stand tall: A search for Hawaiian values.* Honolulu: University of Hawaiʻi Press.

Kanahele, G. S. (1979). *The Hawaiian renaissance.* Polynesian Voyaging Society Archives. Kamehameha Schools. Retrieved from http://kapalama.ksbe.edu/archives/pvsa/primary%202/79%20kanahele/kanahele.htm

Kaʻopua, L. S., Mitschke, D. B., & Kloezeman, K. C. (2008). Coping with breast cancer at the nexus of religiosity and Hawaiian culture: Perspectives of native Hawaiian survivors and family members. *Journal of Religion & Spirituality in Social Work, 27*(3), 275–295. doi:10.1080/15426430802202187

Kawaʻa, E. (2018). A board and stone in every home. In G. K. Miyataki (Ed.), *The journey from within.* Honolulu, Hawaiʻi: Watermark Publishing.

Klest, B., Freyd, J. J., & Foynes, M. M. (2013). Trauma exposure and posttraumatic symptoms in Hawaii: Gender, ethnicity, and social context. *Psychological Trauma, 5*(5), 409–416. doi:10.1037/a0029336

Liu, L., Noone, A. M., Gomez, S. L., Scoppa, S., Gibson, J. T., Lichtensztajn, D., ... Miller, B. A. (2013). Cancer incidence trends among native Hawaiians and other Pacific Islanders in the United States, 1990-2008. *Journal of the National Cancer Institute, 105*(15), 1086–1095. doi:10.1093/jnci/djt156

Look, M. A., Kaholokula, J. K., Carvahlo, A., Seto, T. B., & de Silva, M. (2012). Developing a culturally based cardiac rehabilitation program: The HELA Study. *Progress in Community Health Partnerships: Research, Education, and Action, 6*(1), 103–110. doi:10.1353/cpr.2012.0012

Look, M. A., Maskarinec, G. G., de Silva, M., Seto, T., Mau, M. L., & Kaholokula, J. K. (2014). Kumu hula perspectives on health. *Hawaii Journal of Medicine and Public Health, 73*(12, Suppl. 3), 21–25.

Look, M. A., Trask-Batti, M. K., Agres, R., Mau, M. L., & Kaholokula, J. K. (2013). *Assessment and priorities for health & well-being in native Hawaiians & other Pacific peoples.* Honolulu, Hawaiʻi: Center for Native and Pacific Health Disparities Research.

Lowry, R., Eaton, D. K., Brener, N. D., & Kann, L. (2011). Prevalence of health-risk behaviors among Asian American and Pacific Islander high school students in the U.S., 2001-2007. *Public Health Reports, 126*(1), 39–49. doi:10.1177/003335491112600108

Madan, A., Archambeau, O. G., Milsom, V. A., Goldman, R. L., Borckardt, J. J., Grubaugh, A. L., ... Frueh, B. C. (2012). More than black and white: Differences in predictors of obesity among Native Hawaiian/Pacific Islanders and European Americans. *Obesity, 20*(6), 1325–1328. doi:10.1038/oby.2012.15

Makini, G. K., Jr., Andrade, N. N., Nahulu, L. B., Yuen, N., Yate, A., McDermott, J. F., Jr., ... Waldron, J. A. (1996). Psychiatric symptoms of Hawaiian adolescents. *Cultural Diversity and Mental Health, 2*(3), 183–191. doi:10.1037/1099-9809.2.3.183

Marck, J. (2000). *Topics in Polynesian language and culture history.* Canberra, Australia: Pacific Linguistics.

Maskarinec, G. G., Look, M. A., Tolentino, K., Trask-Batti, M., Seto, T., de Silva, M., & Kaholokula, J. K. (2015). Patient perspectives on Hula Empowering Lifestyle Adaptation Study: Benefits of dancing hula for cardiac rehabilitation. *Health Promotion Practice, 16*(1), 109–114. doi:10.1177/1524839914527451

Mau, M. K., Sinclair, K., Saito, E. P., Baumhofer, K. N., & Kaholokula, J. K. (2009). Cardiometabolic health disparities in Native Hawaiians and other Pacific Islanders. *Epidemiologic Reviews, 31*, 113–129. doi:10.1093/ajerev/mxp004

Mau, M. K, West, M. R., Shara, N. M., Efird, J. T., Alimineti, K., Saito, E., ... Ng, R. (2007). Epidemiologic and clinical factors associated with chronic kidney disease among Asian Americans and Native Hawaiians. *Ethnicity & Health, 12*, 111–127. doi:10.1080/13557850601081720

Mau, M. K., West, M., Sugihara, J., Kamaka, M., Mikami, J., & Cheng, S. F. (2003). Renal disease disparities in Asian and Pacific-based populations in Hawaii. *Journal of the National Medical Association, 95*, 955–963.

Meyer, M. A. (2001). Our own liberation: Reflections on Hawaiian epistemology. *The Contemporary Pacific, 13*(1), 124–148. doi:10.1353/cp.2001.0024

Mokuau, N. (2011). Culturally based solutions to preserve the health of Native Hawaiians. *Journal of Ethnic & Cultural Diversity in Social Work, 20*(2), 98–113. doi:10.1080/15313204.2011.570119

Mokuau, N., Braun, K. L., & Daniggelis, E. (2012). Building family capacity for Native Hawaiian women with breast cancer. *Health & Social Work, 37*(4), 216–224. doi:10.1093/hsw/hls033

Mokuau, N., DeLeon, P. H., Kaholokula, J. K., Soares, S., Tsark, J. U., & Haia, C. (2016). Challenges and promise of health equity for Native Hawaiians. In K. Bogard, V. M. Murry, & C. Alexander (Eds.), *Perspectives on health equity & social determinants of health*. Washington, DC: National Academy of Medicine. Retrieved from https://nam.edu/perspectives-on-health-equity-and-social-determinants-of-health/

Nakagawa, K., Koenig, M. A., Asai, S. M., Chang, C. W., & Seto, T. B. (2013). Disparities among Asians and native Hawaiians and Pacific Islanders with ischemic stroke. *Neurology, 80*(9), 839–843. doi:10.1212/WNL.0b013e3182840797

Nakagawa, K., MacDonald, P. R., & Asai, S. M. (2015). Stroke disparities: Disaggregating Native Hawaiians from other Pacific Islanders. *Ethnicity & Disease, 25*(2), 157–161.

Niheu, K. (2014). Puʻuhonua: Sanctuary and struggle at Makua. In N. Goodyear-Kaʻōpua, I. Hussey, & E. K. Wright (Eds.), *A nation rising: Hawaiian movements for life, land, and sovereignty*. Durham, NC: Duke University Press.

Niheu, K., Turbin, L. M., & Yamada, S. (2007). The impact of the military presence in Hawaiʻi on the health of Na Kānaka Maoli. *Developing Human Resources for Health in the Pacific, 14*(1), 205–212.

Novins, D. K., Aarons, G. A., Conti, S. G., Dahlke, D., Daw, R., Fickenscher, A., ... the Centers for American Indian and Alaska Native Health's Substance Abuse Treatment Advisory Board. (2011). Use of the evidence base in substance abuse treatment programs for American Indians and Alaska Natives: Pursuing quality in the crucible of practice and policy. *Implementation Science, 6*, 63. doi:10.1186/1748-5908-6-63

Office of Hawaiian Affairs. (2017). *Kānehōʻālani—Transforming the health of native Hawaiian men*. Honolulu, Hawaiʻi: Author.

Okamoto, S. K., Helm, S., Pel, S., McClain, L. L., Hill, A. P., & Hayashida, J. K. (2014). Developing empirically based, culturally grounded drug prevention interventions for indigenous youth populations. *Journal of Behavioral Health Services & Research, 41*(1), 8–19. doi:10.1007/s11414-012-9304-0

Oneha, M. F. (2001). Ka mauli o ka ʻoina a he mauli kanaka: An ethnographic study from an Hawaiian sense of place. *Pacific Health Dialog, 8*(2), 299–311

Oneha, M. F., Magnussen, L., & Shoultz, J. (2010). The voices of native Hawaiian women: Perceptions, responses and needs regarding intimate partner violence. *Californian Journal of Health Promotion, 8*(1), 72–81. doi:10.32398/cjhp.v8i1.2032

Osorio, J. (2006). On being Hawaiian. In S. Kanaiaupuni (Ed.), *Hulili: Multi-disciplinary research on Hawaiian well being* (Vol. 3, No. 1, pp. 19–26). Honolulu, Hawaiʻi: Kamehameha Schools.

Papa Ola Lōkahi. (1998). *Ka ʻUhane Lōkahi, 1998 Native Hawaiian health & wellness summit and island ʻaha. Issues, trends and general recommendations*. Honolulu, Hawaiʻi: Papa Ola Lokahi.

Pobutsky, A., Balabis, J., Nguyen, D.-H., & Tottori, C. (2010). *Hawaii Diabetes Report 2010.* Honolulu, Hawai'i: Hawaii State Department of Health, Chronic Disease Management and Control Branch, Diabetes Prevention and Control Program.

Pukui, M. K., & Elbert, S. H. (1986). *Hawaiian dictionary.* Honolulu: University of Hawai'i Press.

Pyett, P., Waples-Crowe, P., & Van Der Sterren, A. (2008). Challenging our own practices in Indigenous health promotion and research. *Health Promotion Journal of Australia, 19*(3), 179–183. doi:10.1071/ HE08179

Rezentes, W. C. (1996). *Ka lama kukui: Hawaiian psychology.* Honolulu, Hawai'i: 'A'ali'i Books.

Schulz, A. J., Israel, B. A., Selig, S. M., Bayer, I. S., & Griffin, C. B. (1998). Development and implementation of principles for community-based research in public health. In R. H. MacNair (Ed.), *Research strategies for community practice.* New York, NY: Haworth Press.

Sentell, T. L., Juarez, D. T., Ahn, H. J., Tseng, C. W., Chen, J. J., Salvail, F. R., Miyamura, J., … Mau, M. K. (2014). Disparities in diabetes-related preventable hospitalizations among working-age Native Hawaiians and Asians in Hawai'i. *Hawai'i Journal of Medicine & Public Health, 73*(12, Suppl. 3), 8–13.

Silva, N. K. (2004). *Aloha betrayed: Native Hawaiian resistance to American colonialism.* Durham, NC: Duke University Press.

Sinclair, K. A., Makahi, E. K., Solatorio, C. S., Yoshimura, S. R., Townsend, C. K. M., & Kaholokula, J. K. (2013). Outcomes from a diabetes self-management intervention for Native Hawaiians and Pacific peoples: Partners in care. *Annals of Behavioral Medicine, 45*(1), 24–32. doi:10.1007/s12160-012-9422-1

Sotero, M. M. (2006). A conceptual model of historical trauma: Implications for public health practice and research. *Journal of Health Disparities Research and Practice, 1*(1), 93–108.

Stannard, D. E. (1989). *Before the horror: The population of Hawai'i on the eve of western contact.* Honolulu: University of Hawai'i Press.

Teaiwa, T. K. (1994). Bikinis and other s/pacific n/oceans. *The Contemporary Pacific, 6*(1), 87–109.

Tengan, T. P. K. (2008). *Native men remade: Gender and nation in contemporary Hawai'i.* Durham, NC: Duke University Press.

Terada, K., Carney, M., Kim, R., Ahn, H. J., & Miyamura, J. (2016). Health disparities in Native Hawaiians and other Pacific Islanders following hysterectomy for endometrial cancer. *Hawai'i Journal of Medicine & Public Health, 75*(5), 137–139.

Trask, H.-K. (1984). Hawaiians, American colonization, and the quest for independence. *Social Process in Hawaii, 31,* 1–35.

Tsark, J. U., & Braun, K. L. (2009). Eyes on the Pacific: Cancer issues of Native Hawaiians and Pacific Islanders in Hawai'i and the US-associated Pacific. *Journal of Cancer Education, 24*(2, Suppl.), S68–S69. doi:10.1080/08858190903404619

U.S. Census Bureau. (2018). *American Community Survey. Native Hawaiian and other Pacific Islander alone or in combination with one or more other races* (TableID: B02012). Retrieved from https://data.census.gov/ cedsci/

Wallerstein, N., Duran, B., Oetzel, J. G., & Minkler, M. (Eds.). (2018). *Community-based participatory research for health: Advancing social and health equity* (3rd ed.). San Francisco, CA: Jossey-Bass.

Walters, K. L., Johnson-Jennings, M., Stroud, S., Rasmus, S., Charles, B., John, S., … Boulafentis, J. (2018). Growing from our roots: Strategies for developing culturally grounded health promotion interventions in American Indian, Alaska Native, and Native Hawaiian communities. *Prevention Science, 21*(Suppl. 1), 54–64. doi:10.1007/s11121-018-0952-z

Warner, S. L. N. (1999). Kuleana: The right, responsibility, and authority of indigenous peoples to speak and make decisions for themselves in language and cultural revitalization. *Anthropology & Education Quarterly, 30*(1), 68–93. doi:10.1525/aeq.1999.30.1.68

Wong, K. A., & Kataoka-Yahiro, M. R. (2017). Nutrition and diet as it relates to health and well-being of Native Hawaiian kūpuna (elders): A systematic literature review. *Journal of Transcultural Nursing, 28*(4), 408–422. doi:10.1177/1043659616649027

World Health Organization. (2013). *Global action plan for the prevention and control of noncommunicable diseases 2013–2020*. Retrieved from http://apps.who.int/iris/bitstream/10665/94384/1/9789241506236_eng.pdf

Wu, Y., Braun, K., Onaka, A. T., Horiuchi, B. Y., Tottori, C. J., & Wilkens, L. (2017). Life expectancies in Hawai'i: A multi-ethnic analysis of 2010 life tables. *Hawai'i Journal of Medicine & Public Health, 76*(1), 9–14. Retrieved from https://www.ncbi.nlm.nih.gov/pubmed/28090398

Ye, D., & Reyes-Salvail, F. (2014). Adverse childhood experiences among Hawai'i adults: Findings from the 2010 behavioral risk factor survey. *Hawai'i Journal of Medicine & Public Health, 73*(6), 181–190. Retrieved from https://www.ncbi.nlm.nih.gov/pmc/articles/PMC4064343/

Yuen, N. Y., Nahulu, L. B., Hishinuma, E. S., & Miyamoto, R. H. (2000). Cultural identification and attempted suicide in Native Hawaiian adolescents. *Journal of the American Academy of Child & Adolescent Psychiatry, 39*(3), 360–367. doi:10.1097/00004583-200003000-00019

WOMEN'S HEALTH EQUITY

LAUREN R. GILBERT ▪ JENNIFER L. NGUYỄN ▪
MARY (DICEY) JACKSON SCROGGINS

LEARNING OBJECTIVES

- Identify the paradox of women living longer but sicker
- Describe differences in health outcomes for diverse groups of women
- Explain how programs and efforts can be designed specifically to achieve health equity for women

INTRODUCTION

Sex is often viewed as a piece of demographic data used as a control variable in analysis. However, when discussing women's health, a much deeper and more nuanced approach is required (Doyal, 2001). Both sex and gender impact health outcomes; however, sex and gender are often incorrectly conflated and used interchangeably. "Sex" refers to a person's biological status as male, female, or intersex; sex is usually assigned at birth and is based on chromosomal, chemical, and anatomical traits. "Gender" refers to the socially constructed meanings, expectations, roles, behaviors, expressions, and identities assigned to a person's status (Bird & Rieker, 2008; Office of Research on Women's Health, 2015). For example, women are socialized and expected to be caregivers to family members, both children and aging parents, which can have negative consequences for their health (see Work and Women's Health box). Men are socialized to mask their pain, both physical and mental, resulting in negative consequences for their health (Courtenay, 2000; Seidler, Dawes, Rice, Oliffe, & Dhillon, 2016). See Heise et al. (2019) for a more detailed description of how gender inequality and restrictive gender norms impact health. For women, both sex (biological factors) and gender (social meanings and expectations) work in conjunction to impact their health. In this chapter, several areas of health disparities will be covered—differences between men and women; differences between groups of women; and the health outcomes of different groups of women. The focus here will be on the gendered experiences of health and ways to address and alleviate some of these differences.

Mortality

Women on average live longer than men. In 2017, the life expectancy at birth was 78.6 years in the United States. When examining the differences between the sexes, females have a life expectancy of 81.1 years, while males have a 5-year lower life expectancy of 76.1 years (Arias & Xu, 2019). A further examination reveals that not all women have the same life expectancy. When compared to the life expectancy of White women, Black women have a life expectancy of about 3 years less, while Hispanic women live more than 3 years longer (see Figure 10.1). This phenomenon is known as the "Hispanic paradox"—Hispanic women live longer than non-Hispanic Whites despite a high prevalence of cardiovascular disease and low socioeconomic status (Medina-Inojosa, Jean, Cortes-Bergoderi, & Lopez-Jimenez, 2014; Smith & Bradshaw, 2006). This phenomenon is discussed in more detail in Chapter 6, Health Equity in U.S. Latinx Populations, but is particularly present for women.

Leading causes of death also vary between men and women. For both men and women, heart disease and cancer were the top two leading causes of death. However, men die from unintentional injuries at a much higher rate than women. Suicide is the eighth leading cause of death among men, but is not a major cause of death for women (Heron, 2019). These numbers are more than likely underreported due to data collection methods and stigma; however, differences are present. Data characterizing suicide attempts are not easily available in the U.S., but survey sources reveal that adult females report suicide attempts 1.5 times the rate of males, and adolescent females report suicide attempts twice the rate of male students (American Foundation for Suicide Prevention, 2020).

When looking at leading causes of death, an intersectional lens highlights even more disparities when comparing different groups of women. Heart disease and cancer are the two leading

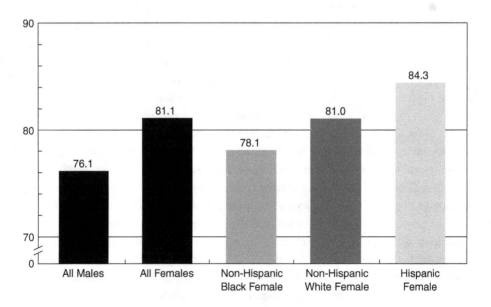

FIGURE 10.1 U.S. life expectancy by race/ethnicity, 2017.

SOURCE: Data from Arias, E., & Xu, J. (2019). United States life tables, 2017. *National Vital Statistics Reports, 68*(7), 1–66. Retrieved from https://www.cdc.gov/nchs/data/nvsr/nvsr68/nvsr68_07-508.pdf

causes of death for all the groups. However, differences emerge in the third leading cause of death. Strokes are the third leading cause of death for non-Hispanic Black women, Hispanic women, and non-Hispanic Asian or Pacific Islander women. However, the third leading cause of death for non-Hispanic White women is chronic lower respiratory disease, while the third leading cause for non-Hispanic American Indian or Alaska Native women is unintentional injuries (Heron, 2019). This disparity most likely reflects fundamental differences in social standing, access to care, and other social determinants of health rather than any biological anomaly or difference in underlying risk-taking.

Morbidity

Women have higher morbidity rates for most acute illnesses and most chronic conditions (Bird & Rieker, 2008; Weiss & Lonnquist, 2017). Part of this may be due to socialization, as it is more acceptable for women to be attentive to and seek help when it comes to their health (Weiss & Lonnquist, 2017). Women also utilize healthcare services more often than men. Women are more likely to visit the doctor, visit the emergency department, participate in preventive case visits, attend dental visits, engage in hospice care, and are more likely to be admitted to the hospital (Pinkhasov et al., 2010).

The origins of our medical knowledge contribute to the disparities between men and women. Women have traditionally been excluded from medical research and clinical trials; hence, men have become the standard benchmark for health and illness. As a result, if women present or experience a health event in a different way, it may take longer to be diagnosed and receive appropriate treatment. For example, women more commonly present with atypical symptoms of ischemic heart disease including fatigue, sleep disturbances, nausea, back pain, dizziness, and heart palpitations as opposed to the typical significant chest pain often reported by men (Berg, Björck, Dudas, Lappas, & Rosengren, 2009; McSweeney et al., 2003). Women are also more likely to report a higher quantity of symptoms than men (Berg et al., 2009). The American College of Cardiology has even recognized this disparity, stating that despite women facing higher mortality rates of cardiovascular disease, stroke, and heart failure, there are known gaps in understanding and management of these conditions (Jackson, 2016).

Furthermore, increased research efforts have included pain experiences, responses, and management between men and women. Large-scale studies show that women report more pain than men and are more likely to report chronic pain (Bartley & Fillingim, 2013). Research has revealed mixed results regarding pain treatment and severity, but gender biases of both the patient and provider influence pain treatment and management. Emerging research reveals biological and psychological processes that interact with gender biases, ultimately affecting pain treatment efficacy (Mogil, 2012; Sorge & Strath, 2018).

Reproductive Health

Women also face health concerns unique to their gender, such as reproductive health concerns. Reproductive health encompasses the diseases, disorders, and conditions that affect the functioning of the male and female reproductive systems during all stages of life. For women, disorders include birth defects, developmental disorders, low birth weight, preterm birth, reduced fertility, and menstrual disorders. Maternal health, pregnancy, and its related concerns and implications for future health are also a unique health concern for women. The potential and ability to bear children, whether or not childbirth occurs, has impacts on a woman's health throughout her lifetime. Healthy People 2020 continues to focus on Maternal, Infant, and Child Health within its 33 main objectives (Office of Disease Prevention and Health Promotion [ODPHP], n.d.). In an example of the ways in which women's health is sometimes marginalized to the health of others, women's health tends to be further scrutinized during pregnancy, when her health choices also have a direct impact on the fetus's well-being.

Prenatal Health

One way to improve pregnancy outcomes is prenatal care, or healthcare received during pregnancy to promote the health and well-being of not only the child but also of the woman. Prenatal visits aim to track the progress and growth of the baby and offer opportunities for testing and early detection of potential issues for the woman or baby. However, not all groups of women receive recommended prenatal care. While a majority (77.1%) of all women do receive recommended prenatal care in the first trimester, only 66.5% of non-Hispanic Black women receive prenatal care during the first trimester, with 10% of Black women receiving late or no prenatal care (Osterman & Martin, 2018). Babies of mothers who do not get prenatal care are three times more likely to have a low birth weight and five times more likely to die than those born to mothers who do get care (Office of Research on Women's Health, 2015). Social determinants of health are strongly tied to lack of prenatal care and represent a major obstacle to achieving health equity for women during the perinatal period.

The limited prenatal care for Black women has significant impacts on birth outcomes. Black women have the highest percentages of preterm (before 37 weeks of pregnancy) births (14% of all births) and the highest percentage of low birth weight babies (14%; Martin, Hamilton, Osterman, Driscoll, & Drake, 2018). These negative health outcomes can lead to further health complications for the baby throughout the life course, including breathing problems, feeding difficulties, cerebral palsy, developmental delay, vision problems, and hearing problems (Martin et al., 2018; Rosenthal & Lobel, 2011). Infant mortality, or the death of a baby before the age of 1, is also the highest for Black babies, at an astounding rate of 11.4 per 100,000 live births, compared to a rate of only 4.9 per 100,000 births for White babies (Martin et al., 2018).

Maternal Mortality

Pregnancy-related mortality rates are even more troubling. These deaths occur during pregnancy or within 1 year of the end of a pregnancy from a pregnancy complication (Centers for Disease Control and Prevention [CDC], n.d.). Maternal deaths began to rise around 1990 and doubled by 2013, going from 7.2 deaths per 100,000 live births to 18 deaths per 100,000 live births in 2014 (Roeder, 2018). Disturbingly, Black women are more heavily burdened by this negative outcome, as seen in Figure 10.2. Black women had a rate of 42.4 deaths per 100,000 live births compared to just 13.0 deaths per 100,000 live births for White women (CDC, n.d.). According to the World Health Organization, Black women have maternal mortality rates comparable to those of women in countries such as Mexico and Uzbekistan, where significant proportions of the population live in poverty (Roeder, 2018).

WHY DO BLACK WOMEN FACE WORSE MATERNAL OUTCOMES?

There are many reasons and these reasons are complex, such as healthcare access and poor quality of care. One of those reasons include the undervaluing of Black women and their experiences. They are not monitored as closely as their White counterparts, and when they do call attention to issues, these tend to be dismissed. One of the famous examples is the world-renowned tennis player Serena Williams. After giving birth to her daughter, she experienced a pulmonary embolism. Recognizing what she was experiencing, she alerted her medical team but was immediately dismissed. After continuing to press her medical team for immediate diagnosis and scan, the CT scan revealed several clots in her lungs. Ms. Williams continues to advocate to reduce maternal morbidity and mortality, especially among Black women.

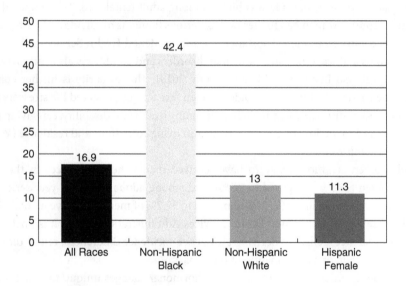

FIGURE 10.2 Maternal mortality: pregnancy mortality ratios per 100,000 live births, 2011 to 2016.

SOURCE: Data from Centers for Disease Control and Prevention. (n.d.). *Pregnancy Mortality Surveillance System*. Retrieved from https://www.cdc.gov/reproductivehealth/maternal-mortality/pregnancy-mortality-surveillance-system.htm

Cancer

Among women, there are approximately 412 new cases (per 100,000 persons) of cancer every year. Of those cases, 134 result in death (U.S. Cancer Statistics Working Group, 2019). African American women have disproportionately higher rates of mortality than all other groups for many cancers, including breast cancer and cervical cancer. While there is some evidence that African American women face higher incidence of certain cancers (e.g., triple-negative breast cancer) due to biological-driven factors, behavioral risk factors frequently tied to social determinants of health also contribute to the cancer disparities seen among women (Dietze, Sistrunk, Miranda-Carboni, O'Regan, & Seewaldt, 2015). Similar theories regarding gene–environment interaction is cited for the high rate of gastric cancer incidence among Asian/Pacific Islanders (Ashktorab, Kupfer, Brim, & Carethers, 2017). Socioeconomic factors, including education, occupations, and living conditions, have stronger associations with cancer mortality rates compared to race/ethnicity alone (Singh & Jemal, 2017). Yet, it is well understood that since minority women are more likely to be of lower socioeconomic status, be medically underserved, and have higher rates of behavioral risk factors (National Cancer Institute, 2016), they are more likely to experience a heavier burden than their counterparts and worse outcomes after diagnosis.

Mental Health

Mental health is another area of health where gender and sex differences are observed. For example, depression and anxiety are more common mental disorders in women (Albert, 2015; National Institute of Mental Health, 2019; Nemeth, Harrell, Beck, & Neigh, 2013; Noble, 2005). Data from the National Survey on Drug Use and Health (NSDUH) in 2017 shows that the prevalence of major depressive episode was higher among adult females (8.7%) compared to males (5.3%). Furthermore, women had higher rates of serious thoughts of suicide and past-year serious mental illness compared to men (Substance Abuse and Mental Health Services Administration, 2019). Symptoms and warning signs of mental disorders and conditions also vary between men and women (National Institute of Mental Health, 2019). This disparity is further complicated when examined across the life course. Older women face unique gendered life stressors that contribute to depressive disorder rates, including declining health and disability, caregiving responsibilities, experiences of maltreatment, and changes in living conditions and residence (Whiteman, Ruggiano, & Thomlison, 2016).

Overall, women are more likely to have received mental health services in the past year compared to men (18.5% compared to 9.9%), and among adults with past-year serious mental illness, women were more likely (71.5% compared to 57.7% of men) to receive mental health services (Substance Abuse and Mental Health Services Administration, 2019). It is unclear to what degree these differences reflect underlying prevalence/incidence differences, reflect differences in help-seeking behavior, or a combination of the two.

Some mental disorders can be attributed to hormonal changes unique to females based on their sex, such as postpartum depression (PPD) and premenstrual dysphoric disorder (PMDD; National Institute of Mental Health, 2019). PPD is a mood disorder that can affect women after birth, making it difficult for them to complete daily care activities for themselves or for others (National Institute of Mental Health, 2013). Approximately 10% to 15% of new mothers may experience PPD, with the greatest risk factor being depression prior to pregnancy (Brummelte & Galea, 2016). However, PPD continues to be under-recognized and undertreated, as many breastfeeding women are reluctant to take medications that may be passed to their babies through breastmilk (Pearlstein, Howard, Salisbury, & Zlotnick, 2009). PMDD, or severe premenstrual symptoms with disabling symptoms, is also believed to be underdiagnosed (Halbreich, Borenstein, Pearlstein, & Kahn, 2003; National Institute of Mental Health, 2019).

Substance Use and Abuse

Although men use substances at higher rates, the gender gap between women and men is narrowing. Women are the fastest growing segment of substance users in the United States, and women experience a more rapid progression of their addiction than men (Ait-Daoud et al., 2019). Women across the life course are drinking more alcohol, engaging in heavier drinking, and are experiencing an increase in alcohol use disorders (Caetano, Ramisetty-Mikler, Floyd, & McGrath, 2006; Epstein, Fischer-Elber, & Al-Otaiba, 2007). Opioid use, both prescription opioids and heroin, has been increasing among women as part of the larger opioid crisis, with the gaps between the rates of past-year heroin use for men and women narrowing (Jones, Logan, Gladden, & Bohm, 2015; Rodriguez & Smith, 2019). Additionally, there has been an overall increase in overdose deaths and emergency department visits related to drug use among women (CDC, 2013; VanHouten, Rudd, Ballesteros, & Mack, 2019).

Substance use during pregnancy is a public health issue, with long-reaching effects. Not only do the drugs have negative health consequences for the woman, but those drugs can be damaging to the developing fetus (Rodriguez & Smith, 2019). Legal and illicit substances can be harmful. Tobacco is the most commonly used substance in pregnancy, followed by alcohol and illicit drugs (Forray & Foster, 2015). Encouraging pregnant women to abstain from legal drugs like tobacco and alcohol can help prevent a variety of complications. It is well known that cigarette exposure is associated with a variety of poor birth outcomes (Bailey, McCook, Hodge, & McGrady, 2012; Rogers, 2008; Secker-Walker & Vacek, 2003). Prenatal exposure to alcohol is the leading preventable cause of birth defects and intellectual and neurodevelopmental disabilities, collectively known as "fetal alcohol syndrome disorder" (FASD; Williams, Smith, & Committee on Substance Abuse, 2015).

Illicit drug use among pregnant women is also a growing concern. Marijuana legalization in several states has contributed to an increase in the use of cannabis during pregnancy, which may increase adverse outcomes for women and babies (Forray & Foster, 2015; Gunn et al., 2016). Newborns exposed to certain substances including opioids during pregnancy can develop the withdrawal syndrome known as "neonatal abstinence syndrome" (NAS; Jilani et al., 2019; Rodriguez & Smith, 2019). The incidence of NAS has been increasing in the U.S. as the opioid crisis continues, resulting in several states mandating the reporting of NAS for public health surveillance (Jilani et al., 2019). Continued attention and surveillance for women using illicit drugs and the associated fetal outcomes remain imperative, as the opioid crisis continues and as marijuana legalization occurs in more states.

Intimate Partner Violence

Intimate partner violence (IPV) may include sexual violence, stalking, physical violence, and psychological aggression by a romantic or sexual partner (Smith et al., 2018). This is a widespread problem, as one in four women report experiencing sexual violence, physical violence, and/or stalking by an intimate partner and reported some form of IPV-related impact (Smith et al., 2018). Acute physical and psychological health impacts of IPV are often seen in emergency departments and primary care clinics (Bonomi, Anderson, Rivara, & Thompson, 2007; Campbell, 2002; Coker, Smith, Bethea, King, & McKeown, 2000; Kramer, Lorenzon, & Mueller, 2004). Women who experience IPV are also at increased risk of self-reported poor health status, depressive symptoms, substance use, chronic disease, chronic mental illness, and injury (Beydoun, Beydoun, Kaufman, Lo, & Zonderman, 2012; Bonomi et al., 2006; Coker et al., 2002). See Clark (2013) for a more detailed description of IPV from a social epidemiologic perspective. Many times, victims of IPV develop posttraumatic stress disorder, which requires additional support (Bradley, Schwartz, & Kaslow, 2005; Koopman et al., 2005).

There are also both physical and mental longer-term consequences of IPV that negatively impact women's overall health (Bonomi et al., 2007). Women who reported IPV also have higher healthcare utilization and costs, even after the IPV has ended (Rivara et al., 2007). IPV also threatens the economic stability of victims when accounting for missing days of paid work and lost productivity in unpaid work (Smith et al., 2018).

While many women experience IPV at some point in their lives, some marginalized groups of women may be at an increased risk but less likely to report or seek help, such as women with disabilities (Barrett, O'Day, Roche, & Carlson, 2009), women living in rural areas (Ragusa, 2017), women who have served in the military (Dichter, Cerulli, & Bossarte, 2011), and immigrant women (Hyman, Forte, Mont, Romans, & Cohen, 2006; Ting & Panchanadeswaran, 2009). These differences can be attributed to the social and structural factors that these groups of women face, including stigma, shame, limited agency, and social norms, as well as structural barriers to reporting and getting help and support (Campbell & Mannell, 2016; McCleary-Sills et al., 2016; Thaggard & Montayre, 2019).

WORK AND WOMEN'S HEALTH

Macro-level policies can also impact women's health, such as maternity leave, by working to alleviate gender inequalities. Maternity leave can improve women's health and well-being by minimizing work–life conflicting responsibilities and also giving women a chance to recover physically from childbirth and bond with the child (Borrell et al., 2014). The U.S. is the only industrialized country without a national paid leave mandate (U.S. Department of Labor Wage and Hour Division, 2012). The federal Family and Medical Leave Act (FMLA) provides 12 weeks of unpaid, job-protected leave to care for newborns or ill family members. Recent studies have demonstrated that maternity leave (unpaid or paid) improves maternal mental health (Borrell et al., 2014), that paid parental leave has specific mental and physical health benefits to mothers and children (Burtle & Bezruchka, 2016; Hewitt, Strazdins, & Martin, 2017; NANDI et al., 2018), and that leave has long-lasting benefits on women's mental health in older age (Avendano, Berkman, Brugiavini, & Pasini, 2015). However, it is clear that socioeconomic realities provide an advantage to certain demographic groups in their ability to take advantage of unpaid leave opportunities. When further examined, there are disparities in paid-leave access and in unpaid-leave utilization, especially when considering factors such as race or ethnicity, education, and employment status (Bartel et al., 2019).

UNPAID WORK

Women carry out at least two and a half times more unpaid housework (such as cooking, cleaning, taking care of children, taking care of the elderly) than men (UN Women, n.d.). As a result, women have less opportunity to pursue paid labor or work much longer hours, especially for women who perform both paid and unpaid work. Yet, society fails to recognize the completion of these tasks as "work" despite valuing anywhere from 10% to 39% of a country's Gross Domestic Product and contributing more to the economy than the manufacturing or transportation sectors (United Nations Economic and Social Council, 2017).

ACHIEVING HEALTH EQUITY—PROGRAMS AND SOLUTIONS

While these are just a small fraction of the health disparities experienced by women in the U.S., there are also solutions at all levels. Policies can change the way research is conducted and by whom. Policies can also influence how prevention programs are funded in communities. Community-level interventions, like the one highlighted in the case study provided later in the chapter, show the impact of empowering community members. Individuals such as primary care and specialty providers can become aware of the disparities facing women and empower themselves to act as advocates for women.

Traditionally, women have been excluded from research, both as scientists and as participants. In 1993, it finally became law that women had to be included in all clinical research after years of exclusion and unenforceable policies (Office of Research on Women's Health, n.d.). Then in 2001, the Institute of Medicine (now, the National Academy of Sciences) confirmed that sex, as an important research variable, is *necessary* when designing and analyzing health research and studies (Wizemann & Pardue, 2001). While hormones may be the cause for some sex differences when considering health and illness, hormones alone cannot account for all the differences seen, and the historical exclusion of women in research has an incalculable effect. Environmental, experiential, and physiological factors also play a role in an individual's response to health and wellness. The National Institutes of Health (NIH) track and report the number of enrolled women in NIH-funded clinical research. As of Fiscal Year 2016, enrollment of women was at 50% or higher (Office of Research on Women's Health, 2017). When researchers examined the inclusion of women in studies focusing on specific disease categories, women were underrepresented in 7 of the 11 categories, including HIV/AIDS, cardiovascular diseases, and chronic kidney diseases (Feldman et al., 2019). Even though there are policies in place to encourage and ensure the inclusion of women in research studies, sex and gender biases still persist.

Primary prevention of IPV is the current focus of the CDC, rather than focusing on victims and rehabilitating perpetrators after the abuse has occurred (Smith et al., 2018). This public health approach includes environmental strategies such as changing social norms and behaviors that accept IPV; developing and evaluating training programs for health professionals; and disseminating strategies that work to prevent IPV (Smith et al., 2018). Policy changes, such as reinstituting the Violence Against Women Act (VAWA), could also make an impact against IPV (Modi, Palmer, & Armstrong, 2014). Providers in primary care and emergency departments, and less traditional screeners, such as providers in substance abuse treatment programs (Fals-Stewart & Kennedy, 2005), can play a role to screen and provide interventions for women who are experiencing IPV.

One solution to address some of the health disparities seen in women is to engage primary care providers more for upstream approaches. These individuals can be engaged to be more aware of women's gender-specific health concerns, thereby empowering them to take active roles in helping all types of women achieve health equity. For example, obstetricians and pediatricians can be leaders in recognizing, screening, diagnosing, and providing treatment to new mothers for PPD (Pearlstein et al., 2009). Addressing the implicit biases that individuals may harbor can also lead to better outcomes.

A public health approach focusing on prevention, screening, and treatment efforts during pregnancy could be effective as pregnancy can be a time when women can be very motivated to change patterns of substance use (Patrick, Schiff, & Committee on Substance Use and Prevention,

2017; Rodriguez & Smith, 2019). Treatment options are available for women depending on the substance of abuse, such as psychosocial interventions, medication-assisted treatments, and other comprehensive treatment services (Hand, Short, & Abatemarco, 2017; Saia et al., 2016; Terplan, Ramanadhan, Locke, Longinaker, & Lui, 2015). However, barriers for pregnant women to participate in these programs exist, such as availability and accessibility, stigma, and legal consequences (Saia et al., 2016; Stone, 2015). Some states have even put policies in place to criminalize pregnant mothers' drug use (Angelotta & Appelbaum, 2017; Harris & Paltrow, 2003; Thomas, Treffers, Berglas, Drabble, & Roberts, 2018). However, punitive policies can prevent a woman from seeking treatment for fear of criminal prosecution and potentially losing custody of her children.

RECOMMENDATION

This chapter touches upon the many broad and complex issues within women's health. Aggregately, data show women to live longer but women suffer from higher morbidity rates than men. From a disaggregated point of view, not all women have the same experiences or outcomes. An intersectional approach provides a more inclusive and extensive perspective when exploring the differences among women. From research, we know and recognize that both biological and social determinants impact a woman's health throughout her lifespan. It is imperative that these perspectives and approaches are considered when designing programs and interventions to address the health disparities and health inequities women face.

INTERSECTIONALITY SPOTLIGHT

Women's reproductive health disparities in particular highlight that an interdisciplinary lens must be utilized when examining health. While pregnancy may be a limited health event for a woman, the multitude of factors that influence the pregnancy are far reaching. Previous research has determined that the adverse birth outcomes experienced by Black women compared to other groups persists when other factors are controlled, including socioeconomic status and prenatal health behaviors. Paradoxically, increased education actually increases the racial disparity in adverse birth outcomes (Rosenthal & Lobel, 2011). Stress is a risk factor for low birthweight and preterm delivery. Stress during the pregnancy and stress accumulated over a lifetime (allostatic load) from repeated exposure to discrimination may culminate during pregnancy to increase Black women's risk of adverse health outcomes (Rosenthal & Lobel, 2011).

While we used race and ethnic categories to explore health outcomes, other factors are just as important. Rural women face unique challenges due to their locations such as access to services, transportation issues, and social isolation (Ragusa, 2017; Warren & Smalley, 2014). A woman's age will impact the pregnancy experience, in terms of both the care she receives and how socially acceptable it is (Diaz & Fiel, 2016; Lean, Derricott, Jones, & Heazell, 2017). Education and social economic status will greatly impact health. Low-paid workers are less likely to have access to paid family leave than those with higher pay, and Hispanic workers have lower rates of paid-leave access and use than their White non-Hispanic counterparts (Bartel et al.,

(continued)

2019). There are other social locations that can impact a woman's health, many of which are discussed in detail in other chapters. An intersectional approach takes all these social locations into consideration, recognizing that health outcomes and consequences are the results of an individual's social location (Brown, Richardson, Hargrove, & Thomas, 2016; Williams, Priest, & Anderson, 2016).

CASE STUDY   WARD 7 NEIGHBORHOOD HEALTH CHAMPIONS

A Community-Based Approach to Increasing Awareness of Gynecologic Cancers, Improving Health Screening Adherence, and Reducing Mortality Toward Achieving Health Equity in Women's Health in a Low-Income, Underserved Ward in Washington, DC.

Through a $35,000 grant from the DC Cancer Consortium to the "Ovarian & Gynecologic Cancer Coalition: Rhonda's Club" and "In My Sister's Care," the DC Neighborhood Health Champions Program was developed to improve early detection of cervical, ovarian, and endometrial cancers by heightening symptom awareness and empowering women living in Ward 7, who are primarily low-income and medically underserved. Primary objectives included the following:

- Creating, training, and empowering a grassroots organization—self-named the Ward 7 Neighborhood Health Champions—to reach out to neighbors and sensitively discuss the need for reproductive health awareness (focused on cervical, ovarian, and endometrial cancers) and the actions women (worried or symptomatic) could take to improve health outcomes

- Educating women on the relationship between these gynecological cancers and a personal or family history of gynecological, breast, colorectal, prostate, and pancreatic cancers

- Starting with Ward 7, initiating the formation of a DC-wide Community Advisory Council initially focused on gynecological cancers

- Continuing existing gynecological cancer outreach and educational programs with a heightened focus in Ward 7

- Fostering public awareness of gynecological cancers using teal, the ribbon color for gynecological cancers

The funding covered October 1, 2008 to September 31, 2009, with a 1-month no-cost extension until October 31, 2009. It is important to note that this funding was supplemented by generous financial and other community support—such as donated food, beverages, and other resources for Champion training and meetings and the signature/culminating event—A Teal Event at Kimball Elementary School on September 26, 2009.

SUMMARY OF SIGNIFICANT ACHIEVEMENTS

The Ward 7 Neighborhood Health Champions Program exceeded expectations in several areas, starting with the number of community members recruited and self-accruing to the program. We proposed recruiting four Champions, each of whom would be expected to conduct at least

(continued)

six outreach activities. We recruited 14 active Champions and always had a core four to six other community members who did not formally join but attended meetings and supported outreach, thus the number of training sessions had to be increased, and monthly educational meetings required more resources. Additionally, in the final quarter of Year 1 funding, the Champions reported more than 30 outreach and educational events/activities.

A major program success was the Teal Event on September 26, highlighting both community support/commitment and community needs. It included the following:

- Support from at least 20 community groups and businesses

- A walk and exercise stations for yoga, dance, and Tai Chi

- Health booths and onsite assessments (e.g., blood pressure tests and counseling, HIV testing, mental health information, gynecologic cancer information, resources for health assistance, and general reproductive health counseling)

- Art tables (in part for younger participants to work on art projects while their parents took advantage of other offerings)

- Performances by local and nationally recognized performers (it is estimated that these performers collectively provided in-kind donations of approximately $19,000)

The event also included information/exhibitors focused on community concerns that went beyond health to include financial planning/solvency and other issues, understanding that these are relevant to community health attainment. Additionally, many community leaders attended the event, acknowledging and supporting the vital work and contribution of the Champions in an area with significant health and other concerns.

PROGRAM MEASURES

A primary measure of program success was the number of women—Champions and those they worked to educate—who were motivated to become current with American Cancer Society screening guidelines for reproductive health. Additionally, Champions encouraged the community to complete general health assessments for concerns most relevant to the population (e.g., hypertension and diabetes). As an element of Champion modeling and leadership in the community, we asked that they each become current with health screening guidelines and that they embed screening messages in their outreach, personally encouraging at least 10 acquaintances and family members to complete screenings. Most Champions did achieve or started to achieve completion, and over a 3-month period, they reported 350 contacts with Ward 7 residents promoting health screenings.

CHALLENGES

There were numerous challenges, including finding the right person to be the Champion leader, a slow start in recruitment, difficulty in activating a DC-wide Community Advisory Council initially focused on gynecological cancers, and identification of resources for worried and/or symptomatic women and families. However, none of the challenges derailed the success of the program and its key goals of creating a community-based force to improve health literacy around gynecologic cancer and perhaps more importantly around general health issues.

(continued)

Funding was a significant issue, partially because the program was so successful in terms of recruiting Champions and attracting others to the program. The original funding was to cover approximately four Champions, and we trained and thus supported 14 plus regular program participants who did not complete the training. An additional orientation/training session was added, and the total spending for the $25 gift card stipend, of course, almost tripled. It is worth noting that we did not advertise the stipend during recruitment.

RECOMMENDATIONS

Before attempting to build community-based programs and engage communities, it is essential to build strong, mutually respectful relationships with formal and informal leaders and representatives. Additionally, trust in the competence and expertise to be found within communities is a must. Residents must be seen as partners in achieving health improvement and equity rather than as causes or impediments. The Ward 7 Neighborhood Health Champions are exceptional, but they are not exceptions.

CURRENT EVENTS

EXPIRATION OF THE VIOLENCE AGAINST WOMEN ACT

The landmark VAWA was signed into law under President Bill Clinton in 1994 and subsequently renewed under both George W. Bush and Barack Obama. However, the Act expired during the 2018 to 2019 government shutdown and has not yet been reinstated despite a bill reauthorizing its passing in the House of Representatives. VAWA provided critical protections for IPV victims including funding prosecution of crimes against women, imposing mandatory restitution, and permitting civil redress. It also provided the legal protection of the federal rape shield law, funded community violence prevention programs, supported immigrant women, and provided legal aid for survivors of domestic violence. While the long-term effects of the lapse of VAWA authorization are still to be seen, it is clear that the loss of this legislation will have a ripple effect throughout the nation.

Discussion Question: How could reinstatement of VAWA help to achieve health equity for women even beyond IPV?

#METOO MOVEMENT

Although coined in 2006 by Tarana Burke, the use of the phrase "Me Too" gained immense popularity in 2017 after actress Alyssa Milano encouraged all women who had been sexually harassed or assaulted to change their social media statuses to "Me Too." The movement took the nation by storm, with more than 5 million Facebook and Twitter mentions within 24 hours, and nearly half of all social media users are estimated to have a friend/follower who posted using the term. The phenomenon has subsequently cast a massive light on issues of sexual violence against women.

Discussion Question: How do large-scale phenomena such as the viral #MeToo movement provide an opportunity to start new programs to support women's health equity?

DISCUSSION QUESTIONS

- How are biological sex and social constructions of gender impacting women's health? How are women's social experiences different than men's? How are these differences manifesting throughout the life course?

- Women report higher rates of suicide attempts, but suicide is a leading cause of death for men. How can we explain that difference? Why is it important to recognize this when we are creating suicide prevention programs and interventions?

- Why do you think the gap between men's and women's substance use is narrowing? What are some factors that women may be using substances more?

- What are other macro-level policies that could be impacting women's health? For example, what are some ways in which the gender wage gap may be impacting women's health? How could we improve these policies to improve women's health?

- Women's health is not only broad but also complex. Are there areas that deserve more attention than others? Which populations of women should receive immediate attention?

REFERENCES

Ait-Daoud, N., Blevins, D., Khanna, S., Sharma, S., Holstege, C. P., & Amin, P. (2019). Women and addiction: An update. *Medical Clinics of North America, 103*(4), 699–711. doi:10.1016/j.mcna.2019.03.002

Albert, P. R. (2015). Why is depression more prevalent in women? *Journal of Psychiatry & Neuroscience, 40*(4), 219–221. doi:10.1503/jpn.150205

American Foundation for Suicide Prevention. (2020, March 1). *Suicide statistics.* Retrieved from https://afsp.org/about-suicide/suicide-statistics

Angelotta, C., & Appelbaum, P. S. (2017). Criminal charges for child harm from substance use in pregnancy. *Journal of the American Academy of Psychiatry and the Law Online, 45*(2), 193–203. Retrieved from http://jaapl.org/content/45/2/193

Arias, E., & Xu, J. (2019). United States life tables, 2017. *National Vital Statistics Reports, 68*(7), 1–66. Retrieved from https://www.cdc.gov/nchs/data/nvsr/nvsr68/nvsr68_07-508.pdf

Ashktorab, H., Kupfer, S. S., Brim, H., & Carethers, J. M. (2017). Racial disparity in gastrointestinal cancer risk. *Gastroenterology, 153*(4), 910–923. doi:10.1053/j.gastro.2017.08.018

Avendano, M., Berkman, L. F., Brugiavini, A., & Pasini, G. (2015). The long-run effect of maternity leave benefits on mental health: Evidence from European countries. *Social Science & Medicine, 132*, 45–53. doi:10.1016/j.socscimed.2015.02.037

Bailey, B. A., McCook, J. G., Hodge, A., & McGrady, L. (2012). Infant birth outcomes among substance using women: Why quitting smoking during pregnancy is just as important as quitting illicit drug use. *Maternal and Child Health Journal, 16*(2), 414–422. doi:10.1007/s10995-011-0776-y

Barrett, K. A., O'Day, B., Roche, A., & Carlson, B. L. (2009). Intimate partner violence, health status, and health care access among women with disabilities. *Women's Health Issues, 19*(2), 94–100. doi:10.1016/j.whi.2008.10.005

Bartel, A. P., Kim, S., Nam, J., Rossin-Slater, M., Ruhm, C., & Waldfogel, J. (2019). Racial and ethnic disparities in access to and use of paid family and medical leave: Evidence from four nationally representative datasets. *Monthly Labor Review.* Retrieved from https://www.bls.gov/opub/mlr/2019/article/racial-and-ethnic-disparities-in-access-to-and-use-of-paid-family-and-medical-leave.htm

Bartley, E. J., & Fillingim, R. B. (2013). Sex differences in pain: A brief review of clinical and experimental findings. *BJA: British Journal of Anaesthesia, 111*(1), 52–58. doi:10.1093/bja/aet127

Berg, J., Björck, L., Dudas, K., Lappas, G., & Rosengren, A. (2009). Symptoms of a first acute myocardial infarction in women and men. *Gender Medicine, 6*(3), 454–462. doi:10.1016/j.genm.2009.09.007

Beydoun, H. A., Beydoun, M. A., Kaufman, J. S., Lo, B., & Zonderman, A. B. (2012). Intimate partner violence against adult women and its association with major depressive disorder, depressive symptoms and postpartum depression: A systematic review and meta-analysis. *Social Science & Medicine, 75*(6), 959–975. doi:10.1016/j.socscimed.2012.04.025

Bird, C. E., & Rieker, P. P. (2008). *Gender and health: The effects of constrained choices and social policies.* New York, NY: Cambridge University Press.

Bonomi, A. E., Anderson, M. L., Rivara, F. P., & Thompson, R. S. (2007). Health outcomes in women with physical and sexual intimate partner violence exposure. *Journal of Women's Health, 16*(7), 987–997. doi:10.1089/jwh.2006.0239

Bonomi, A. E., Thompson, R. S., Anderson, M., Reid, R. J., Carrell, D., Dimer, J. A., & Rivara, F. P. (2006). Intimate partner violence and women's physical, mental, and social functioning. *American Journal of Preventive Medicine, 30*(6), 458–466. doi:10.1016/j.amepre.2006.01.015

Borrell, C., Palència, L., Muntaner, C., Urquía, M., Malmusi, D., & O'Campo, P. (2014). Influence of macrosocial policies on women's health and gender inequalities in health. *Epidemiologic Reviews, 36*(1), 31–48. doi:10.1093/epirev/mxt002

Bradley, R., Schwartz, A. C., & Kaslow, N. J. (2005). Posttraumatic stress disorder symptoms among low-income, African American women with a history of intimate partner violence and suicidal behaviors: Self-esteem, social support, and religious coping. *Journal of Traumatic Stress, 18*(6), 685–696. doi:10.1002/jts.20077

Brown, T. H., Richardson, L. J., Hargrove, T. W., & Thomas, C. S. (2016). Using multiple-hierarchy stratification and life course approaches to understand health inequalities: The intersecting consequences of race, gender, SES, and age. *Journal of Health and Social Behavior, 57*(2), 200–222. doi:10.1177/0022146516645165

Brummelte, S., & Galea, L. A. M. (2016). Postpartum depression: Etiology, treatment and consequences for maternal care. *Hormones and Behavior, 77*, 153–166. doi:10.1016/j.yhbeh.2015.08.008

Burtle, A., & Bezruchka, S. (2016). Population health and paid parental leave: What the United States can learn from two decades of research. *Healthcare, 4*(2), 30. doi:10.3390/healthcare4020030

Caetano, R., Ramisetty-Mikler, S., Floyd, L. R., & McGrath, C. (2006). The epidemiology of drinking among women of child-bearing age. *Alcoholism: Clinical and Experimental Research, 30*(6), 1023–1030. doi:10.1111/j.1530-0277.2006.00116.x

Campbell, C., & Mannell, J. (2016). Conceptualising the agency of highly marginalised women: Intimate partner violence in extreme settings. *Global Public Health, 11*(1/2), 1–16. doi:10.1080/17441692.2015 .1109694

Campbell, J. C. (2002). Health consequences of intimate partner violence. *Lancet, 359*(9314), 1331–1336. doi:10.1016/S0140-6736(02)08336-8

Centers for Disease Control and Prevention. (n.d.). *Pregnancy Mortality Surveillance System.* Retrieved from https://www.cdc.gov/reproductivehealth/maternal-mortality/pregnancy-mortality-surveillance-system .htm

Centers for Disease Control and Prevention. (2013). Vital signs: Overdoses of prescription opioid pain relievers and other drugs among women: United States, 1999–2010. *Morbidity and Mortality Weekly Report, 62*(26), 537–542. Retrieved from https://www.cdc.gov/mmwr/preview/mmwrhtml/mm6226a3. htm

Clark, C. J. (2013). Chapter 48—Intimate partner violence. In M. B. Goldman, R. Troisi, & K. M. Rexrode (Eds.), *Women and health* (2nd ed., pp. 725–733). doi:10.1016/B978-0-12-384978-6.00048-0

Coker, A. L., Davis, K. E., Arias, I., Desai, S., Sanderson, M., Brandt, H. M., & Smith, P. H. (2002). Physical and mental health effects of intimate partner violence for men and women. *American Journal of Preventive Medicine, 23*(4), 260–268. doi:10.1016/S0749-3797(02)00514-7

Coker, A. L., Smith, P. H., Bethea, L., King, M. R., & McKeown, R. E. (2000). Physical health consequences of physical and psychological intimate partner violence. *Archives of Family Medicine, 9*(5), 451–457. doi:10.1001/archfami.9.5.451

Courtenay, W. H. (2000). Constructions of masculinity and their influence on men's well-being: A theory of gender and health. *Social Science & Medicine, 50*(10), 1385–1401. doi:10.1016/S0277-9536(99)00390-1

Diaz, C. J., & Fiel, J. E. (2016). The effect(s) of teen pregnancy: Reconciling theory, methods, and findings. *Demography, 53*(1), 85–116. doi:10.1007/s13524-015-0446-6

Dichter, M. E., Cerulli, C., & Bossarte, R. M. (2011). Intimate partner violence victimization among women veterans and associated heart health risks. *Women's Health Issues, 21*(4 Suppl.), S190–S194. doi:10.1016/j.whi.2011.04.008

Dietze, E. C., Sistrunk, C., Miranda-Carboni, G., O'Regan, R., & Seewaldt, V. L. (2015). Triple-negative breast cancer in African-American women: Disparities versus biology. *Nature Reviews Cancer, 15*(4), 248–254. doi:10.1038/nrc3896

Doyal, L. (2001). Sex, gender, and health: The need for a new approach. *British Medical Journal, 323*(7320), 1061–1063. doi:10.1136/bmj.323.7320.1061

Epstein, E. E., Fischer-Elber, K., & Al-Otaiba, Z. (2007). Women, aging, and alcohol use disorders. *Journal of Women & Aging, 19*(1/2), 31–48. doi:10.1300/J074v19n01_03

Fals-Stewart, W., & Kennedy, C. (2005). Addressing intimate partner violence in substance-abuse treatment. *Journal of Substance Abuse Treatment, 29*(1), 5–17. doi:10.1016/j.jsat.2005.03.001

Feldman, S., Ammar, W., Lo, K., Trepman, E., van Zuylen, M., & Etzioni, O. (2019). Quantifying sex bias in clinical studies at scale with automated data extraction. *JAMA Network Open, 2*(7), e196700. doi:10.1001/jamanetworkopen.2019.6700

Forray, A., & Foster, D. (2015). Substance use in the perinatal period. *Current Psychiatry Reports, 17*(11), 91. doi:10.1007/s11920-015-0626-5

Gunn, J. K. L., Rosales, C. B., Center, K. E., Nuñez, A., Gibson, S. J., Christ, C., & Ehiri, J. E. (2016). Prenatal exposure to cannabis and maternal and child health outcomes: A systematic review and meta-analysis. *BMJ Open, 6*(4), e009986. doi:10.1136/bmjopen-2015-009986

Halbreich, U., Borenstein, J., Pearlstein, T., & Kahn, L. S. (2003). The prevalence, impairment, impact, and burden of premenstrual dysphoric disorder (PMS/PMDD). *Psychoneuroendocrinology, 28*, 1–23. doi:10.1016/S0306-4530(03)00098-2

Hand, D. J., Short, V. L., & Abatemarco, D. J. (2017). Substance use, treatment, and demographic characteristics of pregnant women entering treatment for opioid use disorder differ by United States census region. *Journal of Substance Abuse Treatment, 76*, 58–63. doi:10.1016/j.jsat.2017.01.011

Harris, L. H., & Paltrow, L. (2003). The status of pregnant women and fetuses in US criminal law. *Journal of the American Medical Association, 289*(13), 1697–1699. doi:10.1001/jama.289.13.1697

Heise, L., Greene, M. E., Opper, N., Stavropoulou, M., Harper, C., Nascimento, M., … Gender Equality, Norms, and Health Steering Committee. (2019). Gender inequality and restrictive gender norms: Framing the challenges to health. *The Lancet, 393*(10189), 2440–2454. doi:10.1016/S0140-6736(19)30652-X

Heron, M. (2019). Deaths: Leading causes for 2017. *National Vital Statistics Reports, 68*(6), 1–77. Retrieved from https://www.cdc.gov/nchs/data/nvsr/nvsr68/nvsr68_06-508.pdf

Hewitt, B., Strazdins, L., & Martin, B. (2017). The benefits of paid maternity leave for mothers' post-partum health and well-being: Evidence from an Australian evaluation. *Social Science & Medicine, 182*, 97–105. doi:10.1016/j.socscimed.2017.04.022

Hyman, I., Forte, T., Mont, J. D., Romans, S., & Cohen, M. M. (2006). Help-seeking rates for intimate partner violence (IPV) among Canadian immigrant women. *Health Care for Women International, 27*(8), 682–694. doi:10.1080/07399330600817618

Jackson, E. A. (2016). *Acute myocardial infarction in women: AHA statement.* Retrieved from https://www.acc.org/latest-in-cardiology/ten-points-to-remember/2016/01/26/15/08/acute-myocardial-infarction-in-women

Jilani, S. M., Frey, M. T., Pepin, D., Jewell, T., Jordan, M., Miller, A. M., … Reefhuis, J. (2019). Evaluation of state-mandated reporting of neonatal abstinence syndrome—six states, 2013–2017. *Morbidity and Mortality Weekly Report, 68*, 6–10. doi:10.15585/mmwr.mm6801a2

Jones, C. M., Logan, J., Gladden, R. M., & Bohm, M. K. (2015). Vital signs: Demographic and substance use trends among heroin users — United States, 2002–2013. *Morbidity and Mortality Weekly Report, 64*(26), 719–725. Retrieved from https://www.cdc.gov/mmwr/preview/mmwrhtml/mm6426a3.htm

Koopman, C., Ismailji, T., Holmes, D., Classen, C. C., Palesh, O., & Wales, T. (2005). The effects of expressive writing on pain, depression and posttraumatic stress disorder symptoms in survivors of intimate partner violence. *Journal of Health Psychology, 10*(2), 211–221. doi:10.1177/1359105305049769

Kramer, A., Lorenzon, D., & Mueller, G. (2004). Prevalence of intimate partner violence and health implications for women using emergency departments and primary care clinics. *Women's Health Issues, 14*(1), 19–29. doi:10.1016/j.whi.2003.12.002

Lean, S. C., Derricott, H., Jones, R. L., & Heazell, A. E. P. (2017). Advanced maternal age and adverse pregnancy outcomes: A systematic review and meta-analysis. *PLoS One, 12*(10), e0186287. doi:10.1371/journal.pone.0186287

Martin, J. A., Hamilton, B. E., Osterman, M. J. K., Driscoll, A. K., & Drake, P. (2018). Births: Final data for 2017. *National Vital Statistics Reports, 67*(8), 1–50. Retrieved from https://www.cdc.gov/nchs/data/nvsr/nvsr67/nvsr67_08-508.pdf

McCleary-Sills, J., Namy, S., Nyoni, J., Rweyemamu, D., Salvatory, A., & Steven, E. (2016). Stigma, shame and women's limited agency in help-seeking for intimate partner violence. *Global Public Health, 11*(1/2), 224–235. doi:10.1080/17441692.2015.1047391

McSweeney, J. C., Cody M., O'Sullivan, P., Elberson, K., Moser, D. K., & Garvin, B. J. (2003). Women's early warning symptoms of acute myocardial infarction. *Circulation, 108*(21), 2619–2623. doi:10.1161/01.CIR.0000097116.29625.7C

Medina-Inojosa, J., Jean, N., Cortes-Bergoderi, M., & Lopez-Jimenez, F. (2014). The Hispanic paradox in cardiovascular disease and total mortality. *Progress in Cardiovascular Diseases, 57*(3), 286–292. doi:10.1016/j.pcad.2014.09.001

Modi, M. N., Palmer, S., & Armstrong, A. (2014). The role of Violence Against Women Act in addressing intimate partner violence: A public health issue. *Journal of Women's Health, 23*(3), 253–259. doi:10.1089/jwh.2013.4387

Mogil, J. S. (2012). Sex differences in pain and pain inhibition: Multiple explanations of a controversial phenomenon. *Nature Reviews Neuroscience, 13*(12), 859–866. doi:10.1038/nrn3360

Nandi, A., Jahagirdar, D., Dimitris, M. C., Labrecque, J. A., Strumpf, E. C., Kaufman, J. S., … Heymann, S. J. (2018). The impact of parental and medical leave policies on socioeconomic and health outcomes in OECD countries: A systematic review of the empirical literature. *The Milbank Quarterly, 96*(3), 434–471. doi:10.1111/1468-0009.12340

National Cancer Institute. (2016, August 4). *Cancer disparities*. Retrieved from https://www.cancer.gov/about-cancer/understanding/disparities

National Institute of Mental Health. (2013). *Postpartum depression facts*. Retrieved from Mental Health Information website: https://www.nimh.nih.gov/health/publications/postpartum-depression-facts/postpartum-depression-brochure_146657.pdf

National Institute of Mental Health. (2019). *Women and mental health*. Retrieved from https://www.nimh.nih.gov/health/topics/women-and-mental-health/index.shtml

Nemeth, C. L., Harrell, C. S., Beck, K. D., & Neigh, G. N. (2013). Not all depression is created equal: Sex interacts with disease to precipitate depression. *Biology of Sex Differences, 4*, 8. doi:10.1186/2042-6410-4-8

Noble, R. E. (2005). Depression in women. *Metabolism, 54*(5 Suppl.), 49–52. doi:10.1016/j.metabol.2005.01.014

Office of Disease Prevention and Health Promotion. (n.d.). Maternal, infant, and child health. *Healthy People 2020*. Retrieved https://www.healthypeople.gov/2020/topics-objectives/topic/maternal-infant-and-child-health/objectives

Office of Research on Women's Health. (n.d.). *History of women's participation in clinical research*. Retrieved from https://orwh.od.nih.gov/toolkit/recruitment/history

Office of Research on Women's Health. (2015). *How SEX and GENDER influence health and disease*. Retrieved from https://orwh.od.nih.gov/sites/orwh/files/docs/SexGenderInfographic_11x17_508.pdf

Office of Research on Women's Health. (2017). *Report of the Advisory Committee on Research on Women's Health, Fiscal Years 2015–2016*. Retrieved from https://orwh.od.nih.gov/sites/orwh/files/docs/ORWH_Biennial_Report_WEB_508_FY-15-16.pdf

Osterman, M. J. K., & Martin, J. A. (2018). Timing and adequacy of prenatal care in the United States, 2016. *National Vital Statistics Report, 67*(3), 1–14. Retrieved from https://www.cdc.gov/nchs/data/nvsr/nvsr67/nvsr67_03.pdf

Patrick, S. W., Schiff, D. M., & Committee on Substance Use and Prevention. (2017). A public health response to opioid use in pregnancy. *Pediatrics, 139*(3), e20164070. doi:10.1542/peds.2016-4070

Pearlstein, T., Howard, M., Salisbury, A., & Zlotnick, C. (2009). Postpartum depression. *American Journal of Obstetrics and Gynecology, 200*(4), 357–364. doi:10.1016/j.ajog.2008.11.033

Pinkhasov, R. M., Wong, J., Kashanian, J., Lee, M., Samadi, D. B., Pinkhasov, M. M., & Shabsigh, R. (2010). Are men shortchanged on health? Perspective on health care utilization and health risk behavior in men and women in the United States. *International Journal of Clinical Practice, 64*(4), 475–487. doi:10.1111/j.1742-1241.2009.02290.x

Ragusa, A. T. (2017). Rurality's influence on women's intimate partner violence experiences and support needed for escape and healing in Australia. *Journal of Social Service Research, 43*(2), 270–295. doi:10.1080/01488376.2016.1248267

Rivara, F. P., Anderson, M. L., Fishman, P., Bonomi, A. E., Reid, R. J., Carrell, D., & Thompson, R. S. (2007). Healthcare utilization and costs for women with a history of intimate partner violence. *American Journal of Preventive Medicine, 32*(2), 89–96. doi:10.1016/j.amepre.2006.10.001

Rodriguez, J. J., & Smith, V. C. (2019). Epidemiology of perinatal substance use: Exploring trends in maternal substance use. *Seminars in Fetal and Neonatal Medicine, 24*(2), 86–89. doi:10.1016/j.siny.2019.01.006

Roeder, A. (2018, December 18). America is failing its Black mothers. *Harvard Public Health Magazine*. Retrieved from https://www.hsph.harvard.edu/magazine/magazine_article/america-is-failing-its-black-mothers

Rogers, J. M. (2008). Tobacco and pregnancy: Overview of exposures and effects. *Birth Defects Research Part C: Embryo Today: Reviews, 84*(1), 1–15. doi:10.1002/bdrc.20119

Rosenthal, L., & Lobel, M. (2011). Explaining racial disparities in adverse birth outcomes: Unique sources of stress for Black American women. *Social Science & Medicine, 72*(6), 977–983. doi:10.1016/j.socscimed.2011.01.013

Saia, K. A., Schiff, D., Wachman, E. M., Mehta, P., Vilkins, A., Sia, M., … Bagley, S. (2016). Caring for pregnant women with opioid use disorder in the USA: Expanding and improving treatment. *Current Obstetrics and Gynecology Reports, 5*(3), 257–263. doi:10.1007/s13669-016-0168-9

Secker-Walker, R. H., & Vacek, P. M. (2003). Relationships between cigarette smoking during pregnancy, gestational age, maternal weight gain, and infant birthweight. *Addictive Behaviors, 28*(1), 55–66. doi:10.1016/S0306-4603(01)00216-7

Seidler, Z. E., Dawes, A. J., Rice, S. M., Oliffe, J. L., & Dhillon, H. M. (2016). The role of masculinity in men's help-seeking for depression: A systematic review. *Clinical Psychology Review, 49*, 106–118. doi:10.1016/j.cpr.2016.09.002

Singh, G. K., & Jemal, A. (2017). Socioeconomic and racial/ethnic disparities in cancer mortality, incidence, and survival in the United States, 1950–2014: Over six decades of changing patterns and widening inequalities. *Journal of Environmental and Public Health, 2017*, 19. doi:10.1155/2017/2819372

Smith, D. P., & Bradshaw, B. S. (2006). Rethinking the Hispanic paradox: Death rates and life expectancy for US non-Hispanic White and Hispanic populations. *American Journal of Public Health, 96*(9), 1686–1692. doi:10.2105/AJPH.2003.035378

Smith, S. G., Zhang, X., Basile, K. C., Merrick, M. T., Wang, J., Kresnow, M., & Chen, J. (2018). *The National Intimate Partner and Sexual Violence Survey: 2015 data brief—Updated release*. Retrieved from https://stacks.cdc.gov/view/cdc/60893

Sorge, R. E., & Strath, L. J. (2018). Sex differences in pain responses. *Current Opinion in Physiology, 6*, 75–81. doi:10.1016/j.cophys.2018.05.006

Stone, R. (2015). Pregnant women and substance use: Fear, stigma, and barriers to care. *Health & Justice, 3*, 2. doi:10.1186/s40352-015-0015-5

Substance Abuse and Mental Health Services Administration. (2019). *Behavioral Health Barometer: United States, Volume 5: Indicators as measured through the 2017 National Survey on Drug Use and Health and the National Survey of Substance Abuse Treatment Services* (HHS Publication

No. SMA-19-Baro-17-US., pp. 1–74). Rockville, MD: Author. Retrieved from https://store.samhsa.gov/product/Behavioral-Health-Barometer-Volume-5/sma19-Baro-17-US

Terplan, M., Ramanadhan, S., Locke, A., Longinaker, N., & Lui, S. (2015). Psychosocial interventions for pregnant women in outpatient illicit drug treatment programs compared to other interventions. *Cochrane Database of Systematic Reviews*, (4), CD006037. doi:10.1002/14651858.CD006037.pub3

Thaggard, S., & Montayre, J. (2019). "There was no-one I could turn to because I was ashamed": Shame in the narratives of women affected by IPV. *Women's Studies International Forum, 74*, 218–223. doi:10.1016/j.wsif.2019.05.005

Thomas, S., Treffers, R., Berglas, N. F., Drabble, L., & Roberts, S. C. M. (2018). Drug use during pregnancy policies in the United States from 1970 to 2016: *Contemporary Drug Problems, 45*, 441–459. doi:10.1177/0091450918790790

Ting, L., & Panchanadeswaran, S. (2009). Barriers to help-seeking among immigrant African women survivors of partner abuse: Listening to women's own voices. *Journal of Aggression, Maltreatment & Trauma, 18*(8), 817–838. doi:10.1080/10926770903291795

United Nations Economic and Social Council. (2017). *Commission on the status of women*. Retrieved from https://undocs.org/E/CN.6/2017/3

UN Women. (n.d.). *Redistribute unpaid work*. Retrieved from https://www.unwomen.org/en/news/in-focus/csw61/redistribute-unpaid-work

U.S. Cancer Statistics Working Group. (2019). *U.S. cancer statistics data visualizations tool*. Retrieved from https://gis.cdc.gov/Cancer/USCS/DataViz.html

U.S. Department of Labor Wage and Hour Division. (2012). Fact sheet #28: *The Family and Medical Leave Act*. Retrieved from https://www.dol.gov/whd/regs/compliance/whdfs28.pdf

VanHouten, J. P., Rudd, R. A., Ballesteros, M. F., & Mack, K. A. (2019). Drug overdose deaths among women aged 30–64 years—United States, 1999–2017. *Morbidity and Mortality Weekly Report, 68*, 1–5. doi:10.15585/mmwr.mm6801a1

Warren, J., & Smalley, K. B. (2014). *Rural public health: Best practices and preventive models*. New York, NY: Springer Publishing Company.

Weiss, G. L., & Lonnquist, L. E. (2017). *The sociology of health, healing, and illness* (9th ed., pp. 40–75). New York, NY: Routledge.

Whiteman, K., Ruggiano, N., & Thomlison, B. (2016). Transforming mental health services to address gender disparities in depression risk factors. *Journal of Women & Aging, 28*(6), 521–529. doi:10.1080/08952841.2015.1072027

Williams, D. R., Priest, N., & Anderson, N. B. (2016). Understanding associations among race, socioeconomic status, and health: Patterns and prospects. *Health Psychology, 35*(4), 407–411. doi:10.1037/hea0000242

Williams, J. F., Smith, V. C., & Committee on Substance Abuse. (2015). Fetal alcohol spectrum disorders. *Pediatrics, 136*(5), e1395–e1406. doi:10.1542/peds.2015-3113

Wizemann, T. M., & Pardue, M. L. (2001). *Exploring the biological contributions to human health: Does sex matter?* Washington, DC: National Academies Press. Retrieved from https://www.ncbi.nlm.nih.gov/books/NBK222288

11

ACHIEVING MEN'S HEALTH EQUITY

DEREK M. GRIFFITH

LEARNING OBJECTIVES

- Identify reasons why men's health inequities are frequently overlooked
- Describe the phenomenon of "diseases of despair" and how it relates to men's health inequities
- Define the concept of men's health equity, and discuss how it differs from other terms
- Explain why discussions of men's health equity should inherently take an intersectional lens
- Describe the health of African American men in particular

INTRODUCTION

In most cases, having higher incomes, power, and privilege is associated with better health outcomes (Braveman, Egerter, & Williams, 2011; Pearson, 2008), but this does not always hold true when we compare men's and women's health outcomes (Griffith, Bruce, & Thorpe, 2019). Men make more money, have more social and political power, and do not face sexism, but men also live shorter lives than women in most industrialized countries across the globe (Baker et al., 2014; Thorpe, Griffith, Gilbert, Elder, & Bruce, 2016). Whether measured by rates of premature mortality (World Health Organization, 2014), age-standardized death rates in leading causes of death (e.g., cardiovascular diseases, cancers, diabetes, chronic respiratory diseases; World Health Organization, 2014), life expectancy (National Center for Health Statistics, 2018), or mortality (Bilal & Diez-Roux, 2018), the finding that men live shorter lives than women has been a persistent pattern in the United States and across the globe (Griffith, Bruce, et al., 2019). While the sex difference in life expectancy between men and women is now seen as normal, it is a relatively recent phenomenon that emerged in the 20th century and has persisted into the 21st century (Beltrán-Sánchez, Finch, & Crimmins, 2015).

As differences in health outcomes between men and women emerged in the past century (Beltrán-Sánchez et al., 2015), the differences in health outcomes between groups distinguished by race, ethnicity, and other socially and politically meaningful factors have persisted for more than a century: as long as we have had data in the United States and across the globe (Byrd & Clayton, 2000; De Maio, 2014; Krieger, 1987; Woodward & Kawachi, 2000). Improvements in population health and achieving health equity require an accelerated development of an area of specialization that can explicate how and why inequities among men exist and present evidence that informs efforts to improve the health of men and reduce inequities among them (Griffith, 2018). One useful example of the need to refine our lens is the recent phenomena of "deaths of despair."

HIDDEN IN PLAIN SIGHT: THE NEED TO "GENDER" THE NARRATIVE OF "DEATHS OF DESPAIR"

The increase in "deaths of despair" (Case & Deaton, 2017) or "diseases of despair" (Meit, Heffernan, Tanenbaum, & Hoffmann, 2017) from drug-related mortality, alcohol-related liver disease, and suicide (Masters, Tilstra, & Simon, 2017), particularly among non-Hispanic White men and women aged 45 to 54 years in the United States with a high school degree or less, garnered particular attention. These findings for White Americans were thought to be in sharp contrast to all other race by gender groups in the United States and in other developed countries (e.g., France, Sweden, Germany). While the phenomenon regarding White Americans with this relatively low level of educational attainment has received considerable attention, the coverage has yet to address, highlight, or seek to explain why, among those with a high school degree or less, approximately 40 per 100,000 more non-Hispanic White men than women tend to die earlier (Case & Deaton, 2017).

This gendered story was particularly pronounced in rural areas (Erwin, 2017; Meit et al., 2017), most notably the Appalachian region of the United States: a 205,000-square-mile region that spans the Appalachian Mountains from southern New York to northern Mississippi. As discussed in Chapter 13, Rural, Frontier, and Appalachian Health Equity, the Appalachian region has historically had levels of educational attainment, employment, income, and health outcomes lower than Americans in other regions of the United States. In the Appalachian region of the United States, the highest mortality rate from diseases of despair was among individuals aged 45 to 54 years, at 89.0 deaths per 100,000 population, and the male-to-female mortality ratio in these diseases among those aged 15 to 64 years ranged from 1.96:1 to 2.33:1. What appears to drive the mortality rates from diseases of despair in Appalachia for men is the rate of mortality from alcohol, prescription drug, and illegal drug overdose, particularly among men aged 25 to 34 years (61.9 deaths per 100,000) and 35 to 44 years (61.0 deaths per 100,000; Meit et al., 2017).

However, more recently scholars have noted that the rhetoric around and attention to diseases of despair have masked the fact that these increases may not only be occurring in non-Hispanic Whites. Using data from the National Longitudinal Study of Adolescent to Adult Health, a nationally representative longitudinal study of U.S. residents that began when study participants were adolescents, Gaydosh et al. (2019) found that indicators of despair (e.g., depression, suicidality, heavy drinking, marijuana use) were not limited to Whites with lower educational levels. While the patterns of despair were not limited to these populations and they did not find significant differences in pattern between men and women, Gaydosh et al. (2019) included supplemental tables that showed significant gender differences in each indicator of despair. In addition, Bilal and Diez-Roux (2018) published an article demonstrating that mortality significantly increased in non-Hispanic Black men—for the second year in a row—and significantly decreased only in non-Hispanic White women. This is independent of the fact that non-Hispanic Black men already had the highest rates of mortality of any race by gender group in the United States.

In sum, while it was important for each of these papers to document patterns that varied by race, ethnicity, geography, age, and other factors, gender matters even after considering these factors. Moreover, these studies also highlight how the intersection of factors with gender is important and is often masked by not considering the unique findings that result from combining proxies for social determinants of health like race and gender (Griffith, 2012). Intersecting gender and race in these analyses helps to identify populations that have considerably worse health outcomes, regardless of their potential advantage on one social determinant of health. Most researchers do not regularly report findings that include how gender intersects with other factors and that is significantly hindering our ability to understand determinants of health and our collective ability to achieve health equity.

WHAT IS MEN'S HEALTH EQUITY?

Health equity has been defined as the absence of systematic disparities in health and the determinants of health, coupled with an underlying commitment to eliminate social determinants of health and disparities in health (Braveman, 2014). Braveman (2014) argues that social justice is at the heart of the concept of health equity, but it is unclear what data are driving a focus on health equity when men, across the globe, live shorter and often sicker lives than women. Braveman (2006) argues that "the gender disparity in life expectancy is, albeit an important public health issue, not an appropriate health disparities issue, because in this particular case it is the a priori disadvantaged group—women—who experiences better health" (p. 186). Recent definitions of health disparities from Healthy People 2020 and others have explicitly included the notion that disparities refer to populations whose health is worse based on some social disadvantage or characteristics historically linked to discrimination (Braveman, 2014). The focus of these approaches is to address the determinants of health that impede people's opportunities to be healthy such as poverty, discrimination, pay inequity, and lower access to quality education and housing, safe environments, and health care (Robert Wood Johnson Foundation, 2017).

The fundamental problem with these ways of defining health equity is that they do not consider that groups can be advantaged based on one characteristic (e.g., gender) but disadvantaged based on another (e.g., sexual orientation, race, ethnicity, gender identity, educational attainment). As we have seen across the 20th century and as we are two decades into the new millennium (Beltrán-Sánchez et al., 2015; Bilal & Diez-Roux, 2018; Satcher et al., 2005), closing racial or ethnic gaps does not necessarily close gaps by gender within racial or ethnic groups.

The focus on singular markers of disadvantage and the lack of consideration of the paradox of gender has been problematic in garnering attention and resources to focus on the health of men and accounts for much of the racial and sex difference in mortality globally (World Health Organization, 2014; Satcher et al., 2005; Young, 2009; Young, Meryn, & Treadwell, 2008). Men who are advantaged by their sex or gender but marginalized by race, ethnicity, immigration status, sexual orientation, and other socially meaningful factors discussed throughout this text are critical yet often invisible in efforts to achieve health equity. While useful for identifying factors associated with race and ethnicity that affect health outcomes, a focus on race, ethnicity, socioeconomic status (SES), and even sexual and gender minority status has left a large group of men whose health warrants attention if our goal "… is not to just accurately describe health differences or determine their cause, but to do so in a way that will be useful to making predictions, preventing greater health disparities, and improving human health" (de Melo-Martin & Intemann, 2007, p. 218). Intersectional approaches to men's health offer a way to examine why sex does not have the same meaning and influence within and across all men's lives or health outcomes (Griffith, 2012). Intersectional approaches help to highlight how dynamic cultural factors shape the norms, expectations, stressors, and practices in men's lives. An intersectional approach offers an important lens through which we may further explore how men determine strategies for recreating, reimaging, and redefining masculinities.

Just as behavioral interventions that target racial or ethnic group members of a "health disparity population" (e.g., African Americans) tend to include an overwhelming majority of women (Newton, Griffith, Kearney, & Bennett, 2014), most social determinants of health have not been studied by race/ethnicity and gender, nor have there been a priori hypotheses tested regarding why these differences may exist or emerge over time. These study designs and research strategies homogenize men of health disparity populations, often leading to conclusions that blame men for not being more like women. While there is a need to recognize and consider the common elements and determinants of health of humans who share these sex characteristics, particularly amid the renewed federal interest in examining the effects of sex as a biological variable, gendered social norms, expectations, responsibilities, and obstacles also shape the health risks of people who fit this group (Hankivsky, 2012; Snow, 2008). The social experience of being a cisgender male of a particular age, race, and ethnicity along with environmental, economic, and cultural (ethnic) factors that shape the life context, social experiences, psychological experiences, and health practices reflects macro-level factors linked to disparate health practices and inequities in health outcomes. Thus, not only is the empirical literature linking measures of masculinity to health in its infancy, but it remains dominated by research on Western, Educated, Industrialized, Rich, and Democratic (WEIRD) cultures (Jones, 2010) men's health. The literature linking masculinity and health among Asian, Black, Latino, and Native American men is limited (Griffith, Gunter, & Watkins, 2012). How might the science of men's health progress, however, if we move research on "marginalized" and "subordinated" men from the margins of the literature, or places where they are often invisible or not included in studies, to the center, making "marginalized" and "subordinated" men a more central focus of men's health research?

The field of men's health equity has emerged from gaps in knowledge that exist between health inequities and men's health research. Scholarship on men's health and scholarship on health inequities have grown largely in parallel, although a need remains to examine where these fields intersect. While the scholarly literature in each area has grown exponentially in recent decades, the science of understanding and improving the health of men who are at the margins of each field—yet lie at the nexus of these literatures—has not kept pace with the development of either field (Griffith, 2018). Improvements in population health and achieving health equity require an accelerated development of an area of specialization that can explicate how and why inequities among men exist and that can present evidence that informs efforts to improve the health of men and reduce inequities among them (Griffith, 2018). This emergent field is that of men's health equity.

Men's health equity is a field of research, practice, and policy that seeks to understand and address the needs of men whose poor health is rooted in their underlying social position in society in ways that are sensitive to and congruent with the socially meaningful identities and structures that have implications for individual- and population-level solutions to health inequities

(Srinivasan & Williams, 2014). Men's health equity includes two lines of research: (a) a population-specific approach that focuses on identifying, examining, and developing interventions from the unique biopsychosocial factors that affect the health of socially defined populations (Bediako & Griffith, 2007; Jack & Griffith, 2013) and (b) a comparative approach that is useful for identifying and monitoring gaps between men and women and among groups of men that are unnecessary, avoidable, considered unfair and unjust, and yet are modifiable (Carter-Pokras & Baquet, 2002). Men's health equity includes not only the study of individual- or population-level factors that may exacerbate or lead to worse health outcomes but also the identification of protective factors that may be important foundations for building policy and programmatic interventions at or across biopsychosocial levels and factors (Griffith, 2016). Men's health equity is an effort to move beyond the narrow boundaries and silos of men's health, specific medical specialties, health disparities (and related synonyms), public health, population health, and various social science disciplines and to be an umbrella that includes all who are interested in using scientific methods to inform, address, and eliminate avoidable yet unjust differences in health outcomes among men. While there is considerable attention in men's health to behavior, biology, and other intrapersonal factors that put men at risk for poor health outcomes, men's health equity recognizes and focuses on the premise that men's positions in the social hierarchy are also important for understanding population health (Frohlich & Potvin, 2008).

Beyond the epidemiologic argument about differences in life expectancy and other outcomes or the moral argument that often underlies the desire to achieve health equity, men's health equity highlights real economic and social costs of not focusing on the heterogeneity among men. In their seminal, sobering work, "Economic burden of men's health disparities in the United States," Thorpe, Richard, Bowie, Laveist, and Gaskin (2013) estimated the potential cost-savings from eliminating differences in health disparities among men of color in the United States. Using national data from 2006 to 2009, Thorpe and colleagues found that the total direct medical care expenditures for African American men equaled $447.6 billion, of which $24.2 billion was for excess healthcare expenditures. With regard to indirect costs to the economy from wages lost because of lower productivity and premature death, African American and Hispanic men were associated with $317.6 and $115.0 billion, respectively. In the context of this work, it is important to offer conceptual frameworks and, ultimately, theories and explanations that not only help to explain these phenomena, but that help to inform where and how to intervene. Thus, the goal of men's health disparities is to move beyond a focus on "what" differences exist to "why," "how," or "under what conditions" such differences (or similarities) illuminate modifiable determinants to improve the health and well-being of men (Addis, 2008; Griffith, 2018). These issues become particularly important as we examine health issues in the United States and across the globe.

WHY MASCULINITIES DO NOT SOLELY DETERMINE MEN'S HEALTH

Rose (1985) argues, "The hardest cause to identify is one that is universally present, for then it has no influence on the distribution of disease" (pp. 32–33). In the context of the study of masculinities in men's health, this concept suggests that continued efforts to focus masculinity or masculinities could be problematic without theoretically driven examination of how these factors can be disentangled from other determinants of men's health. The generic term "men" or "men's health," and the homogenizing focus on "what" differences exist between men and women or among men, obscures key aspects of heterogeneity that are essential foundations of interventions and which determine the most beneficial intervention points. Men's health equity is an intersectionality-based health equity lens that highlights that each group of men's experiences are fundamentally different from that of others, based on their unique identity and structural position within systems of inequality and structural impediments (Griffith, 2018; National Academies of Sciences, Engineering, and Medicine, 2017). Using an intersectional lens to study men's health requires researchers to recognize and contextualize the ways that race, class, sexual orientation, disability, and other structures and axes of inequity constitute intersecting systems of oppression and yet take on new meaning when combined with biopsychosocial constructs that are applied to men (e.g., sex, gender, masculinities, manhood; Griffith, 2018).

In some areas of biomedical and public health research and practice, there is a tendency to rely on the demographic boxes that men check as a proxy for their risk, resources, and potential resilience. While these factors have demonstrated how they are defined by others, demographic labels do not capture the complexity of how these men identify and define themselves. Historically, beyond the sex/gender box that signifies economic and sociopolitical power relative to women, many of the demographic and psychosocial boxes that diverse groups of men check have been the markers of subordination or marginalization (Connell, 1987). Groups of males who are marginalized or disadvantaged (e.g., poor men, men of color, uninsured men, gay men; Courtenay, 2002) tend to be invisible when it comes to health policy, yet hypervisible when determining risk and blame for poor health (Griffith, 2015). It is in these populations that we tend to see the greatest need for an intersectional approach to understanding how specific life circumstances and vulnerabilities shape their health profiles and patterns.

While Connell's macrosociological framework of masculinities considers the relations among genders (Connell, 1995), it also prioritizes gender as the lens through which to understand the relevance of other structures that affect men's lives and health. While this may be a useful way to frame the experience of White men from WEIRD cultures (Jones, 2010), for men, Connell characterizes, as subordinated or marginalized, this is less likely to be the case. Connell's masculinities (Connell, 1995) and notions of hegemonic masculinity (Connell, 2012; Connell & Messerschmidt, 2005) remain susceptible to the critique that this lens obscures the ability to locate the individual in larger group practices (Jefferson, 2002; Lusher & Robins, 2009). There is a lack of attention to other dimensions of social structure that play a fundamental role in shaping gender's operation and meaning (Shields, 2008). The structures that shape men's health are interdependent and cut across structures, cultures, and individuals in ways that are embodied in the health and lives of individual men and population groups that they may represent (Lusher & Robins, 2009). The multiple axes of oppression should be fashioned together in ways that consider not only how structures operate in relation to one another but also how intersectionality highlights the ways that structures combine in ways that create new structures that, therefore, shape the experience of men whose lives and health are at the nexus of these structures. And yet, attention to how race, ethnicity, rurality, sexual orientation, gender identity, spiritual practice, religious identity, SES, and other factors combine in ways that force men to negotiate masculinity by drawing upon pieces of hegemonic masculinity that they have the capacity to perform (Coles, 2008), remains at the margins of men's health. More importantly, this framework does not articulate the problem in such way that helps to identify where or how to intervene.

INTERSECTIONALITY SPOTLIGHT

A key aspect of research on social determinants of health disparities is the identification of fundamental social determinants that are antecedents to socioeconomic class and position (Griffith, Metzl, & Gunter, 2011; Kawachi, Daniels, & Robinson, 2005). SES and position contribute heavily to racial and ethnic disparities, but because men are more economically and socially advantaged in most cultures, there is not a socioeconomic theory that explains men's lower life expectancy in relation to women (Lohan, 2007).

Gender, particularly among males, is a fundamental social determinant of health that dramatically illustrates that factors other than SES affect health. Public health professionals must address gender as a fundamental, social determinant of racial and ethnic disparities in health, and intentionally and carefully consider gender in public health interventions. A fundamental determinant of health is one whose implications for health cannot be eliminated by addressing the specific mechanisms and pathways that appear to connect them to poor health (Link & Phelan, 1995). Because fundamental causes involve access to valuable resources that can have implications for many situations and settings, these causes have enduring effects on health outcomes of interest because as one link between the determinant and health declines, another emerges and becomes equally or more prominent (Link & Phelan, 1995). What is often underappreciated about fundamental causes is that their effects are rooted in socially meaningful constructs (e.g., race, ethnicity, social class, education, economic status) that otherwise should not necessarily be significant determinants of health (Dressler, Oths, & Gravlee, 2005). For example, while social class and economic status have significant implications for health in the United States, other countries (e.g., Sweden) have created policies and structures that negate the link between economic resources and health (Marmot & Allen, 2014; Marmot, Friel, Bell, Houweling, & Taylor, 2008).

The literature on masculinities highlights idealized and valued elements that define the gender order; however, race, culture (i.e., religion and spirituality), and age expand our understanding of hegemonic masculinities (Gough, Robertson, & Robinson, 2016) and the intersection of identities and factors that shape gendered experiences and ideals and aspirations of adult males (Griffith & Cornish, 2018). While the literature on fundamental determinants of health has tended to illustrate how socially defined characteristics represent dimensions that consistently advantage one group and disadvantage another (e.g., race, SES), gender is unique as a fundamental determinant of health because of its complex relationship to other fundamental determinants of health such as privilege, resources, and opportunity. For example, while the social and economic benefits of being a man are well documented, so too are the health disadvantages of being male. Further, when gender is combined with race or ethnicity, certain social and economic advantages are negated, particularly in the case of African American men (Jackson & Williams, 2006).

Gender, particularly among males, is a fundamental social determinant of health and, as such, dramatically illustrates that factors other than SES affect health. Because fundamental causes involve access to valuable resources that can have implications for many situations and

(continued)

settings, these causes have enduring effects on the health outcomes of interest: as one link between the determinant and health declines, another emerges and becomes equally or more prominent (Link & Phelan, 1995). Thus, the consideration of men's health inequity inherently takes an intersectional perspective.

TOWARD MEN'S HEALTH EQUITY

Amid a global rise in the interest in men's health and masculinities (see recent reports by World Health Organization, the Pan American Health Organization, and Promundo), there remains an inadequate amount of attention to the heterogeneity in the categories of males and men. The hyperfocus on masculinity, particularly toxic masculinity, as the fundamental cause of men's poor health and the solution to achieving gender equity fails to consider that poor health is not equally distributed among men nor are the benefits that are conferred with being male. Intersectionality has provided an important lens and analytic tool to help researchers "radically contextualize" the complexity of the web of conditions that shape the lives and health of men and either create conditions for health equity or health inequities (National Academies of Sciences, Engineering, & Medicine, 2017). Intersectionality has shed important light on the cultural narratives that frame how we define and explain men's health patterns and the institutional arrangements that create and maintain them (Griffith, Johnson, Ellis, & Schulz, 2010) and has also shed light on the lives of men that remain invisible when we use the generic term men or men's health.

Connell (2012) argues that intersectionality combines a categorical approach on one dimension of difference with a categorical approach to another. This is fundamentally different from how others and I understand and apply the lens of intersectionality. Since its coining more than four decades ago, intersectionality has highlighted how the intersection of structures embodied in populations creates meanings that are fundamentally different from those of the structures that comprise them or the identities that are used to represent them. Using an intersectional lens to study men's health requires researchers to contextualize and recognize the ways that race, class, sexual orientation, disability, and other structures and axes of inequity constitute intersecting systems of oppression when conceptualizing the problem of research interest as well as the intervention. These intersectional approaches and strategies provide a precise tool to facilitate creating well-designed and rigorously supported hypotheses to inform research and policy rather than a broad approach that assumes that all are equally vulnerable and, therefore, all would equally benefit (Frohlich & Potvin, 2008; National Academies of Sciences, Engineering, & Medicine, 2016).

It is critical to consider how sex and gender differences can be analyzed alongside other socially meaningful characteristics (e.g., sexual orientation, gender expression, racial identity, ethnic identity) that are essential to creating more sensitive and salient policy evaluation metrics (Griffith, 2016). Policy and programmatic efforts to pursue health equity that do not consider how sex and gender pattern the impacts of policies that affect health are unlikely to achieve equity because they are not considering key structural factors that shape health. The examples provided in this chapter illustrate how ignoring how gender and race intersect to highlight the unique risks that certain groups of men face undermines the goal of health equity. Men's health equity helps to center the focus of health policy efforts in ways that move away from a deficit-focused conversation and policy around men's health. These efforts also move away from the internal causation and decontextualized approach that locates men's health problems in the men themselves toward new points of programmatic and policy interventions beyond healthcare access and encouraging men to engage in healthier behavior. As opposed to limiting the problem to changing men and masculinity, successfully achieving health equity is likely to require that men's health promotion integrates a gender perspective in exploring the implications of all policies, from a similar social construction of gender as currently occurs in women's health promotion (White & Richardson, 2011).

In addition, it is critical to recognize that health systems and policies that have presumably been gender-neutral or male dominated have failed men and women alike (Broom, 2009). There is a need to incorporate a gendered perspective in all policy processes and spheres, not just in relation to women's health (Varanka, 2008). Both men and women can find common ground in supporting the need for gender-sensitive policies, programs, and evaluation indicators of the effectiveness of these efforts (Broom, 2009). Gender mainstreaming is an approach to writing and evaluating policy that facilitates moving beyond reifying gender differences to look for interconnections that may lead to more effective policy and practice (Griffith, 2016).

Perhaps what distinguishes the science of men's health equity from other areas of health equity is that it is rooted in an intersectional approach. It is critical to approach men's health equity by examining fundamental social determinants that are antecedents to socioeconomic class and position (Griffith, Metzl, et al., 2011; Kawachi et al., 2005), which include race, ethnicity, and gender. While research on health equity has typically focused on demographic characteristics that were markers of disadvantage, it is important to begin by using a framework that considers that these characteristics may not represent the same benefits or harms to all. Even if there are societal, economic, and political benefits to gender and other demographic proxies for the differential allocation of health-harming and health-promoting resources, we cannot assume that they benefit everyone equally or in all cases. It is critical to begin presenting data, designing policies, and monitoring the effects of policies by using an intersectional lens.

The systems and structures that shape differential access to resources that affect individual and population health do so over time, not simply at a point in time (Gee, Hing, Mohammed, Tabor, & Williams, 2019). Researchers have to consider the range of biopsychosocial factors that are at play in the lives of men and those who are shaping the lives of men (Griffith, 2016). Age, developmental phase of life, phase of life-associated role and goal expectations, a life course perspective, and the sociopolitical context of a particular point in time and over time have been fundamental building blocks of men's health equity (Griffith, 2012, 2015, 2016; Thorpe & Archibald, 2019). In sum, time matters as we think about the factors that influence men's individual and population health.

It is critical for research and policy to move beyond identifying how structural locations influence objective life circumstances and health outcomes to considering how the meanings of stressors are shaped by these broader contexts (McLeod, 2012). Structural factors are clearly the foundation of what determines health inequities, but how men understand, explain, and feel about their experiences and status in life also have important implications for health (Griffith, Brinkley-Rubinstein, Thorpe, Bruce, & Metzl, 2015). Particularly for men whose experience includes some form of marginalization, it is critical to consider how they navigate local masculinities and structures where their experience of marginalization (e.g., by race) may be the lens through which they understand their daily experience. For example, Griffith, Ellis, and Allen (2013) found that African American men framed, described, and lived stressful social experiences by characterizing them as racial, rarely if ever highlighting how the intersection of being African American and an adult male played a role in the microsocial experience. If men do or do not appreciate how the racism they experience is gendered, they may have different ways of interpreting, explaining, and responding to it (Ellis, Griffith, Allen, Thorpe, & Bruce, 2015). The precarious nature of manhood, coupled with the chronicity of racism, whether anticipated through vigilance or experienced through microaggressions, suggests that there are added stressors for African American men that have important implications for their health. These added stressors may force African American men to adapt and embody characteristics and ideals that they feel they can benefit from, particularly in work and social settings where stressors are present. Gendered racism includes a broad array of stressors that professional African American men often endure in order to adapt and appeal to masculine norms and to be successful in their chosen careers. Efforts to embody characteristics that reflect good character are often used to counter narratives and experiences that are shaped by the fact that these men were both African American and adult males (Pieterse & Carter, 2007). Because of the intersection of these racial, gender, and age-related identities, presenting themselves as proud, self-reliant, spiritual, family men who embody middle-class values may have positive implications for their mental health and yet negative implications for their physical health (Griffith, Cornish, McKissic, & Dean, 2016).

CASE STUDY   INTERSECTIONALITY AND THE HEALTH OF MIDDLE-AGED AFRICAN AMERICAN MEN

Men's health is based on understanding the social and health implications of gender, a socially defined construct, but it is critical to consider that gender depends on other social categories for meaning (Coles, 2009; Griffith, 2012). This section briefly explores how an intersectional approach can enhance our understanding of the health of middle-aged African American men. For more on middle-aged men's health, please see Griffith, Jaeger, Sherman, and Moore (2019). Figure 11.1 (Griffith, 2012) builds from a model developed by Dr. Thomas LaVeist that helps researchers studying race and ethnicity to be more critical of the way they conceptualize, operationalize, and utilize these terms in empirical research (LaVeist, 1996) and seeks to offer a framework to move beyond identifying *which* social characteristics affect health to articulating *why* those factors affect health, and *how* they come together to influence a population's health. Structural factors, and the physical features that serve as indicators of them, trigger environmental, political, and social determinants of health.

Gendered processes—social relations and practices culturally associated with biological sex—are the complex array of social relations and practices attached to sex that are rooted in biology and shaped by environment and experience (Evans, Frank, Oliffe, & Gregory, 2011; Springer, Mager Stellman, & Jordan-Young, 2012). Gender is both a structural characteristic that helps to define systems of social inequality and an individual-level experience, and it is critical to explore how it is understood, experienced, and practiced daily at both levels (Coles, 2009; Weber & Parra-Medina, 2003). Gendered cultural norms and expectations serve as stressors and psychological strains in men's social contexts and daily lives. Gender affects men's health by triggering physiological and psychological responses that may lead to unconscious and

(continued)

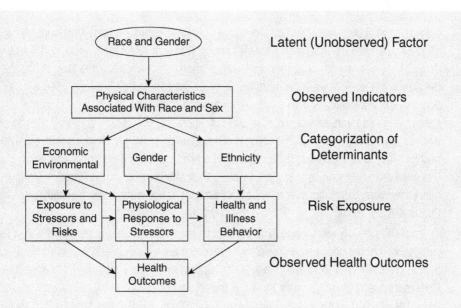

FIGURE 11.1 Intersectional approach to understanding determinants of men's health equity.

SOURCE: Reproduced with permission from Griffith, D. M. (2012). An intersectional approach to men's health. *Journal of Men's Health, 9*(2), 106–112. doi:10.1016/j.jomh.2012.03.003

conscious efforts to reduce the discomfort of experiencing stress (Jackson & Knight, 2006). Men will access culturally acceptable resources within their environments that they may have found "effective" in reducing stress before (Jackson & Knight, 2006), heard, or observed others using these strategies or simply choosing what they see as the best possible resource. These culturally appropriate behaviors are frequently gendered and may help explain the association between men's risky and unhealthy behaviors (Courtenay, 2000).

Lachman (2015)—perhaps the leading scholar on middle-aged adults—argues that midlife is a "pivotal period in the life course." This phase of life can be defined by age, role, responsibility, intrapersonal characteristic, or some combination of these factors. Chronological age may not be the best anchor for identifying what is midlife; midlife may be better considered in terms of roles, timing of events, and life experience (Lachman, Teshale, & Agrigoroaei, 2015). There is evidence that stresses involving multiple role demands or financial pressures may cluster in midlife or take a greater toll in middle age (Aldwin & Levenson, 2001; Lachman et al., 2015). Similarly, Evans et al. (2011) argue that during midlife, "... men construct their masculinity in relation to the physicality of their work and/or the level of income their labor produces. Thus, for men, work defines their status in the masculine hierarchy and has significance as a site for the social production of masculinity" (p. 12). During midlife, changes in the family structure, work status, injuries, and illness may influence both the general outlook on life and the wish and ability to prioritize health-promoting behavior (Wandel & Roos, 2006). It has been demonstrated for some time that disparities—particularly by race and sex—are greatest during middle age

(continued)

(Satcher et al., 2005). Specifically, Satcher et al. (2005) noted that African American men aged 45 to 64 years had the least improvement compared to their White male peers, and it was the decline in health among these men that was primarily responsible for the lack of change in the size of the racial disparity in mortality between the two groups between 1960 and 2000. Some of the masculinities men try to perform when they are younger tend to demonstrate their physical strength, sexual prowess, and risk tolerance, but as men age, they tend to also want to demonstrate more positive aspects of masculinity: being a responsible father, provider, husband, and so on (Bowman, 1989; Hammond & Mattis, 2005). For example, one study found that middle-aged African American men viewed their efforts to be good and active employees, family members, and community members as a barrier to engaging in physical activity (Griffith, Gunter, & Allen, 2011).

Race and ethnicity are sociopolitical constructs, not anthropologically or scientifically based categories, that are useful when the aims of research are to understand how stratification by race influences health (Ford & Harawa, 2010). Critical masculinity scholars have emphasized the importance of locating men's health in the context of class-based, racialized masculinities (Connell, 2000; Crawshaw, 2009; Pease, 2009; Riska, 2006; Robertson, 2007; Schofield, Connell, Walker, Wood, & Butland, 2000). Racially linked factors shape the types of masculinities that men are able to embody because the environments where men live are influenced by the global, national, and local meaning of race (Courtenay, 2002; Ford & Harawa, 2010; Griffith & Cornish, 2018; Pease, 2009). Race is a particularly important determinant of health because it influences social class and economic position in society, not the other way around (Kawachi et al., 2005). Also, African American men may define themselves as middle class based less on economic position and more on values and social behavior (Cole & Omari, 2003).

Ethnicity encompasses aspects of culture, social life, and personal identity that socially defined groups tend to share (Ford & Harawa, 2010). Ethnic groups consist of people assumed to have common cultural and often similar physical traits that distinguish them from other ethnic groups, including primary language, nativity, history, traditions, values, and dietary habits (Smedley & Smedley, 2005). Physical traits, however, are not presumed to distinguish ethnic groups nor assume superior or inferior groups (Smedley & Smedley, 2005). Ethnicity comprises two dimensions: the attributional dimension describes the unique sociocultural characteristics (e.g., culture, diet) of groups, while the relational dimension captures characteristics of the relationship between an ethnically defined group and the society in which it is situated (Ford & Harawa, 2010). In the context of men's health, distinguishing between race and ethnicity can help researchers disentangle health outcomes that may be due to environmental constraints and contexts that vary by race from the cultural traditions, beliefs, habits, and practices that vary by ethnicity. Race and ethnicity are useful markers of one's exposure to health-harming environments and substances, social disadvantage, and health-promoting resources (LaVeist, 2000).

Men's experiences and successes in midlife are strongly influenced by SES and determinants of SES like race and ethnicity (Griffith, 2012; Kawachi et al., 2005), but little work has been done regarding how different socioeconomic groups view progress in age or how these changes over the life course may influence health-promoting habits (Wandel & Roos, 2006).

CONCLUSION

Sex has primarily been used to mark the social, economic, and political disadvantage of women, though this does not translate to women having worse health outcomes than men. While there is a critical need to continue to fund, support, and build the infrastructure necessary to achieve optimal women's health, there is a similar need to achieve not only men's health but also population health equity. Continuing to ignore gender as a fundamental determinant of men's and women's health undermines our ability to achieve health equity. It is also critical to recognize that gender intersects with other social determinants of health in ways that may not be the same for all populations. Research and policy need to be designed to more effectively identify, monitor, and address patterns that exist because of the intersection of more than one structure for which demographic factors serve as useful proxies.

Gender should be a lens used to design, monitor, and determine the effectiveness of all policies, not only ones designed to improve women's health (Varanka, 2008). Gender mainstreaming has been offered as a tool to facilitate moving beyond a discussion that reifies and presumes gender differences in health to looking for interconnections and the diversity among these sex and gender categories that may be fodder for more effective policy and practice. Gender-sensitive policies, programs, and evaluation indicators will benefit women and men alike (Broom, 2009), assuming we do not presume that gender is equally beneficial or harmful for all of a particular sex or gender presentation.

As we move toward policies that consider gender in their framing and in the examination of their impact, it is also critical to bring the biopsychosocial and intersectionality frameworks to bear on these policies (Griffith, 2016; White & Richardson, 2011). It is critical for policy makers to report and evaluate gender differences in health, social, and economic policies without looking to blame the population who seems not to benefit from the policy as much as other populations. Beyond the sex and gender differences in policy effectiveness, it is critical to consider how sex and gender differences can be analyzed alongside other socially meaningful characteristics. Sexual orientation, gender expression, racial identity, ethnic identity, and other factors are essential to integrating with gender and sex to interpret policy evaluation metrics accurately. The goal, therefore, is to understand men's health and men's health equity in their own right, not in comparison to women.

In addition, to achieve men's health equity means dealing with racism. Populations that are not races (e.g., ethnic groups, religious minorities) are becoming racialized in ways that adversely affect their health (LeBrón & Viruell-Fuentes, 2019; Samari, Alcalá, & Sharif, 2019). Came and Griffith (2018) describe racism as the epitome of a "wicked" problem: one that is complex, highly resistant to solutions, and characterized by disagreement about the nature and cause of the problem and their potential solutions. Others have described racism as the defining form of oppression in the United States and the biggest obstacle to achieving health equity (Ford, Griffith, Bruce, & Gilbert, 2019). Gendered racism is even more complex and prone to disagreement, yet it represents and embodies cultural, institutional, and normative factors that are the root causes of men's health inequities.

Finally, there is a critical need to move the U.S. narrative about men's health from such a negative, deficit-based, and intrapersonal one to considering and highlighting the valuable roles males play in family and community life. The gendered ideals of adult men are not synonymous with the rhetoric of "toxic masculinity," which has created a flat, deficit-focused narrative that blames men for their poor health outcomes. There is a critical need to embrace the full range of masculinities, the ones that are harmful and yes the ones that are health and socially beneficial to more accurately contextualize and locate men's health problems. This reframing of masculinity is not only more accurate, but it offers a broader range and a more effective array of options that point to places and opportunities to intervene. These more diverse narratives also reinforce the diverse and intersecting social, economic, cultural, political, and environmental factors that affect men's health. To quote Bell (2018), "If we are to seek new goals for our struggles, we must first reassess the worth of the [gender and] racial assumptions on which, without careful thought, we have presumed too much and relied on too long. Let's begin" (p. 14).

CURRENT EVENTS

MEN'S RIGHTS

An interesting recent cultural phenomenon is the emergence of "men's rights" groups that claim that social changes have begun to marginalize and systematically disadvantage men in comparison to women. To say this view is controversial is an understatement, and opinions range from the thought that the movement is an accurate representation of what it means to be "a man" in today's society, to the thought that the movement is simply a "re-branding" of patriarchy and misogyny. Those who subscribe to the notion, however, believe that this new oppression of men as a whole is to blame for several outcomes for which men face higher rates (e.g., suicide).

Discussion Question: Do the facts regarding disparities in suicide (e.g., higher among men than women, but higher among White men than minority men) align with the statement that oppression of men explains the disparity? Why or why not?

PROSTATE CANCER SCREENING

Prostate cancer screening guidelines change regularly, but regardless of the current set of guidelines at any time, men are very unlikely to accept and receive prostate cancer screening. For many men, the concept of a digital rectal examination (DRE) is something that elicits laughter or even fear. Rates of acceptance of DRE are lower in minority communities than White communities, and prevention initiatives are rarely culturally tailored to the needs of minority men.

Discussion Question: How could a prostate cancer screening initiative be designed to counteract the gender-related and cultural stigma surrounding prostate cancer screening? How could traditional notions of masculinity be utilized to increase a campaign's effectiveness?

DISCUSSION QUESTIONS

- How do the concepts of power and privilege complicate discussion of men's health equity?
- Diseases of despair are unexpectedly higher in non-minority men than in minority men. What cultural processes might impact this?
- What are examples of differences in health that reflect men's health inequalities, as contrasted to examples that represent true men's health inequities?

- In what ways can intersectional identities become even more impactful for men than for women?

- As with women, African American men face higher mortality rates for many of the leading causes of death nationwide. How can prevention messages and initiatives be tailored to the realities and needs of African American men?

ACKNOWLEDGMENTS

This chapter has been supported in part by Vanderbilt University Office of the Vice Provost for Research, the American Cancer Society (RSG-15-223-01-CPPB), and NIMHD (5U54MD010722-02).

REFERENCES

Addis, M. E. (2008). Gender and Depression in Men. *Clinical Psychology: Science and Practice, 15*(3), 153–168.

Aldwin, C. M., & Levenson, M. R. (2001). Stress, coping, and health at mid-life. In M. E. Lachman (Ed.), *The handbook of midlife development* (pp. 188–214). New York, NY: John Wiley & Sons.

Baker, P., Dworkin, S. L., Tong, S., Banks, I., Shand, T., & Yamey, G. (2014). The men's health gap: Men must be included in the global health equity agenda. *Bulletin of the World Health Organization, 92*(8), 618–620. doi: 10.2471/BLT.13.132795

Bediako, S. M., & Griffith, D. M. (2007). Eliminating racial/ethnic health disparities: Reconsidering comparative approaches. *Journal of Health Disparities Research and Practice, 2*(1), 49–62.

Bell, D. (2018). *Faces at the bottom of the well: The permanence of racism.* New York, NY: Basic Books.

Beltrán-Sánchez, H., Finch, C. E., & Crimmins, E. M. (2015). Twentieth century surge of excess adult male mortality. *Proceedings of the National Academy of Sciences, 112*(29), 8993–8998. doi: 10.1073/pnas.1421942112

Bilal, U., & Diez-Roux, A. V. (2018). Troubling trends in health disparities. *New England Journal of Medicine, 378*(16), 1557–1558. doi: 10.1056/NEJMc1800328

Bowman, P. J. (1989). Research perspectives on Black men: Role strain and adaptation across the adult life cycle. In R. L. Jones (Ed.), *Black adult development and aging* (pp. 117–150). Berkeley, CA: Cobb & Henry Publishers.

Braveman, P. (2006). Health disparities and health equity: Concepts and measurement. *Annual Review of Public Health, 27*, 167–194. doi: annurev.publhealth.27.021405.102103

Braveman, P. (2014). What are health disparities and health equity? We need to be clear. *Public Health Reports (Washington, DC: 1974), 129*, 5–8. doi: 10.1177/00333549141291S203

Braveman, P., Egerter, S., & Williams, D. R. (2011). The social determinants of health: Coming of age. *Annual Review of Public Health, 32*, 381–398. doi: 10.1146/annurev-publhealth-031210-101218

Broom, D. H. (2009). Men's health and women's health – Deadly enemies or strategic allies. *Critical Public Health, 19*(3/4), 269–277. doi: 10.1080/09581590902906195

Byrd, W. M., & Clayton, L. A. (2000). *An American health dilemma.* New York, NY: Routledge.

Came, H., & Griffith, D. (2018). Tackling racism as a "wicked" public health problem: Enabling allies in anti-racism praxis. *Social Science & Medicine, 199*, 181–188. doi: 10.1016/j.socscimed.2017.03.028

Carter-Pokras, O., & Baquet, C. (2002). What is a "health disparity"? *Public Health Reports, 117*(5), 426–434.

Case, A., & Deaton, A. (2017). Mortality and morbidity in the 21st century. *Brookings Papers on Economic Activity, 2017*, 397. doi: 10.1353/eca.2017.0005

Cole, E. R., & Omari, S. R. (2003). Race, class and the dilemmas of upward mobility for African Americans. *Journal of Social Issues, 59*(4), 785–802. doi: 10.1046/j.0022-4537.2003.00090.x

Coles, T. (2008). Finding space in the field of masculinity. *Journal of Sociology, 44*(3), 233–248. doi: 10.1177/1440783308092882

Coles, T. (2009). Negotiating the field of masculinity. *Men and Masculinities, 12*(1), 30–44. doi: 10.1177/1097184x07309502

Connell, R. (1987). *Gender and power: Society, the person, and sexual politics.* Stanford, CA: Stanford University Press.

Connell, R. (2012). Gender, health and theory: Conceptualizing the issue, in local and world perspective. *Social Science & Medicine, 74*(11), 1675–1683. doi: 10.1016/j.socscimed.2011.06.006

Connell, R. W. (1995). *Masculinities.* Berkeley, CA: University of California Press.

Connell, R. W. (2000). *The men and the boys.* Sydney, Australia: Allen & Unwin.

Connell, R. W., & Messerschmidt, J. W. (2005). Hegemonic masculinity: Rethinking the concept. *Gender & Society, 19*(6), 829–859. doi: 10.1177/0891243205278639

Courtenay, W. (2002). A global perspective on the field of men's health: An editorial. *International Journal of Men's Health, 1*(1), 1. doi: 10.3149/jmh.0101.1

Courtenay, W. H. (2000). Constructions of masculinity and their influence on men's well-being: A theory of gender and health. *Social Science and Medicine, 50*(10), 1385–1401. doi: 10.1016/S0277-9536(99)00390-1

Crawshaw, P. (2009). Critical perspectives on the health of men: Lessons from medical sociology. *Critical Public Health, 19*(3), 279–285. doi: 10.1080/09581590902941507

De Maio, F. (2014). *Global health inequities: A sociological perspective.* London, UK: Macmillan International Higher Education.

de Melo-Martin, I., & Intemann, K. K. (2007). Can ethical reasoning contribute to better epidemiology? A case study in research on racial health disparities. *European Journal of Epidemiology, 22*(4), 215–221. doi: 10.1007/s10654-007-9108-3

Dressler, W. W., Oths, K. S. & Gravlee, C. C. (2005). Race and ethnicity in public health research: Models to explain health disparities. *Annual Review of Anthropology, 34,* 231–252. doi: 10.1146/annurev.anthro.34.081804.120505

Ellis, K. R., Griffith, D. M., Allen, J. O., Thorpe, R. J., Jr., & Bruce, M. A. (2015). "If you do nothing about stress, the next thing you know, you're shattered": Perspectives on African American men's stress, coping and health from African American men and key women in their lives. *Social Science & Medicine, 139,* 107–114. doi: 10.1016/j.socscimed.2015.06.036

Erwin, P. C. (2017). Despair in the American heartland? A focus on rural health. *American Journal of Public Health, 107*(10), 1533–1534. doi: 10.2105/AJPH.2017.304029

Evans, J., Frank, B., Oliffe, J. L., & Gregory, D. (2011). Health, Illness, Men and Masculinities (HIMM): A theoretical framework for understanding men and their health. *Journal of Men's Health, 8*(1), 7–15. doi: 10.1016/j.jomh.2010.09.227

Ford, C. L., Griffith, D. M., Bruce, M. A., & Gilbert, K. L. (2019). Introduction. In C. L. Ford, D. M. Griffith, M. A. Bruce, & K. L. Gilbert (Eds.), *Racism: Science & tools for the public health professional.* Washington, DC: APHA Press.

Ford, C. L., & Harawa, N. T. (2010). A new conceptualization of ethnicity for social epidemiologic and health equity research. *Social Science & Medicine, 71*(2), 251–258. doi: 10.1016/j.socscimed.2010.04.008

Frohlich, K. L., & Potvin, L. (2008). The inequality paradox: The population approach and vulnerable populations. *American Journal of Public Health, 98*(2), 216–221. doi: 10.2105/AJPH.2007.114777

Gaydosh, L., Hummer, R. A., Hargrove, T. W., Halpern, C. T., Hussey, J. M., Whitsel, E. A., … Harris, K. M. (2019). The depths of despair among US adults entering midlife. *American Journal of Public Health, 109*(5), 774–780. doi: 10.2105/AJPH.2019.305002

Gee, G. C., Hing, A., Mohammed, S., Tabor, D. C., & Williams, D. R. (2019). Racism and the life course: Taking time seriously. *American Journal of Public Health, 109*(S1), S43–S47. doi: 10.2105/AJPH.2018.304766

Gough, B., Robertson, S., & Robinson, M. (2016). Men, 'masculinity' and mental health: Critical reflections. In J. Gideon (Ed.), *Handbook on gender and health* (p. 134). Cheltenham, UK: Edward Elgar.

Griffith, D. M. (2012). An intersectional approach to men's health. *Journal of Men's Health, 9*(2), 106–112. doi: 10.1016/j.jomh.2012.03.003

Griffith, D. M. (2015). I AM a man: Manhood, minority men's health and health equity. *Ethnicity & Disease, 25*(3), 287–293. doi: 10.18865/ed.25.3.287

Griffith, D. M. (2016). Biopsychosocial approaches to men's health disparities research and policy. *Behavioral Medicine, 42*(3), 211–215. doi: 10.1080/08964289.2016.1194158

Griffith, D. M. (2018). "Centering the margins": Moving equity to the center of men's health research. *American Journal of Men's Health, 12*(5), 1317–1327. doi: 10.1177/1557988318773973

Griffith, D. M., Brinkley-Rubinstein, L., Thorpe, R. J., Jr., Bruce, M. A., & Metzl, J. M. (2015). The interdependence of African American men's definitions of manhood and health. *Family & Community Health, 38*(4), 284–296. doi: 10.1097/FCH.0000000000000079

Griffith, D. M., Bruce, M. A., & Thorpe, R. J., Jr. (2019). *Men's health equity: A handbook.* England, UK: Routledge.

Griffith, D. M., & Cornish, E. K. (2018). "What Defines a Man?": Perspectives of African American men on the components and consequences of manhood. *Psychology of Men & Masculinity, 19*(1), 78–88. doi: 10.1037/men0000083

Griffith, D. M., Cornish, E. K., McKissic, S. A., & Dean, D. A. L. (2016). John Henry and the paradox of manhood, fatherhood and health for African American fathers. In L. M. Burton, D. Burton, S. M. McHale, V. King, & J. Van Hook (Eds.), *Boys and men in African American families* (pp. 215–226). Cham, Switzerland: Springer International Publishing.

Griffith, D. M., Ellis, K. R., & Allen, J. O. (2013). Intersectional approach to stress and coping among African American men: Men's and women's perspectives. *American Journal of Men's Health, 7*(4S), 16–27. doi: 10.1177/1557988313480227

Griffith, D. M., Gunter, K., & Allen, J. O. (2011). Male gender role strain as a barrier to African American men's physical activity. *Health Education & Behavior, 38*(5), 482–491. doi: 10.1177/1090198110383660

Griffith, D. M., Gunter, K., & Watkins, D. C. (2012). Measuring masculinity in research on men of color: Findings and future directions. *American Journal of Public Health, 102*(Suppl. 2), S187–S194. doi: 10.2105/AJPH.2012.300715

Griffith, D. M., Jaeger, E. C., Sherman, L. D., & Moore, H. J. (2019). Middle-aged men's health: Patterns and causes of health inequities during a pivotal period in the life course. In D. M. Griffith, M. A. Bruce, & R. J. Thorpe, Jr. (Eds.), *Men's health equity: A handbook* (1st ed., pp. 72–85). New York, NY: Routledge.

Griffith, D. M., Johnson, J., Ellis, K. R., & Schulz, A. J. (2010). Cultural context and a critical approach to eliminating health disparities. *Ethnicity and Disease, 20*(1), 71–76.

Griffith, D. M., Metzl, J. M., & Gunter, K. (2011). Considering intersections of race and gender in interventions that address U.S. men's health disparities. *Public Health, 125*(7), 417–423. doi: 10.1016/j.puhe.2011.04.014

Hammond, W. P., & Mattis, J. S. (2005). Being a man about it: Manhood meaning among African American men. *Psychology of Men and Masculinity, 6*(2), 114–126. doi: 10.1037/1524-9220.6.2.114

Hankivsky, O. (2012). Women's health, men's health, and gender and health: Implications of intersectionality. *Social Science & Medicine, 74*(11), 1712–1720. doi: 10.1016/j.socscimed.2011.11.029

Jack, L., & Griffith, D. M. (2013). The health of African American Men: Implications for research and practice. *American Journal of Men's Health, 7*(4 suppl), 5S–7S.

Jackson, J. S., & Knight, K. M. (2006). Race and self-regulatory health behaviors: The role of the stress response and the HPA axis. In K. W. Schaie & L. L. Carstensten (Eds.), *Social structure, aging and self-regulation in the elderly* (pp. 189–240). New York, NY: Springer Publishing Company.

Jackson, P. B., & Williams, D. R. (2006). The intersection of race, gender and SES: Health paradoxes. In A. J. Schulz & L. Mullings (Eds.), *Gender, race, class & health: Intersectional approaches* (pp. 131–162). San Francisco, CA: Jossey-Bass.

Jefferson, T. (2002). Subordinating hegemonic masculinity. *Theoretical Criminology, 6*(1), 63–88. doi: 10.1177/136248060200600103

Jones, D. (2010). A WEIRD view of human nature skews psychologists' studies. *Science, 328*(5986), 1627. doi: 10.1126/science.328.5986.1627

Kawachi, I., Daniels, N., & Robinson, D. E. (2005). Health disparities by race and class: Why both matter. *Health Affairs, 24*(2), 343–352. doi: 10.1377/hlthaff.24.2.343

Krieger, N. (1987). Shades of difference: Theoretical underpinnings of the medical controversy on black/white differences in the United States, 1830-1870. *International Journal of Health Services, 17*(2), 259–278. doi: 10.2190/DBY6-VDQ8-HME8-ME3R

LaVeist, T. A. (1996). Why we should continue to study race ... but do a better job: An essay on race, racism and health. *Ethnicity & Disease, 6*(1/2), 21–29.

Lachman, M. E. (2015). Mind the gap in the middle: A call to study midlife. *Research in Human Development, 12*(3/4), 327–334. doi: 10.1080/15427609.2015.1068048

Lachman, M. E., Teshale, S., & Agrigoroaei, S. (2015). Midlife as a pivotal period in the life course: Balancing growth and decline at the crossroads of youth and old age. *International Journal of Behavioral Development, 39*(1), 20–31. doi: 10.1177/0165025414533223

LaVeist, T. A. (2000). On the study of race, racism, and health: A shift from description to explanation. *International Journal of Health Services, 30*(1), 217–219. doi: 10.2190/LKDF-UJQ5-W1KU-GLR1

LeBrón, A. M. W., & Viruell-Fuentes, E. A. (2019). Racism and the health of Latina/Latino communities. In C. L. Ford, D. M. Griffith, M. A. Bruce, & K. L. Gilbert. (Eds.), *Racism: Science & tools for the public health professional.* Washington, DC: APHA Press.

Link, B. G., & Phelan, J. (1995). Social conditions as fundamental causes of disease. *Journal of Health & Social Behavior, Spec No,* 80–94. doi: 10.2307/2626958

Lohan,(2007). How might we understand men's health better? Integrating explanations from critical studies on men and inequalities in health. *Social Science & Medicine, 65*(3), 493–504. doi: 10.1016/j.socscimed.2007.04.020

Lusher, D., & Robins, G. (2009). Hegemonic and other masculinities in local social contexts. *Men and Masculinities, 11*(4), 387–423. doi: 10.1177/1097184x06298776

Marmot, M., & Allen, J. J. (2014). Social determinants of health equity. *American Journal of Public Health, 104*(S4), S517–S519. doi: 10.2105/AJPH.2014.302200

Marmot, M., Friel, S., Bell, R., Houweling, T. A., & Taylor, S. (2008). Closing the gap in a generation: Health equity through action on the social determinants of health. *The Lancet, 372*(9650), 1661–1669. doi: 10.1016/S0140-6736(08)61690-6

Masters, R. K., Tilstra, A. M., & Simon, D. H. (2017). Mortality from suicide, chronic liver disease, and drug poisonings among middle-aged U.S. White men and women, 1980–2013. *Biodemography and Social Biology, 63*(1), 31–37. doi: 10.1080/19485565.2016.1248892

McLeod, J. D. (2012). The meanings of stress: Expanding the stress process model. *Society and Mental Health, 2*(3), 172–186. doi: 10.1177/2156869312452877

Meit, M., Heffernan, M., Tanenbaum, E., & Hoffmann, T. (2017). *Appalachian diseases of despair.* Report for the Appalachian Regional Commission. The Walsh Center for Rural Health Analysis–National Opinion Research Center at the University of Chicago. https://www.arc.gov/assets/research_reports/Appalachian DiseasesofDespairAugust2017.pdf

National Academies of Sciences, Engineering, & Medicine. (2016). *The promises and perils of digital strategies in achieving health equity: Workshop summary.* Washington, DC: The National Academies Press.

National Academies of Sciences, Engineering, & Medicine. (2017). *Communities in action: Pathways to health equity.* Washington, DC: National Academies Press.

National Center for Health Statistics. (2018). Deaths: Final data for 2016. *National Vital Statistics Report, 67*(5), 1–76. https://www.cdc.gov/nchs/data/nvsr/nvsr67/nvsr67_05.pdf

Newton, R. L., Jr., Griffith, D. M., Kearney, W., & Bennett, G. G. (2014). A systematic review of physical activity, dietary, and weight loss interventions involving African American men. *Obesity Reviews, 15*(Suppl. 4), 93–106. doi: 10.1111/obr.12209

Pearson, J. A. (2008). Can't buy me whiteness. *Du Bois Review, 5*(1), 27–47. doi: 10.1017/S1742058X0808003X

Pease, B. (2009). Racialised masculinities and the health of immigrant and refugee men. In A. Broom & E. P. Tovey (Eds.), *Men's health: Body, identity and context* (pp. 182–201). Chichester, NH: John Wiley and Sons.

Pieterse, A. L., & Carter, R. T. (2007). An examination of the relationship between general life stress, racism-related stress, and psychological health among Black men. *Journal of Counseling Psychology, 54*(1), 101–109.

Riska, E. (2006). *Masculinity and men's health: Coronary heart disease in medical public discourse.* Oxford, UK: Rowman and Littlefield.

Robertson, S. (2007). *Understanding men and health: Masculinities, identity, and well-being.* Maidenhead, UK: Open University Press.

Rose, G. (1985). Sick individuals and sick populations. *International Journal of Epidemiology*, *14*(1), 32–38. doi: 10.1093/ije/14.1.32

Samari, G., Alcalá, H. E., & Sharif, M. Z. (2019). Racialization of religious minorities. In C. L. Ford, D. M. Griffith, M. A. Bruce, & K. L. Gilbert (Eds.), *Racism: Science & tools for the public health professional*. Washington, DC: APHA Press.

Satcher, D., Fryer, G. E., Jr., McCann, J., Troutman, A., Woolf, S. H., & Rust, G. (2005). What if we were equal? A comparison of the black-white mortality gap in 1960 and 2000. *Health Affairs*, *24*(2), 459–464. doi: 10.1377/hlthaff.24.2.459

Schofield, T., Connell, R., Walker, L., Wood, J., & Butland, D. (2000). Understanding men's health and illness: A gender-relations approach to policy, research, and practice. *Journal of American College Health*, *486*, 247–256. doi: 10.1080/07448480009596266

Shields, S. A. (2008). Gender: An intersectionality perspective. *Sex Roles*, *59*(5-6), 301–311. doi: 10.1007/s11199-008-9501-8

Smedley, A., & Smedley, B. D. (2005). Race as biology is fiction, racism as a social problem is real: Anthropological and historical perspectives on the social construction of race. *American Psychologist*, *60*(1), 16–26. doi: 2005-00117-003

Snow, R. C. (2008). Sex, gender, and vulnerability. *Global Public Health*, *3*(Suppl. 1), 58–74. doi: 10.1080/17441690801902619

Springer, K. W., Mager Stellman, J., & Jordan-Young, R. M. (2012). Beyond a catalogue of differences: A theoretical frame and good practice guidelines for researching sex/gender in human health. *Social science & medicine*, *74*(11), 1817–1824.

Srinivasan, S., & Williams, S. D. (2014). Transitioning from health disparities to a health equity research agenda: The time is now. *Public Health Reports*, *129*(1_suppl2), 71–76.

Thorpe, R. J., Jr., Griffith, D. M., Gilbert, K. L., Elder, K., & Bruce, M. A. (2016). Men's health in 2010s: What is the global challenge? In J. Heidelbaugh (Ed.), *Men's health in primary care* (pp. 1–17). New York, NY: Springer.

Thorpe, R., Richard, P., Bowie, J., Laveist, T., & Gaskin, D. (2013). Economic burden of men's health disparities in the United States. *International Journal of Men's Health*, *12*(3), 195–212. doi: 10.3149/jmh.1203.195

Thorpe, R. J., & Archibald, P. C. (2019). Life course perspective: Implications for men's health equity. In D. M. Griffith, M. A. Bruce, & R. J. Thorpe, Jr. (Eds.), *Men's health equity* (pp. 563–569). New York, NY: Routledge.

Varanka, J. J. (2008). Mainstreaming men into gender sensitive health policies. *Journal of Men's Health*, *5*(3), 189–191. doi: 10.1016/j.jomh.2008.07.004

Wandel, M., & Roos, G. (2006). Age perceptions and physical activity among middle-aged men in three occupational groups. *Social Science & Medicine*, *62*(12), 3024–3034. doi: 10.1016/j.socscimed.2005.11.064

Weber, L., & Parra-Medina, D. (2003). Intersectionality and women's health: Charting a path to eliminating health disparities. In V. Demos & M. T. Segal (Eds.), *Advances in gender research: Gender perspectives on health and medicine* (pp. 181–230). Amsterdam, The Netherlands: Elsevier.

White, A., & Richardson, N. (2011). Gendered epidemiology: Making men's health visible in epidemiological research. *Public Health*, *125*(7), 407–410. doi: 10.1016/j.puhe.2011.04.012

World Health Organization. (2014). *Noncommunicable diseases country profiles 2014*. Geneva, Switzerland: Author. Retrieved from http://apps.who.int/iris/bitstream/handle/10665/128038/9789241?sequence=1

Woodward, A., & Kawachi, I. (2000). Why reduce health inequalities? *Journal of Epidemiology and Community Health*, *54*(12), 923–929. doi: 10.1136/jech.54.12.923

Young, A. M. W. (2009). Poverty and men's health: Global implications for policy and practice. *Journal of Men's Health*, *6*(3), 272. doi: 10.1016/j.jomh.2009.08.176

Young, A. M. W., Meryn, S., & Treadwell, H. M. (2008). Poverty and men's health. *Journal of Men's Health*, *5*(3), 184–188. doi: 10.1016/j.jomh.2008.07.001

LGBTQ HEALTH EQUITY

JACOB C. WARREN ■ K. BRYANT SMALLEY ■ M. ISABEL FERNÁNDEZ

LEARNING OBJECTIVES

- Identify and explain the appropriate terminology when discussing LGBTQ populations
- Describe the common barriers to health experienced by LGBTQ populations that contribute to health disparities
- Discuss the magnitude, risk factors, and prevention strategies of six outcomes of importance for LGBTQ health equity: obesity, cancer, mental health, suicide, substance use, and HIV
- Articulate the ways in which intersectionality impacts LGBTQ health equity
- Explain ways in which programs and services can be LGBTQ-inclusive and affirming

INTRODUCTION

Recent years have seen immense growth in the level of social acceptance of individuals who identify as lesbian, gay, bisexual, transgender, queer, and other sexual and gender minority groups (referred to in this chapter as LGBTQ). Nationally prominent Supreme Court decisions such as *United States v. Windsor* (2013) and *Obergefell v. Hodges* (2015), that together legalized same-sex marriage throughout the United States, have helped to reshape the legal protections of LGBTQ Americans in unprecedented ways. However, decades of historical injustices and discrimination combine with current prejudice to negatively impact the health of LGBTQ people in a variety of outcomes, impacting their ability to achieve health equity.

A surface examination of LGBTQ health readily identifies a host of health behaviors in which LGBTQ people are more likely to engage, ranging from alcohol, cigarette, and drug use (Balsam, Beadnell, & Riggs, 2012; Cabaj, 2014; Green & Feinstein, 2012; Kann et al., 2016; Weber & Dodge, 2017) to poor dietary habits (Diemer, Grant, Munn-Chernoff, Patterson, & Duncan, 2015; Feldman & Meyer, 2007; Gay and Lesbian Medical Association [GLMA], 2001). While these disparate rates of engaging in health risk behaviors are important to understand, a deeper look at the source of disparities reveals that use of the minority stress model—one that recognizes that the discrimination, victimization, and harassment that LGBTQ people face directly impacts their ability to achieve and maintain health in ways that non-LGBTQ people can—provides a much more equity-focused vantage point (Hendricks & Testa, 2012; Meyer, 1995, 2003, 2013).

The result of this accumulative minority stress is profound. Among other things, LGBTQ individuals are more likely to live in poverty, to be homeless, to receive substandard education, and to be uninsured, all of which clearly affect health equity (Burwick, Gates, Baumgartner, & Friend, 2014; McClain, Thomas, & Yehia, 2017; Karpman, Skopec, & Long, 2015). In short, focusing on modifying risky behavior—while important—does not address the underlying societal issues that are truly driving LGBTQ health disparities.

This chapter, therefore, takes a broader, more holistic view of LGBTQ health equity. We begin with a summary of the terminology associated with LGBTQ health, followed by a summary of the recognized barriers that LGBTQ populations face when seeking to achieve health. We then provide a brief overview of the data-driven health disparities that exist within the LGBTQ community, followed by specific discussion of LGBTQ subgroups with their own unique health equity considerations (e.g., transgender men and women). Finally, we provide an overview of recommendations for professionals seeking to improve LGBTQ health equity, illustrated by a case example. For a more detailed look at all of these factors and additional elements affecting the health of LGBTQ individuals, we encourage the reader to refer to the text *LGBT Health: Meeting the Needs of Gender and Sexual Minorities* (Smalley, Warren, & Barefoot, 2017b)—parts of which were adapted for the current chapter.

AFFIRMING TERMINOLOGY

When discussing LGBTQ health, it is important to specifically examine terminology and the remarkable growth in the vocabulary available to describe the immense diversity that exists within the LGBTQ community. The issue of terminology is a vital one when providing affirming programs and services and for a common understanding of the findings in the literature. What follows is a very brief primer of terminology condensed from a more in-depth discussion available in Smalley et al. (2017a).

Fenway Health (2010) defines sexual orientation as "a person's enduring physical, romantic, emotional, and/or spiritual attraction to another person" (p. 11). For the most part, the general public is fairly aware of the concept of sexual orientation, particularly heterosexual/straight, gay, lesbian, and bisexual. Less well-known orientations include queer, pansexual, omnisexual, asexual, and demisexual. While the terms queer, pansexual, and omnisexual are relatively new terms with regards to sexual orientation and do not have precise definitions, people who identify as queer typically reject traditional binary sexual orientation labels, instead preferring to use "queer" as a fluid, umbrella term for all sexual identities outside of the cis/heteronormative majority (Owen, 2014). Often used interchangeably, the terms "omnisexual" and "pansexual" are typically used to describe individuals who have attraction that crosses all gender lines, as contrasted for instance with a bisexual man who may not feel attraction to transgender men. For example, a pansexual individual may be attracted to individuals who identify as female gender, regardless of sex assigned at birth, or to individuals of all genders, also regardless of sex assigned at birth. Persons identifying as asexual report not having sexual/romantic attraction to any gender, and those identifying as demisexual report that they feel sexual attraction only to those with whom they have an emotional connection (typically regardless of gender).

One term that merits specific examination is "queer." Viewed by many as a strongly pejorative noun used to refer to a gay man, the word has been reclaimed by the LGBTQ community, particularly as a global adjective referring to someone who is a gender and/or sexual minority. Increasingly, the term is even coming to represent its own designation as a sexual orientation that rejects prior labels in favor of simply labeling oneself as non-heterosexual. There is ongoing disagreement regarding the acceptability of the word, with many within the LGBTQ community still finding the word to be offensive, and a prevailing intolerance of use of the word by someone outside the LGBT community (Fenway Health, 2010; Human Rights Campaign, 2014; Owen, 2014). However, many individuals strongly identify with the descriptor "queer," and it is clear that the term is now a part of the modern lexicon—the point that it has become the "Q" in LGBTQ.

Although often conflated with sexual orientation, gender identity is a completely separate concept. Gender identity describes an individual's "innate, deeply-felt psychological identification as a man, woman, or something else, which may or may not correspond to the person's external body or assigned sex at birth" (Fenway Health, 2010, pp. 7–8). The most frequently recognized gender minority identity is transgender, which describes an individual whose biological/assigned sex and true gender do not align (e.g., an individual who was assigned female sex at birth, but identifies as male). In contrast, individuals who do identify with their external body and the sex they were assigned at birth are referred to as "cisgender," a term not yet in common use outside the LGBTQ community that is used to describe individuals who do not identify as a gender minority. Other gender identities include genderqueer, nonbinary, androgynous, and two-spirit. While these terms tend to lack precise definitions, individuals identifying with these gender identities typically fall on a spectrum of not identifying exclusively with either the male or female gender (potentially identifying as both or neither), with two-spirit identification typically associated with persons of Native American heritage. One of the most important aspects of gender identity is that it is completely independent of sexual orientation; information about one's sexual orientation or gender identity does not provide any information regarding the other. For instance, a transgender woman may be straight (attracted to men), lesbian (attracted to women), or any other sexual orientation. Thus, both sexual orientation and gender identity must be considered for any individual as a person can be a gender minority without being a sexual minority (and vice versa).

It is worth examining the term "transgender" in a little more detail, as the terminology considered affirming has shifted dramatically over time. Early on, the word transgender tended to be used as both a verb and a noun rather than its current use as an adjective; that is, a person was described as "transgendered" or as "a transgender." The use of either—particularly "a transgender"—is now largely considered inappropriate and offensive. Similarly, the terms "male-to-female transgender" (MtF) and "female-to-male transgender" (FtM) are increasingly falling out of favor. The terms were intended to acknowledge the gender differences within the transgender community (i.e., to allow linguistic separation of transgender men and transgender women), but retained the focus on gender assigned at birth rather than the individual's true gender identity. The terms have been replaced with the simpler and more affirming "transgender woman" (or transgender female) for an individual assigned male at birth but whose true gender identity is female, and "transgender man" (or transgender male) for an individual assigned female at birth but whose true gender identity is male. Correspondingly, an additional recent shift has been away from phrases such as "the sex a person was born" —that is, stating that a transgender woman was "born a man" or "born male"—to the use of the more affirming phrase of "sex assigned at birth" or "gender assigned at birth." Thus, the appropriate phrasing would be to say that a transgender woman was "assigned male at birth." As with sexual orientation, as our understanding of diverse gender identities has evolved, additional terms defined previously such as "genderqueer," "nonbinary," and others have also entered use, but remain largely unknown outside the LGBT community.

For men and women who are transgender, it is also important to utilize affirming language when discussing any history of surgical procedures as part of their transition. The phrase "gender confirmation surgery" is now preferred to "sex change" or "sex reassignment" surgery. Other now outdated terms previously in common use include the distinction of "pre-op" and "post-op." These terms were intended to distinguish between individuals who had not versus had undergone gender confirmation surgeries. While it can be very important to assess a transgender person's surgical history to provide adequate medical care, the use of a specific identifier when referring to a person (e.g., labeling someone a "pre-op transgender man") is considered offensive and perpetuates an assumption that all transgender individuals desire surgery and reifies a notion that a person's external physical makeup is more important than their lived identity. When discussing surgeries, individuals often refer to "top" surgery (e.g., mastectomy, breast implants) and "bottom" surgery (e.g., phalloplasty, vaginoplasty). Again, though, we strongly encourage professionals not query or identify individuals based upon their surgical history unless it is directly relevant to the discussion at hand.

BARRIERS TO HEALTH FOR LGBTQ POPULATIONS

All groups discussed throughout this text face their own unique barriers to achieving and maintaining health. For LGBTQ populations, these barriers often have a troublingly recent origin. It is an often-cited fact that "homosexuality" was listed as a formally diagnosable mental disorder in the U.S. until the late 1970s (Bayer, 1987; Minton, 2002); further, being transgender is (arguably) still diagnosable as a mental disorder. On the other side of diagnosis, however, is the fact that in roughly half of all states, healthcare professionals can legally refuse to provide care to patients based on their sexual orientation and/or gender identity (Lambda Legal, n.d.). Discrimination in the healthcare system is so prevalent that heterosexism, homophobia, cisgenderism, and transphobia are among the most common forms of discrimination reported within healthcare (Albuquerque et al., 2016; Brotman, Ryan, Jalbert, & Rowe, 2002; Dodds, Keogh, & Hickson, 2005; Fish & Bewley, 2010; Grant et al., 2011; Institute of Medicine [IOM], 2011; Kosenko, Rintamaki, Raney, & Maness, 2013; Sinding, Barnhoff, & Grassu, 2004). This frequently leads LGBTQ people to avoid disclosure of their gender identity and/or sexual orientation in medical care situations for fear that they will be treated differently by their providers—a fear reported by three-quarters of transgender individuals (Neville & Henrickson, 2006).

The effects of discrimination extend well beyond the healthcare setting. Fewer than half of states have non-discrimination statutes that protect LGBTQ citizens (Human Rights Campaign, 2015), and ongoing legislative battles persist over issues such as the ability of a transgender man or woman to utilize the bathroom of his or her gender. More than two-thirds of LGBTQ people have experienced discrimination (Sears & Mallory, 2011), and a shocking 90% of transgender people have been harassed, mistreated, or discriminated against at work (Grant et al., 2011). Evidence suggests that LGBTQ individuals experience more hate-motivated violence than any other group, with the transgender community facing even higher rates than their sexual minority counterparts (Grant et al., 2011; Stotzer, 2012). Youth are also particularly impacted. LGBTQ youth are more likely to experience childhood maltreatment, and nearly 60% of sexual minority youth report feeling unsafe at school (Burwick et al., 2014; Kosciw, Greytak, Zongrone, Clark, & Truong, 2018). In perhaps the starkest manifestation of mistreatment of LGBTQ youth, an estimated 40% of homeless youth identify as LGBTQ, the vast majority of whom are homeless because they were kicked out of their homes for being LGBTQ (Durso & Gates, 2012). As a result of these stressors, LGBTQ individuals exhibit high rates of behavioral and exposure-based risk factors including physical inactivity, obesity, tobacco use, unhealthy diet, alcohol consumption, avoidance of care, and high underlying stress that each impact risk for numerous health conditions (Boehmer, Bowen, & Bauer, 2007; Boehmer, Miao, Linkletter, & Clark, 2012, 2014; Booth, Roberts, & Laye, 2012; Diamant et al., 2000; Eliason et al., 2015; McElroy & Brown, 2017; McElroy & Jordan, 2014; McElroy, Wintemberg, Cronk, & Everett, 2016; Minnis et al., 2016; Sturm, 2002).

OVERVIEW OF DISPARATE OUTCOMES

These systemic barriers to health lead to a number of disparities in physical and mental health outcomes. In the following, we specifically examine obesity, cancer, mental health, and HIV. There is limited literature regarding additional outcomes, as the field of LGBTQ health is only just beginning to expand beyond an initial focus on HIV and mental health outcomes (Smalley et al., 2017b).

Obesity

While there is an empirically-supported emphasis on body consciousness and physical appearance that lead to lower rates of obesity and higher rates of eating disorders among gay men (Austin, Nelson, Birkett, Calzo, & Everett, 2013; Bankoff, Richards, Bartlett, Wolf, & Mitchell, 2016; Brown & Keel, 2015; Shearer et al., 2015; VanKim, Porta, Eisenberg, Neumark-Sztainer, & Laska, 2016; Yelland & Tiggemann, 2003), the IOM (2011) specifically identified obesity as one of the most important health issues facing LGBTQ individuals. In particular, lesbians, bisexual women, transgender men, and transgender women face elevated risk for obesity, which in turn contributes to elevated risk in a number of physical health conditions (Cecchini et al., 2010; Mason, Lewis, & Heron, 2017). While the evidence is mixed regarding sexual minority men, there is emerging consistency that bisexual male adolescents and young men are also at increased risk for obesity (Austin et al., 2013; Laska et al., 2015).

Risk factors for obesity among LGBTQ individuals are similar to those seen in non-LGBTQ populations, including older age, rural residence, racial/ethnic minority status, socioeconomic status, eating patterns, physical activity, alcohol use, depression, anxiety, and stress (Mason et al., 2017; Warren, Smalley, & Barefoot, 2016a). When examining culturally-specific factors, evidence suggests that having a larger body size is more socially accepted in lesbian social networks than among cisgender heterosexual women (Bowen, Balsam, Diergaarde, Russo, & Escamilla, 2006; Thayer, 2010; VanKim et al., 2016); interestingly, level of "outness" or disclosure is also associated with obesity, with women who report a higher public identification as a lesbian more likely to be obese (Mason, 2016; Mason & Lewis, 2015). LGBTQ-specific prevention and intervention recommendations include a focus on stress reduction, resilience, affirming language and environment, and the inclusion of LGBTQ "models" in intervention materials (Eliason & Fogel, 2015).

Cancer

Despite being one of the leading causes of death throughout the nation, cancer is an often overlooked outcome of concern among LGBTQ groups. This lack of attention is surprising given the clear disparities that exist in seeking and receiving cancer care and in outcomes themselves. Cancer screening remains one of the most important factors for preventing mortality; however, nearly one in three LGBTQ adults do not have a regular healthcare provider (Buchmueller & Carpenter, 2010; IOM, 2013; Kamen et al., 2014). Even for those who do have a regular provider, LGBTQ cancer patients are more likely to withhold disclosing health concerns that they feel may result in provider discrimination (Boehmer, Miao, & Ozonoff, 2011). This is even moreso the case for women's healthcare, with many LGBTQ women expressing direct concern regarding cervical cancer screening in particular (Johnson, Nemeth, Mueller, Eliason, & Stuart, 2016).

When considering specific cancer sites, the literature produces inconsistent findings regarding breast cancer prevalence. An often-cited source of potential elevated risk centers on LGBTQ women having fewer pregnancies and a less frequent history of breastfeeding (Zaritsky & Dibble, 2010), both of which are risk factors for breast cancer (please note that we fully affirm mothers of all sexual orientations and gender identities, and speak only regarding the demographic profile of LGBTQ women that reveals a decreased likelihood of prior pregnancy). In addition, LGBTQ women report higher body-mass index (BMI), less frequent exercise, and a lower likelihood of engaging in routine breast self-examinations (Zaritsky & Dibble, 2010), all of which are also risk factors for breast cancer. For outcomes, lesbians in particular have been found to have an increased cause-specific breast cancer mortality rate and are more likely to report poor health following diagnosis (Boehmer et al., 2011; Cochran & Mays, 2012). Another area of high importance for LGBTQ health equity is human papillomavirus (HPV)–associated cancers, including anal cancer and cervical cancer. LGBTQ men in particular are at elevated risk for HPV infection overall, which in turn increases the risk of anal cancer (Grulich et al., 2012; Machalek et al., 2012). Unfortunately, knowledge and uptake of the HPV vaccine lags far behind need in the LGBTQ community (Koskan, LeBlanc, & Rosa-Cunha, 2016), presenting an opportune target for intervention. With regards to cervical cancer, there is an abiding assumption that sexual minority women are not at risk for HPV, based on incorrect assumptions regarding the transmissibility of HPV during sexual contact between women and regarding prior histories of sexual contact with men (Gorgos & Marrazzo, 2011; Waterman & Voss, 2015). These misconceptions may affect both the likelihood of women to seek the HPV vaccine and the likelihood of providers of recommending it, resulting in lower vaccine uptake among sexual minority women than among heterosexual women (Bernat, Gerend, Chevallier, Zimmerman, & Bauermeister, 2013). Beyond these studies, little literature is available regarding specific disparities in other cancer sites.

With regards to measures that can be taken to improve outcomes, ensuring that treatment planning, goal-setting, and end-of-life care 1) focuses on patients' wishes and desires, 2) includes patients' partners and families of birth and families of choice, and 3) provides constant affirming support are important considerations (Harding, Epiphaniou, & Chidgey-Clark, 2012; G. P. Quinn, Hudson, Aihe, Wilson, & Schabath, 2017).

Mental Health

As mentioned previously, being gay was diagnosable as a mental disorder until relatively recently (Krajeski, 1996), which has resulted in an understandably complex relationship between the LGBTQ community and the mental health field. While there are a number of mental health diagnoses that are more frequently diagnosed within the community—as presented in the proceeding section of this text—researchers caution against misinterpreting this as sexual orientation and/or gender identity being a "risk factor" for mental health outcomes; rather, the prevailing viewpoint is "that the hostile and tense environment in which [LGBTQ] individuals exist, termed 'minority stress,' results in mental health disparities" (Cohn, Casazza, & Cottrell, 2017, p. 164). This can easily and intuitively be connected to the increased risk of bullying, physical and verbal abuse, and other victimization LGBTQ individuals face (Cohn et al., 2017). We similarly encourage readers to interpret these prevalence disparities as a manifestation of the sociocultural realities of being an LGBTQ person, and not directly related to an individual's sexual orientation and/or gender identity.

Having said that, LGBTQ individuals face increased risk for a number of mental health concerns. Gay men, bisexual men, and transgender men and women are at particular risk for depression, with estimates of major depression up to three times higher for gay and bisexual men; further, over half of transgender men and women meet clinical cutoffs for depression upon screening (Baams, Grossman, Russell, 2015; Bruce, Harper, & Bauermeister, 2015; Cochran, Mays, & Sullivan, 2003; Cohen, Blasey, Taylor, Weiss, & Newman, 2016; Hightow-Weidman et al., 2011). One important note regarding depression is the importance of considering between-group differences. There is a robust literature examining how disclosure (e.g., "outness") affects mental health that reveals complete opposite findings by subgroup: while sexual minority men who are open regarding their sexual orientation have an increased rate of depression compared to cisgender heterosexual individuals, sexual minority women who are open about their sexual orientation have a lower rate of depression (Pachankis, Cochran, & Mays, 2015). Rates of anxiety are approximately 50% higher in the LGBTQ community (Cohen et al., 2016), frequently attributed to internalized homophobia and/or transphobia (when an LGBT person has internalized stereotypes and prejudice they have experienced from others; Lock, 1998; Walch, Ngamake, Bovornusvakool, & Walker, 2016).

There is also evidence that trauma risk is elevated—individuals who have had at least one same-sex partner in their lifetime have nearly double the risk of meeting PTSD criteria, and gender minority individuals have between two to four times the risk of cisgender populations (Shipherd, Maguen, Skidmore, & Abramovitz, 2011). This has been strongly connected in the literature to the increased risk of interpersonal violence, childhood abuse/neglect, bullying, and physical and sexual assault (Balsam & Hughes, 2013; A. L. Roberts, Austin, Corliss, Vandermorris, & Koenen, 2010). To place the magnitude of this risk into perspective, estimates are that 60% to 70% of LGBTQ people have been victimized directly due to bias (Grant et al., 2011; Rose & Mechanic, 2002). Because of the historical discrimination faced within the mental health workforce, the American Psychological Association (2012) has promulgated specific guidelines regarding provision of affirming mental healthcare services, which include increasing clients' sense of safety, reducing overall stress, resolving any residual trauma effects, and empowering clients to combat the stigma and discrimination they experience.

Suicide

It is a stark and consistent fact that LGBTQ people are among the most at risk for suicidal behavior and death by suicide in the nation (Haas et al., 2011; Hawton, Saunders, & O'Connor, 2012; National Action Alliance for Suicide Prevention, 2014; Turecki & Brent, 2016). While it is difficult to arrive at precise prevalence rates due to a variety of challenges (e.g., lack of sexual orientation and gender identity information in death certificates; O'Brien, Liu, Putney, Burke, & Aguinaldo, 2017); estimates that have been made are shocking, including an eight-fold increase in risk between partnered gay couples and married straight couples (Mathy, Cochran, Olsen, & Mays, 2011). Stark disparities also exist in suicidal ideation, with sexual minority individuals having twice the risk as cisgender, heterosexual individuals, and absolute risk among transgender men and women ranging from 32% to 58% (King et al., 2008; Marshall, Claes, Bouman, Witcomb, & Arcelus, 2016; Reisner, White, Bradford, & Mimiaga, 2014). An unfortunate correlate to this is the high rate of suicide attempts among LGBTQ individuals, with a lifetime prevalence of 11% in sexual minority men and women and up to 45% in transgender men and women (as contrasted to 4% in the cisgender, heterosexual population; Haas, Rodgers, & Herman, 2014; Hottes, Bogaert, Rhodes, Brennan, & Gesink, 2016; Marshall et al., 2016).

Key risk factors for suicide include depression, substance abuse, younger age at initiation of sexual behavior, feeling unsafe at school, having inadequate social support, victimization, stress, parental acceptance, family rejection, homelessness, medical discrimination, and early childhood trauma (Clements-Nolle, Marx, & Katz, 2006; D'Augelli et al., 2005; Flynn, Johnson, Bolton, & Mojtabai, 2016; Grossman & D'Augelli, 2007; Haas et al., 2014; IOM, 2011; Ryan, Huebner, Díaz, & Sanchez, 2009). Despite these overwhelming statistics and seemingly intractable risk factors, researchers have also begun to identify important protective factors and intervention targets—these include family connectedness, adult caring, parental and family support (overall), family support of sexual orientation and gender identity, positive disclosure experiences, school support, peer support, early medical transition assistance, and possessing personal documents (e.g., driver's license) that reflect true gender (Bauer, Scheim, Pyne, Travers, & Hammond, 2015; Eisenberg & Resnick, 2006; Mustanski & Liu, 2013; Ryan, Russell, Huebner, Diaz, & Sanchez, 2010; Veale, Saewyc, Frohard-Dourlent, Dobson, & Clark, 2015). Given the external, systemic nature of many of the risk factors for suicide, prevention initiatives focused on increasing these resilience factors have significant potential for reducing the alarming rates previously described.

Substance Use

As with overall mental health, it is important to recognize that the elevated rates of substance use seen within the LGBTQ community have been largely attributed to minority stress and similar processes (Weber & Dodge, 2017). Use patterns have overwhelmingly been viewed as a means of coping with the sociocultural oppression the community experiences (Cabaj, 2014; Cabaj et al., 2012; Keuroghlian et al., 2015). Regardless of origin, however, the fact remains that LGBTQ individuals are more likely to report a history of substance use and are at higher risk for substance abuse disorders than their cisgender, heterosexual counterparts, including having higher rates of substance use and abuse, higher severity of abuse, and longer durations of addictive behavior (Center for Substance Abuse and Treatment, 2012). While population-level estimates are challenging to obtain, estimates are that LGBTQ individuals face two to three times the risk of a substance use history (Cabaj, 2014; Weber & Dodge, 2017). Substance use disorder was among the first health outcomes examined within the LGBTQ community. Early studies published more than 30 years ago report rates of alcohol use at more than 80%, marijuana use at more than 50%, and alcohol use disorder at 29% (McKirnan & Peterson, 1989; Skinner & Otis, 1996; Sorenson & Roberts, 1997). Unfortunately, there has been little movement in these estimates since that time. Transgender men and women are at particularly high risk—those who have experienced physical, sexual, or emotional abuse are three to four times as likely to use alcohol, marijuana, or cocaine and up to eight times as likely to use any drug as cisgender populations (Nuttbrock et al., 2014). Substances that have specifically been linked with abuse among gay men include marijuana, stimulants, sedatives, cocaine, and "party drugs" such as ecstasy—methamphetamine in particular at its peak was seen at a level 10 times higher than the national average (Balsam, Molina, & Lehavot, 2013; Cabaj & Smith, 2012). With the exception of alcohol, use patterns are not as clear for sexual minority women, with sexual minority women reporting more frequent use of alcohol, a higher level of consumption when drinking, and an increased likelihood of experiencing alcohol-related problems (Balsam et al., 2013).

Identified risk factors for substance use include prejudice, discrimination, victimization, cultural rejection (e.g., cultural strain between LGBTQ identity and racial/ethnic identity), accessibility of affirming services, family response to LGBTQ identity, and comorbid health conditions (Cabaj, 2014). As with other mental health issues, creating a prevention and treatment environment that is affirming and supportive is critical. The literature shows that while LGBTQ individuals are more likely to seek substance use treatment in comparison to non-LGBTQ populations, their needs are less likely to be met (Flentje, Livingston, Roley, & Sorenson, 2015; Senreich, 2010). This is attributed partially to lack of provider knowledge of the unique mental health pressures faced by LGBTQ individuals (such as homophobia and transphobia; Cabaj, 2014). Establishing a sense of safety in the treatment environment—including affirming practices such as the use of gender-inclusive intake forms—is a critical first step (Weber & Dodge, 2017). Other recommendations include offering group sessions that are specific to LGBTQ individuals and not being afraid to discuss lack of cultural knowledge with the therapeutic client (Weber & Dodge, 2017).

HIV and Other Sexually Transmitted Diseases

Since its emergence in the early 1980s, HIV and AIDS have been associated with the LGBTQ community in both scientific circles and general public perception. The disproportionate effect of HIV on sexual minority men and transgender women in particular is stark and undeniable, with sexual minority men representing roughly half of all newly diagnosed cases in Western/Central Europe and North America (UNAIDS, 2016). Unfortunately, after many years of decline, recent trends show an increase in new HIV infections among sexual minority men, particularly young men, despite a significant decrease in that same time span among heterosexual men and women and injection drug users (Centers for Disease Control and Prevention [CDC], 2018; Horvath, Yared, Lammert, Lifson, & Kulasingam, 2017). More than 1.25 million current U.S. residents have been diagnosed with HIV, with nearly three-quarters of men attributing their HIV infection to male-to-male sexual contact or male-to-male sexual contact and injection drug use (CDC, 2019). While data on HIV infection among transgender women is not as robust, prevalence estimates are as high as 28% overall and a staggering 56% among African American transgender women (Herbst et al., 2008).

The literature on risk and protective factors for HIV is decades-long and challenging to summarize concisely; however, key factors include a greater number of sexual partners, substance use, participation in certain LGBTQ subcultures (e.g., leathermen), homelessness, decreased access to medical care, sociocultural stigma and oppression, anxiety (Bird, LaSala, Hidalgo, Kuhns, & Garofalo, 2016; de Vries, 2014; Horvath, Yared, Lammert, Lifson, & Kulasingam, 2017; Kidder, Wolitski, Pals, & Campsmith, 2008; Lelutiu-Weinberger et al., 2013; Meyer, 2003; Moskowitz, Seal, Rintamaki, & Rieger, 2011; Operario, Yang, Reisner, Iwamoto, & Nemoto, 2014; Smith, Grierson, Wain, Pitts, & Pattison, 2004). The interconnected role of many of these risk factors has led to the emergence of what is termed "syndemic theory," recognizing that attempts to intervene in one risk factor must take into account the ways in which many of the risk factors for HIV relate to one another. Specifically, substance abuse, mental health disorders, victimization, and abuse have all been identified as complexly interwoven risk factors with HIV infection that should be considered as a larger, conglomerated disparity process (Mustanski, Garofalo, Herrick, & Donenberg, 2007). Specific recommendations for prevention programs and interventions include a focus on the continuum of care for individuals with HIV, increasing a focus on viral suppression, use of pre-exposure prophylaxis (PrEP), HIV-testing initiatives, condom distribution, and culturally-tailored interventions (Horvath et al., 2017). The HIV epidemic and related public health response have created an astonishingly robust community-engaged, affirming, inclusive response that should serve as a model for the collaborative creation and testing of prevention initiatives for other health outcomes among LGBTQ populations.

HIV AMONG SEXUAL MINORITY MEN OF COLOR

The HIV epidemic has hit sexual minority men who are also members of a racial or ethnic minority group particularly hard. In fact, the proportion of new HIV diagnoses among White sexual minority men decreased from 33% to 28% between 2010 and 2016, during which time it increased from 24% to 29% among Hispanic/Latino sexual minority men and stayed constant at 38% among African American men (CDC, 2018). Put plainly, that means that nearly two-thirds of new HIV diagnoses among sexual minority men are among those who are members of just these two racial and ethnic minority groups. Should prevention efforts fail to stop these trends, it has been estimated that 50% of all African American sexual minority men and 25% of Hispanic/Latino sexual minority men will be diagnosed with HIV in their lifetime, contrasted to less than 10% of White sexual minority men (Hess, Hu, Lansky, Mermin, & Hall, 2016). There is an urgent need to expand the use of culturally-tailored, or preferably, culturally-specific intervention programs to curb this alarming trend.

SPECIAL CONSIDERATIONS FOR TRANSGENDER MEN AND WOMEN

The majority of this chapter has focused on the sexual minority aspects of the LGBTQ community due largely to the limited literature available focused on transgender health. While the literature on the health needs of transgender men and women is not as robust as for sexual minority individuals, there are a number of consistent findings and population-specific recommendations that professionals can use to guide work with transgender groups. First, transgender men and women face increased sociocultural oppression even beyond their cisgender sexual minority counterparts (Conron, Mimiaga, & Landers, 2010; dickey, Budge, Katz-Wise, & Garza, 2016; dickey & Keo-Meier, 2017). This blatant discrimination and violence extends even into the medical community, in which there are alarmingly frequent reports of traumatic treatment to the extent that transgender men and women sometimes avoid all aspects of medical care due to fear of victimization (dickey et al., 2016; Grant et al., 2011). While not all transgender individuals utilize medical care as part of their transition, the literature on transgender health has focused mostly on the medical aspects of the transition process (see dickey & Keo-Meier, 2017 for a complete discussion), leaving much room for additional inquiry into the broader health needs of transgender men and women.

Among transgender adults, medical interventions often include hormone treatment and gender confirmation surgeries to masculinize or feminize the body to match the individual's true gender (dickey & Keo-Meier, 2017). For children who identify as transgender, a common medical intervention is pubertal suppression at the first sign of puberty. This process simply halts puberty associated with the sex assigned at birth in a way that is reversible, but without initiating a hormonal puberty of the child's true gender (Delemarre-van de Waal & Cohen-Kettenis, 2008). There is strong evidence that pubertal suppression reduces the risk of anxiety, depression, and substance use and is often considered more "acceptable" to parents because it is temporary and reversible (dickey & Keo-Meier, 2017; Edwards-Leeper & Spack, 2012; J. Olson, Schrager, Belzer, Simons, & Clark, 2015; Steensma, Kreukels, de Vries, & Cohen-Kettenis, 2013). Pubertal suppression allows children, parents, and providers to "pause" puberty until a child's gender identity crystallizes more fully and a decision can be made about which puberty (feminizing or masculinizing) is best for the child (Deutsch, 2016).

Barriers to broader health equity in transgender men and women are numerous. Transgender individuals experience higher rates of discrimination in employment, housing, healthcare, and public accommodations/services delivery, with nearly two-thirds of transgender men and women reporting they have experienced at least one major discriminatory experience that severely affected their financial well-being, their emotional well-being, and/or their overall quality of life (Conron, Scott, Stowell, & Landers, 2012; Grant et al., 2011). The issue of violence reaches crisis levels—one out of four transgender men and women have been physically assaulted because of their gender identity and one in ten have been sexually assaulted (Grant et al., 2011). In other health disparities, as summarized in dickey & Keo-Meier (2017), transgender individuals report higher rates of each of the following: depression, anxiety, stress, and other mental health concerns (Bockting, Miner, Swinburne Romine, Hamilton, & Coleman, 2013; Budge, Adelson, & Howard, 2013; Dargie et al., 2014; Fredriksen-Goldsen et al., 2013; Su et al., 2016; Warren, Smalley, Barefoot, 2016b); self-injury and suicide (dickey, Reisner, & Juntunen, 2015; Grant et al., 2011); alcohol and illicit drug use (Benotsch et al., 2013; Keuroghlian, Reisner, White, & Weiss, 2015; Reback & Fletcher, 2014; Reisner, Greytak, Parsons, & Ybarra, 2015; Santos et al., 2014); HIV (Grant et al., 2011; Herbst et al., 2008; Poteat, Reisner, & Radix, 2014); poor dietary quality and less active exercise habits (Smalley et al., 2015); obesity (Conron et al., 2012; Fredriksen-Goldsen et al., 2013; VanKim et al., 2014; Warren et al., 2016a); and poor physical health and disability among older adults (Fredriksen-Goldsen et al., 2013).

In terms of prevention and intervention, providing emotional support to transgender youth is critically important, as the majority of transgender youth will be bullied, harassed, and/or assaulted by students, teachers, and school staff and very few report someone coming to their defense (Kosciw et al., 2018; Toomey, Ryan, Diaz, & Russell, 2011). When considering protective factors, one of the most important buffers for children is having parental acceptance, support, and understanding (dickey & Keo-Meier, 2017; K. Olson, Durwood, DeMeules, & McLaughlin, 2016). Adults who lacked this support show higher risk for HIV, homelessness, substance abuse, depression, self-injury, and suicide (dickey et al., 2015).

On a final note, there is an important yet delicate balance between providing affirming care that completely validates an individual's true identity, and ensuring that medical professionals—when appropriate and indicated—are aware that an adult in particular may possess organ systems or other physical factors that do not align with their gender (dickey & Keo-Meier, 2017; T. K. Roberts & Fantz, 2014). This becomes a very fine line for providers and other health professionals to walk—finding the best way to assess for and treat the organ systems present, without invalidating the person's gender, is an area of great need in LGBTQ health research.

RECOMMENDATIONS FOR PRACTITIONERS

In designing health promotion programs and in providing clinical care, there are a number of best practices that have been developed. Capriotti and Flentje (2017) offer an in-depth discussion of these factors, which are summarized in Table 12.1. These include overall guiding principles and specific recommendations when implementing programs and/or healthcare.

TABLE 12.1 Implementing LGBTQ-Affirming Programs and Services

GUIDING PRINCIPLES	SPECIFIC RECOMMENDATIONS
▪ Competent care affirms all sexualities and genders as valid, important, and non-pathological. ▪ Competent care appreciates institutional and societal context. ▪ Competent providers recognize themselves as fallible and biased, catch mistakes, attend to ruptures, and check in with patients. ▪ Competent care recognizes patients as unique individuals. ▪ Competent care appreciates intersectionality of LGBTQ identity and other identities.	▪ Make LGBTQ inclusion visually salient ▪ Modify paperwork to be LGBTQ-inclusive ▪ Use affirmative and inclusive language in all communications ▪ Openly, proactively express your LGBTQ-affirmative stance ▪ Thoroughly discuss confidentiality and privacy policies ▪ Conceptualize LGBTQ participants' experience through a systematic framework that accounts for variability among individuals ▪ Query history of LGBTQ-related stressors with an interested and inquisitive stance ▪ Consider the relationship between LGBTQ-related issues and the program/service's focus

INTERSECTIONALITY SPOTLIGHT

As discussed throughout this chapter, the role of intersectionality in LGBTQ health equity cannot be overstated. In nearly every outcome discussed, members of other health disparity populations (e.g., racial/ethnic minority, rural) face stark outcome disparities linked in large part to increased risk for the various factors previously discussed (e.g., discrimination, access to care). Despite the widely-recognized impact of intersectionality in LGBTQ health, the literature on intersectionality among LGBTQ populations has been criticized as focusing on the additional differences in outcomes rather than focusing on the fundamental process and system that leads to these increased disparities—in essence, viewing intersectionality descriptively and largely ignoring the actual intersectionality itself as a specifically studied component (Toomey, Huynh, Jones, Lee, & Revels-Macalinao, 2016; Wade & Harper, 2015; Warren, Smalley, & Barefoot, 2017).

While limited, the work that has been done with this process-focused perspective reveals that the overlapping levels of discrimination are a major factor—for example, African American and Hispanic LGBTQ individuals report more rejection, discrimination, and social isolation from their racial/ethnic community than do White LGBTQ individuals (Balaji et al., 2012; Ryan et al., 2009; Stokes & Peterson, 1998), which has been shown to lead to a longer coming out process with more selective disclosure (Jimenez, 2003; Kennamer, Honnold, Bradford, & Hendricks, 2000; Millett, Flores, Peterson, & Bakeman, 2007; Moradi et al., 2010; Parks, Hughes, & Matthews, 2004; Rosario, Schrimshaw, & Hunter, 2004). Among Asian LGBTQ youth, those who report lower levels of family acceptance and support regarding their LGBTQ identity have lower levels of self-esteem and greater psychological distress (Homma & Saewyc, 2007). As discussed throughout the chapter, these factors are related to a great number of the disparate outcomes seen in the LGBTQ community as a whole. Additionally, the more prevalent role of religion in racial/ethnic minority groups increases risk for social rejection, leading some minority LGBTQ individuals to maintain ties even with churches that reject them because of the strong role faith plays within the community (K. Quinn, Dickson-Gomez, & Kelly, 2016; Woody, 2014).

Unfortunately, the layered nature of discrimination and rejection for intersectional LGBTQ individuals extends far into the LGBTQ community itself. Two-thirds of sexual minority men report that they are "stressed" because of racism they have experienced from other LGBTQ individuals, leading to a sense of being invisible within the community itself (Giwa & Greensmith, 2012; Han et al., 2015). This tension between two communities represents an important core aspect of intersectionality—racial/ethnic minority LGBTQ individuals often find themselves reconciling conflicting messaging and pressures from their racial/ethnic community and the LGBTQ community in order to "fit in" (Nabors et al., 2001), leading many to feel the need to code-switch (alter behaviors, speech, and even clothing) based upon which social context they are in at the time (Balaji et al., 2012). This dual (or higher, depending on number of intersectional factors) strain is an important factor to consider when developing interventions for LGBTQ populations.

CASE STUDY THE TREVOR PROJECT

In 1995, an obscure short film named *Trevor* won an Oscar for Best Short Subject Live-Action film. By today's standards, the 23-minute film may not seem groundbreaking, but at the time a film about a 13-year-old boy's crush on another boy, and the life-threatening effects of that crush becoming discovered, was nothing short of revolutionary. Following the award, the producers sought to secure an airing of the film, which they eventually achieved on HBO. Given the film's serious subject matter of teen suicide, the producers started researching what resources they could highlight during the airing that LGBTQ youth could access. Finding none, they launched what has come to be the largest crisis intervention and suicide prevention resource for LGBTQ youth and young adults. The initiative has grown to include the Trevor Lifeline, TrevorChat, TrevorText, TrevorSpace, and Trevor Education Workshops. Trevor Lifeline (1-866-488-7386) is the initiative's core crisis and suicide prevention lifeline, which helps to ensure that all LGBTQ youth have access to an affirming resource when finding themselves in crisis. TrevorChat is a companion online instant messaging platform that allows an alternate access point, as is TrevorText (text START to 678678). TrevorSpace is an online community that allows LGBTQ youth to connect with peers around the world to enhance community and belongingness. Trevor Education has expanded the reach of the initiative beyond crisis support to target structural change. Its Trevor Lifeguard program provides video, curriculum, and resources for teachers in middle and high school designed to teach educators about the challenges faced by LGBTQ youth, the warning signs of suicide, and how to respond to someone who may be in crisis. This preliminary exposure can be expanded through Trevor Ally trainings and intensive CARE (Connect, Accept, Respond, Empower) trainings. The Trevor Project represents a true multilevel initiative designed not only to intervene at the point of crisis but also to help change the structural issues that increase the risk of suicide in the first place. More information on the Trevor Project can be found at www.thetrevorproject.com

CURRENT EVENTS

ACCESS TO PRE-EXPOSURE PROPHYLAXIS

The use of PrEP has immense potential for reducing new HIV infections among LGBTQ populations, in particular for sexual minority men and for transgender women. PrEP is a combination of drugs originally developed to treat HIV infection that have been found to also reduce acquisition if taken prior to exposure (tenofovir and emtricitabine, brand name Truvada). When taken correctly, PrEP has been shown to reduce the risk of acquiring HIV by 99% (CDC, n.d.). While the use of PrEP has been hailed as the next frontier of HIV prevention, there are significant concerns regarding its equity implications. The cost of PrEP is estimated at $1,300 per month for those without insurance, and when not taken exactly as prescribed, the effectiveness drops from 99% to an estimated 44% reduction in risk (Costa-Roberts, 2015).

(continued)

Discussion Question: If the rates of new HIV infections are increasing in groups with lower access to healthcare, insurance, and the socioeconomic privilege that allows an individual to take Truvada as prescribed, how do we develop programs that mitigate these factors and ensure this powerful prevention option reaches those at highest need?

"BATHROOM BILLS"

There is ongoing debate and controversy nationwide regarding what have been come to be referred to as "bathroom bills." In a number of cases at various levels throughout the country, transgender youth have brought cases in attempts to ensure their ability to utilize bathroom and locker facilities that align with their true gender. The core argument has been that Title IX provisions, which protect students from discrimination based on sex, extend protections to transgender students as well. The issue has drawn conflicting rulings nationwide, even at the level of the Supreme Court. In 2017, following the withdrawal of President Obama's guidance on Title IX transgender protections, the Supreme Court refused to hear the case of Gavin Grimm, who had sued to ensure his ability to utilize male bathroom facilities. This left in place a ruling that forced him to utilize a segregated, single-stall facility. However, in 2019, the Supreme Court also refused to hear a case brought by cisgender students arguing that a school's policy allowing transgender youth to utilize gender-consistent bathrooms violated *their* privacy rights. This leaves patchwork protection for transgender students throughout the U.S. and high uncertainty regarding the ways in which transgender rights are viewed at the federal level.

Discussion Question: How does having patchwork policy—typically providing protections to students who already reside in more affirming communities—impact the known risk factors for negative health outcomes among transgender youth, and which populations would be most affected?

DISCUSSION QUESTIONS

- How does the use of offensive terminology and the misgendering of transgender youth increase the risk for the disparities discussed throughout this chapter?

- Describe a program that could help to address barriers to health equity for LGBTQ populations across multiple social-ecological levels.

- What are some common risk factors across LGBTQ health disparity outcomes, and what are strategies that could be employed to address their widespread impact?

- Intersectionality is often viewed as "complicating" prevention and intervention approaches; how could knowledge of intersectionality be used in a way that specifically improves the effectiveness of a program to reduce substance abuse among bisexual African American women?

- Envision the entire process of attending a routine medical checkup from calling to schedule to paying at the end of the visit, and identify all the ways in which a person's sexual orientation could be intentionally or unintentionally invalidated during that process. What steps could be taken to make the process more inclusive and affirming?

REFERENCES

Albuquerque, G. A., de Lima Garcia, C., da Silva Quirino, G., Alves, M. J. H., Belém, J. M., dos Santos Figueiredo, F. W., ... de Abreu, L. C. (2016). Access to health services by lesbian, gay, bisexual, and transgender persons: Systematic literature review. *BMC International Health and Human Rights*, *16*(1), 2. doi:10.1186/s12914-015-0072-9

American Psychological Association. (2012). Guidelines for psychological practice with lesbian, gay, and bisexual clients. *American Psychologist*, *67*(1), 10–42. doi:10.1037/a0024659

Austin, S. B., Nelson, L. A., Birkett, M. A., Calzo, J. P., & Everett, B. (2013). Eating disorder symptoms and obesity at the intersections of gender, ethnicity, and sexual orientation in US high school students. *American Journal of Public Health*, *103*, e16–e22. doi:10.2105/AJPH.2012.301150

Baams, L., Grossman, A. H., & Russell, S. T. (2015). Minority stress and mechanisms of risk for depression and suicidal ideation among lesbian, gay, and bisexual youth. *Developmental Psychology*, *51*(5), 688–696. doi:10.1037/a0038994

Balaji, A. B., Oster, A. M., Viall, A. H., Heffelfinger, J. D., Mena, L. A., & Toledo, C. A. (2012). Role flexing: How community, religion, and family shape the experiences of young Black men who have sex with men. *AIDS Patient Care and STDs*, *26*(12), 730–737. doi:10.1089/apc.2012.0177

Balsam, K. F., Beadnell, B., & Riggs, K. (2012). Understanding sexual orientation health disparities in smoking: A population-based analysis. *The American Journal of Orthopsychiatry*, *82*(4), 482–493. doi:10.1111/j.1939-0025.2012.01186.x

Balsam, K. F., & Hughes, T. (2013). Sexual orientation, victimization, and hate crimes. In C. J. Patterson & A. R. D'Augelli (Eds.), *Handbook of psychology and sexual orientation* (p. 267–280). New York, NY: Oxford University Press.

Balsam, K. F., Molina, Y., & Lehavot, K. (2013). Alcohol and drug use in lesbian, gay, bisexual, and transgender (LGBT) youth and young adults. In P. M. Miller (Ed.), *Principles of addiction* (pp. 563–573). San Diego, CA: Elsevier. doi:10.1016/B978-0-12-398336-7.00058-9

Bankoff, S. M., Richards, L. K., Bartlett, B., Wolf, E. J., & Mitchell, K. S. (2016). Examining weight and eating behavior by sexual orientation in a sample of male veterans. *Comprehensive Psychiatry*, *68*, 134–139. doi:10.106/j.comppsych.2016.03.007

Bauer, G. R., Scheim, A. I., Pyne, J., Travers, R., & Hammond, R. (2015). Intervenable factors associated with suicide risk in transgender persons: A respondent driven sampling study in Ontario, Canada. *BMC Public Health*, *15*, 525. doi:10.1186/s12889-015-1867-2

Bayer, R. (1987). *Homosexuality and American psychiatry: The politics of diagnosis* (Rev. ed.). Princeton, NJ: Princeton University Press.

Benotsch, E. G., Zimmerman, R., Cathers, L., McNulty, S., Pierce, J., Heck, T., ... Snipes, D. (2013). Non-medical use of prescription drugs, polysubstance use, and mental health in transgender adults. *Drug and Alcohol Dependence*, *132*, 391–394. doi:10.1016/j.drugalcdep.2013.02.027

Bernat, D. H., Gerend, M. A., Chevallier, K., Zimmerman, M. A., & Bauermeister, J. A. (2013). Characteristics associated with initiation of the human papillomavirus vaccine among a national sample of male and female young adults. *The Journal of Adolescent Health*, *53*(5), 630–636. doi:10.1016/j.jadohealth.2013.07.035

Bird, J. D., LaSala, M. C., Hidalgo, M. A., Kuhns, L. M., & Garofalo, R. (2016). "I had to go to the streets to get love": Pathways from parental rejection to HIV risk among young gay and bisexual men. *Journal of Homosexuality*, *64*, 321–342. doi:10.1080/00918369.2016.1179039

Bockting, W., Miner, M., Swinburne Romine, R., Hamilton, A., & Coleman, E. (2013). Stigma, mental health, and resilience in an online sample of the US transgender population. *American Journal of Public Health*, *103*, 943–951. doi:10.2105/AJPH.2013.301241

Boehmer, U., Bowen, D. J., & Bauer, G. R. (2007). Overweight and obesity in sexual-minority women: Evidence from population-based data. *American Journal of Public Health*, *97*(6), 1134–1140. doi:10.2105/AJPH.2006.088419

Boehmer, U., Miao, X., Linkletter, C., & Clark, M. A. (2012). Adult health behaviors over the life course by sexual orientation. *American Journal of Public Health*, *102*(2), 292–300. doi:10.2105/AJPH.2011.300334

Boehmer, U., Miao, X., Linkletter, C., & Clark, M. A. (2014). Health conditions in younger, middle, and older ages: Are there differences by sexual orientation? *LGBT Health, 1*(3), 168–176. doi:10.1089/lgbt.2013.0033

Boehmer, U., Miao, X., & Ozonoff, A. (2011). Cancer survivorship and sexual orientation. *Cancer, 117*(16), 3796–3804. doi:10.1002/cncr.25950

Booth, F. W., Roberts, C. K., & Laye, M. J. (2012). Lack of exercise is a major cause of chronic diseases. *Comprehensive Physiology, 2*(2), 1143–1211. doi:10.1002/cphy.c110025

Bowen, D. J., Balsam, K. F., Diergaarde, B., Russo, M., & Escamilla, G. M. (2006). Healthy eating, exercise, and weight: Impressions of sexual minority women. *Women & Health, 44*(1), 79–93. doi:10.1300/J013v44n01_05

Brotman, S., Ryan, B., Jalbert, Y., & Rowe, B. (2002). The impact of coming out on health and health care access: The experiences of gay, lesbian, bisexual, and two-spirit people. *Journal of Health and Social Policy, 15*(1), 1–29. doi:10.1300/J045v15n01_01

Brown, T. A., & Keel, P. K. (2015). Relationship status predicts lower restrictive eating pathology for bisexual and gay men across 10-year follow-up. *International Journal of Eating Disorders, 48*(6), 700–707. doi:10.1002/eat.22433

Bruce, D., Harper, G. W., & Bauermeister, J. A. (2015). Minority stress, positive identity development, and depressive symptoms: Implications for resilience among sexual minority male youth. *Psychology of Sexual Orientation and Gender Diversity, 2*(3), 287–296. doi:10.1037/sqd0000128

Buchmueller, T., & Carpenter, C. S. (2010). Disparities in health insurance coverage, access, and outcomes for individuals in same-sex versus different-sex relationships, 2000–2007. *American Journal of Public Health, 100*(3), 489–495. doi:10.2105/ajph.2009.160804

Budge, S. L., Adelson, J. L., & Howard, K. S. (2013). Anxiety and depression in transgender individuals: The roles of transition status, loss, social support, and coping. *Journal of Consulting and Clinical Psychology, 81*, 545–557. doi:10.1037/a0031774

Burwick, A., Gates, G., Baumgartner, S., & Friend, D. (2014). *Human services for low-income and at-risk LGBT populations: An assessment of the knowledge base and research needs.* Washington, DC: U.S. Department of Health and Human Services. Retrieved from https://www.acf.hhs.gov/sites/default/files/opre/lgbt_hsneeds_assessment_reportfinal1_12_15.pdf

Cabaj, R. P. (2014). Substance use issues among gay, lesbian, bisexual, and transgender people. In M. Galanter, H. D. Kleber, & K. T. Brady (Eds.), *Textbook of substance abuse treatment* (pp. 707–721). Washington, DC: American Psychiatric Association.

Cabaj, R. P., Gorman, M., Pellicio, W. J., Ghindia, D. J., & Neisen, J. H. (2012). An overview for providers treating LGBT clients. In *A provider's introduction to substance abuse treatment for lesbian, gay, bisexual, and transgender individuals* (HHS Publication No. (SMA) 12-4104, pp. 1–14). Rockville, MD: U.S. Department of Health and Human Services.

Cabaj, R. P., & Smith, M. (2012). Overview of treatment approaches, modalities, and issues of accessibility in the continuum of care. In Center for Substance Abuse Treatment (Ed.), *A provider's introduction to substance abuse treatment for lesbian, gay, bisexual, and transgender individuals* (HHS Publication No. (SMA) 12-4104, pp. 49–60). Rockville, MD: U.S. Department of Health and Human Services.

Capriotti, M. R., & Flentje, A. (2017). Recommendations for practitioners for providing competent care to gender and sexual minority individuals. In K. B. Smalley, J. C. Warren, & K. N. Barefoot (Eds.), *LGBT health* (pp. 382–401). New York, NY: Springer Publishing Company.

Cecchini, M., Sassi, F., Lauer, J. A., Lee, Y. Y., Guajardo-Barron, V., & Chisholm, D. (2010). Chronic diseases: Chronic diseases and development 3 tackling of unhealthy diets, physical inactivity, and obesity: Health effects and cost-effectiveness. *Lancet, 376*, 1775–1784. doi:10.1016/S0140-6736(10)61514-0

Center for Substance Abuse Treatment. (2012). *A provider's introduction to substance abuse treatment for lesbian, gay, bisexual, and transgender individuals* (HHS Publication No. (SMA) 12-4104). Rockville, MD: U.S. Department of Health and Human Services.

Centers for Disease Control and Prevention. (n.d.). *Pre-exposure prophylaxis (PrEP).* Retrieved from https://www.cdc.gov/hiv/risk/prep/index.html

Centers for Disease Control and Prevention. (2018). *HIV surveillance—Men who have sex with men (MSM).* Retrieved from https://www.cdc.gov/hiv/pdf/library/slidesets/cdc-hiv-surveillance-slides-msm-2017.pdf

Centers for Disease Control and Prevention. (2019). *HIV surveillance report: Diagnoses of HIV Infection in the United States and Dependent Areas, 2018 (Preliminary)* (Vol. 30). Retrieved from https://www.cdc.gov/hiv/pdf/library/reports/surveillance/cdc-hiv-surveillancereport-2018-vol-30.pdf

Clements-Nolle, K., Marx, R., & Katz, M. (2006). Attempted suicide among transgender persons: The influence of gender-based discrimination and victimization. *Journal of Homosexuality, 51*(3), 53–69. doi:10.1300/J082v51n03_04

Cochran, S. D., & Mays, V. M. (2012). Risk of breast cancer mortality among women cohabiting with same sex partners: Findings from the National Health Interview Survey, 1997–2003. *Journal of Women's Health, 21*(5), 528–533. doi:10.1089/jwh.2011.3134

Cochran, S. D., Mays, V. M., & Sullivan, J. G. (2003). Prevalence of mental disorders, psychological distress, and mental health services use among lesbian, gay, and bisexual adults in the United States. *Journal of Consulting and Clinical Psychology, 71*(1), 53–61. doi:10.1037/0022-006X.71.1.53

Cohen, J. M., Blasey, C., Taylor, C. B., Weiss, B. J., & Newman, M. G. (2016). Anxiety and related disorders and concealment in sexual minority young adults. *Behavioral Therapy,46*, 91–101. doi:10.1016/j.beth.2015.09.006

Cohn, T. J., Casazza, S. P., & Cottrell, E. M. (2017). The mental health of gender and sexual minority groups in context. In K. B. Smalley, J. C. Warren, & K. N. Barefoot (Eds.), *LGBT health* (pp. 161–180). New York, NY: Springer Publishing Company.

Conron, K. J., Mimiaga, M. J., & Landers, S. J. (2010). A population-based study of sexual orientation identity and gender differences in adult health. *American Journal of Public Health, 100*(10), 1953–1960. doi:10.2105/AJPH.2009.174169

Conron, K. J., Scott, G., Stowell, G. S., & Landers, S. J. (2012). Transgender health in Massachusetts: Results from a household probability sample of adults. *American Journal of Public Health,102*(1), 118–122. doi:10.2105/AJPH.2011.300315

Costa-Roberts, D. (2015). 8 things you didn't know about Truvada. *PBS NewsHour Weekend.* Retrieved from https://www.pbs.org/newshour/health/8-things-didnt-know-truvadaprep

D'Augelli, A. R., Grossman, A. H., Salter, N. P., Vasey, J. J., Starks, M. T., & Sinclair, K. O. (2005). Predicting the suicide attempts of lesbian, gay, and bisexual youth. *Suicide and Life-Threatening Behavior, 35*(6), 646–660. doi:10.1521/suli.2005.35.6.646

Dargie, E., Blair, K. L., Pukall, C. F., & Coyle, S. M. (2014). Somewhere under the rainbow: Exploring the identities and experiences of trans persons. *Canadian Journal of Human Sexuality, 23*, 60–74. doi:10.3138/cjhs.2378

de Vries, H. J. (2014). Sexually transmitted infections in men who have sex with men. *Clinics in Dermatology,32*(2), 181–188. doi:10.1016/j.clindermatol.2013.08.001

Delemarre-van de Waal, H., & Cohen-Kettenis, P. (2008). Clinical management of gender identity disorder in adolescents: A protocol on psychological and paediatric endocrinology aspects. *European Journal of Endocrinology, 155*, S131–S137. doi:10.1530/eje.1.02231

Deutsch, M. B. (Ed.). (2016). *Guidelines for the primary and gender-affirming care of transgender and gender nonbinary people* (2nd ed.). San Francisco: Center for Excellence in Transgender Health, Department of Family and Community Medicine, University of California, San Francisco. Retrieved from http://transhealth.ucsf.edu/trans?page=guidelines-home

Diamant, A. L., Wold, C., Spritzer, K., Gelberg, L., Diamant, A. L., Wold, C., … Gelberg, L. (2000). Health behaviors, health status, and access to and use of health care: A population-based study of lesbian, bisexual, and heterosexual women. *Archives of Family Medicine, 9*(10), 1043–1051. doi:10.1001/archfami.9.10.1043

dickey, l. m., Budge, S. A., Katz-Wise, S., & Garza, M. V. (2016). Health disparities in the transgender community: Exploring differences in insurance coverage. *Psychology of Sexual Orientation and Gender Diversity, 3*(3), 275–282. doi:10.1037/sgd0000169

dickey, l. m., & Keo-Meier, C. (2017). Gender minority health: Affirmative care for the community. In K. B. Smalley, J. C. Warren, & K. N. Barefoot (Eds.), *LGBT health* (pp. 247–268). New York, NY: Springer Publishing Company.

dickey, l. m., Reisner, S. L., & Juntunen, C. L. (2015). Non-suicidal self-injury in a large online sample of transgender adults. *Professional Psychology: Research & Practice, 46*(1), 3–11. doi:10.1037/a0038803

Diemer, E. W., Grant, J. D., Munn-Chernoff, M. A., Patterson, D. A., & Duncan, A. E. (2015). Gender identity, sexual orientation, and eating-related pathology in a national sample of college students. *Journal of Adolescent Health, 57*(2), 144–149. doi:10.1016/j.jadohealth.2015.03.003

Dodds, C., Keogh, P., & Hickson, F. (2005). *It makes me sick: Heterosexism, homophobia and the health of gay and bisexual men.* London, UK: Sigma Research. Retrieved from http://sigmaresearch.org.uk/files/report2005a.pdf

Durso, L. E., & Gates, G. J. (2012). *Serving our youth: Findings from a national survey of service providers working with lesbian, gay, bisexual, and transgender youth who are homeless or at risk of becoming homeless.* Los Angeles, CA: The Williams Institute with True Colors Fund and The Palette Fund. Retrieved from http://williamsinstitute.law.ucla.edu/wp-content/uploads/Durso-Gates-LGBT-Homeless-Youth-Survey-July-2012.pdf

Edwards-Leeper, L., & Spack, N. P. (2012). Psychological evaluation and medical treatment of transgender youth in an interdisciplinary "Gender Management Service" (GeMS) in a major pediatric center. *Journal of Homosexuality, 59,* 321–336. doi:10.1080/00918369.2012.653302

Eisenberg, M. E., & Resnick, M. D. (2006). Suicidality among gay, lesbian and bisexual youth: The role of protective factors. *Journal of Adolescent Health, 39*(5), 662–668. doi:10.1016/j.jadohealth.2006.04.024

Eliason, M. J., & Fogel, S. C. (2015). An ecological framework for sexual minority women's health: Factors associated with greater body mass. *Journal of Homosexuality, 62,* 845–882. doi:10.1080/00918369.2014.1003007

Eliason, M. J., Ingraham, N., Fogel, S. C., McElroy, J. A., Lorvick, J., Mauery, D. R., & Haynes, S. (2015). A systematic review of the literature on weight in sexual minority women. *Women's Health Issues, 25*(2), 162–175. doi:10.1016/j.whi.2014.12.001

Feldman, M. B., & Meyer, I. H. (2007). Eating disorders in diverse lesbian, gay, and bisexual populations. *International Journal of Eating Disorders, 40*(3), 218–226. doi:10.1002/eat.20360

Fenway Health. (2010). *Glossary of gender and transgender terms.* Retrieved from http://fenwayhealth.org/documents/the-fenway-institute/handouts/Handout_7-C_Glossary_of_Gender_and_Transgender_Terms__fi.pdf

Fish, J., & Bewley, S. (2010). Using human rights–based approaches to conceptualise lesbian and bisexual women's health inequalities. *Health & Social Care in the Community, 18*(4), 355–362. doi:10.1111/j.1365-2524.2009.00902.x

Flentje, A., Livingston, N. A., Roley, J., & Sorenson, J. L. (2015). Mental and physical health needs of lesbian, gay, and bisexual clients in substance abuse treatment. *Journal of Substance Abuse Treatment, 58,* 78–83. doi:10.1016/j.jsat.2015.06.022

Flynn, A. B., Johnson, R. M., Bolton, S. L., & Mojtabai, R. (2016). Victimization of lesbian, gay, and bisexual people in childhood: Associations with attempted suicide. *Suicide and Life-Threatening Behavior, 46*(4), 457–470. doi:10.1111/sltb.12228

Fredriksen-Goldsen, K. I., Cook-Daniels, L., Kim, H.-J., Erosheva, E. A., Emlet, C. A., Hoy-Ellis, C., ... Muraco, A. (2013). Physical and mental health of transgender older adults: An at-risk and underserved population. *The Gerontologist,54,* 488–500. doi:10.1093/geront/gnt021

Gay and Lesbian Medical Association. (2001). *Healthy People 2010: Companion document for lesbian, gay, bisexual, and transgender (LGBT) health.* San Francisco, CA: Author. Retrieved from http://glma.org/_data/n_0001/resources/live/HealthyCompanionDoc3.pdf

Giwa, S., & Greensmith, C. (2012). Race relations and racism in the LGBTQ community of Toronto: Perceptions of gay and queer social service providers of color. *Journal of Homosexuality, 59*(2), 149–185. doi:10.1080/00918369.2012.648877

Gorgos, L. M., & Marrazzo, J. M. (2011). Sexually transmitted infections among women who have sex with women. *Clinical Infectious Diseases, 53*(Suppl. 3), S84–S91. doi:10.1093/cid/cir697

Grant, J. M., Mottet, L. A., Tanis, J., Harrison, J., Herman, J. L., & Keisling, M. (2011). *Injustice at every turn: A report of the national transgender discrimination survey.* Retrieved from http://endtransdiscrimination.org/PDFs/NTDS_Report.pdf

Green, K. E., & Feinstein, B. A. (2012). Substance use in lesbian, gay, and bisexual populations: An update on empirical research and implications for treatment. *Psychology of Addictive Behaviors, 26*(2), 265–278. doi:10.1037/a0025424

Grossman, A. H., & D'Augelli, A. R. (2007). Transgender youth and life-threatening behaviors. *Suicide and Life-Threatening Behavior, 37*(5), 527–537. doi:10.1521/suli.2007.37.5.527

Grulich, A. E., Poynten, I. M., Machalek, D. A., Jin, F., Templeton, D. J., & Hillman, R. J. (2012). The epidemiology of anal cancer. *Sexual Health,9*(6), 504–508. doi:10.1071/SH12070

Haas, A. P., Eliason, M., Mays, V. M., Mathy, R. M., Cochran, S. D., D'Augelli, A. R., … Clayton, P. J. (2011). Suicide and suicide risk in lesbian, gay, bisexual, and transgender populations: Review and recommendations. *Journal of Homosexuality, 58*, 10–51. doi:10.1080/00918369.2011.534038

Haas, A. P., Rodgers, P. L., & Herman, J. L. (2014). *Suicide attempts among transgender and gender non-conforming adults: Findings of the National Transgender Discrimination Survey.* Retrieved from http://williamsinstitute.law.ucla.edu/wp-content/uploads/AFSP-Williams-Suicide-Report-Final.pdf

Han, C. S., Ayala, G., Paul, J. P., Boylan, R., Gregorich, S. E., & Choi, K. H. (2015). Stress and coping with racism and their role in sexual risk for HIV among African American, Asian/Pacific Islander, and Latino men who have sex with men. *Archives of Sexual Behavior,44*(2), 411–420. doi:10.1007/s10508-014-0331-1

Harding, R., Epiphaniou, E., & Chidgey-Clark, J. (2012). Needs, experiences, and preferences of sexual minorities for end-of-life care and palliative care: A systematic review. *Journal of Palliative Medicine,15*(5), 602–611. doi:10.1089/jpm.2011.0279

Hawton, K., Saunders, K. E. A., & O'Connor, R. C. (2012). Self-harm and suicide in adolescents. *Lancet, 379*, 2373–2382. doi:10.1016/S0140-6736(12)60322-5

Hendricks, M. L., & Testa, R. J. (2012). A conceptual framework for clinical work with transgender and gender-nonconforming clients: An adaptation of the Minority Stress Model. *Professional Psychology: Research and Practice, 43*, 460–487. doi:10.1037/a0029597

Herbst, J. H., Jacobs, E. D., Finlayson, T. J., McKleroy, V. S., Neumann, M. S., & Crepaz, N. (2008). Estimating HIV prevalence and risk behaviors of transgender persons in the United States: A systematic review. *AIDS and Behavior,12*(1), 1–17. doi:10.1007/s10461-007-9299-3

Hess, K., Hu, X., Lansky, A., Mermin, J., & H. Hall, I. (2016, February). *Estimating the lifetime risk of a diagnosis of HIV infection in the United States* (Abstract 52). Paper presented at the Conference on Retroviruses and Opportunistic Infections (CROI), Boston, MA. Retrieved from https://www.croiconference.org/sessions/estimating-lifetime-risk-diagnosis-hiv-infection-united-states

Hightow-Weidman, L. B., Phillips, G., Jones, K. C., Outlaw, A. Y., Fields, S. D., & Smith, J. C. (2011). Racial and sexual identity-related maltreatment among minority YMSM: Prevalence, perceptions, and the association with emotional distress. *AIDS Patient Care and STDs, 25*(Suppl. 1), S39–S45. doi:10-1089/apc.2011.9877

Homma, Y., & Saewyc, E. M. (2007). The emotional well-being of Asian-American sexual minority youth in school. *Journal of LBGT Health Research,3*(1), 67–78. doi:10.1300/J463v03n01_08

Horvath, K. J., Yared, N., Lammert, S., Lifson, A., & Kulasingam, S. (2017). HIV and other sexually transmitted infections within the gender and sexual minority community. In K. B. Smalley, J. C. Warren, & K. N. Barefoot (Eds.), *LGBT health* (pp. 215–246). New York, NY: Springer Publishing Company.

Hottes, T. S., Bogaert, L., Rhodes, A. E., Brennan, D. J., & Gesink, D. (2016). Lifetime prevalence of suicide attempts among sexual minority adults by study sampling strategies: A systematic review and meta-analysis. *American Journal of Public Health, 106*(5), e1–e12. doi:10.2105/AJPH.2016.303088

Human Rights Campaign. (2014, June). *HRC officially adopts the use of "LGBTQ" to reflect diversity of own community.* Retrieved from http://www.hrc.org/blog/hrc-officially-adopts-use-of-lgbtq-to-reflect-diversity-of-own-community

Human Rights Campaign. (2015). *Beyond marriage equality: A blueprint for federal non-discrimination protections.* Washington, DC: Author.

Institute of Medicine. (2013). *Collecting sexual orientation and gender identity data in electronic health records: Workshop summary.* Washington, DC: National Academies Press. Retrieved from https://www.ncbi.nlm.nih.gov/books/NBK132859

Institute of Medicine, Committee on Lesbian, Gay, Bisexual, and Transgender Health Issues and Research Gaps and Opportunities. (2011). *The health of lesbian, gay, bisexual, and transgender people: Building a foundation for better understanding.* Washington, DC: National. Retrieved from https://www.ncbi.nlm .nih.gov/books/NBK64806

Jimenez, A. D. (2003). Triple jeopardy: Targeting older men of color who have sex with men. *Journal of Acquired Immune Deficiency Syndromes, 33*(Suppl. 2), S222–S225. doi:10.1097/00126334-200306012-00020

Johnson, M. J., Nemeth, L. S., Mueller, M., Eliason, M. J., & Stuart, G. W. (2016). Qualitative study of cervical cancer screening among lesbian and bisexual women and transgender men. *Cancer Nursing, 39*(6): 455–463. doi:10.1097/NCC.0000000000000338

Kamen, C., Palesh, O., Gerry, A. A., Andrykowski, M. A., Heckler, C., Mohile, S., … Mustian, K. (2014). Disparities in health risk behavior and psychological distress among gay versus heterosexual male cancer survivors. *LGBT Health, 1*(2), 86–92. doi:10.1089/lgbt.2013.0022

Kann, L., O'Malley Olsen, E., McManus, T., Harris, W. A., Shanklin, S. L., Flint, K. H., . . . Zaza, S. (2016). Sexual identity, sex of sexual contacts, and health-related behaviors among students in grades 9–12— United States and selected sites, 2015. *MMWR Surveillance Summary, 65*(SS09), 1–202. doi:10.15585/ mmwr.ss6509a1

Karpman, M., Skopec, L., & Long, S. K. (2015). *QuickTake: Uninsurance rate nearly halved for lesbian, gay, and bisexual adults since mid-2013.* Retrieved from http://hrms.urban.org/quicktakes/Uninsurance-Rate -Nearly-Halved-for-Lesbian-Gay-and-Bisexual-Adults-since-Mid-2013.html

Kennamer, J., Honnold, J., Bradford, J., & Hendricks, M. (2000). Differences in disclosure of sexuality among African American and White gay/bisexual men: Implications for HIV/AIDS prevention. *AIDS Education and Prevention, 12*(6), 519–531.

Keuroghlian, A. S., Reisner, S. L., White, J. M., & Weiss, R. D. (2015). Substance use and treatment of substance use disorders in a community sample of transgender adults. *Drug and Alcohol Dependence, 152,* 139–146. doi:10.1016/j.drugalcdep.2015.04.008

Kidder, D. P., Wolitski, R. J., Pals, S. L., & Campsmith, M. L. (2008). Housing status and HIV risk behaviors among homeless and housed persons with HIV. *Journal of Acquired Immune Deficiency Syndromes, 49*(4), 451–455. doi:10.1097/QAI.0b013e31818a652c

King, M., Semlyen, J., Tai, S. S., Killaspy, H., Osborn, D., Popelyuk, D., & Nazareth, I. (2008). A systematic review of mental disorder, suicide, and deliberate self harm in lesbian, gay and bisexual people. *BMC Psychiatry, 8,* 70. doi:10.1186/1471-244X-8-70

Kosciw, J. G., Greytak, E. A., Zongrone, A. D., Clark, C. M., & Truong, N. L. (2018). *The 2017 National School Climate Survey: The experiences of lesbian, gay, bisexual, transgender, and queer youth in our nation's schools.* New York, NY: GLSEN. Retrieved from https://www.glsen.org/sites/default/files/2019-10/GLSEN-2017- National-School-Climate-Survey-NSCS-Full-Report.pdf

Kosenko, K., Rintamaki, L., Raney, S., & Maness, K. (2013). Transgender patient perceptions of stigma in health care contexts. *Medical Care, 51*(9), 819–822. doi:10.1097/MLR.0b013e31829fa90d

Koskan, A. M., LeBlanc, N., & Rosa-Cunha, I. (2016). Exploring the perceptions of anal cancer screening and behaviors among gay and bisexual men infected with HIV. *Cancer Control, 23*(1), 52–58. doi:10.1177/ 107327481602300109

Krajeski, J. (1996). Homosexuality and the mental health professions: A contemporary history. In R. P. Cabaj & T. S. Stein (Eds.), *Textbook of homosexuality and mental health* (pp. 17--31). Arlington, VA: American Psychiatric Association.

Lambda Legal. (n.d.). *In your state: Public accommodations.* Retrieved from http://www.lambdalegal.org/ states-regions/in-your-state

Laska, M. N., VanKim, N. A., Erickson, D. J., Lust, K., Eisenberg, M. E., & Rosser, B. S. (2015). Disparities in weight and weight behaviors by sexual orientation in college students. *American Journal of Public Health, 105,* 111–121. doi:10.2105/AJPH.2014.302094

Lelutiu-Weinberger, C., Pachankis, J. E., Golub, S. A., Walker, J. J., Bamonte, A. J., & Parsons, J. T. (2013). Age cohort differences in the effects of gay-related stigma, anxiety and identification with the gay community on sexual risk and substance use. *AIDS and Behavior, 17*(1), 340–349. doi:10.1007/s10461-011-0070-4

Lock, J. (1998). Treatment of homophobia in a gay male adolescent. *American Journal of Psychotherapy, 52*(2), 202–214. doi:10.1176/appi.psychotherapy.1998.52.2.202

Machalek, D. A., Poynten, M., Jin, F., Fairley, C. K., Farnsworth, A., Garland, S. M., … Grulich, A. E. (2012). Anal human papillomavirus infection and associated neoplastic lesions in men who have sex with men: A systematic review and meta-analysis. *The Lancet Oncology, 13*(5), 487–500. doi:10.1016/s1470-2045(12)70080-3

Marshall, E., Claes, L., Bouman, W. P., Witcomb, G. L., & Arcelus, J. (2016). Non-suicidal self-injury and suicidality in trans people: A systematic review of the literature. *International Review of Psychiatry, 28,* 58–69. doi:10.3109/09540261.2015.1073143

Mason, T. B. (2016). Binge eating and overweight and obesity among young adult lesbians. *LGBT Health, 3,* 6. doi:10.1089/lgbt.2015.0119

Mason, T. B., & Lewis, R. J. (2015). Minority stress, depression, relationship quality, and alcohol use: Associations with overweight and obesity among partnered young adult lesbians. *LGBT Health, 2,* 333–340. doi:10.1089/lgbt.2014.0053

Mason, T. B., Lewis, R. J., & Heron, K. (2017). Obesity in gender and sexual minority groups. In K. B. Smalley, J. C. Warren, & K. N. Barefoot (Eds.), *LGBT health* (pp. 45–62). New York, NY: Springer Publishing Company.

Mathy, R. M., Cochran, S. D., Olsen, J., & Mays, V. M. (2011). The association between relationship markers of sexual orientation and suicide: Denmark, 1990–2001. *Social Psychiatry and Psychiatric Epidemiology, 46,* 111–117. doi:10.1007/s00127-009-0177-3

McClain, Z., Thomas, R., & Yehia, B. (2017). Sociocultural and systemic barriers to health for gender and sexual minority populations. In K. B. Smalley, J. C. Warren, & K. N. Barefoot (Eds.), *LGBT health* (pp. 15–26). New York, NY: Springer Publishing Company.

McElroy, J. A., & Brown, M. T. (2017). Chronic illnesses and conditions in gender and sexual minority individuals. In K. B. Smalley, J. C. Warren, & K. N. Barefoot (Eds.), *LGBT health* (pp. 83–102). New York, NY: Springer Publishing Company.

McElroy, J. A., & Jordan, J. (2014). Disparate perceptions of weight between sexual minority and heterosexual female college students. *LGBT Health,1*(2), 122–130. doi:10.1089/lgbt.2013.0021

McElroy, J. A., Wintemberg, J. J., Cronk, N. J., & Everett, K. D. (2016). The association of resilience, perceived stress and predictors of depressive symptoms in sexual and gender minority youths and adults. *Psychology and Sexuality, 7*(2), 116–130. doi:10.1080/19419899.2015.1076504

McKirnan, D. J., & Peterson, P. L. (1989). Alcohol use and drug use among homosexual men and women: Epidemiology and population characteristics. *Addictive Behaviors, 14*(5), 545–553. doi:10.1016/0306-4603(89)90075-0

Meyer, I. H. (1995). Minority stress and mental health in gay men. *Journal of Health and Social Behavior, 36,* 38–56. doi:10.2307/2137286

Meyer, I. H. (2003). Prejudice, social stress, and mental health in lesbian, gay, and bisexual populations: Conceptual issues and research evidence. *Psychological Bulletin, 129*(5), 674–697. doi:10.1037/0033-2909.129.5.674

Meyer, I. H. (2013). Prejudice, social stress, and mental health in lesbian, gay, and bisexual populations: Conceptual issues and research evidence. *Psychology of Sexual Orientation and Gender Diversity, 1*(Suppl.), 3–26. doi:10.1037/2329-0382.1.S.3

Millett, G. A., Flores, S. A., Peterson, J. L., & Bakeman, R. (2007). Explaining disparities in HIV infection among Black and White men who have sex with men: A meta-analysis of HIV risk behaviors. *AIDS, 21*(15), 2083–2091. doi:10.1097/QAD.0b013e3282e9a64b

Minnis, A. M., Catellier, D., Kent, C., Ethier, K. A., Soler, R. E., Heirendt, W., … Rogers, T. (2016). Differences in chronic disease behavioral indicators by sexual orientation and sex. *Journal of Public Health Management Practice, 22*(Suppl. 1), S25–S32. doi:10.1097/PHH.0000000000000350

Minton, H. L. (2002). *Departing from deviance: A history of homosexual rights and emancipatory science in America.* Chicago, IL: University of Chicago Press.

Moradi, B., Wiseman, M. C., DeBlaere, C., Goodman, M. B., Sarkees, A., Brewster, M. E., & Huang, Y. P. (2010). LGB of color and White individuals' perceptions of heterosexist stigma, internalized homophobia, and outness: Comparisons of levels and links. *The Counseling Psychologist, 38*(3), 397–424. doi:10.1177/0011000009335263

Moskowitz, D. A., Seal, D. W., Rintamaki, L., & Rieger, G. (2011). HIV in the leather community: Rates and risk-related behaviors. *AIDS and Behavior, 15*(3), 557–564. doi:10.1007/s10461-009-9636-9

Mustanski, B., Garofalo, R., Herrick, A., & Donenberg, G. (2007). Psychosocial health problems increase risk for HIV among urban young men who have sex with men: Preliminary evidence of a syndemic in need of attention. *Annals of Behavioral Medicine, 34*(1), 37–45. doi:10.1080/08836610701495268

Mustanski, B., & Liu, R. T. (2013). A longitudinal study of predictors of suicide attempts among lesbian, gay, bisexual, and transgender youth. *Archives of Sexual Behavior, 42*(3), 437–448. doi:10.1007/s10508-012-0013-9

Nabors, N. A., Hall, R. L., Miville, M. L., Nettles, R., Pauling, M. L., & Ragsdale, B. L. (2001). Multiple minority group oppression: Divided we stand? *Journal of the Gay and Lesbian Medical Association, 5*(3), 101–105. doi:10.1023/A:1011652808415

National Action Alliance for Suicide Prevention. (2014). *A prioritized research agenda for suicide prevention: An action plan to save lives.* Rockville, MD: National Institute of Mental Health and the Research Prioritization Task Force. Retrieved from https://www.sprc.org/resources-programs/prioritized-research-agenda-suicide-prevention-action-plan-save-lives

Neville, S., & Henrickson, M. (2006). Perceptions of lesbian, gay and bisexual people of primary healthcare services. *Journal of Advanced Nursing, 55*(4), 407–415. doi:10.1111/j.1365-2648.2006.03944.x

Nuttbrock, L., Bockting, W., Rosenblum, A., Hwahng, S., Mason, M., Macri, M., & Becker, J. (2014). Gender abuse, depressive symptoms, and substance use among transgender women: A 3-year prospective study. *American Journal of Public Health, 104*(11), 2199–2206. doi:10.2105/AJPH.2014.302106

Obergefell v. Hodges, 135 S.Ct. 2071 (2015).

O'Brien, K. H. M., Liu, R. T., Putney, J. M., Burke, T. A., & Aguinaldo, L. D. (2017). Suicide and self-injury in gender and sexual minority populations. In K. B. Smalley, J. C. Warren, & K. N. Barefoot (Eds.), *LGBT health* (pp. 181–198). New York, NY: Springer Publishing Company.

Olson, J., Schrager, S. M., Belzer, M., Simons, L. K., & Clark, L. F. (2015). Baseline psychologic and psychosocial characteristics of transgender youth seeking care for gender dysphoria. *Journal of Adolescent Health, 57*(4), 374–380. doi:10.1016/j.jadohealth.2015.04.027

Olson, K., Durwood, L., DeMeules, M., & McLaughlin, K. (2016). Mental health of transgender children who are supported in their identities. *Pediatrics,137*, e20153223. doi:10.1542/peds.2015-3223

Operario, D., Yang, M.-F., Reisner, S. L., Iwamoto, M., & Nemoto, T. (2014). Stigma and the syndemic of HIV-related health risk behaviors in a diverse sample of transgender women. *Journal of Community Psychology, 42*(5), 544–557. doi:10.1002/jcop.21636

Owen, L. (2014, October). About the Q. *PFLAG.* Retrieved from https://www.pflag.org/blog/about-q

Pachankis, J. E., Cochran, S. D., & Mays, V. M. (2015). The mental health of sexual minority adults in and out of the closet: A population-based study. *Journal of Consulting and Clinical Psychology, 83*(5), 890–901. doi:10.1037/ccp0000047

Parks, C. A., Hughes, T. L., & Matthews, A. K. (2004). Race/ethnicity and sexual orientation: Intersecting identities. *Cultural Diversity and Ethnic Minority Psychology,10*(3), 241. doi:10.1037/1099-9809.10.3.241

Poteat, T., Reisner, S. L., & Radix, A. (2014). HIV epidemics among transgender women. *Current Opinion in HIV and AIDS, 9*(2), 168–173. doi:10.1097/COH.0000000000000030

Quinn, G. P., Hudson, J. N., Aihe, M. T., Wilson, L. E., & Schabath, M. B. (2017). Cancer in gender and sexual minority groups. In K. B. Smalley, J. C. Warren, & K. N. Barefoot (Eds.), *LGBT health* (pp. 63–82). New York, NY: Springer Publishing Company.

Quinn, K., Dickson-Gomez, J., & Kelly, J. A. (2016). The role of the Black Church in the lives of young Black men who have sex with men. *Culture, Health & Sexuality, 18*(5), 524–537. doi:10.1080/13691058.2015.1091509

Reback, C. J., & Fletcher, J. B. (2014). HIV prevalence, substance use, and sexual risk behaviors among transgender women recruited through outreach. *AIDS and Behavior, 18*(7), 1359–1367. doi:10.1007/s10461-013-0657-z

Reisner, S. L., Greytak, A., Parsons, J. P., & Ybarra, M. (2015). Gender minority social stress in adolescence: Disparities in adolescent bullying and substance use by gender identity. *Journal of Sex Research, 52*, 243–256. doi:10.1080/00224499.2014.886321

Reisner, S. L., White, J. M., Bradford, J. B., & Mimiaga, M. J. (2014). Transgender health disparities: Comparing full cohort and nested matched-pair study designs in a community health center. *LGBT Health*, *1*, 177–184. doi:10.1089/lgbt.2014.0009

Roberts, A. L., Austin, S. B., Corliss, H. L., Vandermorris, A. K., Koenen, K. C. (2010). Pervasive trauma exposure among US sexual orientation minority adults and risk of posttraumatic stress disorder. *American Journal of Public Health*, *100*(12), 2433–2441. doi:10.2105/AJPH.2009.168971

Roberts, T. K., & Fantz, C. R. (2014). Barriers to quality health care for the transgender population. *Clinical Biochemistry*, *47*, 983–987. doi:10.1016/j.clinbiochem.2014.02.009

Rosario, M., Schrimshaw, E. W., & Hunter, J. (2004). Ethnic/racial differences in the coming-out process of lesbian, gay, and bisexual youths: A comparison of sexual identity development over time. *Cultural Diversity and Ethnic Minority Psychology*, *10*(3), 215–228. doi:10.1037/1099-9809.10.3.215

Rose, S. M., & Mechanic, M. B. (2002). Psychological distress, crime features, and help-seeking behaviors related to homophobic bias incidents. *American Behavioral Scientist*, *46*, 14–26. doi:10.1177/0002764202046001003

Ryan, C., Huebner, D., Díaz, , R. M., & Sanchez, J. (2009). Family rejection as a predictor of negative health outcomes in White and Latino lesbian, gay, and bisexual young adults. *Pediatrics*, *123*(1), 346–352. doi:10.1542/peds.2007-3524

Ryan, C., Russell, S. T., Huebner, D., Diaz, R., & Sanchez, J. (2010). Family acceptance in adolescence and the health of LGBT young adults. *Journal of Child and Adolescent Psychiatric Nursing*, *23*(4), 205–213. doi:10.1111/j.1744-6171.2010.00246.x

Santos, G. M., Rapues, J., Wilson, E. C., Macias, O., Packer, T., Colfax, G., & Raymond, H. F. (2014). Alcohol and substance use among transgender women in San Francisco: Prevalence and association with human immunodeficiency virus infection. *Drug and Alcohol Review*, *33*, 287–295. doi:10.1111/dar.12116

Sears, B., & Mallory, C. (2011). *Documented evidence of employment discrimination & its effects on LGBT people*. Los Angeles, CA: The Williams Institute. Retrieved from http://williamsinstitute.law.ucla.edu/wp-content/uploads/Sears-Mallory-Discrimination-July-20111.pdf

Senreich, E. (2010). Are specialized LGBT program components helpful for gay and bisexual men in substance abuse treatment? *Substance Use and Misuse*, *45*(7-8), 1077–1096. doi:10.3109/10826080903483855

Shearer, A., Russon, J., Herres, J., Atte, T., Kodish, T., & Diamond, D. (2015). The relationship between disordered eating and sexuality amongst adolescents and young adults. *Eating Behaviors*, *19*, 115–119. doi:10.106/j.eatbeh.2015.08.001

Shipherd, J. C., Maguen, S., Skidmore, W. C., & Abramovitz, S. M. (2011). Potentially traumatic events in a transgender sample: Frequency and associated symptoms. *Traumatology*, *17*(2), 56–67. doi:10.1177/1534765610395614

Sinding, C., Barnhoff, L., & Grassu, P. (2004). Homophobia and heterosexism in cancer care: The experiences of lesbians. *Canadian Journal of Nursing Research*, *36*(4), 170–188. Retrieved from https://cjnr.archive.mcgill.ca/article/view/1917

Skinner, W. F., & Otis, M. D. (1996). Drug and alcohol use among lesbian and gay people in a southern U.S. sample: Epidemiological, comparative, and methodological findings from the Trilogy Project. *Journal of Homosexuality*, *30*(3), 59–92. doi:10.1300/J082v30n03_04

Smalley, K. B., Warren, J. C., & Barefoot, K. N. (2015). Differences in health risk behaviors across understudied LGBT subgroups. *Health Psychology*, *35*(2), 103–114. doi:10.1037/hea0000231

Smalley, K. B., Warren, J. C., & Barefoot, K. N. (2017a). Gender and sexual minority health: History, current state, and terminology. In K. B. Smalley, J. C. Warren, & K. N. Barefoot (Eds.), *LGBT health* (pp. 3–14). New York, NY: Springer Publishing Company.

Smalley, K. B., Warren, J. C., & Barefoot, K. N. (2017b). *LGBT health: Meeting the needs of gender and sexual minorities*. New York, NY: Springer Publishing Company.

Smith, A. M., Grierson, J., Wain, D., Pitts, M., & Pattison, P. (2004). Associations between the sexual behaviour of men who have sex with men and the structure and composition of their social networks. *Sexually Transmitted Infections*, *80*(6), 455–458. doi:10.1136/sti.2004.010355

Sorenson, L., & Roberts, S. J. (1997). Lesbian uses of and satisfaction with mental health services: Results from the Boston Lesbian Health Project. *Journal of Homosexuality*, *33*(1), 35–49. doi:10.1300/J082v33n01_03

Steensma, T. D., Kreukels, B. P., de Vries, A. L., & Cohen-Kettenis, P. T. (2013). Gender identity development in adolescence. *Hormones & Behavior, 64*(2), 288–297. doi:10.1016/j.yhbeh.2013.02.020

Stokes, J. P., & Peterson, J. L. (1998). Homophobia, self-esteem, and risk for HIV among African American men who have sex with men. *AIDS Education and Prevention, 10*(3), 278–292.

Stotzer, R. (2012). *Comparison of hate crime rates across protected and unprotected groups—An update.* Los Angeles, CA: The Williams Institute. Retrieved from http://williamsinstitute.law.ucla.edu/wp-content/uploads/Stotzer-Hate-Crime-Update-Jan-2012.pdf

Sturm, R. (2002). The effects of obesity, smoking, and drinking on medical problems and costs. *Health Affairs, 21*(2), 245–253. doi:10.1377/hlthaff.21.2.245

Su, D. Irwin, J. A., Fisher, C., Ramos, A., Kelley, M., Mendoza, D. A. R., & Coleman, J. D. (2016). Mental health disparities within the LGBT population: A comparison between transgender and nontransgender individuals. *Transgender Health, 1*(1), 12–20. doi:10.1089/trgh.2015.0001

Thayer, A. N. (2010). *Community matters: The exploration of overweight and obesity within the lesbian population* (Doctoral dissertation). Retrieved from Proquest. (Accession No. DP19730).

Toomey, R. B., Huynh, V. W., Jones, S. K., Lee, S., & Revels-Macalinao, M. (2016). Sexual minority youth of color: A content analysis and critical review of the literature. *Journal of Gay & Lesbian Mental Health, 21*(1), 3–31. doi:10.1080/19359705.2016.1217499

Toomey, R. B., Ryan, C., Diaz, R. M., & Russell, S. T. (2011). High school Gay-Straight Alliances (GSAs) and young adult well-being: An examination of GSA presence, participation, and perceived effectiveness. *Applied Developmental Science, 15*(4), 175–185. doi:10.1080/10888691.2011.607378

Turecki, G., & Brent, D. A. (2016). Suicide and suicidal behaviour. *Lancet, 387*, 1227–1239. doi:10.1016/S0140-6736(15)00234-2

UNAIDS. (2016). *Global AIDS update, 2016.* Retrieved from http://www.who.int/hiv/pub/arv/global-AIDS-update-2016_en.pdf?ua=1

United States v. Windsor, 133 S.Ct. 2675 (2013).

VanKim, N. A., Erickson, D. J., Eisenberg, M. E., Lust, K. E., Rosser, B. R., & Laska, M. N. (2014). Weight-related disparities for transgender college students. *Health Behavior and Policy Review, 1*(2), 161–171. doi:10.14485/HBPR.1.2.8

VanKim, N. A., Porta, C. M., Eisenberg, M. E., Neumark-Sztainer, D., & Laska, M. N. (2016). Lesbian, gay and bisexual college student perspectives on disparities in weight-related behaviours and body image: A qualitative analysis. *Journal of Clinical Nursing, 25*, 3676–3686. doi:10.1111/jocn.13106

Veale, J., Saewyc, E., Frohard-Dourlent, H., Dobson, S., & Clark, B. (2015). *Being safe, being me: Results of the Canadian Trans Youth Health Research Survey.* Retrieved from https://apsc-saravyc.sites.olt.ubc.ca/files/2018/03/SARAVYC_Trans-Youth-Health-Report_EN_Final_Web2.pdf

Wade, R. M., & Harper, G. W. (2015). Young Black gay/bisexual and other men who have sex with men: A review and content analysis of health-focused research between 1988 and 2013. *American Journal of Men's Health, 11*, 1388–1405. doi:10.1177/1557988315606962

Walch, S. E., Ngamake, S. T., Bovornusvakool, W., & Walker, S. V. (2016). Discrimination, internalized homophobia, and concealment in sexual minority physical and mental health. *Psychology of Sexual Orientation and Gender Diversity, 3*(1), 37–48. doi:10.1037/sgd0000146

Warren, J. C., Smalley, K. B., & Barefoot, K. N. (2016a). Differences in psychosocial predictors of obesity among LGBT subgroups. *LGBT Health, 3*, 283–291. doi:10.1089/lgbt.2015.0076

Warren, J. C., Smalley, K. B., & Barefoot, K. N. (2016b). Psychological well-being among transgender and genderqueer individuals. *International Journal of Transgenderism, 17*(3/4), 114–123. doi:10.1080/15532739.2016.1216344

Warren, J. C., Smalley, K. B., & Barefoot, K. N. (2017). The health of racial and ethnic minority gender and sexual minority populations. In K. B. Smalley, J. C. Warren, & K. N. Barefoot (Eds.), *LGBT health* (pp. 269–292). New York, NY: Springer Publishing Company.

Waterman, L., & Voss, J. (2015). HPV, cervical cancer risks, and barriers to care for lesbian women. *The Nurse Practitioner, 40*(1), 46–53. doi:10.1097/01.NPR.0000457431.20036.5c

Weber, G., & Dodge, A. (2017). Substance use among gender and sexual minority youth and adults. In K. B. Smalley, J. C. Warren, & K. N. Barefoot (Eds.), *LGBT health* (pp. 199–-214). New York, NY: Springer Publishing Company.

Woody, I. (2014). Aging out: A qualitative exploration of ageism and heterosexism among aging African American lesbians and gay men. *Journal of Homosexuality, 61*(1), 145–165. doi:10.1080/00918369.2013.835603

Yelland, C., & Tiggemann, M. (2003). Muscularity and the gay ideal: Body dissatisfaction and disordered eating in homosexual men. *Eating Behaviors, 4,* 107–116. doi:10.1016/S1471-0153(03)00014-X

Zaritsky, E., & Dibble, S. L. (2010). Risk factors for reproductive and breast cancers among older lesbians. *Journal of Women's Health, 19*(1), 125–131. doi:10.1089/jwh.2008.1094

RURAL, FRONTIER, AND APPALACHIAN HEALTH EQUITY

K. BRYANT SMALLEY ■ JACOB C. WARREN ■ JEAN R. SUMNER

LEARNING OBJECTIVES

- Describe the complexities of defining "rurality"
- Name specific rural health disparities in the areas of mental/behavioral health, obesity, and chronic disease
- Discuss how access to healthcare impacts the health of rural residents
- Describe the importance of integrated care and telehealth to rural practice
- Convey the ways in which intersectionality affects rural residents who are African American, Hispanic, and/or LGBTQ

INTRODUCTION

While all societies have their ultimate roots in rural living, the continued urbanization of industrialized nations has shifted the dominant lifestyle from rural to urban. As populations, institutions of higher learning, tax bases, and health research enterprises have correspondingly become more urban, a stark gap in risk factors and health status has emerged. While the unique health needs of rural communities have been recognized for some time, the vast majority of health promotion and prevention strategies are designed, implemented, and evaluated in urban communities (Warren & Smalley, 2014c). While a decreasing proportion of U.S. residents live in rural areas, the fact remains that nearly one in five Americans lives in a rural area, and three-quarters of the nation's counties are classified as rural (Hart, Larson, & Lishner, 2005; U.S. Census Bureau, 2020). While the overall research literature is comparatively limited, there is strong consistency that rural residents face disparities in outcomes ranging from diabetes to suicide and increased risk associated with everything from fundamental access to care to levels of discrimination experienced by rural residents who are also members of racial/ethnic minority groups. This chapter provides a summary of the ways in which rurality is defined, an overview of specific health disparities experienced by rural groups, a discussion of the barriers to rural health equity, and concludes with a summary of strategies and solutions being implemented to improve rural health.

DEFINING RURALITY

On the surface, the issue of defining what a rural area is may seem simple. The word "rural" conjures images of hay fields, roaming horses, mountain streams, and desert winds. In reality, though, the study of rural health is greatly complicated by the fundamentally subjective nature of rurality that often produces varying study findings. Varying definitions focus on characteristics, such as population size, population density, proximity to urban centers, and proximity of healthcare. For example, the federal Office of Management and Budget (OMB) defines rural counties on a binary, with rural counties designated as those in which there is no urbanized area of more than 50,000 inhabitants. A core challenge with the OMB definition is that it classifies many suburban areas as rural, despite the fact that its residents commute on a daily basis and thus have regular access to the resources of a large urban center. As a response to this issue, the Health Resources and Services Administration (HRSA) developed the Rural-Urban Commuting Area (RUCA) codes, which take into account urbanization, population density, and daily commuting to urban centers. Currently, recognizing the challenges of both sets of definitions, the HRSA functionally combines the OMB definition with its RUCA codes to determine rurality (see more at HRSA, 2018). Yet, another definition is employed by the U.S. Census Bureau, which examines the population size of individual census tracts in the absence of the additional considerations that HRSA's RUCA codes integrate.

One major problem, though, is that all quantitative measures of rurality share one common flaw: the notion that there is a hard and fast cutoff between what is rural versus what is urban, and in the case of county-level definitions, the assumption that functional population centers are contained within a single county. For instance, as with the OMB, many state legislatures define rural counties as ones with populations below a certain size, for example, 35,000 residents. Beyond the issues of density (counties have wildly varying sizes, diminishing the validity of examining population numbers) and cities that span more than one county, such a bright line definition inherently implies that a community that previously had 34,999 residents and now has 35,001 is no longer rural simply because of the addition of two people. The sensitivity of rural definitions to relatively small variations in the location and density of populations is perhaps best illustrated by the fact that nearly 20% of counties in the United States are classified as rural by either OMB or Census, but not the other (Hart et al., 2005).

In reality, the core consideration in defining "rurality" is that, when broken down to the most impactful aspects of rurality, population size is not what makes an area rural—rather, it is qualitative factors that truly constitute what it means to be rural. When you ask a rural or urban resident what makes an area rural, they do not say a specific population size. Rather, they describe the flavor and culture of rural. The most commonly discussed aspects are remoteness, isolation, self-reliance, agriculture, poverty, religiosity, behavioral norms, and health stigma (Smith & Parvin, 1973; Warren & Smalley, 2014c). The tie between rurality and agriculture is so strong that one of the earliest discussions of rural health argued that all rural cultural and economic conditions find their roots in agriculture (Jordan & Hargrove, 1987), and early researchers proposed the percentage of residents employed in agriculture as a proxy for the rurality of a community (Stewart, 1958). Rural areas are more likely to be in persistent poverty, which impacts a variety of outcomes as documented throughout this text—in fact, poverty has long been one of the largest focal areas of those working on health equity and social justice because of its pervasive effect on the ability to achieve and maintain health (Murali & Oyebode, 2004; Patrick, Stein, Porta, Porter, & Ricketts, 1988). Religion plays a very prominent role in rural areas, particularly in the South—rural residents are more likely to regularly attend church, which provides an excellent structural partner in pursuing rural health equity, but can also lead to complications in seeking needed help (e.g., rural religious individuals are more likely to believe that the Church can answer all of life's problems that that mental health issues should be handled within the Church; Farley & Ruesink, 1997; Fox, Merwin, & Blank, 1995; Glenna, 2003). Particularly in the mental health realm, rural areas exhibit much higher levels of stigma, impacting the willingness of rural residents to not only seek care, but even to continue care after it has been initiated (Parr & Philo, 2003).

Overall, these qualities are much more difficult to measure, however, leading the majority of rural health researchers employing a quantitatively based definition. Still, the immense variations between definitions create a complicated literature that is often-times conflicting due to differences in the definition of rurality employed in an individual study. Despite these variations, there are still a number of outcomes for which there is consistency regarding the presence not only of rural/urban disparities but also of disparities within rural communities.

RURAL HEALTH DISPARITIES

Mental and Behavioral Health

There are persistent issues of severely limited access to care, elevated levels of risk factors, and a high degree of mental health stigma in rural areas that result in rural residents being more likely to suffer from a variety of mental health concerns. The vast majority (85%) of mental health professional shortage areas (MHPSAs) are located in rural areas (Bird, Dempsey, & Hartley, 2001), reflecting the fact that more than half of all the counties in the United States do not have a single psychologist, psychiatrist, or clinical social worker (American Psychological Association, 2001; National Advisory Committee on Rural Health, 1993). The shortage is so severe that it would take an estimated 1,500 new mental health professionals practicing exclusively in rural areas to meet the national need (American Psychological Association, 2001; National Advisory Committee on Rural Health, 1993). Shortages in the mental health workforce have been linked to perceptions of lower salaries, fewer social/cultural opportunities, and an elevated risk of professional burnout related to often being the only provider in a region (HRSA, 2007). The issue of stigma in rural areas is twofold: not only does the overall level of stigma increase the smaller a community is, rural residents must also seek care in a context that provides much less anonymity (e.g., having to park in a psychologist's parking lot in a small community inherently discloses receipt of mental health services; HRSA, 2007; Helbok, 2003; Hoyt, Conger, Valde, & Weihs, 1997). This combination of stigma and lack of anonymity makes rural residents less likely to seek mental healthcare than their urban counterparts (Wagenfeld & Buffum, 1983). While the literature is conflicting regarding the presence of disparities in many mental health issues, there is strong agreement regarding two areas of inequity: substance use and suicide.

Illicit drug use is often perceived to be an "urban" problem, but methamphetamines and opioids in particular have hit rural America very hard (Gfroerer, Larson, & Colliver, 2008). Rural youth also exhibit increased risk for substance use, including alcohol, tobacco, prescription drugs, inhalants, marijuana, methamphetamines, and cocaine (Foster, 2000; Lambert, Gale, & Hartley, 2008;

Substance Abuse and Mental Health Services Administration, 2001). Battling rural substance use is difficult—as described earlier, there are substantial shortages of mental health providers in general in rural communities—but the availability of substance use disorder treatment providers is even more limited, impacting the ability to access both outpatient and inpatient services (American Society of Addiction Medicine, 2001, 2005; Center for Substance Abuse Treatment, 2000; Sowers & Rohland, 2004). These shortages are particularly troubling because an estimated 40% of rural residents with mental illness have a comorbid substance use disorder (Gogek, 1992).

Rural areas of the United States also exhibit higher rates of death by suicide, with both more suicide deaths and a higher likelihood of suicide completion than in urban areas (Goldsmith, Pellmar, Kleinman, & Bunney, 2002; Ivey-Stephenson et al., 2017; President's New Freedom Commission on Mental Health, 2003). These differences can be as high as a 3-fold increase in risk among adults and an alarming 15-fold increase among rural adolescents (Forrest, 1988; Mulder et al., 2001). Identified risk factors for rural suicide include increased access to lethal means (e.g., firearms), social isolation, mental health stigma, and limited access to mental health services (Smalley & Warren, 2014).

RURAL OPIOIDS

The ongoing opioid crisis in the United States has become more and more prominent to the general public, and for good reason. It is estimated that every day, more than 130 people in the United States die from opioid overdose (CDC, 2018). The epidemic has hit rural America exceedingly hard, especially rural Appalachia. Appalachian counties have a nearly unbelievable opioid prescription rate of 84 prescriptions per 100 residents and an opioid overdose death rate that is over 70% higher than that seen in non-Appalachian counties (National Association of Counties and the Appalachian Regional Commission, 2019). Georgia, a state with 37 Appalachian counties, has seen the crisis unfold in striking fashion. From 1999 to 2017, the opioid overdose mortality rate in rural counties increased from 0.5 deaths per 100,000 people to 9.5 per 100,000 people, representing a staggering 19-fold increase (see Figure 13.1).

Obesity and Chronic Disease

Rural children and adults are more likely to be obese than their urban counterparts (Jackson, Doescher, Jerant, & Hart, 2005; Liu et al., 2007; Patterson, Moore, Probst, & Shinogle, 2004; Scott & Wilson, 2011b). The reasons for this are varied and multilevel, as summarized in Table 13.1.

The increased rates of obesity in rural areas unsurprisingly lead to increased rates of heart disease and diabetes, two of the most robustly studied disparities in rural communities. Rural areas have higher rates of hypertension and death from cardiovascular diseases (Bale, 2010; Pearson & Lewis, 1998), with rates even higher among minority residents (Rimando, Warren, & Smalley, 2014). Despite representing only 20% of the nation's population, rural residents make up over one-third of hypertension diagnoses; shockingly, nearly one-quarter of all hypertension diagnoses in the U.S. is in rural African Americans (Mainous, King, Garr, & Pearson, 2004). Appalachian

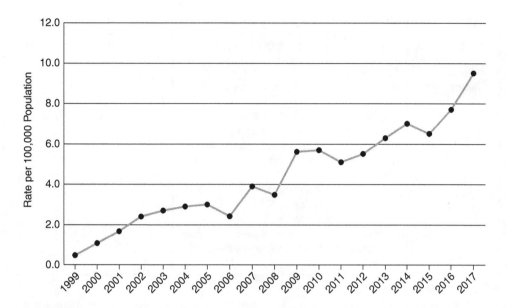

FIGURE 13.1 Opioid overdose death rate in rural Georgia, 1999 to 2017.

SOURCE: Data from Georgia Department of Public Health, Office of Health Indicators for Planning, Online Analytical Statistical Information System (OASIS).

TABLE 13.1 Factors Linked to Rural Obesity

LEVEL	DOMAIN AND RELATED FACTORS	RECOMMENDED ACTIONS
Individual factors	**Gender** Rural women are more likely to be obese Rural women have higher fat diets **Race and Ethnicity** Non-Hispanic Black and Mexican American women and Hispanic children and adolescents are more likely to be obese **Stress and Depression** Maladaptive coping Limited access to care Social isolation	Stress-reduction interventions Nutrition education initiatives Addressing social determinants of health Creating a sense of community and support
Family and household factors	**Poverty and Food Insecurity** Rural households have lower incomes and are more likely to exhibit food insecurity **Financial Constraints and Eating Patterns** Rural mothers are more likely to skip meals and eat smaller portions Rural residents consume more sugar-sweetened beverages and fewer fruits and vegetables	Parenting programs Teaching children nutritional limits

(continued)

TABLE 13.1 Factors Linked to Rural Obesity (*continued*)

LEVEL	DOMAIN AND RELATED FACTORS	RECOMMENDED ACTIONS
Community factors	**Food Access** Rural areas are more likely to be food deserts **Opportunities for Physical Activity** Rural residents are more likely to be inactive in both daily living and leisure Rural residents have longer commuting distances Rural residents have more sedentary jobs (farm automation) **School Environment** Rural schools face financial pressures that may compromise nutritional quality of meals	Implementing farmer's markets Delivery of WIC food Increasing availability of telehealth-based programs

WIC: women, infants, and children.
SOURCE: Greder, K., Ihmels, M., Burney, J., & Doudna, K. (2014). Obesity in rural America. In J. C. Warren & K. B. Smalley (Eds.), *Rural public health* (pp. 139–154). New York, NY: Springer Publishing Company.

residents also exhibit particularly high rates of stroke and heart attack (Odoi, 2009). In addition to the increased prevalence, a key factor in heart disease and stroke deaths is the increased response and transit time for emergency medical services (EMS) in rural communities (Gebhardt & Norris, 2006).

The rural South is the core of the Centers for Disease Control and Prevention's designated "diabetes belt" (Warren & Smalley, 2014a). Even after adjusting for age, body mass index, insurance coverage, and demographic characteristics, rural residents exhibit higher rates of diabetes in self-report data and medical expenditure data (Krishna, Gillespie, & McBride, 2010; Warren & Smalley, 2014a). Reflecting the overall lack of access to care (discussed in more detail in the next section), rural diabetics receive less care than their urban counterparts and are specifically less likely to receive a recommended annual eye examination or a foot check, placing them at increased risk for vision loss and amputation (Andrus, Kelley, Murphey, & Herndon, 2004; Krishna et al., 2010). These effects are particularly pronounced among rural African Americans, who have a higher age-adjusted death rate from diabetes than urban Whites, rural Whites, and even urban African Americans (Slifkin, Goldsmith, & Ricketts, 2000). Key contributing factors include lack of diabetes education in rural areas (Krishna et al., 2010), lack of exercise opportunities (Kegler, Escoffery, Alcantara, Ballard, & Glanz, 2008), cost of care (Boyle, Thompson, Gregg, Barker, & Williamson, 2010), and the cost-related inability to remain adherent to treatment regimens (Bell et al., 2007; Skelly et al., 2005).

ACCESS TO HEALTHCARE

While the ability of rural residents to achieve and maintain health is impacted by much more than medical care, the fundamental lack of access to medical care undergirds the entire health system in rural areas. A commonly discussed model of issues related to healthcare in rural areas is that of the availability, accessibility, and acceptability of care. Rural areas have fewer healthcare providers with increased average distance between patient and provider, which leads many rural residents to avoid care until no longer physically able to ignore symptoms (Connor, Kralewski, & Hillson, 1994; HRSA, 2007; Weinert & Boik, 1995). The reasons for this lack of care include a variety of social, economic, and geographic factors that make rural residents arguably the group in the United States with the lowest level of access to healthcare (Ziller, 2014). As a result, despite having higher medical needs due to the disparities discussed throughout this chapter, rural residents see a medical provider fewer times in any given year than their urban counterparts (Larson & Fleishman, 2003). Correspondingly, rural residents are less likely to have an annual physical, receive preventive care, and have routine screenings for cholesterol, colorectal cancer, breast cancer, and cervical cancer (Ziller, Coburn, Loux, Hoffman, & McBride, 2003), in turn leading rural patients to be diagnosed with cancer on average at a later stage of disease than urban patients.

Three of the largest barriers in access to care include health insurance coverage, local availability of primary care providers and specialists, and related challenges with transportation. Rural residents are more likely to be uninsured, are more likely to be on public insurance programs, and are more likely to be underinsured than their urban counterparts (Ziller, 2014; Ziller, Coburn, & Yousefian, 2006). These differences have been attributed to the older age of rural residents, the increased likelihood of living in poverty, and the larger proportion of the rural workforce that is either self-employed (e.g., farmer) or employed by small businesses that do not offer health insurance (Coburn, Kilbreth, Long, & Marquis, 1998; Lenardson, Ziller, Coburn, & Anderson, 2009; Ziller, Lenardson, & Coburn, 2012). The lack of insurance leaves rural residents less likely to have a medical home, leads them to travel farther in order to receive care, and often forces them to forego needed medical care because of inability to pay—directly leading to higher mortality rates in rural residents (Bennett, Olatosi, & Probst, 2008; Probst, Bellinger, Walsemann, Hardin, & Glover, 2011; Ziller et al., 2012). Even if rural residents do have insurance and the financial means to seek care, there is a stark lack of providers in rural communities. More than three-quarters of all rural counties in the United States are federally designated primary care health professional shortage areas (HPSAs), indicating they do not have a sufficient number of primary care providers to meet the area's needs (Fordyce, Chen, Doescher, & Hart, 2007). The availability of specialty care in rural areas is even lower, leading to fragmented care with limited ability for local follow-up and support (Fordyce et al., 2007; Jones, Parker, & Ahearn, 2009). Access is further impacted by the fact that rural residents have less opportunity to receive after-hours or weekend care due to lack of providers who offer such services and an increased likelihood of being employed in non-flexible shift work (Lenardson et al., 2009; Ziller et al., 2012). Further complicating all aspects of accessibility is the substantial transportation barrier present in rural communities. Rural areas typically do not have public transportation infrastructure, leaving residents without an inherent ability to physically travel to appointments (even if all other barriers—e.g., insurance—have been removed). This has a significant impact—rural residents without a driver's license have half the number of regular checkup visits and chronic care follow-up visits as those with driver's licenses (Arcury, Preisser, Gesler, & Powers, 2006). The systemic effect of lack of transportation crosses into other social determinants of health—for example, transportation has been identified as one of the largest barriers to successful employment for rural low-income families (Fletcher, Garasky, Jensen, & Nielsen, 2010).

STRATEGIES AND SOLUTIONS

Integrated Care

While not limited to rural settings, the model of integrated care—wherein an individual accesses physical and mental health services through a partnership between physical and mental health providers—has emerged as a best practice in improving rural health outcomes. Because the majority of people with a mental health condition are treated by a primary care provider and not a mental health provider, integrating mental health into primary care is a natural extension of the primary care environment (Regier, Goldberg, & Taube, 1978; Reiger et al., 1993). There are varying levels of integration delineated by Doherty, McDaniel, and Baird (1996), as summarized in Table 13.2.

When examining rural-specific implementation, four general approaches have been identified: diversification, in which mental health services are provided directly by an employee of the consolidated health center; linkage/colocation, in which mental health services are provided on-site by a nonemployee; referral, in which care is provided off-site by a nonemployee but under a formal agreement; and enhancement, in which primary care practitioners receive additional training to provide mental healthcare themselves (Bird, Lambert, Hartley, Coburn, & Beeson, 1998). While diversification, linkage, and referral map back to the overall integrated care framework in Table 13.2, enhancement reflects a reality of rural mental health provider shortages, which may lead primary care providers to seek to themselves provide both aspects of care, but with improved training and competence.

Integrated care—regardless of model—has a consistent evidence base to support its implementation. An Agency for Healthcare Research and Quality (AHRQ) literature review (Butler et al., 2008) concluded that integrated care improves symptom severity, has an increased overall treatment response, and enhances full recovery when implemented. However, despite this evidence, there remain a number of barriers to widespread implementation of integrated care that have been summarized in five domains as presented in Table 13.3 (Butler et al., 2008; Gale & Lambert, 2009; Institute of Medicine, 2005; Lambert & Gale, 2014; Lambert & Hartley, 1998).

Telehealth

Despite biases held by urban residents that rural populations are technologically disconnected or lack technological literacy, the use of telehealth has long been associated with rural areas (in fact, the federal Office for the Advancement of Telehealth is located within HRSA's Office of Rural

TABLE 13.2 Levels of Integrated Care

LEVEL 1	LEVEL 2	LEVEL 3	LEVEL 4	LEVEL 5
Separate Systems and Facilities (standard)	Basic Collaboration from a Distance (referral relationship)	Basic Collaboration on Site (warm handoff)	Close Collaboration through Partially Integrated System (case collaboration)	Fully Integrated Systems (team-based healthcare)

TABLE 13.3 Barriers to Implementation of Integrated Care and Potential Solution

LEVEL	EXAMPLES	POTENTIAL SOLUTIONS
National and System	Limited supply of mental health professionals Misdistribution of providers Separation of funding streams for physical vs. behavioral health	Increase rural training programs Create regional incentives Consolidate oversight of physical and mental health
Regulatory	State-level licensing laws Scope of practice variations Facility licensure issues	Create composite health license boards National credentialing standards Unification of facility licensure process
Reimbursement	Specific exclusions of integrated services (e.g., "double-billing") Variations in coverages across insurances Differences in billing and coding practices Mental health carveouts	Codify the ability of more than one provider to bill for a single encounter Regulate integrated care coverage Create unified billing codes Eliminate carveouts
Practice and Culture	Differences in practice styles, terminology, and treatment approaches between physical and mental health providers	Increase interprofessional training opportunities; create integrated training workshops and certifications
Patient	Financial resources for multiple co-pays Limitations in number of mental health sessions covered Stigma regarding mental health	Create business arrangement to share revenue Enforce parity laws; create efficient treatment plans Implement individual and public awareness campaigns

Health Policy). As with integrated care, telehealth is not a model exclusively for rural; however, its ability to address numerous rural health barriers makes it an ideal approach for improving rural health outcomes. By utilizing technology—be it video, telephone, or sophisticated remote diagnostic equipment—telehealth allows rural residents the ability to access at-a-distance care (minimizing travel burden) while also helping address barriers associated with insufficient local volume to sustain providers (in particular, specialty care). Telehealth has also been expanded into broader health promotion efforts, providing otherwise unavailable services ranging from smoking cessation and 12-step program to chronic disease self-management (see Case Study; Warren & Smalley, 2014b).

Telehealth is a particularly impactful rural health intervention because it addresses the three core barriers to health within rural communities: availability, accessibility, and acceptability of care. By providing the ability to access providers and programs not available locally, telehealth directly improves the availability of care (both clinical and prevention). Similarly, by removing the travel burden necessary to reach providers, telehealth increases the accessibility of care. Finally, with thoughtful implementation, telehealth can increase acceptability of care as well. For instance, connecting a mental health provider into a "physical health" exam room can help rural residents feel more like mental health is actually a part of their medical care.

As with integrated care, there are a number of factors that currently limit its broader implementation; however, many of these challenges are subject to nationwide advocacy and are likely to change in the near future. Two issues merit particular focus: billing and licensure. Billing codes are continually updated to provide for the unique nature of telehealth. Structurally, a telehealth encounter is typically broken into two charges: a presentation charge and a provision of care charge. This allows the location where the patient is physically located to receive compensation for the cost of presenting the patient to the remote provider and for the distance provider to receive compensation for the clinical encounter. Coverage provisions still vary widely from state to state, and centralization or coordination of this process across states could be beneficial. Finally, the state-level nature of licenses currently limits the ability of telehealth to reach its full potential, as providers cannot practice telehealth across state lines unless licensed in both states. One proposed solution is national licensure of healthcare providers, but there is little overall traction for this level of change. Instead, states have begun to explore compacts and reciprocal licensure that can help providers more easily become licensed in multiple states.

INTERSECTIONALITY SPOTLIGHT

Because rurality is tied to geography and not directly to personal characteristics, intersectionality becomes a very important consideration for rural health equity initiatives. In essence, rural communities are a microcosm of the rest of the United States, and within them possess all the types of diversity discussed throughout this book. Correspondingly, rural America faces the same health disparities as the rest of the nation, and unfortunately, these disparities are often magnified. For example, rural African American residents are more likely to have diagnoses of several chronic diseases (e.g., diabetes and heart disease), but also have a higher age-adjusted death rate from those diseases than both rural Whites and urban African Americans (Slifkin et al., 2000).

While all groups are represented in rural, three groups have received the most attention: African American, Hispanic, and lesbian, gay, bisexual, transgender, or queer (LGBTQ). Studies show rural African Americans are less likely to have health insurance, see a physician less frequently, are more likely to be obese, are less likely to meet physical activity recommendations, receive preventive screenings less frequently, and are at increased risk for heart disease, diabetes, stroke, and both colorectal and breast cancer (Bennett et al., 2008; Connolly, Unwin, Sherriff, Belous, & Kelly, 2000; Housing Assistance Council, 2012; Howard, Labarthe, Hu, Yoon, & Howard, 2007; Hueston & Hubbard, 2000; Kochanek, Xu, Murphy, Miniño, & Kung, 2011; Kung, Hoyert, Xu, & Murphy, 2008; Lemacks, Wells, Ilich, & Ralston, 2013; Mainous et al., 2004; Middleton, 2009; O'Connor & Wellenius, 2012; Saydan & Lochner, 2010; Scott & Wilson, 2011a; Wilson-Anderson, Williams, Beacham, & McDonald, 2013). Specific recommendations for improving health within rural African American populations include focusing on community-based (and especially church-based) prevention programs and ensuring interventions are culturally tailored to not only rural and African American

(continued)

populations but specifically to rural African American populations (Frank & Grubbs, 2008; Lemacks et al., 2013; Warren et al., 2014).

Rural Hispanic populations have higher levels of non-benefited employment, lower educational attainment, and are less likely to be English speakers (Effland & Kassel, 1998; Saenz, 2008; United States Department of Agriculture [USDA], 2003, 2005), all of which affect the ability to seek out and receive not only healthcare, but preventive and supportive services as well. These and other factors leave rural Hispanic populations at increased risk for diabetes, undiagnosed hypertension, diabetes, death by stroke, and colorectal and cervical cancer (Brown et al., 2011; Cohen & Ingram, 2005; Coughlin et al., 2006; Mainous, Koopman, & Geesey, 2004; Mier et al., 2012; Singh, 2012; Swenson et al., 2002). Specific recommendations for improving these outcomes include a focus on health literacy, improving access to care, ensuring services are available in the language of preference for individuals, and incorporating economic support initiatives such as General Education Diploma (GED) courses (Bennett et al., 2008; Vitale & Bailey, 2012; Warren et al., 2014).

Residents of rural areas who also identify as LGBTQ also face elevated risks for poor health. The broader sociocultural oppression of LGBTQ individuals (see Chapter 12, LGBTQ Health Equity) is often exacerbated in rural communities due to an emphasis on conformity to social and gender norms, a generally conservative political climate, and fundamental religiosity (Round, 1988). As a result, stigma and discrimination toward LGBTQ individuals and overall heterosexism and cisgenderism are more prevalent in rural areas (Edwards, 2005; Leedy & Connolly, 2007; Swank, Fahs, & Frost, 2013). While the literature is limited, rural LGBTQ residents face elevated risk for substance use disorder, sexual risk-taking, HIV, mental health concerns, and obesity (CDC, 2000; Cohn, 1997; Cohn & Leake, 2012; Preston, D'Augelli, Kassab, & Starks, 2007; Rostosky, Owens, Zimmerman, & Riggle, 2003; Steinberg & Fleming, 2000). Specific recommendations for intervention include supporting legislation and public policy related to financial resource and healthcare access; providing public education on the impact of homophobia, discrimination, and victimization; and increasing community resources to connect local LGBTQ individuals together to create a rural support system (Oswald & Culton, 2003).

CASE STUDY   TELEPARAMEDICINE

As discussed throughout this chapter, the fundamental availability, accessibility, and acceptability of medical care are a major driving force in the presence of rural health disparities. Because of its ability to address these barriers, the use of telehealth has emerged as a best practice in improving access to care for rural residents throughout the country. At the same time, however, issues of volume and payer mix complicate the viability and sustainability of emergency medical service (EMS) in rural communities, and rural hospitals face significant financial issues surrounding utilization of emergency departments (EDs) for primary care. Recently, telehealth advocates have worked to address the triple issue of access to primary care, sustainability of EMS, and financial stabilization of EDs in a model that completely changes the paradigm of how telehealth is delivered.

(continued)

The concept of community paramedicine—wherein the scope of services offered via ambulance is expanded to include primary care and/or patient navigation services—has gained significant traction in the field of rural health. There are two main models: the primary health care model, wherein paramedics provide postdischarge evaluation, monitor chronic illnesses, and specifically focus on known high-risk patients, and the community coordination model, wherein paramedics take on, in part, the role of a navigator for patients (helping to coordinate care and connect to other social and medical services; Pearson, Gale, & Shaler, 2014). Many rural community paramedicine programs combine aspects of both models. The core concept is that allowing paramedics to provide nonemergency access to basic care that they are already trained to do (e.g., administer immunizations), not only expands access to care, it also presents a new revenue stream for the EMS system.

A core challenge in the ability of community paramedicine to achieve its full potential is (understandable) limits to scope of practice. Paramedics are trained in emergency medicine protocols rather than primary care, preventing them from being able to provide comprehensive primary care services and from being able to robustly implement ED diversion approaches for nonemergent cases (that may necessitate consultation with a provider with a higher license).

Up until recently, the concept of telehealth was largely viewed as a model whereby patients at one doctor's office could connect to another doctor's office for a consultation or visit with a specialist. The core issue of accessibility remains in place—what happens with individuals who do not have access to a doctor's office in the first place?

A powerful solution lies in *teleparamedicine*: Make ambulances official telehealth presentation sites, allowing paramedics to present patients for primary care from within an ambulance. Such a model instantly makes primary care mobile—expanding access to care—improves the sustainability of EMS—providing a new revenue stream—and assists with ED diversion, allowing paramedics to receive a physician consult if needed. In essence, it allows ambulances to always have a physician on-site.

In partnership between the Mercer University School of Medicine, the Georgia Department of Community Health, the Centers for Medicare and Medicaid Services, and local hospitals, rural practitioners worked not only to receive state funding to implement a community teleparamedicine initiative but also to receive a formal waiver to change the fundamental policy necessary to make the ambulances billable presentation sites. This model of combining innovative strategies with financial sustainability and policy change serves as an example of the complexity of addressing rural health equity issues, but also of the truly innovative ways that multiple challenges can be addressed within a single initiative.

CURRENT EVENTS

RURAL HOSPITAL CLOSURES

The U.S. is in the midst of a rural hospital closure crisis, with more than 100 rural hospitals closing in the past 10 years. These closures nearly exclusively related to financial insolvency, with EDs and labor and delivery units seen as two of the largest financial drains on a hospital when there is insufficient volume to recoup the inherent cost of running the service lines. There is ongoing debate about the best way to stabilize the remaining hospital infrastructure, ranging from increasing reimbursement rates to strategically/proactively closing certain hospitals to improve the financial viability of other nearby hospitals.

Discussion Question: How could it be that closing a rural hospital could in turn stabilize nearby hospitals? What criteria would need to be considered when choosing which hospitals to close?

NALOXONE

The ready availability of overdose-reversing agents such as Narcan hold great promise for reducing deaths due to opioid overdose. These drugs are controlled and available only by prescription, however. To ensure the broadest possible reach, many states have implemented standing orders wherein each resident of the state has a functional prescription (typically "officially" written by the public health commissioner for the state). This allows any resident to walk into a pharmacy and request a prescription be filled for Narcan.

Discussion Question: While standing orders for Narcan are an important step in ensuring equal access to overdose-reducing agents, what other barriers remain in place? How could those barriers be removed in combination with the standing order to ensure equal access to all?

DISCUSSION QUESTIONS

- How do varying definitions of "rurality" complicate both the research literature and the distribution of resources to address rural health equity?

- What specific strategies could be employed to combat some of the sources of the suicide disparity seen in rural areas?

- Why would simply establishing a new clinic in a rural setting still potentially fail to meet the access needs of rural residents?

- How can telehealth be used to improve access to integrated care, and what are the barriers to implementing such a program?

- What are ways in which intervention programs can be specifically designed to meet the needs of African American rural residents?

REFERENCES

American Psychological Association. (2001). *Caring for the rural community: 2000–2001 report*. Retrieved from https://www.apa.org/practice/programs/rural/2000-2001-report.pdf

American Society of Addiction Medicine. (2001). Preface. In D. Mee-Lee (Ed.), *ASAM patient placement criteria for the treatment of substance-related disorders* (2nd ed.). Chevy Chase, MD: Author.

American Society of Addiction Medicine. (2005). *Public policy statement on treatment for alcoholism and other drug dependencies*. Chevy Chase, MD: Author.

Andrus, M. R., Kelley, K. W., Murphey, L. M., & Herndon, K. C. (2004). A comparison of diabetes care in rural and urban medical clinics in Alabama. *Journal of Community Health*, *29*, 29–44. doi:10.1023/B:JOHE.0000007443.96138.03

Arcury, T. A., Preisser, J. S., Gesler, W. M., & Powers, J. M. (2006). Access to transportation and health care utilization in a rural region. *The Journal of Rural Health*, *21*, 1, 31–38. doi:10.1111/j.1748-0361.2005.tb00059.x

Bale, B. (2010). Optimizing hypertension management in underserved rural populations. *Journal of the National Medical Association*, *102*, 10–17. doi:10.1016/S0027-9684(15)30470-3

Bell, R. A., Arcury, T. A., Stafford, J. M., Golden, S. L., Snively, B. M., & Quandt, S. A. (2007). Ethnic and sex differences in ownership of preventive health equipment among rural older adults with diabetes. *Journal of Rural Health*, *23*, 332–338. doi:10.1111/j.1748-0361.2007.00111.x

Bennett, K. J., Olatosi, B., & Probst, J. C. (2008). *Health disparities: A rural-urban chartbook*. Columbia: South Carolina Rural Health Research Center. Retrieved from https://www.ruralhealthresearch.org/publications/676

Bird, P. C., Dempsey, P., & Hartley, D. (2001). *Addressing mental health workforce needs in underserved rural areas: Accomplishments and challenges*. Portland: Maine Rural Health Research Center. Retrieved from http://muskie.usm.maine.edu/Publications/rural/wp23.pdf

Bird, D. C., Lambert, D., Hartley, D., Coburn, A. F., & Beeson, P. G. (1998). Integrating primary care and mental health in rural America: A policy review. *Administration and Policy in Mental Health and Mental Health Services Research*, *25*(3), 287–308. doi:10.1023/A:1022291306283

Boyle, J. P., Thompson, T. J., Gregg, E. W., Barker, L. E., & Williamson, D. F. (2010). Projection of the year 2050 burden of diabetes in the US adult population: Dynamic modeling of incidence, mortality, and prediabetes prevalence. *Population Health Metrics*, *8*, 29. doi:10.1186/1478-7954-8-29

Brown, S. A., Garcia, A. A., Winter, M., Silva, L., Brown, A., & Hanis, C. L. (2011). Integrating education, group support, and case management for diabetic Hispanics. *Ethnicity and Disease*, *21*(1), 20–26. Retrieved from https://www.ncbi.nlm.nih.gov/pmc/articles/PMC3153083/

Butler, M., Kane, R., McAlpine, D., Kathol, R. G., Fu, S. S., Hagedorn, H., & Wilt, T. J. (2008). *Integration of mental health/substance abuse and primary care (AHRQ Publication No. 09-E003)*. Rockville, MD: Agency for Healthcare Research and Quality. Retrieved from https://www.ahrq.gov/downloads/pub/evidence/pdf/mhsapc/mhsapc.pdf

Center for Substance Abuse Treatment. (2000). *Changing the conversation: Improving substance abuse treatment*. Rockville, MD: U.S. Department of Health and Human Services. Retrieved from https://atforum.com/documents/Natxplan%201.pdf

Centers for Disease Control and Prevention. (2000). HIV/AIDS in urban and nonurban areas of the United States. *HIV/AIDS Surveillance Supplemental Report*, *6*(2), 1–16. doi:. Retrieved from https://www.cdc.gov/hiv/pdf/library/reports/surveillance/cdc-hiv-surveillance-supplemental-report-vol-6-2.pdf

Centers for Disease Control and Prevention. (2011). Health disparities and inequalities report—United States, 2011. *Morbidity and Mortality Weekly Report*, *60*(Suppl.), 1–113. Retrieved from https://www.cdc.gov/mmwr/pdf/other/su6001.pdf

Centers for Disease Control and Prevention. (2018). *Mortality: CDC WONDER*. Atlanta, GA: U.S. Department of Health and Human Services.

Coburn, A. F., Kilbreth, E. H., Long, S. H., & Marquis, M. S. (1998). Urban-rural differences in employer-based health insurance coverage of workers. *Medical Care Research Review*, *55*(4), 484–496. doi:10.1177/107755879805500406

Cohen, S. J., & Ingram, M. (2005). Border health strategic initiative: Overview and introduction to a community-based model for diabetes prevention and control. *Preventing Chronic Disease, 2*(1), A05. Retrieved from https://www.ncbi.nlm.nih.gov/pmc/articles/PMC1323308

Cohn, S. E. (1997). AIDS in rural America. *Journal of Rural Health, 13,* 237–239. doi:10.1111/j.1748-0361.1997 .tb00847.x

Cohn, T. J., & Leake, V. S. (2012). Affective distress among adolescents who endorse same-sex sexual attraction: Urban versus rural differences and the role of protective factors. *Journal of Gay & Lesbian Mental Health, 16*(4), 291–305. doi:10.1080/19359705.2012.690931

Connolly, V., Unwin, N., Sherriff, P., Belous, R., & Kelly, W. (2000). Diabetes prevalence and socioeconomic status: A population-based study showing increased prevalence of type 2 diabetes mellitus in deprived areas. *Journal of Epidemiological Community Health, 54,* 173–177. doi:10.1136/jech.54.3.173

Connor, R. A., Kralewski, J. E., & Hillson, S. D. (1994). Measuring geographical access to health care in rural areas. *Medical Care Review, 51*(3), 337–377. doi:10.1177/107755879405100304

Coughlin, S. S., Richards, T. B., Thompson, T., Miller, B. A., VanEenwyk, J., Goodman, M. T., & Sherman, R. L. (2006). Rural and nonrural differences in colorectal cancer incidence in the United States, 1998–2001. *Cancer, 107*(5), 1181–1188. doi:10.1002/cncr.22015

Doherty, W., McDaniel, S., & Baird, M. (1996). Five levels of primary care/behavioral health-care collaboration. *Behavioral Healthcare of Tomorrow, 5,* 25–27.

Edwards, J. (2005). Invisibility, safety and psycho-social distress among same-sex attracted women in rural South Australia. *Rural and Remote Health, 5*(1), 343. Retrieved from https://www.rrh.org.au/journal/ article/343

Effland, A. B., & Kassel, K. (1998). Hispanics in rural America: The influence of immigration and language on economic well-being. *USDA Economic Research Service.* Retrieved from https://www.ers.usda.gov/ webdocs/publications/40678/32996_aer731h_002.pdf?v=0

Farley, G. E., & Ruesink, D. C. (1997). Churches. In G. A. Goreham (Ed.), *Encyclopedia of rural America: The Land and People* (pp. 102–105). Santa Barbara, CA: ABC-CLIO.

Fletcher, C. N., Garasky, S. B., Jensen, H. H., & Nielsen, R. (2010). Transportation access: A key employment barrier for rural low-income families. *Journal of Poverty, 14*(2), 123–144. doi:10.1080/10875541003711581

Fordyce, M. A., Chen, F. M., Doescher, M. P., & Hart, L. G. (2007). *2005 physician supply and distribution in rural areas of the United States.* Seattle, WA: WWAMI Rural Health Research Center. Retrieved from https://depts.washington.edu/uwrhrc/uploads/RHRC%20FR116%20Fordyce.pdf

Forrest, S. (1988). Suicide and the rural adolescent. *Adolescence, 23,* 341–346.

Foster, S. E. (2000). *No place to hide: Substance abuse in mid-size cities and rural America.* New York, NY: National Center on Addiction and Substance Abuse.

Fox, J., Merwin, E., & Blank, M. (1995). De facto mental health services in the rural South. *Journal of Health Care for the Poor and Underserved, 6,* 434–468. doi:10.1353/hpu.2010.0003

Frank, D., & Grubbs, L. (2008). A faith-based screening and education program for diabetes, CVD, and stroke in rural African Americans. *The Association of Black Nursing Faculty Journal, 19*(3), 96–101.

Gale, J., & Lambert, D. (2009). *Maine barriers to integration study: The view from Maine on the barriers to integrated care and recommendations for moving forward.* Portland: University of Southern Maine. Retrieved from *Maine barriers to integration study: The view from Maine on the barriers to integrated care and recommendations for moving forward.*

Gebhardt, J. G., & Norris, T. E. (2006). Acute stroke care at rural hospitals in Idaho: Challenges in expediting stroke care. *Journal of Rural Health, 22*(1), 88–91. doi:10.1111/j.1748-0361.2006.00004.x

Gfroerer, J. C., Larson, S. L., & Colliver, J. D. (2008). Drug use patterns and trends in rural communities. *Journal of Rural Health, 23*(S1), 10–15. doi:10.1111/j.1748-0361.2007.00118.x

Glenna, L. (2003). Religion. In D. L. Brown & L. E. Swanson (Eds.), *Challenges for rural America in the twenty-first century* (pp. 262–272). University Park: The Pennsylvania State University Press.

Gogek, L. B. (1992). Dr. Gogek replies. *American Journal of Psychiatry, 149,* 1286. doi:10.1176/ajp.149 .9.1286

Goldsmith, S., Pellmar, T., Kleinman, A., & Bunney, W. (2002). *Reducing suicide: A national imperative.* Washington, DC: National Academies Press. Retrieved from https://www.nap.edu/read/10398/chapter/1

Greder, K., Ihmels, M., Burney, J., & Doudna, K. (2014). Obesity in rural America. In J. C. Warren & K. B. Smalley (Eds.), *Rural public health* (pp. 139–154). New York, NY: Springer Publishing Company.

Hart, L. G., Larson, E. H., & Lishner, D. M. (2005). Rural definitions for health policy and research. *American Journal of Public Health*, *95*(7), 1149–1155. doi:10.2105/AJPH.2004.042432

Health Resources and Services Administration. (2007). *Mental health and rural America: 1994-2005.* Rockville, MD: Author. Retrieved from https://www.ruralhealthresearch.org/mirror/6/657/RuralMentalHealth.pdf

Health Resources and Services Administration. (2018). *Defining rural population*. Retrieved from https://www.hrsa.gov/rural-health/about-us/definition/index.html

Helbok, C. M. (2003). The practice of psychology in rural communities: Potential ethical dilemmas. *Ethics and Behavior*, *13*, 367–384. doi:10.1207/S15327019EB1304_5

Housing Assistance Council. (2012). *HAC rural research brief: Race and ethnicity in rural America* (HAC tabulations of 2010 Census of Population and housing, Summary File 1). Retrieved from http://www.ruralhome.org/storage/research_notes/rrn-race-and-ethnicity-web.pdf

Howard, G., Labarthe, D. R., Hu, J., Yoon, S., & Howard, V. J. (2007). Regional differences in African Americans' high risk for stroke: The remarkable burden of stroke for southern African Americans. *Annals of Epidemiology*, *17*(9), 689–696. doi:10.1016/j.annepidem.2007.03.019

Hoyt, D. R., Conger, R. D., Valde, J. G., & Weihs, K. (1997). Psychological distress and help seeking in rural America. *American Journal of Community Psychology*, *25*(4), 449–470. doi:10.1023/A:1024655521619

Hueston, W., & Hubbard, E. (2000). Preventive services for rural and urban African American adults. *Archives of Family Medicine*, *9*, 262–266. doi:10.1001/archfami.9.3.263

Institute of Medicine. (2005). *Quality through collaboration: The future of rural health*. Washington, DC: National Academies Press. Retrieved from https://www.nap.edu/read/11140/chapter/1

Ivey-Stephenson, A. Z., Crosby, A. E., Jack, S. P. D., Haileyesus, T., & Kresnow-Sedacca, M. (2017). Suicide trends among and within urbanization levels by sex, race/ethnicity, age group, and mechanism of death - United States, 2001-2015. *Morbidity and Mortality Weekly Report*, *66*(18), 1–16.

Jackson, J. E., Doescher, M. P., Jerant, A. F., & Hart, L. G. (2005). A national study of obesity prevalence and trends by type of rural county. *Journal of Rural Health*, *21*, 140–148. doi:10.1111/j.1748-0361.2005.tb00074.x

Jones, C. A., Parker, T. S., & Ahearn, M. (2009). Taking the pulse of rural health care: New health information technologies hold promise for improving health care in remote areas. *Amber Waves*, *7*(3), 10–15. Retrieved from https://www.ers.usda.gov/amber-waves/2009/september/taking-the-pulse-of-rural-health-care

Jordan, S. A., & Hargrove, D. S. (1987). Implications of an empirical application of categorical definitions of rural. *Journal of Rural Community Psychology*, *8*, 14–29.

Kegler, M. C., Escoffery, C., Alcantara, I., Ballard, D., & Glanz, K. (2008). A qualitative examination of home and neighborhood environments for obesity prevention in rural adults. *International Journal of Behavior, Nutrition, and Physical Activity*, *5*, 65–74. doi:10.1186/1479-5868-5-65

Krishna, S., Gillespie, K. N., & McBride, T. M. (2010). Diabetes burden and access to preventive care in the rural United States. *Journal of Rural Health*, *26*, 3–11. doi:0.1111/j.1748-0361.2009.00259.x

Kung, H.-C., Hoyert, D., Xu, J., & Murphy, S. (2008). Deaths: Final data for 2005. *National Vital Statistics Reports*, *56*(10), 1–120. Retrieved from https://www.cdc.gov/nchs/data/nvsr/nvsr56/nvsr56_10.pdf

Lambert, D., & Gale, J. A. (2014). Integrated care in rural areas. In J. C. Warren & K. B. Smalley (Eds.), *Rural public health* (pp. 67–84). New York, NY: Springer Publishing Company.

Lambert, D., Gale, J. A., & Hartley, D. (2008). Substance abuse by youth and young adults in rural America. *Journal of Rural Health*, *24*(3), 221–228. doi:10.1111/j.1748-0361.2008.00162.x

Lambert, D., & Hartley, D. (1998). Linking primary care and mental health: Where have we been? Where are we going? *Psychiatric Services*, *49*(7), 965–967. doi:10.1176/ps.49.7.965

Larson, S. L., & Fleishman, J. A. (2003). Rural-urban differences in usual source of care and ambulatory service use: Analyses of national data using Urban Influence Codes. *Medical Care*, *41*, III65–III74. doi:10.1176/ps.49.7.965

Leedy, G., & Connolly, C. (2007). Out of the cowboy state: A look at lesbian and gay lives in Wyoming. *Journal of Gay & Lesbian Social Services: Issues in Practice, Policy & Research*, *19*(1), 17–34. doi:10.1300/J041v19n01_02

Lemacks, J., Wells, B., Ilich, J., & Ralston, P. (2013). Interventions for improving nutrition and physical activity behaviors in African American populations: A systematic review, January 2000 through December 2011. *Preventing Chronic Disease, 10*, 120256. doi:10.5888/pcd10.120256

Lenardson, J. D., Ziller, E. C., Coburn, A. F., & Anderson, N. J. (2009). *Profile of rural health insurance coverage: A chartbook*. Portland: University of Southern Maine. Retrieved from https://www.ruralhealthresearch.org/publications/688

Liu, J., Bennett, K. J., Harun, N., Zheng, X., Probst, J. C., & Pate, R. R. (2007). *Overweight and physical inactivity among rural children aged 10–17: A national and state portrait*. Retrieved from https://www.ruralhealthresearch.org/publications/556

Mainous, A., King, D., Garr, D., & Pearson, W. (2004). Race, rural residence, and control of diabetes and hypertension. *Annals of Family Medicine, 2*(6), 563–568. doi:10.1370/afm.119

Mainous, A. G., Koopman, R., & Geesey, M. E. (2004). Diabetes & hypertension among rural Hispanics: Disparities in diagnostics and disease management. *South Carolina Rural Health Research Center*. Retrieved from https://www.ruralhealthresearch.org/mirror/1/141/%284-4%29+Diabetes+and+Hypertension+among+Rural+Hispanics.pdf

Middleton, J. (2009). A proposed new model of hypertensive treatment behavior in African Americans. *Journal of the National Medical Association, 101*(1), 12–17. doi:10.1016/S0027-9684(15)30805-1

Mier, N., Wang, X., Smith, M. L., Irizarry, D., Trevino, L., Alen, M., & Ory, M. G. (2012). Factors influencing health care utilization in older Hispanics with diabetes along the Texas-Mexico border. *Population Health Management, 15*(3), 149–156. doi:10.1089/pop.2011.0044

Mulder, P. L., Kenken, M. B., Shellenberger, S. Constantine, M. G., Streigel, R., Sears, S. F., … Hager, A. (2001). The behavioral health care needs of rural women. Retrieved from https://www.apa.org/pubs/info/reports/rural-women.pdf

Murali, V., & Oyebode, F. (2004). Poverty, social inequality, and mental health. *Advances in Psychiatric Treatment, 10*, 216–224. doi:10.1192/apt.10.3.216

National Advisory Committee on Rural Health. (1993). *Sixth annual report on rural health*. Rockville, MD: Office of Rural Health Policy.

National Association of Counties and Appalachian Regional Commission. (2019). *Opioids in Appalachia: The role of counties in reversing a regional epidemic*. Washington, DC: Author. Retrieved from https://www.naco.org/sites/default/files/documents/Opioids-Full.pdf

O'Connor, A., & Wellenius, G. (2012). Rural-urban disparities in the prevalence of diabetes and coronary heart disease. *Public Health, 126*, 813–820. doi:10.1016/j.puhe.2012.05.029

Odoi, A. (2009). Needs-based population health planning: Identifying barriers to health care services in the Appalachian region of East Tennessee. *Veterinary Vision, 8*(1), 10–11.

Oswald, R. F., & Culton, L. S. (2003). Under the rainbow: Rural gay life and its relevance for family. *Family Relations, 52*(1), 72–81. doi:10.1111/j.1741-3729.2003.00072.x

Parr, H., & Philo, C. (2003). Rural mental health and social geographies of caring. *Social and Cultural Geography, 4*(4), 471–488. doi:10.1080/1464936032000137911

Patrick, D. L., Stein, J., Porta, M., Porter, C. Q., & Ricketts, T. C. (1988). Poverty, health services, and health status in rural America. *Milbank Quarterly, 66*(1), 105–136. doi:10.2307/3349987

Patterson, P. D., Moore, C. G., Probst, J. C., & Shinogle, J. A. (2004). Obesity and physical activity in rural America. *Journal of Rural Health, 20*, 151–158. doi:10.1111/j.1748-0361.2004.tb00022.x

Pearson, K., Gale, J., & Shaler, G. (2014). *The evidence for community paramedicine in rural areas: State and local findings and the role of the State Flex Program* (Flex Monitoring Team Briefing Paper No. 34). Retrieved from http://www.flexmonitoring.org/wp-content/uploads/2014/03/bp34.pdf

Pearson, T. A., & Lewis, C. (1998). Rural epidemiology: Insights form a rural population laboratory. *American Journal of Epidemiology, 148*(10), 949–957. doi:10.1093/oxfordjournals.aje.a009571

President's New Freedom Commission on Mental Health. (2003). *Subcommittee on rural issues*. Retrieved from http://govinfo.library.unt.edu/mentalhealthcommission/subcommittee/Sub_Chairs.htm

Preston, D., D'Augelli, A. R., Kassab, C. D., & Starks, M. T. (2007). The relationship of stigma to the sexual risk behavior of rural men who have sex with men. *AIDS Education & Prevention, 19*(3), 218–230. doi:10.1521/aeap.2007.19.3.218

Probst, J. C., Bellinger, J. D, Walsemann, K. M., Hardin, J., & Glover, S. H. (2011). Higher risk of death in rural Blacks and Whites than urbanites is related to lower incomes, education, and health coverage. *Health Affairs, 30*(10), 1872–1879. doi:10.1377/hlthaff.2011.0668

Regier, D., Goldberg, I., & Taube, C. (1978). The de facto US mental health services system: A public health perspective. *Archives of General Psychiatry, 35*, 685–693. doi:10.1001/archpsyc.1978.01770300027002

Reiger, D. A., Narro, W. E., Rae, D. S., Manderscheid, R. W., Locke, B. Z., & Goodwin, F. K. (1993). The de facto US mental and addictive disorders service system. Epidemiologic catchment area prospective 1-year prevalence rates of disorders and services. *Archives of General Psychiatry, 50*(2), 85–94. doi:10.1001/archpsyc.1993.01820140007001

Rimando, M., Warren, J. C., & Smalley, K. B. (2014). Heart disease in rural areas. In J. C. Warren & K. B. Smalley (Eds.), *Rural public health* (pp. 115–138). New York, NY: Springer Publishing Company.

Rostosky, S. S., Owens, G. P., Zimmerman, R. S., & Riggle, E. D. (2003). Associations among sexual attraction status, school belongingness, and alcohol and marijuana use in rural high school students. *Journal of Adolescence, 26*, 741–751. doi:10.1016/j.adolescence.2003.09.002

Round, K. A. (1988). AIDS in rural areas: Challenges to providing care. *Social Work, 33*, 257–261. doi:10.1093/sw/33.3.257

Saenz, R. (2008). *A profile of Latinos in rural America* (Fact sheet no. 10). Durham: University of New Hampshire, Carsey Institute. Retrieved from https://scholars.unh.edu/cgi/viewcontent.cgi?referer=&httpsredir=1&article=1034&context=carsey

Saydan, S., & Lochner, K. (2010). Socioeconomic status and risk of diabetes-related mortality in the United States. *Public Health Reports, 125*, 377–388. doi:10.1177/003335491012500306

Scott, A., & Wilson, R. F (2011a). Social determinants of health among African Americans in a rural community in the Deep South: An ecological exploration. *Rural and Remote Health, 11*, 1634. Retrieved from http://www.rrh.org.au/articles/subviewnew.asp?ArticleID=1634

Scott, A., & Wilson, R. F. (2011b). Upstream ecological risks for overweight and obesity among African American youth in a rural town in the Deep South. *Preventing Chronic Disease, 8*(1), A17. Retrieved from https://www.cdc.gov/pcd/issues/2011/jan/09_0244.htm

Singh, G. K. (2012). Rural-urban trends and patterns in cervical cancer mortality, incidence, stage, and survival in the United States, 1950–2008. *Journal of Community Health, 37*(1), 217–223. doi:10.1007/s10900-011-9439-6

Skelly, A. H., Arcury, T. A., Snively, B. M. Bell, R. A., Smith, S. L., Wetmore, L. K., & Quandt, S. A. (2005). Self-monitoring of blood glucose in a multiethnic population of rural older adults with diabetes. *Diabetes Educator, 31*, 84–90. doi:10.1177/0145721704273229

Slifkin, R. T., Goldsmith, L. J., & Ricketts, T. (2000). *Race and place: Urban-rural differences in health for racial and ethnic minorities* (NC Rural Health Research and Policy Analysis Center Working Paper Series, No. 66). Chapel Hill: University of North Carolina. Retrieved from https://www.shepscenter.unc.edu/rural/pubs/finding_brief/fb61.pdf

Smalley, K. B., & Warren, J. C. (2014). Mental health in rural areas. In J. C. Warren & K. B. Smalley (Eds.), *Rural public health* (pp. 85–94). New York, NY: Springer Publishing Company.

Smith, B. J., Parvin, D. W. (1973). Defining and measuring rurality. *Southern Journal of Agricultural Economics, 5*(1), 109–113. doi:10.1017/S008130520001089X

Sowers, W. E., & Rohland, B. (2004). American Association of Community Psychiatrists' principles for managing transitions in behavioral health systems. *Psychiatric Services, 55*(11), 1271–1275. doi:10.1176/appi.ps.55.11.1271

Steinberg, S., & Fleming, P. (2000). The geographic distribution of AIDS in the United States: Is there a rural epidemic? *The Journal of Rural Health, 16*(1), 11–19. doi:10.1111/j.1748-0361.2000.tb00432.x

Stewart, C. T. (1958). The urban-rural dichotomy. *American Journal of Sociology, 64*, 52–58. doi:10.1086/222422

Substance Abuse and Mental Health Services Administration Office of Applied Studies. (2001). *Results from the 2001 National Household Survey on Drug Abuse: Volume 1. Summary of national findings*. Rockville, MD: Author.

Swank, E., Fahs, B., & Frost, D. M. (2013). Region, social identities, and disclosure practices as predictors of heterosexist discrimination against sexual minorities in the United States: Region, social identities, and disclosure practices as predictors of heterosexist discrimination against. *Sociological Inquiry, 83*(2), 238–258. doi:10.1111/soin.12004

Swenson, C. J., Trepka, M. J., Rewers, M. J., Scarbro, S., Hiatt, W. R., & Harmann, R. F. (2002). Cardiovascular disease mortality in Hispanics and non-Hispanic Whites. *American Journal of Epidemiology, 156*(10), 919–928. doi:10.1093/aje/kwf140

U.S. Census Bureau. (2020). *Explore census data.* Retrieved from https://data.census.gov/cedsci/

U.S. Department of Agriculture, Economic Research Service. (2003). *Rural education at a glance* (Rural Development Research Report Number 98). Retrieved from https://www.ers.usda.gov/webdocs/publications/47074/30684_rdrr98_lowres_002.pdf?v=0

U.S. Department of Agriculture, Economic Research Service. (2005). *Rural Hispanics at a glance* (Economic Information Bulletin Number 8). Retrieved from https://www.ers.usda.gov/webdocs/publications/44570/29568_eib8full.pdf?v=41305

Vitale, M., & Bailey, C. (2012). Assessing barriers to health care services for Hispanic residents in rural Georgia. *Journal of Rural Social Sciences, 27*(3), 17–45. Retrieved from http://journalofruralsocialsciences.org/pages/Articles/JRSS%202012%2027/3/JRSS%202012%2027%203%2017-45.pdf

Wagenfeld, M. O., & Buffum, W. E. (1983). Problems in, and prospects for, rural mental health services in the United States. *International Journal of Rural Health, 12*, 89–107. doi:10.1080/00207411.1983.11448938

Warren, J. C., & Smalley, K. B. (2014a). Diabetes in rural areas. In J. C. Warren & K. B. Smalley (Eds.), *Rural public health* (pp. 155–168). New York, NY: Springer Publishing Company.

Warren, J. C., & Smalley, K. B. (2014b). Future directions in rural public health. In J. C. Warren & K. B. Smalley (Eds.), *Rural public health* (pp. 255–262). New York, NY: Springer Publishing Company.

Warren, J. C., & Smalley, K. B. (2014c). What is rural? In J. C. Warren & K. B. Smalley (Eds.), *Rural public health* (pp. 1–10). New York, NY: Springer Publishing Company.

Warren, J. C., Smalley, K. B., Rimando, M., Barefoot, K. N., Hatton, A., & LeLeux-Labarge, K. (2014). Rural minority health: Race, ethnicity, and sexual orientation. In J. C. Warren & K. B. Smalley (Eds.), *Rural public health* (pp. 203–226). New York, NY: Springer Publishing Company.

Weinert, C., & Boik, R. J. (1995). MSU rurality index: Development and evaluation. *Research in Nursing and Health, 18*(5), 453–464. doi:10.1002/nur.4770180510

Wilson-Anderson, K., Williams, P., Beacham, T., & McDonald, N. (2013). Breast health teaching in predominantly African American Rural Mississippi Delta. *The Association of Black Nurse Faculty Journal, 24*, 28–33.

Ziller, E. (2014). Access to medical care in rural America. In J. C. Warren & K. B. Smalley (Eds.), *Rural public health* (pp. 11–28). New York, NY: Springer Publishing Company.

Ziller, E. C., Coburn, A. F., Loux, S. L., Hoffman, C., & McBride, T. D. (2003). *Health insurance coverage in rural America: Chartbook.* Washington, DC: The Kaiser Commission. Retrieved from https://www.kff.org/wp-content/uploads/2013/01/health-insurance-coverage-in-rural-america-pdf.pdf

Ziller, E. C., Coburn, A. F., & Yousefian, A. E. (2006). Out-of-pocket health spending and the rural underinsured. *Health Affairs, 25*(6), 1688–1699. doi:10.1377/hlthaff.25.6.1688

Ziller, E. C., Lenardson, J. D., & Coburn, A. F. (2012). Health care access and use among the rural uninsured. *Journal of Healthcare for the Poor and Underserved, 23*(3), 1327–1345. doi:10.1353/hpu.2012.0100

HEALTH EQUITY IN IMMIGRANT AND REFUGEE POPULATIONS

MARK EDBERG

LEARNING OBJECTIVES

- Contrast the terms "migrant," "immigrant," and "refugee"
- Describe the experiential factors and social determinants of health that are particularly present in migrant populations
- Name specific health disparities faced by migrant populations
- Explain both the Trajectory Approach and the Transnational Continuum Approach for conceptualizing migrant health disparities
- Discuss how intersectionality affects migrant populations

INTRODUCTION

According to the *World Migration Report 2018* from the International Organization for Migration (IOM, 2018), as of 2015 there were an estimated 244 million international migrants and 740 million internal migrants worldwide. This is an important global issue, given the recent refugee crises in Europe, the Middle East, the Americas, and Myanmar, and the prominence of immigration in the political landscape of so many countries, including the United States, where immigrants and their children are becoming an increasingly significant segment of the U.S. population. Immigrants constitute 13.7% of the total U.S. population (U.S. Census Bureau, 2015), and immigrants and their U.S.-born children now number approximately 89.4 million people, or 28% of the overall U.S. population (Migration Policy Institute, 2019). While the interaction between migration and health inequities is complex, it is clear that progress in this area is an important component of the overall effort to achieve health equity for racial/ethnic minority populations.

Migrants, the broader category that includes both immigrants and refugees, leave their home countries "for a variety of reasons, including conflict, natural disasters or environmental degradation, political persecution, poverty, discrimination and lack of access to basic services and the search for new opportunities, particularly in terms of work or education" (IOM, 2013, p. 7). Their circumstances may include exposure to multiple health risks, from communicable and non-communicable diseases, stress and trauma, physical or sexual abuse, violence and injury, loss of family and social support, loss of possessions, and mental health conditions including depression.

Immigrants and refugees may come to the U.S. with a range of health conditions as well as health risk practices. In addition to any of the diseases affecting the U.S. born, conditions particularly affecting immigrants and refugees include:

- *Tuberculosis:* This disease is more prevalent among migrant populations, especially among foreign-born Asians and Pacific Islanders and foreign-born persons of African descent (Centers for Disease Control and Prevention [CDC], 2013; Yang & Hwang, 2016). It is also seen in combination with HIV/AIDS as a co-occurring condition. It requires a long treatment protocol, which presents difficulties for underserved migrants and which may have been unavailable in the home country or during migration (Migrant Clinicians Network, 2018).

- *Hepatitis:* Some migrants may be at increased risk for Hepatitis A due to a lack of access to clean water and sanitation facilities while traveling as well as substandard housing situations. According to the World Health Organization (WHO, 2018), in developing countries with poor sanitary conditions and hygienic practices, most children (90%) are infected with the Hepatitis A virus before the age of 10 years. However, those infected as children do not typically experience symptoms, and epidemics or outbreaks are uncommon because older children and adults are generally immune. For Hepatitis B, high-endemic areas include Southeast Asia and the Pacific Basin (excluding Japan, Australia, and New Zealand), sub-Saharan Africa, the Amazon Basin, parts of the Middle East, the Central Asian Republics and some countries in Eastern Europe (CDC, 2018). With respect to Hepatitis C, the top five prevalence countries are China, Pakistan, India, Egypt, and Russia (Polaris Observatory HCV Collaborators, 2017). Notably, the U.S. is itself the sixth highest-prevalence country.

- *Cardiovascular disease (CVD) and diabetes:* CVD has been on the rise globally for some time, and thus it is not entirely surprising that it is a factor among some immigrant and refugee populations as well. A recent study examining National Health Interview Survey (NHIS) data (Commodore-Mensah et al., 2018) found that both obesity and diabetes were highest among immigrants from Mexico/Central America/Caribbean and the Indian subcontinent, while hypertension was highest among Russian and Southeast Asian immigrants. African and Middle Eastern immigrants also had a higher prevalence of diabetes than European immigrants, but without the corresponding higher prevalence of obesity/overweight.

- *Mental health:* While there is generally a lower prevalence of mental health issues among immigrants, this varies by population and circumstance. Immigrants and refugees can experience a range of mental health issues that may include depression due to loss of social support, economic deprivation, or changes in their social status and roles. Immigrants, and in particular refugees, are likely to experience post-traumatic stress disorder (PTSD) and chronic pain or other somatic syndromes (Kirmayer et al., 2011) as a result of violence victimization or witnessing violence, fleeing from war, civil conflict, natural disasters, loss of family and friends, and extreme conditions during migration—among other experiences. Substance abuse may also be an issue. It is also important to recognize that mental health and psychiatric disorders are conceptualized, understood, and experienced in different ways across cultures—the Western biomedical system and its diagnostic categories are not necessarily applicable across immigrant cultures (Edberg, 2013; Kirmayer et al., 2011).

■ *Other infectious diseases:* These may range from Zikavirus to other long-standing and endemic conditions found in home countries or *en route.*

There are a few other consistent issues as well:

■ *Refugees tend to be older than immigrants,* and in comparison to immigrants, the odds of refugees rating their health status as fair or poor, and of having a chronic condition were higher. Specific conditions included arthritis, behavioral health problems, heart disease, hypertension, and stroke. Additionally, refugees report greater pain of the kind that limits their usual activities (Yun, Fuentes-Afflick, & Desai, 2012).

■ *Foreign-born children have a lower rate of immunization than U.S.-born immigrants.* In part, this is because programs, resources, and records vary by country (Kandula, 2008; Strine et al., 2002; Yang & Hwang, 2016).

On top of the health issues that are specific to or accentuated among immigrants and refugees, both these populations experience multiple barriers to accessing healthcare and prevention, including a lack of insurance (see Figure 14.1).

Immigrant "health paradox." There has been, for a long time, reference in the literature to a phenomenon called the immigrant or Latino health paradox in which immigrant and refugee populations typically arrive in the U.S. with better health status than the average native-born but lose this health status advantage after a number of years (Singh & Miller, 2004; Teruya & Bazargan-Hejazi, 2013). For example, while most Mexican immigrants living in the U.S. come to the country healthier than the average American, this changes—about 7% of immigrants living in the U.S. for 10 years or less have fair or poor health, after 15 years this rises to 15% (Kaiser Family Foundation, 2005; Singh & Miller, 2004). There are many possible reasons—one may be self-selection for healthiness among those who emigrate (explaining better health status at time of immigration), combined with a trajectory in the United States that entails certain difficulties and barriers to health. There have

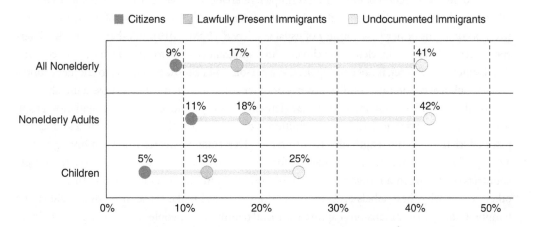

FIGURE 14.1 Uninsured rates among nonelderly adults and children by immigration status (2015).

SOURCE: Data from Kaiser Family Foundation March 2016 (reported in Cunningham, 2017).

been numerous critiques of this hypothesis, addressing sample selection bias and other factors. At the same time, many immigrant and refugee groups also come to the U.S. after fleeing or otherwise leaving traumatic and severe crises, presenting with significant health inequities as a result.

DEFINITIONS

Before going any further, it is important to review definitions of "immigrant" and "refugee" because the differences between these two categories have implications for health equity. Both categories fall within a broader definition of "migrant." The IOM defines a migrant as "an umbrella term, not defined under international law, reflecting the common lay understanding of a person who moves away from his or her place of usual residence, whether within a country or across an international border, temporarily or permanently, and for a variety of reasons. The term includes a number of well-defined legal categories of people, such as migrant workers; persons whose particular types of movements are legally defined, such as smuggled migrants; as well as those whose status or means of movement are not specifically defined under international law, such as international students" (IOM, 2019). This definition, however, leaves some ambiguity in distinguishing between types of migrants—immigrants, refugees, asylees, internal versus external migrants, and expats—noting that the categories "refugee" and "asylee" are often treated separately from other kinds of migrants. Generally, a refugee is a person who, "owing to a well-founded fear of persecution for reasons of race, religion, nationality, membership of a particular social group or political opinions, is outside the country of his nationality and is unable or, owing to such fear, is unwilling to avail himself of the protection of that country" (from Article. 1(A)(2), Convention relating to the Status of Refugees, 1951 as modified by the 1967 Protocol). The 1984 Cartagena Declaration states that refugees also include persons who flee their country "because their lives, safety or freedom have been threatened by generalised violence, foreign aggression, internal conflicts, massive violations of human rights or other circumstances which have seriously disturbed public order" (United Nations High Commissioner for Refugees, 1984, p. 36). Under international law, refugees require international protection and cannot be forced to return home (see United Nations, 1951).

The common definition of immigrant is simpler, referring to "a person who moves into a country other than that of his or her nationality or usual residence, so that the country of destination effectively becomes his or her new country of usual residence" (IOM, 2019). In other words, the difference is in part framed as an element of choice—an immigrant chooses to relocate in another country. The distinction, however, is not entirely clear, as a person could choose to relocate to another country because political conditions, conflict, poverty or other risks, and circumstances pose a threat.

Any definition has *temporal* and *spatial* elements involving movement of a population group over time and across space. The IOM definition is open-ended with respect to time and does not place restrictions on the length of stay within any given state. Someone who is an immigrant, or a refugee for that matter, may be a migrant for some period of time—traveling through multiple countries or staying in a refugee camp—before resettling in one specific country. This is yet another reason why these labels and categories do not always make sense. Moreover, neither the temporal nor spatial dimensions capture the *social* definition of people who are migrating. There is a dimension of power, class, and political interest implicated in the several definitions. If a medical doctor moves with his/her family from the U.S. to, for example, Thailand, will this person be referred to as an "immigrant" or a "migrant"? If a global development professional from the

UK takes up permanent residence in East Africa, are the immigrant or migrant labels applied? Or even if a retiree from a developed nation moves to a tropical nation to live his or her last years, will they be called an immigrant or migrant? These individuals will typically be called "expats." There are also individuals who move to another country for extended but limited periods of time, such as temporary work visa holders or student visa recipients. These individuals, at least in the U.S., are not legally considered immigrants as they are expected to leave once their permit expires. Yet their stay might be several years long and they may experience many of the realities of immigrant life. Such definitional issues have been recognized as problematic for public health, public policy, and regulatory frameworks (Gushulak, Weekers, & MacPherson, 2010).

TWO APPROACHES FOR UNDERSTANDING HEALTH INEQUITIES AMONG IMMIGRANTS AND REFUGEES

The following are two selected approaches for understanding the determinants of health equity among immigrant and refugee populations and thus also frameworks for structuring interventions. Both approaches draw from a broad social-ecological model (Bronfenbrenner, 1979, 2005; Stokols, 1992) increasingly used as a central orientation for public health efforts. They are not the only frameworks or approaches, but represent a range of factors that should be considered.

The Trajectory Approach

Numerous factors contributing to racial/ethnic health inequities overall have been identified, including factors relevant to immigrant and refugee populations. However, these contributing factors likely do not operate as distinct factors, but in a co-occurring and interactive fashion that creates a *pathway* or *trajectory* with respect to the health of a population (see Edberg, Cleary, & Vyas, 2011; Starfield, 2007). As noted in the previous discussion of intersectionality, socioeconomic status, for example, is often linked to discrimination and exclusion, shaping a way of life with respect to health that may include limitations on access to and quality of care, as well as higher exposure to community and environmental health risk. As noted by Edberg et al. (2011, p. 580), "these objective conditions, over time, may generate behavior patterns and community norms that follow from expectations of high risk and limited care options, and a particular relationship to the healthcare system. For immigrant and refugee populations, such trajectories can also be shaped by cultural patterns related to health, the immigration experience itself and the dislocations and traumas that may be associated with it, as well as socioeconomic status." The resulting health inequities are thus an outcome of particular patterns of vulnerability, circumstances, and response.

The idea of a trajectory means that the social ecology of contributing factors operates as a dynamic system over time, shaping an ongoing relationship between a population and the health-related system, where the term "health-related system" is a holistic construct, referring to the combination of health services per se together with the economic, community, social, and cultural supports necessary for their effective delivery, and for a population to be able to engage in healthy behavior. For immigrants and refugees in the U.S., this trajectory might entail a progression from relatively good health status when entering the country to decreasing (and then slightly increasing) status over time as a function of marginalization from health and supporting resources, driven by multiple contributing factors.

The following domains were proposed by Edberg et al. (2011) as one framework for identifying the multiple aspects of health inequities as a trajectory—in this case, for immigrants, but broadly relevant to refugees as well:

Migration Experience

Includes the home-country situation at time of emigration (e.g., crises, civil war, famine, disasters, patterns of health behavior and social relationships), the migration experience, including difficult or lengthy migration periods (e.g., exposure to violence, robbery, rape; extended exposure to severe conditions; extended time in refugee camps before and during migration).

Social Adjustment

Length of time in the U.S., acculturation, differences from home-country social status, challenges to traditional gender roles and parental authority, change in available social supports, intergenerational conflict, and in general stressors created by the acculturation/adjustment process itself, regardless of migration experience.

Socioeconomic Status

Economic, employment, and housing status, including economic supports (or lack of) for healthcare, such as insurance, employment with benefits, types and availability of employment (and change over time in any of these factors). As of October 2014, 28% of immigrant children lived in poverty, compared to 19% of U.S.-born children (Child Trends, 2018).

Social Supports

Linked to cultural identity, extended family, neighborhood, cultural, employment, and other important social network systems, and the degree to which any of these networks facilitate access to healthcare (social capital), healthy/unhealthy behavior, and healing.

Neighborhood Characteristics

Other community and neighborhood supports or barriers for health, including community organizations, faith organizations, recreation sites, parks, sources of healthy food (restaurants, grocery stores). This category also includes the presence/absence of environmental risks such as water/sanitation problems, sources of pollution, crime, and violence. The level of *community efficacy* (Sampson, 2003; Sampson, Morenoff, & Gannon-Rowley, 2002; Sampson, Raudenbush, & Earls 1997) also fits in this category.

Health Status

Health status (self-report) referring to general assessments of a person's health as well as specific conditions.

Health Knowledge and Practices

Knowledge, attitudes, and practices with respect to health, how health is defined, disease etiologies and treatments, and healthcare utilization. This includes knowledge connected to indigenous *ethnomedical systems* (Edberg, 2013; Foster, 1976). This category should also include any differences between home-country healthcare practices and current/U.S. practices.

Access to Care

Actual and perceived physical availability of and access to healthcare services and the relative location of services. Actual and perceived availability of culturally competent care at service delivery settings—including language interpretation services, healthcare practices that recognize client cultural patterns, healthcare staff who are diverse.

Perceived Discrimination

This is important because experiences of discrimination affect willingness to seek care and adherence to treatment. It can include perceived level of discrimination and racism in daily experience, frequency of these experiences or events, as well as perceived acceptance, integration, and involvement in various community settings (e.g., neighborhood, school, work, healthcare).

The domains of this trajectory approach also incorporate a process of migration beginning with a home-country situation and health-related patterns, then impacted by the nature of the migration experience itself and by an often complex and extended adjustment to life in the United States (see Edberg, Benavides, Rivera, Shaikh, & Mattiola, 2018; Edberg, Wong, Park, & Corey, 2002).

Following the trajectory model, the combination of factors just listed may, over time, increase or decrease the "distance" between a population trajectory and the mainstream health-related system—which can be viewed as degree of *marginalization*. At the same time, factors that may operate within a context of marginality can be protective (e.g., social cohesion), such that marginalization in itself may include positive and negative aspects. In general, when assessing health inequities among immigrants and refugees, the trajectory approach suggests that an increase in *negative marginality*, represented by the presence or degree of negative factors in the preceding domains, will be associated with a decrease in health status vis-a-vis the general population.

The Transnational Continuum Approach

As noted, the trajectory approach just detailed encompasses an understanding of health inequities among immigrants and refugees as a *transnational continuum*. It is very common in the current literature on migrant health in the U.S. to employ a vocabulary of health risk factors that are analogous to those applied to domestic population groups. Thus, as Castañeda et al. (2015) have noted, factors such as language, norms, behaviors, cultural beliefs, acculturation, and acculturative stress are typically correlated with health outcomes in the same way that norms, behaviors, attitudes, and so on are similarly correlated for domestic populations. But these are often treated as "border up" considerations—factors connected to life patterns and situations in the U.S., not explicitly connected to the broader context of migration and its transnational nature. It is, however, more accurate to posit that health determinants for immigrants and refugees integrate or "collapse" their experience across the following three key domains (Castañeda et al., 2015; Edberg et al., 2011, 2018), forming an ecology of health determinants that spans time and space.

Home Country

This domain includes how people lived in their home country and their health risks and status in that setting. It also includes home country, socioeconomic status, gender relationships, household configuration, family structure, diet and exercise, social status, access to resources, access to education, and access to healthcare. Additionally, the domain includes the often-complex set of reasons driving people to leave their homes—civil strife, political oppression, crime and gang violence, natural disasters, famine, lack of economic opportunity, hunger, and discrimination—the latter against a particular ethnic group, religious, or sexual minority, for example.

Migration Experience

This domain encompasses a wide range of experiences—fleeing in the middle of the night or leaving via an organized process; sometimes traveling by precarious, dangerous means (a rubber raft, an overcrowded fishing boat, running and hiding by land, or crossing multiple countries); and having little control and being robbed and otherwise victimized. It also includes long periods in transit countries or refugee camps for months, even years, before finding sponsors to bring the individuals and families to a new country.

Resettlement in the New Country

Again, a vast range of experience is captured here—unfamiliar language, unfamiliar institutions, confusion about how to access any services or conduct basic tasks like buying food, the high cost of housing, the necessity of living in an area that may not be safe and may not have easy access to markets or transportation, and lack of social support. Even trying to understand how to place children in school can be difficult. Finding work can be difficult. Maintaining family structure as it was in the home country may be difficult, as gender patterns typically change and both male and female adults often have to work, potentially disrupting gendered authority and "breadwinner" roles. Moreover, there are different modes of acculturation between parents and children (Telzer, 2010). In one of these modes, children acculturate and learn the language faster than parents, causing additional stress on family authority patterns.

Most important to think about in the transnational continuum model is that *these domains are not discrete*, they flow into and impact each other, and to understand what is going on with any particular health situation, it is important to assess the possible aggregation of factors across the three domains. For example, consider a man who was head of the family in his home country and who held a position of some respect in his community. Because of increasing political violence, he flees with his family and others, but becomes separated during the process. During his flight, he is robbed of his valuables, and loses a sibling. He reunites with his family in a refugee camp, but in the meantime his wife has found a job out of necessity in the camp. He, on the other hand, does not find a job and is experiencing trauma from the loss of his sibling. When they get to the new country, his wife is already more adept at securing work, and again, she finds work and he does not, at least right away. He is depressed and angry at the role he finds himself in, and begins drinking, causing health problems. As you can see, all three domains, functioning together, affect the nature of his health condition.

The integration of health determinants across migration domains as described in the transnational continuum approach is echoed in several other approaches that seek to address phases

TABLE 14.1 Factors Contributing to Health Inequities (Trajectory and Transnational Continuum Approaches)

APPROACH	DOMAINS
Trajectory Approach	Migration experience Social adjustment Socioeconomic status Social supports Neighborhood characteristics Health status Health knowledge and practices Access to care Perceived discrimination
Transnational Continuum Approach	Home country (situation) Migration experience Resettlement in the new country

of a migrant's situation. Zimmerman, Kiss, and Hossain (2011), for example, have proposed a framework with five phases: pre-departure phase, travel phase, destination phase, and for some, interception phase, and return phase (see Table 14.1).

RECOMMENDATIONS FOR PRACTITIONERS

Given what has been outlined in this chapter, here are a few basic crosscutting aspects of the immigrant/refugee health inequities described, as well as common approaches to developing solutions:

- Almost any immigrant or refugee population will present with some inequities related to access, unfamiliarity, trauma from multiple domains of the migration experience, and social adjustment issues. There are a wide range of situations and legal issues across different populations that shape unique trajectories.

- There is no single experience or trajectory that is true for any group of immigrants or refugees. There are indeed likely to be patterns, but these will vary by the intersectional experience of subcategories and subgroups, by community receptivity to new immigrants, and by other factors. Be careful of easy assumptions.

- Assessing needs and understanding health inequities among immigrants and refugees requires a broad social-ecological focus, which can include the two specific approaches previously discussed—the Trajectory Approach and the Transnational Continuum Approach. Because of the range and complexity of factors contributing to inequities, this may take time.

- By all means, collaboration with the immigrant or refugee communities is essential. As part of such collaboration, trust building and an investment in time are keys.

- There may not always be programs to address health equities that are tailored to a specific refugee/immigrant community. In that case, collaboration will again be necessary in order to conduct an *assessment* of factors contributing to the problem and to *develop* and *implement* a tailored program or programs. There are, however, some commonalities across immigrant/refugee communities such that a program addressing, for example, mental health and social support needs in one community may be useful for another—particularly if there are similarities in the migration continuum.

■   Where differences in *ethnomedical systems* and practices exist, it is useful to reach out and collaborate with indigenous healers in the community for the implementation of prevention or healthcare services. This will help in establishing trust and help bridge cultural gaps.

INTERSECTIONALITY SPOTLIGHT

As with any label, the designation of "immigrant" or "refugee" masks multiple differences that have an impact on health status. Domains of difference within the category of, for example, "immigrants/refugees from country X" may include:

■   *Ethnicity and race:* There may be a wide variation from any country. Because of its colonial history, for example, immigrants from Mexico into the U.S. can include people who are of predominantly European ancestry (often called "gueros"), mestizos who are of mixed European and indigenous ancestry, and indigenous peoples such as the Zapotec, Mixtec, and Maya—who may not speak Spanish or don't speak it as their first language. Immigrants and refugees from Central or Latin America, and from the Caribbean, may have these differences, but also have varying degrees of African ancestry. Immigrants from South Africa, as another example, may be of African, South Asian, or European descent. Immigrants from Lebanon or other Arab countries may be classified as "racially White," yet treated very differently. These variations have a clear impact on the way in which immigrants experience social determinants of health within the U.S.

■   *Class:* The ethnic/racial categories just described are inevitably linked to class as well—not surprisingly, particularly where lighter skin/European ancestry is most often associated with class-derived power. There are also other ways in which class enters in to immigrant/refugee trajectories, including the "wave" of immigration. When there is civil war or revolution in the home country, the first to flee are often those with money and powerful positions who fear that those assets will be taken and they will face imprisonment or worse when a new government takes power. Later "waves" are more likely to include people who are simply fleeing the violence or who can no longer make a living and survive under crisis conditions. They come with few material assets.

■   *Gender and sexual identity:* For some, leaving the home country may be prompted by intolerance or violence towards LGBT persons, or rejection by family and community members for their sexual identity. For women, leaving home may be necessary in order to escape gender-based violence, from partner violence to honor killings.

The key is that these categories intersect (Viruell-Fuentes, Miranda, & Abdulrahim, 2012)—ethnicity/racial category typically overlaps with class, class overlaps with immigrant wave, gender and sexual identities intersect with class and the likelihood of violent victimization, and so

(continued)

on. Health and social trajectories are shaped by these multiple subjectivities. Moreover, these distinctions and any negative consequences associated with them in the home country may be replicated in the U.S.While these variations are recognized and important, intersectionality—particularly among immigrant populations—is frequently overlooked.

CASE STUDIES

The following are two case examples of selected immigrant and refugee communities that experience health inequities, how these occur in trajectories, and how they are outcomes of a transnational domain continuum. In each case, there is a discussion of strategies for addressing the health inequities in that population group drawing from the two models presented previously.

CASE STUDY: RECENT CENTRAL AMERICAN IMMIGRANTS TO THE U.S. IN THE WASHINGTON, DC METRO AREA—A COMPLEX TRAJECTORY OF INEQUITIES

This first case is an example of immigrant health inequities that are the outcome of multiple, interacting factors affecting a population and community.

The Situation

The Washington, DC metropolitan area has long been a destination for an increasing number of immigrants and refugees from multiple countries. Mirroring national trends, and particularly the most recent Census data, Latino immigrants are the largest of these populations (Krogstad & Keegan, 2015). Specifically, the metro area is one of the three largest U.S. population centers for Central American immigrants (Zong & Batalova, 2015). This population is distinct from other Latino/Hispanic groups, including those Latino subgroups (e.g., Mexican-American, Puerto Rican) that have been established for generations in the U.S. More recent immigrant groups represent a significant proportion of Latino population increases—a 137% increase in Central Americans between 2000 and 2010 and 104% for South Americans, compared to a 54% increase from Mexico over the same period (Ennis, Ríos-Vargas, & Albert, 2011). This population suffers disproportionately from multiple health inequities, lower rates of insurance coverage than the majority population, and significant barriers with respect to prevention and care.

A microcosm of this immigrant population can be found in a community near Washington, DC that is majority Latino and also home to immigrants from multiple countries. For purposes of this case example we will call this community "Global Town." In recent years, health and other risks for youth in Global Town have increased for a number of reasons, outcomes of a complex trajectory that includes the following characteristics.

Community dynamics connected to youth and families fleeing from home-country conditions. In recent years, several factors have been prominent: (a) An influx of youth immigrating to Global Town as a result of extreme violence as well as poverty in their home Central American countries (primarily El Salvador, Guatemala, and Honduras) where gang activity has intensified. Many of these youth have been victimized and/or traumatized during their migration

(continued)

journeys and also face difficulties in social/school adjustment and reuniting with family members in Global Town. (b) At the same time, there has been a recent, significant increase in gang violence–related incidents in or near Global Town, bringing the issue very close to home for many youth. (c) Increasing and disproportionate exposure to multiple health risks for youth linked to a spectrum of contributing factors, including language and social barriers, family conflict, low levels of physical activity/poor nutrition, primacy of immediate survival needs over other risks, and economic constraints.

Limited access to social and health services, for several reasons, including legal barriers, language barriers, reticence and mistrust on the part of many residents, and a lack of services in general. While more organizations and services have come into the community in recent years, health services remain minimal. According to one recent local health assessment (Urban Institute study, Scott et al., 2014), as well as a Community Asset Inventory undertaken by research staff at the Avance Center for the Advancement of Immigrant/Refugee Health (n.d.), there are no medical specialists, pediatricians, or psychiatrists in the zip codes for Global Town. The ratios of primary care physicians and nurse practitioners per person, compared to the county at large, are exceedingly low. For example, in Global Town, the ratio of primary care physicians is 5/100,000 people, compared to 54/100,000 in the surrounding county as a whole (Scott et al., 2014), or less than 1/10 the average county access level. In addition, nearly 60% of Global Town residents do not have health insurance (Scott et al., 2014).

Poverty and resulting priorities. Often, the most immediate focus for households living in poverty is on securing income to cover rent, food, and basic expenses. This may take precedence over school attendance or even school completion, and it contributes to a wide range of household stressors and conflicts that we have seen as influencers on mental health outcomes, among others. According to U.S. Census data, the per capita income in Global Town was about half the region's average (U.S. Census Bureau, 2018a, 2018b). At schools within the Global Town boundary, an overwhelming majority of elementary (85%), middle (73%), and high school students (55%) are eligible for free and reduced price meals or free milk (National Center for Educational Statistics, 2016).

Community safety. Global Town families also experience constant threats to their safety. Local data compilations by zip code rate Global Town as a 41.1 out of 100 with respect to violent crime (national average is 22.7) and 64.3 for property crime (national average is 35.4; BestPlaces, n.d.). As noted earlier, the community has also been struggling with increasingly high rates of gang activity that has made life dangerous particularly for adolescents and youth.

Low levels of community efficacy and readiness to change. As Sampson (Sampson, 2003; Sampson et al., 1997) and others have argued, a limited belief among residents that there are resources or that other community members are willing to take action to improve community circumstances is associated with poor health outcomes. A recent community boundary study provided qualitative data suggesting that a common community attitude is that Global Town is the "bottom rung" on an immigrant trajectory (Edberg et al., 2015), which may be associated with a low level of investment in the community.

(continued)

Cultural and language factors. These include limited proficiency in English. For instance, almost 82% of households are primarily Spanish-speaking (U.S. Census Bureau, 2018a), and some residents from Guatemala do not even speak Spanish as a first language, but Mayan languages such as Mam. In addition to language, accessing mental health services is not always culturally familiar to this population and is stigmatized as well, at times inhibiting open discussion and use of services even if available.

Because Global Town has experienced a large increase in the number of immigrant youth in the past 2 years (an increase of 500 new students in the local high school in 2016), the Avance Center for the Advancement of Immigrant/Refugee Health, a partnership between the George Washington University Milken Institute School of Public Health and multiple Global Town community organizations, conducted a pilot survey (n = 104) among a convenience sample of youth to assess levels of trauma, anxiety, and depression. Immigrant youth reported experiencing traumatic experiences in their home country (60%), during the immigration process (22%), and after arriving in the U.S. (21%). Overall 64% of the youth showed clinical signs of depression based on the PHQ-9 scale, with 16% scoring in the moderate-to-severe categories. All measures of anxiety and trauma during the immigration process or after being in the U.S. were associated with greater depressive symptoms (see Edberg et al., 2017). This pilot data empirically support the observed association between chronic stress and mental health outcomes.

An additional pilot study is now being completed that lends depth to an understanding of the kinds of trauma-related experience extant in the community. This study involved the conduct of life-history interviews with 75 Central American immigrants to assess social determinants of health in the three major domains of the transnational continuum mentioned previously—home country situation, migration experience, and adjustment in the U.S. (the Transnational Continuum domains). The data are partially analyzed and already show a high percentage of immigrants who have experienced or witnessed serious traumatic events, from violence in the home country, to physical and sexual abuse as well as forced confinement during migration, to economic and other stressors in the U.S. Among the results emerging from the analysis (ongoing) to date are as follows: (a) The two primary reasons for leaving respondents' home country were to escape imminent violence victimization and poverty with few opportunities. Those escaping violence were fleeing from gangs or domestic violence. Respondents paid smugglers (coyotes) from $5,000 to $20,000 for the journey. (b) More than two-thirds of respondents whose interviews have been analyzed so far experienced migration stress, including experiencing or witnessing violence or sexual assault, imprisonment for ransom, temporary incarceration, and difficulties crossing the desert. Almost half experienced health problems during migration and more than half reported stress in the U.S. (Edberg et al., 2018).

There is yet another consideration—a "circular" transnational history that must be understood as integral to the determinants of health for these immigrants. Before the 1970s, Central American migration patterns were seasonal and intraregional (Castles, de Haas, & Miller, 2014). However, by the late 1970s and early 1980s, migration was a direct outcome of civil wars and authoritarian regimes notorious for violent repression, including the Somozas in Nicaragua, Efrain Rios-Montt in Guatemala, and the military junta and several successive regimes in

(continued)

El Salvador (Castles et al., 2014; Economic Commission for Latin America and the Caribbean, 2011). Ironically, it is these migrants, fleeing from violence, who founded the MS-13 gang, and appropriated the 18th Street gang, in Los Angeles (where there was and is a gang-rich environment necessitating a protective structure), both of which were subsequently exported back to El Salvador, Guatemala, and Honduras via deportations. In turn, these two gangs are responsible for the violence from which youth are now, once again, fleeing, and once again entering the U.S. where the political climate is difficult.

Solutions: Implementing Multi-Level Participatory Community Interventions

Given the multiplicity of factors contributing to a social ecology of vulnerability for this population, and hence to a range of health inequities, no single, targeted solution will be sufficient. As an illustration, the Avance Center for the Advancement of Immigrant/Refugee Health has developed, implemented, and tested several multi-levelcommunity approaches that seek to address the *social ecology of vulnerability*.

- In 2005, SAFER Latinos (funded by the Centers for Disease Control and Prevention) was implemented in response to the increasing level of youth and gang-related violence in the Global Town intervention community. A multi-level, prevention intervention was developed, working with community organizations, that identified five key factors (*family cohesion, school-related barriers, community cohesion, community efficacy and alienation, and gang presence*) held to be concurrent mediators of youth violence, and thus targets of the SAFER Latinos intervention. The intervention included: (a) social *promotores*—Latino, "lay facilitators" who conducted outreach to families; (b) peer advocates—immigrant Latino students recruited from the high school to support other Latino immigrant students in negotiating the school environment and preventing dropout; (c) a community Drop-In Center located in central Global Town that offered academic support, General Education Diploma (GED) classes, recreational activities, and limited counseling services; and (d) multiple community events with appropriate messaging and themes (Edberg, Cleary, Andrade, et al., 2010; Edberg, Cleary, Klevens, et al., 2010). Data from the pilot intervention showed some promise; for example, young adults who participated in Drop-In Center activities and reported higher levels of gang knowledge (a rough proxy for gang involvement), showed a reduction in favorable attitudes towards violence after program participation. Community violence data also indicated a decline in several violence variables over the study period in the intervention versus comparison community (Edberg, Cleary, Andrade, et al., 2010; Edberg, Cleary, Klevens, et al., 2010).

- Building on this work, the Avance Center (under a grant from the National Institute on Minority Health and Health Disparities) sought to address the complex factors contributing to co-occurring health issues among youth—including family/partner violence, sexual risk, substance use, and interpersonal violence. The multi-level *Adelante* intervention was first developed using a community-based

(continued)

participatory research model tailored to the Latino community, which incorporated evidence-based components drawn from SAFER Latinos and global work (Andrade et al., 2016; Edberg et al., 2015, 2017), and using a Positive Youth Development (PYD) approach (Edberg et al., 2017; Lerner, 2005; Lerner & Lerner, 2011; Lerner et al., 2005; Silbereisen & Lerner 2007) intended to build youth capacities to manage health risks as well as a supportive environment (family, community). Adelante component pre-post tests indicated significant improvement in PYD constructs, including a positive (>40%) increase in: school and community *connection*, *confidence*, and school/work *competence*. There was also a 70% increase in outcomes-related prevention knowledge and a 15% increase in prevention skills. Parents participating in the Parents as Leaders component improved with respect to PYD constructs between 2% and 33%. Both youth and parents in the Family Dinner component significantly increased their *competence* with respect to family communication/relations. Preliminary analysis of intervention risk behavior outcomes demonstrated a significant, inverse effect on reported sexual activity (as one example of a risk behavior outcome) during the 3 months after involvement for both the Adelante intervention ($b = -0.01$, $p = .09$) and higher risk Adelante case management ($b = -0.65$, $p < .05$) samples.

In 2014, the Avance Center was awarded a REACH (Racial and Ethnic Approaches to Community Health) grant, and has implemented, with significant community participation including a community advisory board (CAB), an environmental intervention (Water Up!) to promote water consumption as opposed to sugar-sweetened beverages, a major cause of diabetes and obesity in the Latino community. This project is built extensively on the relationships and trust gained from the two previous projects (Barrett et al., 2017; Colon-Ramos, Cremm, Rivera, & Edberg, 2016).

CASE STUDY: HMONG COMMUNITIES IN CENTRAL CALIFORNIA— A CLASH OF HEALTH BELIEF SYSTEMS AND PRACTICES
The Situation
While the first case example described a complex set of factors causing health inequities for Central American immigrants, this example focuses more on disparities that can arise when an immigrant population arrives with a system of beliefs and practices related to health (known as an "*ethnomedical system*"—see Edberg, 2013; Foster, 1976) that is very different from the predominant Western biomedical system. The Hmong are a unique Southeast Asian population with historical origins in China but primarily live in the mountainous regions of Laos, Thailand, and Vietnam. Prior to the Vietnam War, the Hmong lived in relatively isolated small-village communities, with no written language until a Romanized alphabet was developed by missionaries in the 1950s. As a direct consequence of the war, large numbers of Hmong people came to U.S. Because of their intimate knowledge of the mountainous regions where they lived, the U.S. had trained a secret Hmong army to disrupt supply lines coming down the Ho Chi Minh trail from North Vietnam (Ely, 1990), which passed through remote mountainous areas in Laos, and to

(*continued*)

rescue downed American pilots. The Hmong army was highly regarded for its courage against the much-better equipped North Vietnamese (Edberg, 2013; Fadiman, 1997).

When the communists took over in Vietnam, then Laos in 1975, both governments persecuted the Hmong as collaborators, and many Hmong tried to flee across the borders to refugee camps in Thailand. Thus from 1976 on, Hmong from these camps were resettled in the U.S., primarily in Central California, Minnesota, and Wisconsin, though there are resettled Hmong in San Diego, CA, Providence, RI, and other locations as well. There are now approximately 260,073 Hmong in the U.S., as of the 2010 Census (Pfeifer, Sullivan, Yang, & Yang, 2012), a 40% increase from 2000, with the largest Hmong population in California. Until he passed away in 2011, Vang Pao, leader of the Hmong Army in Laos during the Vietnam War, resettled to San Diego, CA where he remained a leader of the Hmong community.

The Hmong that first arrived had little experience with either Western culture or the Western/biomedical health system. Most Hmong were not literate, and finding work was difficult—though they did receive refugee assistance and other benefits. Moreover, the Hmong who first came to the U.S. were accustomed to extended-family, patriarchal clan-based living arrangements, and were primarily *animist* with respect to spiritual orientation (belief in multiple spirits that are part of the daily life environment), with an emphasis on supernatural forces and ancestor worship. While the Hmong have since become more religiously diverse, at the time they first immigrated, Hmong people were predominantly adherents to these indigenous traditions (Cobb, 2010).

Very importantly, the Hmong believed in the existence of multiple souls within each individual, a belief that played (and still plays) an important role in the etiology of disease and in healing. *Shamans* (indigenous healers) are central to healing because they are seen as capable of interacting with the world of spirits to identify the cause of a person's illness and to promote curative action. Children are connected to the Hmong cosmology because they are inhabited by souls from the spirit realm who are waiting to be born. Three days after birth, a Hmong baby is given a "soul-calling" ceremony in which the baby is first given a name. A necklace is placed around the baby's neck to keep the soul (called a "plig").

When someone is sick, a shaman is typically called to perform a different kind of soul-calling ceremony. A shaman goes into trance in order to reinstate a wandering soul, which is seen as a possible cause of the illness. Other illnesses may require a ritual excision of a bad spirit from the patient's body or restorative treatment with herbs.

As summed up by one California health policy research institute, "Hmong residents face multiple barriers to accessing quality healthcare services—economic, linguistic, and cultural. Economic barriers include: underinsured or uninsured status. Some of the linguistic barriers include: lack of proficiency in English, lack of trained medical interpreters, and lack of medical terminology in their native language. The cultural barriers include: lack of knowledge about the Western healthcare delivery system, skepticisms about Western medicine, and lack of respect by healthcare providers for their culture including their beliefs about health and illness. Most refugees had minimal exposure to Western medicine in their homeland. They used the services

(*continued*)

of traditional healers who successfully practiced healing rituals for centuries. These challenges affect their ability to access effective health care that could prevent, delay, or diagnose diseases" (Bengiamin, Chang, & Capitaman, 2011, p. 5).

One of the most widely documented cases of a clash between the Hmong ethnomedical system and Western biomedicine was chronicled in *The Spirit Catches You and You Fall Down: A Hmong Child, Her American Doctors, and the Collision of Two Cultures* (Fadiman, 1997). In this case, a young Hmong girl named Lia Lee was diagnosed with severe epilepsy at a hospital in Fresno, California. In the Hmong *ethnomedical system*, however, epileptic symptoms meant something very different than they did to biomedical practitioners. According to Hmong belief, epileptic symptoms were viewed as the result of *soul loss*, where a soul must have been frightened out of Lia's body by a sudden or dramatic situation. The Hmong called this condition *qaub dab peg*, or, literally, *a spirit catches you and you fall down*. The precipitating event identified by the Lee family was a loud door slam, which caused her soul to flee and led to her seizures. At the same time, epileptic seizures were also viewed by the Hmong as a kind of blessing, as evidence that the person can perceive things other people cannot, and therefore a special, spiritual capability. To cure the seizures and return Lia's soul to her, a shaman (called a *txiv neeb*) was needed to perform a soul calling.

The difference between the treatment prescribed by doctors at the hospital and the treatment prescribed under the Hmong system was dramatic. While the Lee family did think that something should be done to stop Lia's increasingly severe seizures, the communication barriers, misunderstanding, and frustration on both sides impeded treatment. The Lee family did not always understand the regimen of medications for their daughter, and they believed that some of the medications were in fact causing harm—which was not unfounded, since Lia suffered from side effects including, eventually, an infection that caused a coma and eventual vegetative state. In turn, the doctors did not understand the Hmong ethnomedical beliefs about epilepsy and viewed the Lee family as resistant, even to the point that Lia was taken from her family for a period of time by social services (Fadiman, 1997).

At the time, few resources were available to bridge the gap in understanding. Even though both the biomedical doctors and the Lee family came to some understanding of each other's treatment approach and reasons, this did not really occur until the story reached its tragic conclusion. It is a case in point for the need to understand the diversity in health beliefs and practices and to take a collaborative approach to treatment that recognizes the legitimacy of different systems.

Solutions: Collaborative Cultural Approaches

Because the gap in health beliefs and practices was significant between the Hmong and Western biomedicine (though that gap is closing over time), and because the Hmong population in Central California is large, several hospitals and other organizations have begun incorporating a collaborative approach to healthcare:

- Mercy Medical Center in Merced, California, instituted a Hmong shaman policy in 2009, because of the relatively high proportion of Hmong who seek services there

(continued)

(Brown, 2009). The hospital now formally recognizes the cultural role of traditional healers, who are certified as practitioners and can perform nine approved treatment ceremonies in the hospital, including the "soul-calling" ritual. As part of the policy, the hospital also provides a training program to introduce Hmong shamans to Western biomedicine and counter some of the fears that Hmong people have regarding biomedicine. This training includes visits to operating rooms, use of microscopes, introduction to germ theory, and other elements. But perhaps most important, the presence of shamans appears to have increased Hmong trust in hospital treatment, a significant change. The program is called "*Partners in Healing*" and it has attracted interest from other communities in the U.S. and globally where there are Hmong immigrant populations.

- The Central Valley Health Policy Institute at California State University, Fresno (see Bengiamin et al., 2011) conducted a mixed-methods study to: assess prenatal healthcare beliefs, practices, utilization, and needs of the Hmong men and women from three of the highest Hmong-populated counties in Central California; gain a better understanding of traditional Hmong prenatal and healthcare practices; identify barriers to prenatal care for Hmong; and use the findings to inform next steps. The study was conducted in several communities in partnership with the Hmong Health Collaborative (Valley Vision, n.d.), and interviews were conducted by Hmong bilingual graduate students. Findings included a high degree (45%) of dissatisfaction with respondents' experience of Western medicine (including 60% who reported a disconnect between Western and Hmong medicine), and issues with language access and lack of cultural competence training. The study concluded that Hmong residents utilize and rely on Western healthcare, yet cannot abandon their cultural and traditional healthcare practices in the new cultural setting, and that equitable and effective care will require that clinicians be able to function effectively within the context of the cultural beliefs, behaviors, and needs of these communities.

CURRENT EVENTS

MIGRANT FAMILY SEPARATION

Few issues have sparked such intense public scrutiny in recent years as with the case of migrant family separation. The practice, implemented by the Trump administration, led to the forced separation of thousands of migrant children from their families. In some cases, children were held in detention centers akin to prisons. In others, children were placed in foster homes where they may have had substantial language barriers and little to no contact with their parents. While it will take decades for the full effects of these separations to become evident, it is clear that the mental and physical health and well-being of the children has not been a primary concern within the policy. Preliminary reports suggest symptoms

(continued)

of post-traumatic stress disorder (PTSD) in children and parents, inadequate pediatric care (including vaccinations), and lack of formal schooling during critical formative times.

Discussion Question: How could the forced separation of migrant families ultimately exacerbate the underlying factors contributing to health disparities in migrant populations?

ICE RAIDS AND MIGRANT FARMWORKERS

The increased frequency of official "raids" by Immigration and Custom Enforcement has left migrant and seasonal farmworkers (both documented and undocumented) in constant fear of deportation. In many states, this has led to decreased utilization of migrant-specific health services such as 330(g) programs. In turn, many farmers are reporting a decrease in the migrant farmworker circuit. Levels of prejudice toward farmworkers appear to be increasing, with several elected legislators running on platforms that include "rounding up" undocumented workers and personally deporting them. Should the flow of migrant farmworkers stop, many have argued the entire farming industry would grind to a halt and could lead to nationwide food shortages.

Discussion Questions: What would the long-term economic effects of a continually decreasing migrant farmworker flow be? In what ways could making migrant farmworkers less likely to access available healthcare exacerbate the problem?

DISCUSSION QUESTIONS

- How do American stereotypes and prejudices of migrants, immigrants, and refugees differ? How does this affect health disparities?

- Many of the factors that migrants seek to escape are themselves social determinants of health that continue to affect them in the U.S.—how does this complicate elimination of health disparities for migrant populations?

- How do living conditions in migrant camps and during the immigration process contribute to health disparities seen in migrant populations?

- How do the Trajectory Approach and the social determinants of health model interface with each other? Does one represent an expansion/application of the other?

- How do factors such as religion and socioeconomic status play a major role in the experience of migrants upon reaching the U.S.?

REFERENCES

Andrade, E. I., Cubilla, I. C., Sojo-Lara, G., Cleary, S. D., Edberg, M. C., & Simmons, L. K. (2016). Where PYD meets CBPR: A photovoice program for Latino immigrant youth. *Journal of Youth Development*, *11*(2). doi:10.5195/JYD.2016.450

Avance Center for the Advancement of Immigrant/Refugee Health. (n.d.). Retrieved from http://www.avancegw.org

Barrett, N., Colón-Ramos, U., Elkins, A., Rivera, I., Evans, W. D., & Edberg, M. (2017). Formative research to design a promotional campaign to increase drinking water among Central American Latino youth in an urban area. *Journal of Health Communication/International Perspectives*, *22*, 459–468. doi:10.1080/10810730.2017.1303557

Bengiamin, M., Chang, X., & Capitaman, J. A. (2011). *Understanding traditional Hmong health and prenatal care beliefs, practices, utilization and needs*. Fresno: California State University Fresno. Retrieved from http://www.fresnostate.edu/chhs/cvhpi/documents/hmong-report.pdf

BestPlaces. (n.d.). *Crime in zip 20783 (Langley Park, MD)*. Retrieved from https://www.bestplaces.net/crime/zip-code/maryland/langley_park/20783

Bronfenbrenner, U. (1979). *The ecology of human development: Experiments by nature and design*. Cambridge, MA: Harvard University Press.

Bronfenbrenner, U. (2005). *Making human beings human: Bioecological perspectives on human development*. Thousand Oaks, CA: Sage Publications.

Brown, P. L. (2009, September 19). A doctor for the disease, a shaman for the soul. *New York Times*. Retrieved from https://www.nytimes.com/2009/09/20/us/20shaman.html

Castañeda, H., Holmes, S. M., Madrigal, D. S., DeTrinidad Young, M., Beyeler, N., & Quesada, J. (2015). Immigration as a social determinant of health. *Annual Review of Public Health, 36*, 375–392. doi:10.1146/annurev-publhealth-032013-182419

Castles, S., de Haas, H., & Miller, M. M. (2014). *The age of migration: International population movements in the modern world* (5th ed.). New York, NY: The Guilford Press.

Centers for Disease Control and Prevention. (2013). CDC health disparities and inequalities report—United States, 2013. *Morbidity and Mortality Weekly Report, 62*(Suppl. 3), 1–187. Retrieved from https://www.cdc.gov/mmwr/pdf/other/su6203.pdf

Child Trends. (2018). *Immigrant children*. Retrieved from http://www.childtrends.org/indicators/immigrant-children

Cobb, T. (2010). Strategies for providing cultural competent health care for Hmong Americans. *Journal of Cultural Diversity, 17*: 79–83.

Colon-Ramos, U., Cremm, E., Rivera, I., & Edberg, M. (2016, April). Barriers, facilitators and strategies to promote healthy eating among recent Hispanic immigrant mothers living in a food swamp. *Federation of American Societies for Experimental Biology Journal, 30*(1 Suppl.), 901.8. Retrieved from https://www.fasebj.org/doi/abs/10.1096/fasebj.30.1_supplement.901.8

Commodore-Mensah, Y., Selvin, E., Aboagye, J., Turkson-Ocran, R. A., Li, X., Himmelfarb, C. D., … Cooper, L. A. (2018). Hypertension, overweight/obesity and diabetes among immigrants in the United States: An analysis of the 2010–2016 National Health Interview Survey. *BMC Public Health, 18*, 773. doi:10.1186/s12889-018-5683-3

Cunningham, P. W. (2017, September 6). The Health 202: Immigrants' health care problems are about to get worse. *Washington Post*. Retrieved from https://www.washingtonpost.com/news/powerpost/paloma/the-health-202/2017/09/06/the-health-202-immigrants-health-care-problems-are-about-to-get-worse/59aeffdf30fb04264c2a1ceb/

Economic Commission for Latin America and the Caribbean. (2011). *Social panorama of Latin America 2011*. Santiago, Chile: Author.

Edberg, M. (2013). *Culture, health and diversity: Understanding people, reducing disparities*. Boston, MA: Jones & Bartlett.

Edberg, M., Benavides, J., Rivera, I., Shaikh, H., & Mattiola, R. (2018, October). Trauma and other health determinants among recent Central American immigrants: Implications for youth and young adults. *NEOS, 10*(2), 16–17.

Edberg, M., Cleary, S, Andrade, E., Evans, W. D., Simmons, L. K., & Cubilla-Batista, I. (2017). Applying ecological positive youth development theory to address co-occurring health disparities among immigrant Latino youth. *Health Promotion Practice, 18*(4), 488–496. doi:10.1177/1524839916638302

Edberg, M., Cleary, S., Andrade, E., Leiva, R., Bazurto, M., Rivera, M. I., … Calderon, M. (2010). SAFER Latinos: A community partnership to address contributing factors for Latino youth violence. *Progress in Community Health Partnerships, 4*(3), 221–233. doi:10.1353/cpr.2010.0009

Edberg, M., Cleary, S., Klevens, J., Collins, E., Leiva, R., Bazurto, M., … Calderon, M. (2010). The SAFER Latinos project: Addressing a community ecology underlying Latino youth violence. *Journal of Primary Prevention, 31*, 247–257. doi:10.1007/s10935-010-0219-3

Edberg, M., Cleary, S., Simmons, L., Cubilla-Batista, I., Andrade, E. L., & Gudger, G. (2015). Defining the "community": An application of ethnographic methods for a Latino immigrant health disparities intervention. *Human Organization, 74*(1), 27–41. doi:10.17730/humo.74.1.6561p4u727582850

Edberg, M., Cleary, S., & Vyas, A. (2011). A trajectory model for understanding and assessing health disparities in immigrant/refugee communities. *Journal of Immigrant and Minority Health, 13*(3), 576–584. doi:10.1007/s10903-010-9337-5

Edberg, M., Wong, F., Park, R., & Corey, K. (2002, July). Preliminary qualitative results from an ongoing study of HIV risk in three Southeast Asian communities. *Proceedings of the XIV International AIDS Conference,* Barcelona, Spain

Ely, J. (1990). The American war in Indochina. *Stanford Law Review, 42*(5), 1093–1148. doi:10.2307/1228968

Ennis, S. R., Ríos-Vargas, M., & Albert, N. G. (2011). *The Hispanic population 2010* (Table 1, Hispanic or Latino Origin by Type, 2000-2010). Suitland, MD: U.S. Census Bureau. Retrieved from https://www.census.gov/prod/cen2010/briefs/c2010br-04.pdf

Fadiman, A. (1997). *The spirit catches you and you fall down: A Hmong child, her American doctors, and the collision of two cultures.* New York, NY: Farrar, Straus, and Giroux.

Foster, G. M. (1976). Disease etiologies in non-Western medical systems. *American Anthropologist, 78*(4), 773–782. doi:10.1525/aa.1976.78.4.02a00030

Gushulak, B. D., Weekers, J., & MacPherson, D. W. (2010). Migrants and emerging public health issues in a globalized world: Threats, risks and challenges, an evidence-based framework. *Emerging Health Threats Journal, 2,* e10. doi:10.3402/ehtj.v2i0.7091

Harris, A. M. (2018). Travel-related infectious diseases: Hepatitis B. In Centers for Disease Control and Prevention. *Yellow book 2018.* Retrieved from https://wwwnc.cdc.gov/travel/yellowbook/2018/infectious-diseases-related-to-travel/hepatitis-b

International Organization for Migration. (n.d.). *Key migration terms.* Retrieved from https://www.iom.int/key-migration-terms

International Organization for Migration. (2011). *Glossary on migration* (2nd ed., International Migration Law Series No. 25). Geneva, Switzerland: Author. Retrieved from https://publications.iom.int/system/files/pdf/iml25_1.pdf

International Organization for Migration. (2013). *International migration, health and human rights.* Geneva, Switzerland: International Organization for Migration. Retrieved from https://publications.iom.int/system/files/pdf/iom_unhchr_en_web.pdf

International Organization for Migration. (2018). *World migration report 2018.* Geneva, Switzerland: Author. Retrieved from https://www.iom.int/sites/default/files/country/docs/china/r5_world_migration_report_2018_en.pdf

International Organization for Migration. (2019). *Key migration terms.* Retrieved from https://www.iom.int/key-migration-terms

Kaiser Family Foundation. (2005). Mexican immigrants' health status worsens after living in the U.S., study finds. *Daily health policy report.* San Francisco, CA: Author.

Kandula, N. (2008). Immigrant and refugee health issues. In S. Boslaugh & L. McNutt (Eds.), *Encyclopedia of epidemiology* (pp. 525–528). Thousand Oaks, CA: Sage Publications.

Kirmayer, L. J., Lavanya, N. L., Munoz, M., Rashid, M., Ryder, A. G., Guzder, J., … Pottie, K. (2011). Common mental health problems in immigrants and refugees: General approach in primary care. *Canadian Medical Association Journal, 183*(12), E959–E967. doi:10.1503/cmaj.090292

Krogstad, J. M., & Keegan, M. (2015). From Germany to Mexico: How America's source of immigrants has changed over a century. *Pew Research Center.* Retrieved from http://www.pewresearch.org/fact-tank/2015/10/07/a-shift-from-germany-to-mexico-for-americas-immigrants

Lerner, R. M. (2005, September 9). *Promoting positive youth development: Theoretical and empirical bases.* White paper prepared for a Workshop on the Science of Adolescent Health and Development, National Research Council, Washington, DC.

Lerner, R. M., & Lerner, J. (2011). *The positive development of youth: Report of the findings from the first seven years of the 4-H study on positive youth development.* Medford, MA: Tufts University Institute for Applied Research in Positive Youth Development and the National 4-H Council.

Lerner, R. M., Lerner, J., Almerigi, J. B., Theokas, C., Phelps, E., Gestsdottir, S., ... von Eye, A. (2005). Positive youth development, participation in community youth development programs, and community contributions of fifth grade adolescents: Findings from the first wave of the 4-H study of positive youth development. *Journal of Early Adolescence, 25,* 17–71. doi:10.1177/0272431604272461

Migrant Clinicians Network. (2018). *Migrant health issues.* Retrieved from https://www.migrantclinician.org/issues/migrant-info/health-problems.html

Migration Policy Institute. (2019). *Frequently requested statistics on immigrants and immigration in the United States.* Washington, DC: Migration Policy Institute. Retrieved from https://www.migrationpolicy.org/article/frequently-requested-statistics-immigrants-and-immigration-united-states-8

National Center for Educational Statistics. (2016). *Statistics.* Retrieved from http://nces.ed.gov/ccd/schoolsearch

Pfeifer, M. E., Sullivan, J., Yang, K., & Yang, W. (2012). Hmong population and demographic trends in the 2010 Census and 2010 American Community Survey. *Hmong Studies Journal, 13*(2), 1–31. Retrieved from http://hmongstudies.org/PfeiferSullivanKYangWYangHSJ13.2.pdf

Polaris Observatory/HCV Collaborators. (2017). Global prevalence and genotype distribution of hepatitis C virus infection in 2015: A modelling study. *The Lancet Gastroenterology and Hepatology, 2*(3), 161–176. doi:10.1016/S2468-1253(16)30181-9

Sampson, R. J. (2003). The neighborhood context of well-being. *Perspectives in Biology and Medicine, 46*(3S), S53–S64. doi:10.1353/pbm.2003.0073

Sampson, R. J., Morenoff, J. D., & Gannon-Rowley, T. (2002). Assessing neighborhood effects: Social processes and new directions in research. *Annual Review of Sociology, 28*(1), 443–478. doi:10.1146/annurev.soc.28.110601.141114

Sampson, R. J., Raudenbush, S., & Earls, F. (1997). Neighborhoods and violent crime: A multilevel study of collective efficacy. *Science, 277,* 918–924. doi:10.1126/science.277.5328.918

Scott, M. M., MacDonald, G., Collazos, J., Levinger, B., Leighton, E., & Ball, J. (2014). *From cradle to career: The multiple challenges facing immigrant families in Langley Park Promise Neighborhood.* Washington, DC: Urban Institute. Retrieved from https://www.urban.org/sites/default/files/alfresco/publication-pdfs/413164-From-Cradle-to-Career-The-Multiple-Challenges-Facing-Immigrant-Families-in-Langley-Park-Promise-Neighborhood.PDF

Silbereisen, R. K., & Lerner, R. M. (2007). *Approaches to positive youth development.* London, UK: Sage Publications.

Singh, G. K., & Miller, B. A. (2004). Health, life expectancy, and mortality patterns among immigrant populations in the United States. *Canadian Journal of Public Health, 95*(3), I14–I21. doi:10.1007/BF03403660

Starfield, B. (2007). Pathways of influence on equity in health. *Social Science and Medicine, 64,* 1355–1362. doi:10.1016/j.socscimed.2006.11.027

Stokols, D. (1992). Establishing and maintaining healthy environments: Toward a social ecology of health promotion. *American Psychologist, 47*(1), 6–22. doi:10.1037/0003-066X.47.1.6

Strine, T., Barker, L. E., Mokdad, A. H., Luman, E. T., Sutter, R. W., & Chu, S. (2002). Vaccination coverage of foreign-born children 19 to 35 months of age: Findings from the National Immunization Survey, 1999–2000. *Pediatrics, 110*(2), 1–5. doi:10.1542/peds.110.2.e15

Telzer, E. H. (2010). Expanding the acculturation gap-distress model: An integrative review of research. *Human Development, 53,* 313–340. doi:10.1159/000322476

Teruya, S. A., & Bazargan-Hejazi, S. (2013). The immigrant and Hispanic paradoxes: A systematic review of their predictions and effects. *Hispanic Journal of Behavioral Science, 35*(4), 486–509. doi:10.1177/0739986313499004.

United Nations. (1951). United Nations convention relating to the status of refugees, Geneva, 28 July 1951. In *United Nations Treaty Series* (Vol. 189, p. 137). Retrieved from https://treaties.un.org/pages/ViewDetailsII.aspx?src=IND&mtdsg_no=V-2&chapter=5&Temp=mtdsg2&clang=_en

United Nations High Commissioner for Refugees. (1984). *Declaration of Cartagena*. Retrieved from https://www.unhcr.org/en-us/about-us/background/45dc19084/cartagena-declaration-refugees-adopted-colloquium-international-protection.html

U.S. Census Bureau. (2015). *American community survey*. Retrieved from https://www.census.gov/programs-surveys/acs.html

U.S. Census Bureau. (2018a). *Quickfacts: Langley Park CDP, Maryland*. Retrieved from https://www.census.gov/quickfacts/fact/table/langleyparkcdpmaryland/PST045218

U.S. Census Bureau (2018b). *Washington-Arlington-Alexandria, DC-VA-MD-WV Metro Area*. Retrieved from https://censusreporter.org/profiles/31000US47900-washington-arlington-alexandria-dc-va-md-wv-metro-area/

Valley Vision. (n.d.). *Project: Hmong health collaborative*. Retrieved from https://valleyvision.org/projects/hmong-health-collaborative

Viruell-Fuentes, E. A., Miranda, P. Y., & Abdulrahim, S. (2012). More than culture: Structural racism, intersectionality theory, and immigrant health. *Social Science & Medicine, 75*, 2099–2106. doi:10.1016/j.socscimed.2011.12.037

World Health Organization. (2018, September 19). *Hepatitis A*. Retrieved from http://www.who.int/news-room/fact-sheets/detail/hepatitis-a

Yang, P. Q., & Hwang, S. H. (2016). Explaining immigrant health service utilization: A theoretical framework. *Sage Creative Commons, 6*, 1–15. doi:10.1177/2158244016648137

Yun, K., Fuentes-Afflick, E., & Desai, M. M. (2012). Prevalence of chronic disease and insurance coverage among refugees in the United States. *Journal of Immigrant and Minority Health, 14*(6), 933–940. doi:10.1007/s10903-012-9618-2

Zimmerman, C., Kiss, L., & Hossain, M. (2011). Migration and health: A framework for 21st century policymaking. *PLoS Medicine, 8*(5), e1001034. doi:10.1371/journal.pmed.1001034

Zong, J., & Batalova, J. (2015). Frequently requested statistics on immigrants and immigration in the United States. *Migration Policy Institute*. Retrieved from http://www.migrationpolicy.org/article/frequently-requested-statistics-immigrants-and-immigration-united-states

HEALTH EQUITY IN VETERAN POPULATIONS

DONNA L. WASHINGTON ■ IFEOMA STELLA IZUCHUKWU ■
CHRISTINA E. HARRIS

LEARNING OBJECTIVES

- Describe the demographic characteristics of the Veteran population
- Articulate the differences in health risks and needs among military service eras
- Discuss the ways in which social determinants of health differ between Veteran and non-Veteran populations
- Describe differences between Veterans who use the U.S. Department of Veterans Affairs (VA) healthcare system and those who do not, and how this affects health equity
- Describe the ways in which intersectionality impacts Veteran health outcomes

INTRODUCTION

Veterans of the U.S. military are a unique population, with military service–related experiences and exposures conferring increased medical and mental health risks. In 2018, there were an estimated 20 million living U.S. Veterans (National Center for Veterans Analysis and Statistics [NCVAS] 2019). The Veterans Health Administration (VHA) is the largest integrated healthcare system in the U.S., with approximately six million Veteran enrollees using VA healthcare services each year. However, a larger number of Veterans use healthcare settings outside of VA for some or all of their healthcare (Frayne et al., 2018). Therefore, both VA and non-VA healthcare providers must be proficient in addressing the healthcare needs of U.S. Veterans.

HEALTHCARE PROVIDERS IN COMMUNITY (NON-VA) HEALTHCARE SETTINGS: IDENTIFYING VETERANS AND OBTAINING A MILITARY HEALTH HISTORY

For healthcare providers outside of the VA, screening patients about military service (current or past) at initial healthcare visits is important, because many Veterans will not volunteer information about military service, and some will not identify as Veterans.

This screening may be accomplished by asking, "Have you ever served in the military (e.g., on active duty in the U.S. Armed Forces, Reserves, or National Guard)?"

To facilitate obtaining information to help understand patients' military service–related health problems and concerns, VA has developed online resources for obtaining a military health history—Military Health History Pocket Card for Clinicians (Office of Academic Affiliations, 2019).

DEMOGRAPHIC CHARACTERISTICS AND USE OF VA HEALTHCARE

The composition of the U.S. military and the nature of military service have changed over time. Accordingly, the Veteran population is heterogeneous across periods of military service with respect to demographic characteristics, military exposures and sequelae, and their use of VA and non-VA healthcare services. Veterans' demographic characteristics by period of military service are given in Table 15.1. The largest cohort of Veterans, comprising one-third of the Veteran population, are those who served during the Vietnam Era. The median age of Veterans overall, 64 years in 2016, is 20 years older than the median age of non-Veterans. Overall, the size of the Veteran population has declined over time due to aging and military downsizing, decreasing by 23% since 1995 (Eibner et al., 2015). While the overall Veteran population is projected to continue to decrease, the number who served in Iraq or Afghanistan post-9/11 is projected to increase, from 12% in 2014 to 19% to 24% by 2024 (Eibner et al., 2015). The proportionate representation of women has increased and is also expected to continue increasing. Women comprised 8.6% of the 2016 Veteran population and are projected to increase to 11% by 2024 (Eibner et al., 2015). Racial/ethnic minorities comprise 22.3% of all Veterans, but are a steadily growing proportion of Veterans of each of the recent military eras (see Table 15.1). Women Veterans are younger and more racial/ethnically diverse than male Veterans (Frayne et al., 2018; Washington, Bean-Mayberry, Hamilton, Cordasco, & Yano, 2013).

Despite the decreasing size of the Veteran population, the use of VA healthcare has increased over time. For example, between 2005 and 2015, the annual number of Veterans using VA increased from 4.8 million to 5.9 million (Frayne et al., 2018). Overall, 34.9% of Veterans use VA healthcare, though with variation in VA use by military service era cohort (see Table 15.1). With this increase in VA use, the demographic characteristics of VA users have been changing. Women are the fasting growing group, with a 90% increase in the number of women using VA services between 2005 and 2015 in contrast to a 19% increase in the number of men using VA in that time frame.

VETERANS' UNIQUE HEALTH RISKS BY MILITARY SERVICE ERA

The current U.S. Veteran population served in the military during military service periods spanning from World War II to the ongoing Gulf War (Operations Enduring Freedom, Iraqi Freedom,

TABLE 15.1 Veterans Demographic Characteristics by Period of Military Service, 2016

MILITARY SERVICE ERA*	NUMBER (MILLIONS)	AGE, MEDIAN (YEARS)	SEX, % FEMALE	RACE/ETHNICITY, % RACIAL/ETHNIC MINORITY	USE OF VA HEALTHCARE, % USING VA HEALTHCARE
Post-9/11	2.6	35	17.0	34.6	36.4
Gulf War 1 Era	3.2	47	14.3	30.4	29.4
Vietnam Era	6.7	68	3.2	17.3	40.7
Korean Conflict	2.0	83	2.7	12.0	38.2
World War II	1.6**	91	4.5	8.3	36.3
Peacetime only	5.4***	59	9.4	21.0	26.8
All Veterans		64	8.6	22.3	34.9
All Non-Veterans		44	54.7	37.9	0.4

*Gulf War 1 Era 8/02/1990—10/06/2001 (includes Persian Gulf War [8/02/1990—4/06/1991]); Vietnam Era 8/04/1964—1/27/1973; Korean Conflict 6/25/1950—7/27/1953; World War II 12/07/1941—12/31/1946.
**Number includes pre–Korean Conflict peacetime.
***Pre–Vietnam peacetime 2.1 million; post–Vietnam peacetime 3.3 million.
SOURCE: Adapted from NCVAS, "Key Statistics by Veteran Status and Period of Service." 2016 American Community Survey Public Use Microdata Sample.

and New Dawn [OEF/OIF/OND]). Table 15.2 lists unique health risks for each U.S. period of military service, and cross-cutting military environmental exposures and occupational hazards.

The World War II Veterans who are alive today are over 90 years old, and Korean War Veterans are in their mid-80s or older. Three to five percent of military personnel during those service periods were female, compared to 17% today. These Veterans, as well as those who served in the early part of the Cold War, experienced unique health risks related to cold injury (e.g., frostbite), chemical warfare agent experiments, and nuclear weapons testing or cleanup. Long-term and delayed sequelae include peripheral neuropathy, skin cancer in frostbite scars, arthritis in involved areas of cold injuries, and increased malignancy risk for those with significant exposure to ionizing radiation. Similar to non-Veterans in their age cohort, Veterans of those military eras are also subject to the health conditions of aging.

Vietnam-Era Veterans are now approximately 65 to 75 years of age. Near the end of the Vietnam War, compulsory enlistment in the military ended, the 2% cap on the percentage of women allowed in the military was eliminated (Public Law 90-130), and participation of women in the military began a steady increase that continues to this day (Washington et al., 2013). Military personnel serving in Vietnam were exposed to many environmental hazards, including Agent Orange and other herbicides. These exposures have been linked to several types of malignancies, porphyria cutanea tarda, peripheral neuropathy, and spina bifida in offspring. The nature of the combat and military environment during the Vietnam Era significantly increased risk for

TABLE 15.2 U.S. Period of Military Service Eras and Associated Health Risks

PERIOD OF SERVICE	HEALTH RISKS
Any military service era	*Military environmental exposures*: asbestos; burn pit smoke; cold injuries; contaminated water (benzene, trichloroethylene, vinyl chloride); endemic diseases; heat stroke/exhaustion; hexavalent chromium; lead; military sexual trauma; mustard gas; nerve agents; pesticides; radiation (ionizing and nonionizing); sand, dust, smoke, and particulates; TCDD and other dioxins *Occupational hazards*: asbestos, industrial solvents, lead, radiation, fuels, polychlorinated biphenels (PCBs), noise/vibration, chemical agent resistant coating (CARC)
World War II: 12/07/1941–12/31/1946	*Unique health risks*: cold injury; chemical warfare agent experiments; nuclear weapons testing or cleanup
Cold War: 1945–1990s	*Unique health risks*: chemical warfare agent experiments; nuclear weapons testing or cleanup
Korean Conflict: 6/25/1950–7/27/1953	*Unique health risks*: cold injury; chemical warfare agent experiments; nuclear weapons testing or cleanup
Vietnam Era: 8/04/1964–1/27/1973	*Unique health risks*: agent orange exposure; hepatitis C; cold injury
Gulf War (Other): 8/02/1990–10/06/2001 (includes Persian Gulf War [8/02/1990–4/06/1991])	Gulf War (OEF/OIF/OND): Unique health risks: animal bites/rabies; blunt trauma; burn injuries (blast injuries); chemical or biological agents; chemical munitions demolition; combined penetrating injuries; depleted uranium (DU); dermatologic issues; embedded fragments (shrapnel); mental health issues; multi-drug resistant Acinetobacter; oil well fires; reproductive health issues; spinal cord injury; traumatic amputation; traumatic brain injury; vision loss *Immunizations*: anthrax, botulinum toxoid, smallpox, yellow fever, typhoid, cholera, hepatitis B, meningitis, whooping cough, polio, tetanus *Infectious diseases/pathogens*: malaria, brucellosis, *Campylobacter jejuni*, *Coxiella burnetii*, Mycobacterium tuberculosis, nontyphoid Salmonella, Shigella, visceral Leishmaniasis, West Nile virus
Gulf War (OEF/OIF/OND): 10/07/2001—ongoing	*Unique health risks*: same as Gulf War (other), plus malaria prevention: Mefloquine—Lariam *Immunizations*: same as Gulf War (other) *Infectious diseases*: same as Gulf War (other)

OEF/OIF/OND, Operation Enduring Freedom/Operation Iraqi Freedom/Operation New Dawn; TCDD, tetrachlorodibenzodioxin.

SOURCE: Adapted from Office of Academic Affiliations, Department of Veterans Affairs. (2019). Military health history pocket card for clinicians. Retrieved from: https://www.va.gov/OAA/pocketcard

post-traumatic stress disorder (PTSD) and substance use disorder. The Vietnam War was the first U.S. war in which Veterans returned home to a hostile civilian environment, which contributed to readjustment problems and exacerbation of mental health disorders.

Gulf War Veterans, both those who served prior to 2001 and those who served in southeast Asia (Afghanistan, Kuwait, Iraq) in OEF/OIF/OND, are subject to several unique health risks related to combat, the military environment, and mental health sequelae (see Table 15.2). Physical injuries due to combat include amputations, spinal cord injury, and traumatic brain injury (TBI). TBI is an injury to the structure or functioning of the brain from head trauma that immediately results in loss of consciousness, loss of memory for events before or after the event, neurologic deficit or intracranial lesion, or altered mental state (VA, 2016). In contrast to amputations and spinal cord injury, which are generally readily apparent, mild TBI may be missed initially. Common symptoms of TBI may be vague and include cognitive (e.g., poor concentration, difficulty completing tasks), neurosensory (e.g., paresthesia, visual or hearing problems), physical (e.g., dizziness, headache), and psychological (e.g., insomnia, anxiety) effects (VA, 2016).

CHARACTERISTICS OF VETERANS COMPARED TO NON-VETERANS

Veterans differ from U.S. adults who have not served in the military on many social determinants of health, behavioral health risk factors, and prevalence and severity of health conditions that are also present in the general U.S. population. At the time of selection into the military and after completing basic training, military personnel are generally healthier than their same age civilian counterparts, a phenomenon known as the "healthy soldier effect" (McLaughlin, Nielsen, & Waller, 2008). However, after separation from military service, Veterans have a decline in their health over time, such that there is a crossover effect, where their health status is worse than that of non-Veterans (Waller & McGuire, 2011). This crossover effect has been demonstrated in both male and female Veteran populations (Washington, Bird, et al., 2016; Wilmoth, London, & Parker, 2010). Risks for declines in Veterans' health include adverse sociodemographic characteristics and behavioral risk factors, along with the effects of military service. In addition, characteristics of military culture that may be strengths or adaptive behavior while deployed may contribute to vulnerabilities that adversely affect physical or mental health after reintegration into civilian life (Table 15.3). Overall, compared with non-Veterans, Veterans are disproportionately older, male, and less healthy (Eibner et al., 2015).

Social Determinants of Health

Veterans who use VA healthcare, compared with non-Veterans, are more likely to be unemployed (12.6% male Veterans, 12.2% female Veterans, vs. 10.3% male non-Veterans, 9.1% female non-Veterans). College educational attainment was similar for males (percent with college degrees: 30.3% male Veterans; 31.5% male non-Veterans), but female Veterans had higher educational attainment than non-Veterans (percent with college degrees: 48.1% female Veterans; 33.9% female non-Veterans). Veterans using VA are less likely than non-Veterans to have income below the federal poverty level (8.5% male Veterans; 12.3% female Veterans; 12.9% male non-Veterans; 15.3% female non-Veterans; Eibner et al., 2015).

TABLE 15.3 Impact of Military Culture and Healthcare

STRENGTH	GUIDING IDEA	VULNERABILITY
Placing welfare of others above one's own welfare	Selflessness	Not seeking help for health problems because personal health is not a priority
Commitment to accomplishing missions and protecting comrades in arms	Loyalty	Survivor guilt and complicated bereavement after loss of friends
Toughness and ability to endure hardships without complaint	Stoicism	Not acknowledging significant symptoms and suffering after returning home
Following an internal moral compass to choose "right" over "wrong"	Moral code	Feeling frustrated and betrayed when others fail to follow a moral code
Becoming the best and most effective professional possible	Excellence	Feeling ashamed (denial or minimization) of imperfections

SOURCE: U.S. Department of Veterans Affairs. (2015). Military culture: Core competencies for healthcare professionals: Self-assessment and introduction to military ethos (Module 1). Retrieved from https://www.ptsd.va.gov/professional/continuing_ed/military_culture_competencies_hcp.asp

Though several socioeconomic characteristics are more favorable for Veterans compared with non-Veterans, Veterans are over-represented among the homeless population (NCVAS, 2012). In 2010, Veterans accounted for 10% of the U.S. adult homeless population. With VA and federal attention to homelessness, by 2014, the overall number of homeless Veterans declined by 33%; however, the number of homeless women did not show the same decline (U.S. Department of Housing and Urban Development [HUD], 2014). Women Veterans are three to four times more likely to become homeless than non-Veteran women, with risk factors including unemployment, disability, poor physical and mental health, and sexual assault during military service (Washington et al., 2010).

Behavioral Risk Factors

The Behavioral Risk Factor Surveillance System (BRFSS) is an annual national population-based telephone survey that collects data on Veteran status, and several measures of sociodemographic, health, and healthcare utilization characteristics. The 2010 BRFSS found that after adjusting for differences in sociodemographic factors, both male and female Veterans were more likely than non-Veterans to report tobacco use, whereas only male Veterans were more likely to report heavy alcohol use (Hoerster et al., 2012; Lehavot, Hoerster, Nelson, Jakupcak, & Simpson, 2012). Veterans had modestly more physical activity than non-Veterans; however, a longitudinal analysis of women Veterans in the Women's Health Initiative found that Veterans, compared with non-Veterans, had steeper declines over time in their level of physical activity (Bouldin & Reiber, 2012; Washington, Gray, et al., 2016). A majority of both Veterans and non-Veterans were overweight or obese, but this was reported more often in both male (75%) and female (64%) Veterans compared with non-Veterans (70% of males, 57% of females). However, after adjusting for sociodemographic differences, Veteran status was not independently associated with obesity.

Health Conditions

The Medical Expenditure Panel Survey (MEPS), which collects nationally representative data on health conditions and other characteristics of individual households and their members, provides evidence on differences between Veterans and non-Veterans in the prevalence of diagnosed health conditions (MEPS, n.d.-a, n.d.-b). In the 2006 to 2012 MEPS, hypertension (#1) and lipid disorders (#2) were the top two conditions in both groups. Other commonly diagnosed conditions in Veterans (by rank: 1-hypertension; 2-lipid disorders; 3-diabetes mellitus; 4-mental health conditions; 5-cancer; 6-ischemic heart disease; 7-low back pain; 8-gastroesophageal reflux disease) were also among the top ten diagnosed conditions in non-Veterans, though the rank ordered differed somewhat (rank in non-Veterans: 1-hypertension; 2-lipid disorders; 5-diabetes; 3-mental health conditions; 8-cancer; 9-ischemic heart disease; 4-low back pain; 6-gastroesophageal reflux disease).

Veterans had higher diagnosed rates of all conditions except mental health conditions (see Figure 15.1). Compared with non-Veterans, Veterans had double the prevalence of diagnosed

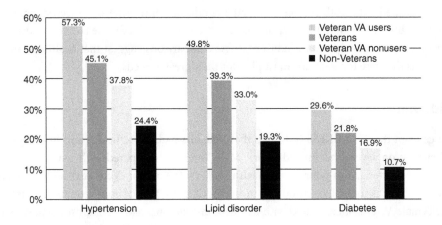

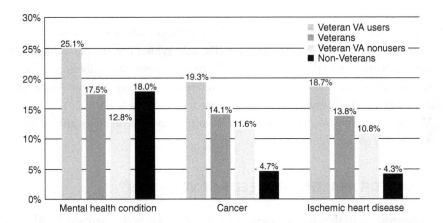

FIGURE 15.1 Comparisons between Veterans and non-Veterans and between Veteran VA healthcare users and non-users in prevalence of common health conditions.

SOURCE: Data from RAND analysis of MEPS 2006–2012 data. Eibner C, RAND Health, 2015.

hypertension, lipid disorders, and diabetes mellitus, and triple the prevalence of diagnosed cancer and ischemic heart disease. Though diagnosed prevalence of mental health conditions in the MEPS survey was similar between Veterans and non-Veterans, there were differences in prevalence of specific mental health conditions. For example, PTSD was diagnosed in 3% of Veterans, in contrast to less than 1% of non-Veterans. Other data sources, that incorporate physical examinations and screeners for active conditions, have identified a higher diagnosed prevalence of physical and mental health conditions among Veterans.

These differences in diagnosed prevalence rates reflect differences between Veterans and non-Veterans in demographic characteristics, healthcare access, and effects of military service. Veterans are older (median age 64 vs. 44) and are comprised of a higher proportion of men (93% vs. 40% in MEPS 2006–2012 data), and therefore would be expected to have higher rates of chronic conditions associated with aging. VA healthcare is available to Veterans with reduced financial barriers to healthcare use compared with healthcare in the broader U.S.; therefore, VA users, to the extent that their eligibility translates into greater healthcare use, may have greater opportunity than non-Veterans to have conditions diagnosed. As noted previously, military service is associated with both service-connected conditions and onset or exacerbations of other chronic conditions. Though it is unclear the extent to which each of these factors contributes to a higher prevalence of diagnosed conditions, these comparisons suggest that healthcare providers and systems that care for Veterans must plan for their greater needs.

Health Status

Findings from the 2010 BRFSS indicated that Veterans had worse health and functioning than non-Veterans on several health indicators. Male Veterans, compared with male non-Veterans, more often reported fair or poor overall health (21% vs. 14% of non-Veterans), and limited activities due to physical, mental, or emotional problems (30% vs. 17% of non-Veterans; Hoerster et al., 2012). Female Veterans, compared with female non-Veterans, had similar proportions with fair or poor overall health (each 18%), greater proportions with limited activities (30% vs. 22%), and more often had frequent poor physical health (15% vs. 12%) and mental distress (16% vs. 12%; Lehavot et al., 2012).

There were variations by race/ethnicity in these Veteran/non-Veteran comparisons. Among respondents to the 2007 to 2009 BRFSS, non-Hispanic White, non-Hispanic Black, American Indian/Alaska Native, and Hispanic Veterans all reported more physically unhealthy days than their race/ethnicity-concordant non-Veteran counterparts (comparisons for Asians and Native Hawaiian/Other Pacific Islanders were not reported; Luncheon & Zack, 2012). Non-Hispanic White Veterans and Hispanic Veterans also more often reported mentally unhealthy days than non-Veterans of those race/ethnicity groups.

SCREENING FOR HEALTHCARE NEEDS OF VETERANS

Clinicians providing healthcare to Veterans must screen for both common health conditions and military-related conditions. As noted above, common conditions such as hypertension, and behavioral risk factors such as tobacco use, may occur more frequently among Veterans. The VA in collaboration with the Department of Defense (DoD) and other leading professional organizations has developed clinical practice guidelines for selected issues affecting military service members and Veterans (www.healthquality.va.gov/; see Discussion Questions for information). Subject areas covered by the guidelines include chronic diseases in primary care, mental health, military-related conditions, pain, rehabilitation, and women's health. Postdeployment health assessments should include screening for combat-related physical injury including TBI, mental health sequelae of military service, chronic pain, substance use disorder (SUD), military sexual trauma, infectious diseases, environmental hazards, and social stressors (Olenick, Flowers, & Diaz, 2015; Roy & Perkins, 2018; Sessums & Jackson, 2013).

POST-DEPLOYMENT AND NEW PATIENT HEALTH ASSESSMENTS

- Physical injury due to combat
  - Amputations and phantom limb pain
  - Traumatic brain injury (TBI) and postconcussion syndrome
- Mental health sequelae:
  - PTSD; depression; generalized anxiety disorder
  - Suicide
  - Chronic multisymptom illness
- Chronic pain
- Substance use disorder
- Military sexual trauma (MST)
- Infectious diseases: Malaria, tuberculosis
- Environmental hazards: Noise-related hearing loss and tinnitus; toxins
- Social stress: Intimate partner violence; divorce; homelessness

Suicide Screening

- Are you feeling hopeless about the present/future?
- If yes, have you had thoughts about taking your life?

TBI is "an injury to the structure or functioning of the brain by an outside physical force that immediately results in one of more of: loss of consciousness, loss of memory for events either before or after the event, neurologic deficit or intracranial lesion, or altered mental state" (VA/DoD TBI clinical practice guideline). Mild TBI has been described by some as the signature event of the current war. Symptoms of TBI (poor concentration, memory problems, dizziness, headache, anxiety, insomnia) overlap with other conditions and may emerge after years; therefore, all Veterans should be screened for this as part of their initial intake.

PTSD is characterized by intrusive thoughts, nightmares, and flashbacks of past traumatic events, avoidance of reminders of trauma, hypervigilance, and sleep disturbance. Several brief screening instruments are available for rapid assessment during the clinical encounter (e.g., the 4-item Primary Care PTSD screen; see Discussion Questions). Veterans who screen positive for PTSD or depression should be asked about suicidal ideation and intent (see Post-Deployment and New Patient Health Assessments box).

Military sexual trauma (MST) is defined as sexual harassment that is threatening in character or physical assault that is sexual in nature that occurred in the military. The prevalence of MST is much higher in women than men, though given the large proportion of men in the military, the absolute number of Veterans who have experienced MST is similar between men and women. MST is associated with a higher risk of developing PTSD than is combat.

CHARACTERISTICS OF VETERAN VA HEALTHCARE USERS COMPARED TO VETERAN VA NON-USERS

VA provides comprehensive medical, mental health, and social services with no insurance premium. Visit and pharmacy copayments are required only for Veterans whose household income is above the VA's low-income threshold and who do not have military service–related conditions or enrollment priority factors. Given these reduced financial barriers to VA healthcare use, not surprisingly, demographic factors and health status influence use of VA healthcare (Dursa, Barth, Bossarte, & Schneiderman, 2016; Washington, Villa, Brown, Damron-Rodriguez, & Harada, 2005; Washington, Yano, Simon, & Sun, 2006). Veterans who use VA for healthcare are typically older, sicker, and have greater barriers to accessing healthcare in non-VA settings compared with other Veterans. These healthcare access barriers include having lower income, being uninsured, and residing in rural areas where community non-VA services may be limited. Compared with non-Hispanic White Veterans, racial/ethnic minority Veterans are more likely to use VA for some or all of their healthcare (Dursa et al., 2016; Washington et al., 2005; Washington, Farmer, et al., 2015).

Military service–connected disabilities are medical or mental health conditions that developed during or were exacerbated by military service. Veterans with service-connected disabilities may use VA healthcare without a copayment, and often preferentially seek VA care because they may get specialized care for their conditions, whereas that expertise may not necessarily be available in their local areas. The prevalence of diagnosed health conditions differs significantly by VA healthcare user status, with Veteran VA users having higher rates of all common diagnoses examined (Figure 15.1). These may include both military service–related as well as other health conditions.

RECOMMENDATIONS FOR ACHIEVING HEALTH EQUITY FOR VETERANS

Veterans of the U.S. military are a distinctive population, with strengths developed or honed over the course of their military service, as well as vulnerabilities and military service–related exposures that increase their health risks. Collectively, U.S. Veterans have a higher prevalence than non-Veterans of diagnosed chronic health conditions. Though the older age and male predominance of Veterans may account for many of these differences, these unadjusted comparisons reflect the populations and health conditions that healthcare providers caring for Veterans will need to address. Military service also confers increased risk for physical injury related to combat, and "invisible wounds of war," such as TBI, PTSD, MST, SUD, and suicide. It is essential for healthcare providers in both VA and community (non-VA) settings to screen Veterans for these "invisible wounds of war" and to be aware of medical services and referrals for Veterans. Education of healthcare professionals should incorporate a Veteran-centered care curriculum to prepare future healthcare providers to address the needs of their Veteran patients (Ross, Ravindranath, Clay, & Lypson, 2015; Lypson, Ravindranath, & Ross, 2014).

Veterans who use VA healthcare are a particularly vulnerable group. Large differences in socioeconomic status, behavioral risk factors, and health status are present between VA users and both Veteran VA non-users and the general U.S. population. The prevalence of diagnosed chronic health conditions is also highest in this group. VA provides comprehensive medical, mental health, and social services to address the complex needs of this group. As VA makes greater use of community care in the future to deliver services to Veterans, providers at those sites should plan for the needs of this group.

RESOURCES FOR VETERANS

- U.S. Department of Veterans Affairs (www.va.gov/)
- Women Veterans Health Care (www.womenshealth.va.gov/; 1-855-829-6636)
- VA/DoD Clinical Practice Guidelines (www.healthquality.va.gov/)
- VA National Center for PTSD (www.ptsd.va.gov/)
- Psychological Health Center of Excellence (PHCoE) (www.pdhealth.mil)
- VA Office of Academic Affiliations (https://www.va.gov/OAA/pocketcard/)

INTERSECTIONALITY SPOTLIGHT

Equitable access to high-quality care for all Veterans is a major tenet of the VA healthcare mission (VHA Office of Health Equity [OHE], 2016). With its reduced financial barriers to healthcare use and its provision of social services, VA care can address some of the barriers to health equity that are present in the broader U.S. In addition, advances over time in the organization and delivery of VA care have been designed to improve overall care quality, which some theorize could reduce disparities (Washington et al., 2017). Examples of such advances include early implementation of electronic health records, and nationwide implementation of patient-centered medical homes (PCMH). While monitoring of VA care quality and outcomes has revealed narrowing of disparities in some areas (Saha et al., 2008; Trivedi, Grebla, Wright, & Washington, 2011), evidence exists for ongoing disparities for several vulnerable Veteran groups (Breland et al., 2017; May, Yano, Provenzale, Steers, & Washington, 2019; Washington et al., 2017; Wong et al., 2019).

Racial and ethnic disparities in the VA were the subject of a 2008 systematic review (Saha et al., 2008). Most of the studies examined differences between African American and White Veterans. That review identified that disparities were most prevalent for medication adherence, surgery and other invasive procedures, and processes of care that are likely to be affected by provider communication and shared decision-making. A study that focused on Black–White differences in achievement of quality of care measures from 2000 to 2009 found that for most processes of care, disparities were no longer present, whereas for clinical measures of hypertension

(continued)

control and diabetes control, disparities persisted (Trivedi et al., 2011). A subsequent study that included all racial/ethnic groups evaluated whether these racial/ethnic disparities in hypertension and diabetes control persisted with VA implementation of PCMHs (Washington et al., 2017). It found that despite modest improvements in overall quality, racial/ethnic disparities narrowed somewhat for Hispanics, but persisted for African American, American Indian/Alaska Native, and Native Hawaiian Other Pacific Islander groups.

Racial/ethnic disparities in mortality across the VA were also evaluated and contrasted to racial/ethnic mortality disparities in the U.S. (Wong et al., 2019). A key finding was that patterns in disparities differed between VA and U.S. populations. Black–White disparities in all-cause mortality were present for men in both populations, though disparities were lower in the VA. Black–White disparities in all-cause mortality that were present for women in the U.S. were not evident in the VA. For American Indian/Alaska Native male Veterans, disparities in all-cause mortality were present in the VA, but not the U.S. population. In sum, these findings suggest that "equal-access" type healthcare systems such as VA may partially address health disparities, but that other non-healthcare factors should also be explored.

Among Veteran VA users, there are sizable sex differences in the prevalence of diagnosed conditions (Frayne et al., 2018; VHA OHE, 2016). Though hypertension, lipid disorders, and diabetes are leading diagnoses among men, for women Veteran VA users, conditions associated with musculoskeletal pain were most common. The VA promotes evidence-based complementary and integrative health (CIH) therapies as nonpharmacologic approaches for chronic pain. Among Veterans ages 18 to 54 with chronic musculoskeletal pain, women are more likely than men to use CIH therapies (Evans et al., 2018). At the same time, Black women are less likely than women of other races/ethnicities to use these nonopioid therapies to treat chronic pain (Evans et al., 2018). Sex and gender differences in Veterans' health and VA care has been examined for several other conditions and was the subject of a June 2019 supplement to *Women's Health Issues*.

CASE STUDY — LONG-STANDING IMPACT OF WAR ON A VETERAN'S MENTAL HEALTH

A 64-year-old man presents for a follow-up visit with a chief complaint of feeling more tired and worsening back pain. He has been your patient for the past 5 years, but you note that he has not been in the office for the past 9 months despite having poorly controlled diabetes mellitus and hypertension. He was laid off from his job last year and since that time he has been struggling with feeling sad and has isolated himself from his friends and family. He mentions his sleep has also been poor and that he has been having nightmares and flashbacks that remind him of his time spent in Vietnam. You ask him more about his time in the service including where he was stationed, military occupation, environmental exposures such as Agent Orange, and lastly about his combat experience. Upon further questioning he was in combat for 2 years and he witnessed many of his friends being killed. When he returned home he did not find that any of his friends or family were able to relate to his experiences, and therefore he suppressed these memories. He recently saw a news story about the ongoing fighting in the Middle East, and since that time he has felt his mood and anxiety heighten. He is coming to you to ask you for assistance.

DISCUSSION QUESTION

■ What are good options for approaching this patient's worsening mood and social isolation?

CURRENT EVENTS

ACCESS TO VA SERVICES

In recent years, there has been significant public attention drawn to wait times and true accessibility of VA healthcare services. Issues of wait times and distance to care are particularly salient for rural Veterans, who may have no other access point to receive healthcare. The VA has responded by supporting transportation networks and increased presence of telehealth-based VA clinics in local communities.

Discussion Question: What other approaches could be used to increase access to care for rural Veterans? What other groups may be particularly affected by challenges in accessing care?

DISCUSSION QUESTIONS

- Why should health professionals ask about military service?

- What are common health problems affecting returning military personnel?

- Where can Veterans obtain information about accessing and managing their VA benefits and healthcare?

- Where can community (non-VA) healthcare providers learn about medical services for Veterans and obtain Veteran-related health information?

REFERENCES

Bouldin, E. D., & Reiber, G. E. (2012). Physical activity among Veterans and non-Veterans with diabetes. *Journal of Aging Research, 2012,* 135192. doi:10.1155/2012/135192

Breland, J. Y., Phibbs, C. S., Hoggatt, K. J., Washington, D. L., Lee, J., Haskell, S., ... Frayne, S. M. (2017). The obesity epidemic in the Veterans Health Administration: Prevalence among key populations of women and men veterans. *Journal of General Internal Medicine, 32*(Suppl. 1), 11–17. doi:10.1007/s11606-016-3962-1

Dursa, E. K., Barth, S. K., Bossarte, R. M., & Schneiderman, A. I. (2016). Demographic, military, and health characteristics of VA health care users and nonusers who served in or during Operation Enduring Freedom or Operation Iraqi Freedom, 2009–2011. *Public Health Reports, 131*(6), 839–843. doi:10.1177/0033354916676279

Eibner, C., Krull, H., Brown, K., Cefalu, M., Mulcahy, A. W., Pollard, M., ... Farmer, C. M. (2015). *Current and projected characteristics and unique health care needs of the patient population served by the Department of Veterans Affairs.* Santa Monica, CA: RAND Corporation. Retrieved from: https://www.rand.org/pubs/research_reports/RR1165z1.html

Evans, E. A., Herman, P. M., Washington, D. L., Lorenz, K. A., Yuan, A., Upchurch, D. M., ... Taylor, S. L. (2018). Gender differences in use of complementary and integrative health by U.S. military veterans with chronic musculoskeletap pain. *Women's Health Issues, 28*(5), 379–386. doi:10.1016/j.whi.2018.07.003

Frayne, S. M., Phibbs, C. S., Saechao, F., Friedman, S. A., Shaw, J. G., Romodan, Y., ... & Haskell, S. (2018) *Sourcebook: Women veterans in the Veterans Health Administration. Volume 4: Longitudinal trends in sociodemographics, utilization, health profile, and geographic distribution.* Washington, DC: U.S. Department of Veterans Affairs. Retrieved from: https://vaww.infoshare.va.gov/sites/womenshealth/whsra/repres/WHS_Sourcebook_Vol-IV_508c.pdf

Hoerster, K. D., Lehavot, K., Simpson, T., McFall, M., Reiber, G., & Nelson, K. M. (2012). Health and health behavior differences: U.S. Military, veteran, and civilian men. *American Journal of Preventive Medicine, 43*(5), 483–489. doi:10.1016/j.amepre.2012.07.029

Lehavot, K., Hoerster, K. D., Nelson, K. M., Jakupcak, M., & Simpson, T. L. (2012). Health indicators for military, veteran, and civilian women. *American Journal of Preventive Medicine, 42*(5), 473–480. doi:10.1016/j.amepre.2012.01.006

Luncheon, C., & Zack, M. (2012). Health-related quality of life among US veterans and civilians by race and ethnicity. *Preventing Chronic Disease, 9*, E108. doi:10.5888/pcd9.110138

Lypson, M. L., Ravindranath, D., & Ross, P. T. (2014). Developing skills in veteran-centered care: Understanding where soldiers really come from. Retrieved from: http://www.mededportal.org/publication/9818

May, F. P., Yano, E. M., Provenzale, D., Steers, W. N., & Washington, D. L. (2019). Race, poverty, and mental health drive colorectal cancer screening disparities in the Veterans Health Administration. *Medical Care, 57*(10), 773–780. doi:10.1097/MLR.0000000000001186

McLaughlin, R., Nielsen, L., & Waller, M. (2008). An evaluation of the effect of military service on mortality: Quantifying the healthy soldier effect. *Annals of Epidemiology, 18*, 928–936. doi:10.1016/j.annepidem.2008.09.002

Medical Expenditure Panel Survey. (n.d.-a). *Data overview.* Retrieved from: http://meps.ahrq.gov/mepsweb/data_stats/data_overview.jsp

Medical Expenditure Panel Survey. (n.d.-b). *Survey background.* Retrieved from: https://meps.ahrq.gov/mepsweb/about_meps/survey_back.jsp

National Center for Veterans Analysis and Statistics. (2012). *Profile of sheltered homeless veterans for fiscal years 2009 and 2010.* Washington, DC: U.S. Department of Veterans Affairs.

National Center for Veterans Analysis and Statistics (2019). Population Tables. Table 1L: VetPop2016 Living veterans by age group, gender, 2015–2045. Retrieved from: https://www.va.gov/vetdata/Veteran_Population.asp

Office of Academic Affiliations, Department of Veterans Affairs. (2019). Military health history pocket card for clinicians. Retrieved from: https://www.va.gov/OAA/pocketcard

Olenick, M., Flowers, M., & Diaz, V. J. (2015). US veterans and their unique issues: Enhancing health care professional awareness. *Advances in Medical Education and Practice, 6*, 635–639. doi:10.2147/AMEP.S89479

Ross, P. T., Ravindranath, D., Clay, M., & Lypson, M. L. (2015). A greater mission: Understanding military culture as a tool for serving those who have served. *Journal of Graduate Medical Education, 7*(4), 519–522. doi:10.4300/JGME-D-14-00568.1

Roy, M. J., & Perkins, J. G. (2018). Medical care of the returning veteran. In M. D. Aronson (Ed.), *UpToDate.* Retrieved from https://www.uptodate.com/contents/medical-care-of-the-returning-veteran

Saha, S., Freeman, M., Toure, J., Tippens, K. M., Weeks, C., & Ibrahim, S. (2008). Racial and ethnic disparities in the VA health care system: A systematic review. *Journal of General Internal Medicine, 23*(5), 654–671. doi:10.1007/s11606-008-0521-4

Sessums, L. L., & Jackson, J. L. (2013). In the clinic. Care of returning military personnel. *Annals of Internal Medicine, 159*(1), ITC1–ITC15. doi:10.7326/0003-4819-159-1-201307020-01001

Trivedi, A. M., Grebla, R. C., Wright, S. M., & Washington, D. L. (2011). Despite improved quality of care in the Veterans Affairs health system, racial disparity persists for important clinical outcomes. *Health Affairs, 30*(4), 707–715. doi:10.1377/hlthaff.2011.0074

U.S. Department of Housing and Urban Development. (2014). *The 2014 annual homeless assessment report (AHAR) to Congress.* Washington, DC. Retrieved from https://files.hudexchange.info/resources/documents/2014-AHAR-Part1.pdf

U.S. Department of Veterans Affairs. (2015). Military culture: Core competencies for healthcare professionals: Self-assessment and introduction to military ethos (Module 1). Retrieved from https://www.ptsd.va.gov/professional/continuing_ed/military_culture_competencies_hcp.asp

U.S. Department of Veterans Affairs. (2016). VA/DoD clinical practice guideline for management of concussion/mild traumatic brain injury. Retrieved from: https://www.healthquality.va.gov/guidelines/Rehab/mtbi

VA Office of Health Equity. (2016). *National veteran health equity report—FY2013*. US Department of Veterans Affairs, Washington, DC. Available online at http://www.va.gov/healthequity/NVHER.asp

Waller, M., & McGuire, A. C. L. (2011). Changes over time in the "healthy solider effect." *Population Health Metrics, 9*, 7. doi:10.1186/1478-7954-9-7

Washington, D. L., Bean-Mayberry, B., Hamilton, A. B., Cordasco, K. M., & Yano, E. M. (2013). Women veterans' healthcare delivery preferences and use by military service era: Findings from the National Survey of Women Veterans. *Journal of General Internal Medicine, 28*(Suppl. 2), S571–S576. doi:10.1007/s11606-012-2323-y

Washington, D. L., Bird, C. E., LaMonte, M. J., Goldstein, K. M., Rillamas-Sun E., Stefanick M. L., . . . Weitlauf J. C. (2016). Military generation and its relationship to mortality in women veterans in the Women's Health Initiative. *Gerontologist, 56*(Suppl. 1), S126-S137. doi:10.1093/geront/gnv669

Washington, D. L., Farmer, M. M., Mor, S. S., Canning, M., & Yano, E. M. (2015). Assessment of the healthcare needs and barriers to VA use experienced by women veterans: Findings from the National Survey of Women Veterans. *Medical Care, 53*(4 Suppl. 1), S23-S31. doi:10.1097/MLR.0000000000000312

Washington, D. L., Gray, K., Hoerster, K. D., Katon, J. G., Cochrane, B. B., LaMonte, M. J., . . . Tinker, L. (2016). Trajectories in physical activity and sedentary time among women veterans in the Women's Health Initiative. *Gerontologist, 56*(Suppl. 1), S27–S39. doi:10.1093/geront/gnv676

Washington, D. L., Steers, W. N., Huynh, A. K., Frayne, S. M., Uchendu, U. S., Riopelle, D., ... & Hoggatt, K. J. (2017). Racial and ethnic disparities persist at Veterans Health Administration Patient-Centered Medical Homes. *Health Affairs, 36*(6), 1086–1094.

Washington, D. L., Villa, V., Brown, A., Damron-Rodriguez, J., & Harada, N. (2005). Racial/ethnic variations in veterans' ambulatory care use. *American Journal of Public Health, 95*(12), 2231–2237.

Washington, D. L., Yano, E. M., McGuire, J., Hines, V., Lee, M., & Gelberg, L. (2010). Risk factors for homelessness among women veterans. *Journal of Health Care for the Poor and Underserved, 21*(1), 82–91.

Washington, D. L., Yano, E. M., Simon, B., & Sun, S. (2006). To use or not to use: What influences why women veterans choose VA health care. *Journal of General Internal Medicine, 21*(Suppl. 3), S1–S8.

Wilmoth, J. M., London, A. S., & Parker, W. M. (2010). Military service and men's health trajectories in later life. *The Journals of Gerontology, Series B: Psychological Sciences and Social Sciences. 65*, 744–755.

Wong, M. S., Hoggatt, K. J., Steers, W. N., Frayne, S. M., Huynh, A. K., Yano, E. M., ... & Washington, D. L.. (2019). Racial/ethnic disparities in mortality across the Veterans Health Administration. *Health Equity, 3*(1), 99–108.

HEALTH EQUITY IN POPULATIONS WITH DISABILITIES

ERIN VINOSKI THOMAS ■ EMILY GRAYBILL ■ MARGARET MURRAY

LEARNING OBJECTIVES

- Describe the types of disabilities that exist and the general prevalence of disabilities in the United States
- Identify the types of health disparities that individuals with disabilities experience
- Describe how systemic oppression serves as a barrier to achieving health equity among individuals with disabilities
- Contrast the medical model, social model, and biopsychosocial model of disabilities, and describe the ways in which those models affect achievement of health equity
- Describe how community-based participatory research (CBPR) and Universal Design serve as best practices in achieving health equity for individuals with disabilities

INTRODUCTION

Disability is a broad category that is defined differently across academic and clinical disciplines, federal agencies, and federal legislation (Krahn, Walker, & Correa-De-Araujo, 2015). Disability refers to congenital (i.e., from birth) or acquired (e.g., sustained via injury, health condition, or as a result of aging) structural impairments, activity limitations, or participation restrictions that reflect the interaction between a person's body and the society in which they live (World Health Organization [WHO], 2001). The term "disability" encompasses many conditions, including physical or mobility disabilities; intellectual disabilities; developmental disabilities; vision, hearing, and other sensory disabilities; and other conditions such as chronic medical or mental health conditions that influence limitations in self-care and/or independent living. Some disabilities are "visible" in that they are observable or perceivable to others, and others "invisible" or not immediately apparent to others. Approximately 25% of adults living in the United States have some type of disability (Okoro, Hollis, Cyrus, & Griffin-Blake, 2018), and the estimated prevalence of disability across the globe is approximately 15% (WHO, 2011). The prevalence of disability is expected to rise over the next several decades due to increased global prevalence of chronic disease and advances in medical technology and related longer life expectancy of adults living in developed countries (Iezzoni, Kurtz, & Rao, 2014).

HEALTH DISPARITIES IN INDIVIDUALS WITH DISABILITIES

Individuals with disabilities of all types face substantial disparities in health access, quality, and outcomes across almost all health indicators compared to those without disabilities (Altman & Bernstein, 2008). Adults with disabilities are four times more likely to report poor to fair health, have higher prevalence of cardiovascular disease (12.4% vs. 3.4% [ages 18–44] and 27.7% vs. 9.7% [ages 45–64]), and have an approximately three times higher incidence of type 2 diabetes than adults without disabilities (Altman & Bernstein, 2008; Krahn et al., 2015). Adults with disabilities are more likely to engage in no leisure-time physical activity and to smoke than those without disabilities (28.8% vs. 18.0%) and are more than twice as likely as those with no disabilities to go without needed healthcare due to financial barriers (Havercamp, Scandlin, & Roth, 2004; Krahn et al., 2015). Adults with disabilities also have heightened risk for mental health concerns such as anxiety and depression compared with those without disabilities, partially due to their having inadequate social and emotional supports and experiencing persistent stigma and discrimination (Chevarley, Thierry, Gill, Ryerson, & Nosek, 2006; Krahn et al., 2015).

Health disparities among people with disabilities persist throughout the life course. For example, children and youth with disabilities experience inequities in accessing adequate healthcare (Cheak-Zamora & Thullen, 2017), are at increased risk for developing mental health conditions (Einfeld, Ellis, & Emerson, 2011; Hysing, Elgen, Gillberg, Lie, & Lundervold, 2007), and have increased exposure to and experience disproportionately adverse outcomes following violence, disaster, terrorism, and other traumatic events (Stough, Ducy, & Kang, 2017). Youth and young adults with disabilities experience gaps in healthcare while transitioning from pediatric services to adult care, resulting in the development and worsening of chronic conditions, increased use of emergency services, and increased risk of death (McPheeters et al., 2014; White & Cooley, 2018). On the other end of the spectrum, older adults with intellectual and developmental disabilities experience poorer health outcomes compared to older adults without such disabilities (Perkins & Moran, 2010).

FACTORS THAT INFLUENCE DISABILITY HEALTH DISPARITIES

Factors influencing health inequities among people with disabilities are well documented and exist at all levels of the social–ecological model (McLeroy, Bibeau, Steckler, & Glanz, 1988). Some of the causes of poorer health among people with disabilities are attributable to the person's primary disability itself; however, the widespread discrimination and exclusion of individuals with disabilities, particularly within healthcare systems, also influences these disparities (Krahn et al., 2015). It is important to consider which health disparities are unavoidable due to the nature of the disability and those that are avoidable due to inequitable health access for individuals with disabilities (Krahn et al., 2015).

Systemic oppression that influences disability health disparities is evident within public health and healthcare systems. For example, individuals with disabilities receive inadequate screening and preventive services due to shortages of adequately trained providers and a dearth of accessible facilities (WHO, 2018). Discrimination toward individuals with disabilities by healthcare providers is another influential factor leading to reduced healthcare-seeking behavior (Moscoso-Porras & Alvarado, 2018). The healthcare profession makes harmful assumptions about individuals with disabilities that perpetuate health disparities, including (a) the assumption that individuals with disabilities differ in a meaningful way from individuals without disabilities, (b) that individuals with disabilities have a lower level of cognitive ability than individuals without disabilities, and (c) that health disparities among people with disabilities result simply from having a disability. This third assumption in particular results in fewer and less aggressive treatment options being presented to individuals with disabilities who need medical and healthcare (National Academies of Sciences, Engineering, and Medicine [NASEM], 2018).

Deficient epidemiologic surveillance of health issues among people with disabilities also indirectly affects these health disparities. Without conducting population-based research that is inclusive of those with disabilities, researchers and clinicians cannot reliably compare health issues among people with and without disabilities, therefore precluding their ability to adequately address disability health disparities (Williams & Moore, 2011). Although Healthy People 2020 specifically aims to increase the number of national data systems by incorporating the six standardized disability identification questions (U.S. Department of Health and Human Services [DHHS], 2011b, 2014), this increased population-level surveillance has not instigated broader awareness of disability inclusion nor uptake of disability demographic questions by independent investigators conducting health research (Rios, Magasi, Novak, & Harniss, 2016). Correspondingly, people with disabilities are severely underrepresented in mainstream health studies (National Council on Disability, 2009).

A unique and persistent form of "ableism" (i.e., the belief that people with disabilities are inferior to those without disabilities; Linton, 1998) that may influence disability health disparities is evidenced in the way the impact of disease is measured within public health systems. The disability-adjusted life years (DALY) metric is used in academic, policy, nonprofit, and economic settings to quantitatively measure, using a combination of morbidity and mortality estimates, the impact of disease on the productivity of a population (Parks, 2014). The DALY metric is problematic in that (a) it is rooted in the premise that a disabled person's life is less valuable and thus less cost-effective than the life of a person without disability, and (b) disability weights are established by comparing the productivity and quality of life for people with different disabilities, which underestimates the abilities and quality of life of people with disabilities (NASEM, 2018). The systematic use of the DALY metric to quantify the impact of disease may result in disproportionately low health-related resource allocation for persons with disabilities.

Beyond the healthcare system, individuals have experienced systematic discrimination, from institutionalization, to sterilization, to legal exclusion from education throughout history. Today, individuals with disabilities are less likely to access post-secondary education (Newman, 2005), secure meaningful employment that pays a living wage and provides private health insurance (Krahn et al., 2015), and have access to reliable transportation (Krahn et al., 2015). These disparities are reinforced through inadequate systems of support (Krahn et al., 2015). Even within studies of health disparity and inequity, people with disabilities have received substantially less attention than other historically marginalized groups. Disability also has been largely absent from sociological studies of inequality (Shandra, 2018). With federal anti-discrimination legislation, a move toward school inclusion, block grant funding requiring state-level services and supports for individuals with disabilities, and increased attention to disability inequity issues in federal health initiatives, access to needed supports for individuals with disabilities has increased (Krahn et al., 2015), yet disparities persist.

DISABILITY-SPECIFIC MODELS OF HEALTH DISPARITIES AND HEALTH EQUITY

Frameworks that support the study of health disparities and health equity among individuals with disabilities are constantly developing (Emerson & Hatton, 2014). Several prominent models of disability inform research, advocacy, and clinical practice around issues of disability and health.

The Medical Model

The medical model remains the dominant framework for understanding disability within many health-related disciplines (Donoghue, 2003) and in most high-income and many low-and middle-income countries (Emerson, Fujiura, & Hatton, 2007). This model characterizes the inequities experienced by individuals with disabilities as inevitable and resulting from limitations or "deficits" in personal capability. As such, the "solutions" to disability health disparities that derive from the medical model emphasize the importance of curing or preventing the conditions that cause these limitations, both at the individual and broader societal levels.

Social Model

Scholars have more recently moved toward adopting a social model of disability, prompted in part by the disability rights movement of the 1970s and beyond (Beaudry, 2016). The social model presents disability as a social construct rising from dominant sociocultural attitudes about disability, an inflexible social or physical environment, and the resulting oppression of people with disabilities, rather than a result of individual "limitations" (Oliver, 1990). The "solutions" to issues of disability health inequities that derive from the social model emphasize the importance of modifying the built and social environments to increase access and inclusion.

The Biopsychosocial Model

The WHO merged tenets of the medical and social models to inform their International Classification of Functioning, Disability and Health (ICF), which is the most widely adopted disability classification system (WHO, 2002). The ICF recognizes that structural impairments and limitations in participation, *and* external environmental factors and societal attitudes, influence the concept and experience of disability (WHO, 2002; see Figure 16.1). The ICF aligns with the more holistic biopsychosocial model, which emerged in the mid-20th century in response to reductionist and molecular views of health that attempted to separate individuals, with all of their identities and experiences, from the health conditions they faced (Engel, 1980). The goal of the ICF is to serve as a common framework through which the multidimensionality of the experiences of people with disabilities can be understood (Emerson & Hatton, 2014).

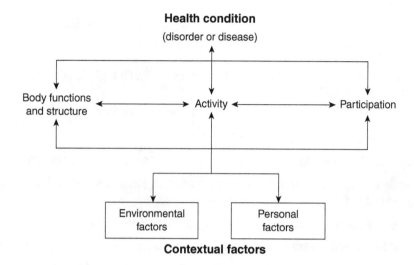

FIGURE 16.1 The WHO international classification of functioning, disability, and health.

SOURCE: World Health Organization. (2002). *Towards a common language for functioning, disability and health.* Geneva, Switzerland: Author. Retrieved from http://www.who.int/classifications/icf/training/icfbeginnersguide.pdf

ACHIEVING HEALTH EQUITY FOR INDIVIDUALS WITH DISABILITIES

Krahn and colleagues (2015) describe five broad actions under which ongoing initiatives exist with the goal of achieving health equity for persons with disabilities.

1. Improve Access to Healthcare

Increasing access to healthcare for people with disabilities requires initiatives at the organizational, community, and policy levels. Increasing access to and within healthcare facilities can be realized through improved public transit systems, implementing standards for accessible medical equipment (e.g., exam tables and scales), and improving the monitoring and enforcement of Americans with Disabilities Act (ADA) compliance (WHO, 2018). Organizations such as the National Center on Health, Physical Activity and Disability (NCHPAD) have compiled assessment tools specifically for healthcare environments to assess and improve physical accessibility (NCHPAD, n. d.). Health reform at the policy level, such as upholding provisions of the Affordable Care Act that disallow denial of coverage due to preexisting conditions and Medicaid expansion, is also a critical step toward achieving this goal.

2. Collect Data to Drive Policy and Practice

DHHS has recently achieved the goal of including six standardized disability questions (see Box 16.1) in all federal health surveys (Centers for Disease Control and Prevention, n.d.; DHHS, 2011b). Data collected through these standardized self-report items will allow for researchers to understand and begin to address health issues faced by individuals within the disability community as a whole and among specific disability subgroups.

BOX 16.1

SIX STANDARDIZED DISABILITY IDENTIFYING QUESTIONS USED ON ALL FEDERAL HEALTH SURVEYS

U.S. Department of Health and Human Services: Six Standardized Disability Questions

1. Are you deaf or do you have serious difficulty hearing?

2. Are you blind or do you have serious difficulty seeing, even when wearing glasses?

3. Because of a physical, mental, or emotional condition, do you have serious difficulty concentrating, remembering, or making decisions? (5 years or older)

4. Do you have serious difficulty walking or climbing stairs? (5 years or older)

5. Do you have difficulty dressing or bathing? (5 years or older)

6. Because of a physical, mental, or emotional condition, do you have difficulty doing errands alone, such as visiting a doctor's office or shopping? (15 years or older)

SOURCE: U.S. Department of Health and Human Services. (2011b). *Implementation guidance on data collection standards for race, ethnicity, sex, primary language, and disability status.* Retrieved from http://aspe.hhs.gov/datacncl/standards/ACA/4302

It will be important for scholars to advocate for routinely analyzing data by disability status and type, just as it has become common to analyze data by race and ethnicity. It is equally important that researchers make efforts to include people with disabilities in their research studies and refrain from creating disability exclusion criteria unless it is scientifically or medically necessary to do so (Williams & Moore, 2011).

3. Strengthen the Health and Human Services Workforce Capacity

The National Council on Disability (2009) indicates that the absence of adequate disability-related training for healthcare professionals is one of the most pressing barriers to health equity for people with disabilities. Repeated recommendations exist for improving training of the public health and clinical workforces on disability issues. Three necessary areas of training include (a) disability awareness training for all public health workers and clinicians, (b) discipline-specific training on relevant aspects of disability, and (c) building infrastructure for core leadership training of health professionals to address disability issues across the life span.

Healthy People 2020 included a goal to increase the number of U.S. Master of Public Health–granting public health training programs that offer coursework in disability from 50% to 55% by 2020 (DHHS, 2010). Even if this goal is realized, just over half of the public health workforce will have the *option* to complete disability-related coursework—such courses would not be required. Additional efforts to infuse disability concepts into public health education accreditation standards are needed so that *all* public health students are required to receive content on disability.

4. Include People With Disabilities in All Public Health Programs and Services

Public health entities, such as local and state health departments, are often remiss to explicitly and intentionally include individuals with disabilities in mainstream programs, services, and research. The use of the term "mainstream" refers to programs and services designed to reach the general population, rather than specific or targeted programs examining issues related to disability (Office of Disease Prevention and Health Promotion, n.d.). Including people with disabilities within program policies and services offered by local health departments is an important step toward achieving disability health equity (Lyons, Hoglind, & Vinoski Thomas, 2019). The National Association of County and City Health Officials' (NACCHO) Health and Disability Program offers an annual, no-cost technical assistance program to which local health departments who are interested or need assistance in improving their disability inclusion can apply (NACCHO, n.d.).

5. Ensure Preparedness for Emergencies to Protect Health and Save Lives

During anthropogenic and natural emergencies, individuals with disabilities are less likely to be evacuated and more likely to die (WHO, 2013). There are structural issues to evacuation, such as lacking specialized evacuation equipment, and insufficient preparation for individual issues that arise based on individual needs of people with disabilities. Federal initiatives such as a 2004 executive order that established the Interagency Coordinating Council on Emergency Preparedness and Individuals with Disabilities have set precedent for increasing attention to the needs of people with disabilities, older adults, and others with functional and access needs within emergency preparedness and response planning. The NACCHO technical assistance program mentioned previously also actively assists local health departments with revising their emergency preparedness plans to be more inclusive and connecting health department staff with local disability-serving organizations (e.g., University Centers for Excellence on Developmental Disabilities, Statewide Independent Living Council, State Council on Developmental Disabilities) to better understand the needs of their constituents.

BEST PRACTICES FOR DESIGNING PROGRAMS TO ADDRESS DISABILITY HEALTH DISPARITIES

As researchers, clinicians, and practitioners develop initiatives to address health disparities faced by people with disabilities, it is important that *community-based approaches* that are responsive to needs identified by individuals with disabilities and initiatives that leverage emerging technologies that promote the *full inclusion* of people with disabilities in all programs and services are considered.

Best-Practice Approach: Community-Based Participatory Research

Community-based participatory research (CBPR) is a framework that emphasizes the importance of equal involvement among researchers and community members in all phases of the research and program development process (Freire, 1970; Lewin, 1947; Minkler, 2005). Although CBPR approaches are most commonly used in research and program development initiatives with racially and ethnically diverse communities, CBPR has been successfully used within various disability communities, including individuals with intellectual and developmental disabilities (e.g., Ham et al., 2004; Nicolaidis et al., 2015) and people with autism (e.g., Nicolaidis et al., 2011). The overarching goal of CBPR is to ensure all research and programming is inclusive of and responsive to the needs of communities.

As discussed in more detail in Chapter 4, Health Equity Research and Collaboration Approaches, the key components of a CBPR approach to research and program development include (a) considering the community as a unit of identity; (b) leveraging the strengths and resources of the community in program development; (c) promoting shared learning and decision-making among research partners; (d) striking a balance between research and community action that benefits the scientific community and the individuals with lived experience; (e) emphasizing the relevance of community-defined, rather than researcher-defined, problems; (f) using iterative processes to develop and maintain community–research relationships; (g) disseminating knowledge gained from CBPR projects back to and by all involved partners; and (h) establishing long-term commitment from all partners (Holkup, Tripp-Reimer, Salois, & Reinert, 2004; Israel et al., 2003). The approach aligns well with the phrase "nothing about us without us," which is foundational to disability advocacy (Charlton, 1998) and refers to the fundamental right people with disabilities have to be centered in all processes that involve their well-being.

Best-Practice Approach: Universal Design

Many researchers develop health education and promotion programs that are specifically targeted toward the disability community, with varying degrees of success in improving health outcomes among the disability population. Although some types of programs (particularly those at the pilot and feasibility phases) might benefit from this exclusive approach, it is considered a best practice to develop health programs that are fully *inclusive of*, but not *specific to*, individuals with disabilities. A promising framework to support inclusive program design is Universal Design. Universal Design (Mace, Hardie, & Place, 1991; Story, Mueller, & Mace, 1998) is a framework aimed to guide advances in access and equity for individuals with disabilities. The framework guides the creation of structures, environments, and products in a way that maximizes their utility by all people and reduces or removes the need for adaptation, modification, or specialized design (Center for Universal Design, 1997), thereby eliminating barriers considered by the social model to produce disability. Universal Design is rooted in the field of architecture and has been applied within education systems to maximize outcomes for students with disabilities (Bowe, 2000; Mole, 2012) and within research to guide the successful recruitment and retention of participants with disabilities (Williams & Moore, 2011). It is becoming increasingly important for researchers and clinicians to consider aspects of Universal Design in the development of health programs to reach and adequately serve individuals with disabilities and other groups who experience access issues. Universally designed health programs aimed to improve health equity for persons with disabilities should ensure recruitment of potential participants who meet the program inclusion criteria, regardless of their disability status; provide multiple, flexible pathways by which participants can participate in and benefit from the program; and include individuals with disabilities living in the community and people who have expertise working in the area of disability research in the design and evaluation of programs (Williams & Moore, 2011).

INTERSECTIONALITY SPOTLIGHT

People with disabilities comprise the largest minority group in the U.S. and include people representing all historically disadvantaged and underrepresented racial, ethnic, gender, and geographic groups. Among the broad and heterogeneous population of people with disabilities, further disparities exist among people who have disabilities *and* identify with other intersectional identities. Indeed, disability is considered a phenomenon that amplifies the magnitude of health disparities experienced by individuals from minority groups (Blick, Franklin, Ellsworth, Havercamp, & Kornblau, 2015). The experience of living with disability and belonging to another marginalized group has been described as experiencing a "double burden" due to the compounding of health inequities experience by these groups (DHHS, 2011a).

For example, Black and Latinx populations experience higher prevalence of disability than non-Hispanic White greater populations, and Black and Latinx individuals with disabilities have greater health disparities than Black and Latinx individuals without disabilities (Blick et al., 2015). Data from the 2011 Behavioral Risk Factor Surveillance System show that people from diverse racial and ethnic groups with disabilities are disproportionately more likely to report having fair or poor health, have a chronic health condition, and have poorer access to healthcare than individuals from racial and ethnic minority groups who do not have disabilities (Drum, McClain, Horner-Johnson, & Taitano, 2011).

Similarly, the prevalence of disability is high in transgender communities (nearly 40% of the population report having some type of disability), and people who identify as transgender *and* have a disability experience poorer health access and outcomes than those who are transgender and do not have a disability and those who have a disability and do not identify as transgender (James et al., 2016). For example, the National Center for Transgender Equality's 2015 survey suggested that transgender respondents with disabilities were nearly twice as likely as transgender respondents without disabilities to report experiencing psychological distress (59% vs. 31%; James et al., 2016). Contributing to this and other disparities faced by this population is likely the alarmingly high rates of interpersonal violence experienced by both people who are transgender and people with disabilities (Kattari, Walls, & Speer, 2017).

National data suggest the prevalence of all types of disability is higher in rural U.S. counties than in urban counties, and that these disparities persist across race, gender, and age subgroups (Seekins & Greiman, 2014; von Reichert, Greiman, & Myers, 2017). People with disabilities who live in rural areas have increased difficulty accessing healthcare (University of Montana Rural Research & Training Center on Disability in Rural Communities [UMRTC], 2017). They also have lower employment rates and have more difficulty finding accessible housing and transportation compared with those with disabilities who live in urban and suburban areas, which may further compound existing health disparities (UMRTC, 2017).

It will be important for researchers, clinicians, and community members to continue to advocate for including people with disabilities in health disparities research and programs and to conduct research and develop programs aimed at reducing health disparities among people with disabilities who are members of other historically disadvantaged groups. Although the National Institute on Minority Health and Health Disparities (NIMHD) does not currently

(*continued*)

recognize individuals with disabilities as a health disparity population, the institute recently released a statement indicating their interest in funding proposals that explore health disparities at the intersections of disability and other disadvantaged identities (NIMHD, 2019). This may serve as an important step toward improving resource allocation to address health disparities faced by individuals living at the intersections of multiple marginalized identities.

CASE STUDY   ADDRESSING HEALTHCARE BARRIERS FOR INDIVIDUALS WITH DISABILITIES

Individuals with disabilities experience difficulty accessing the care they need to be healthy. One woman with a visual impairment described specific challenges she faces when searching for health information and when visiting healthcare providers. She first discussed the lack of adequate digital health information that is accessible to people with visual impairments. She described that although many people can find useful health information on the web, it can be more difficult for people with visual impairments to access this same information due to widespread use of inaccessible web formats. She also discussed the need to ensure that online patient portals that are designed to facilitate scheduling appointments, viewing test results, and contacting providers are broadly accessible to people with visual impairments and other disabilities.

Another point this woman discussed was, when providers do not use online portals or when online portals are inaccessible to her, she is asked to fill out paperwork when she arrives at the provider's office. Providers do not always have large print versions of their patient paperwork on hand. As an accommodation, she is usually paired with a staff member who can help her complete the paperwork. A major barrier she has faced in these scenarios is that she is often asked to answer the questions out loud in the provider's waiting room, where other patients may be able to hear her answers. She has been hesitant to fully describe symptoms or answer all questions in these scenarios due to the lack of privacy provided. Asking these questions out loud where others are present may also be a violation of the Health Information Portability and Accountability Act of 1996 (HIPAA).

The concept of *Universal Design*, discussed earlier in this chapter, can be used to develop solutions to the healthcare barriers this individual described. All individuals and organizations who provide digital health information should ensure the accessibility of the information to the broadest possible populations. This can be realized by using larger print and less complex language, which can benefit many groups (e.g., older adults, youth, young adults) in addition to people with disabilities. Increasing access to digital health information can also be realized by following the guidelines set forth within Section 504 of the Rehabilitation Act of 1973 and in the Web Content Accessibility Guidelines (WCAG) 2.0, which are referenced in the Patient Protection and Affordable Care Act of 2010. Web designers can access free web-based tools, or receive technical assistance, to assess website accessibility. Web Accessibility In Mind (WebAIM, n.d.) is one example of an organization that provides these services.

Other *Universal Design* solutions in this context would be for providers to consider offering a small private space for all individuals and families requiring assistance in completing their

(continued)

health paperwork and/or for providers to offer the option of completing health questionnaires using Audio Computer-Assisted Self-Interview (ACASI) software. These services would benefit individuals with many types of disabilities—and may also benefit those who use English as a second language, families with young children, those with low literacy, older adults, and others.

CURRENT EVENT

FAIR LABOR STANDARDS ACT

Under Section 14(c) of the Fair Labor Standards Act, employers can receive waivers that allow them to pay workers with disabilities less than the federal minimum wage if the disability affects their job performance. Department of Labor data reveal that over 150,000 U.S. workers are covered under the 14(c) exemption. Because of emerging concerns regarding not only abuse of the system, but its fundamental assertion that individuals with disabilities are "inferior" workers, several states have subsequently banned the exemption, implementing laws that require minimum wage be paid to all workers. Many legislators have called for a phase-out of the initiative nationwide, with supporters stating it would create parity for workers with disabilities and opponents stating it would limit employment opportunities for individuals with disabilities.

Discussion Question: Does allowing a federal exemption to pay workers with disabilities less than minimum wage inherently devalue individuals themselves? What alternative ways could policies encourage employment of individuals with disabilities?

DISCUSSION QUESTIONS

- Which model of disability health disparities/health equity identified in this chapter aligns most closely with your professional values? With your personal values? Describe why.

- Think about a health education/promotion initiative that you are familiar with (e.g., a program you have read about, worked on, seen a news story about). Describe two ways you could modify this program to make it more inclusive of and accessible to people with disabilities.

- List and describe three factors that influence health disparities for people with disabilities in a specific area of health that you are interested in (e.g., sexual health, environmental health).

- Select one of the five identified actions under which ongoing initiatives exist to improve health equity. Identify and discuss another initiative that could help improve disability health equity in that action area.

- How could you apply one of the best practices identified in designing programs to improve health equity within an intersectional population of people with disabilities (e.g., people with disabilities from communities of color, people with disabilities who are gender nonconforming)?

REFERENCES

Altman, B. M., & Bernstein, A. (2008). *Disability and health in the United States, 2001–2005.* Hyattsville, MD: National Center for Health Statistics. Retrieved from https://www.cdc.gov/nchs/data/misc/disability2001-2005.pdf

Beaudry, J. (2016). Beyond (models of) disability? *Journal of Medicine and Philosophy, 41,* 210–228. doi:10.1093/jmp/jhv063

Blick, R. N., Franklin, M. D., Ellsworth, D. W., Havercamp, S. M., & Kornblau, B. L. (2015). *The double burden: Health disparities among people of color living with disabilities.* Retrieved from https://nisonger.osu.edu/sites/default/files/u4/the_double_burden_health_disparities_among_people_of_color_living_with_disabilities.pdf

Bowe, F. G. (2000). *Universal design in education: Teaching nontraditional students.* Westport, CT: Bergin and Garvey.

Center for Universal Design. (1997). *The principles of universal design, version 2.0.* Raleigh: North Carolina State University. Retrieved from https://projects.ncsu.edu/ncsu/design/cud/about_ud/udprinciplestext.htm

Centers for Disease Control and Prevention. (n.d.). *Disability datasets.* Retrieved from https://www.cdc.gov/ncbddd/disabilityandhealth/datasets.html

Charlton, J. I. (1998). *Nothing about us without us: Disability, oppression and empowerment.* Berkeley: University of California Press.

Cheak-Zamora, N. C., & Thullen, M. (2017). Disparities in quality and access to care for children with developmental disabilities and multiple health conditions. *Maternal and Child Health Journal, 21,* 36–44. doi:10.1007/s10995-016-2091-0

Chevarley, F. M., Thierry, J. M., Gill, C. J., Ryerson, A. B., & Nosek, M. A. (2006). Health, preventive health care, and health care access among women with disabilities in the 1994–1995 National Health Interview Survey, Supplement on Disability. *Women's Health Issues, 16,* 297–312. doi:10.1016/j.whi.2006.10.002

Donoghue, C. (2003). Challenging the authority of the medical definition of disability: An analysis of the resistance to the social constructionist paradigm. *Disability & Society, 18*(2), 199–208. doi:10.1080/0968759032000052833

Drum, C., McClain, M. R., Horner-Johnson, W., & Taitano, G. (2011). *Health disparities chart book on disability and racial and ethnic status in the United States.* Durham: Institute on Disability, University of New Hampshire. Retrieved from https://iod.unh.edu/sites/default/files/media/Project_Page_Resources/HealthDisparities/health_disparities_chart_book_080411.pdf

Einfeld, S. L., Ellis, L. A., & Emerson, E. (2011). Comorbidity of intellectual disability and mental disorder in children and adolescents: A systematic review. *Journal of Intellectual and Developmental Disabilities, 36,* 137–143. doi:10.1080/13668250.2011.572548

Emerson, E., Fujiura, G. T., & Hatton, C. (2007). International perspectives. In S. L. Odom, R. H. Horner, M. Snell, & J. Blacher (Eds.), *Handbook on developmental disabilities* (pp. 593–613). New York, NY: Guilford Press.

Emerson, E., & Hatton, C. (2014). *Health inequalities and people with intellectual disabilities.* New York, NY: Cambridge University Press.

Engel, G. (1980). The clinical application of the biopsychosocial model. *American Journal of Psychiatry, 137,* 535–544. doi:10.1093/jmp/6.2.101

Freire, P. (1970). *Pedagogy of the oppressed.* New York, NY: Herder & Herder.

Ham, M., Jones, N., Mansell, I., Northway, R., Price, L., & Walker, G. (2004). 'I'm a researcher!' Working together to gain ethical approval for a participatory research study. *Journal of Learning Disabilities, 8*(4), 397–407. doi:10.1177/1469004704047507

Holkup, P. A., Tripp-Reimer, T., Salois, E. M., & Weinert, C. (2004). Community-based participatory research: An approach to intervention research with a Native American community. *Advances in Nursing Science, 27*(3), 162–175. doi:10.1097/00012272-200407000-00002

Hysing, M., Elgen, I., Gillberg, C., Lie, S. A., & Lundervold, A. J. (2007). Chronic physical illness and mental health in children: Results from a large-scale population study. *Journal of Child Psychology and Psychiatry, 48*, 785–792. doi:10.1111/j.1469-7610.2007.01755.x

Iezzoni, L. I., Kurtz, S. G., & Rao, S. R. (2014). Trends in US adult chronic disability rates over time. *Disability and Health Journal, 7*(4), 402–412. doi:10.1016/j.dhjo.2014.05.007

Israel, B. A., Schulz, A. J., Parker, E. A., Becker, A. B., Allen III, A. J., & Guzman, J. R. (2003). Critical issues in developing and following community-based participatory research principles. In M. Minkler & N. Wallerstein (Eds.), *Community-based participatory research for health* (pp. 53–76). San Francisco, CA: Jossey-Bass.

James, S. E., Herman, J. L., Rankin, S., Keisling, M., Mottet, L., & Anafi, M. (2016). *The report of the 2015 U.S. transgender survey.* Washington, DC: National Center for Transgender Equality. Retrieved from https://transequality.org/sites/default/files/docs/usts/USTS-Full-Report-Dec17.pdf

Kattari, S. K., Walls, N. E., & Speer, S. R. (2017). Differences in experiences of discrimination in accessing social services among transgender/gender nonconforming individuals by (dis)ability. *Journal of Social Work in Disability & Rehabilitation, 116*, 125–126. doi:10.1080/1536710X.2017.1299661

Krahn, G. L., Klein Walker, D., & Correa-de-Araujo, R. (2015). Persons with disabilities as an unrecognized health disparity population. *American Journal of Public Health, 105*, S198–S206. doi:10.2105/ajph.2014.302182

Lewin, K. (1947). Frontiers in group dynamics: II. Channels of group life; social planning and action research. *Human Relations, 1*(2), 143–153. doi:10.1177/001872674700100201

Linton, S. (1998). *Claiming disability: Knowledge and identity.* New York: New York University Press.

Lyons, S., Hoglind, T., & Vinoski Thomas, E. (2019). NACCHO's follow-up assessment of disability inclusion within local health departments. *Journal of Public Health Management and Practice, 25*(6), 616–618. doi:10.1097/PHH.1085

Mace, R. L., Hardie, G. J., & Place, J. P. (1991). Accessible environments: Toward universal design. In W. E. Presier, J. C. Vischer, & E. T. White (Eds.), *Design intervention: Toward a more human architecture.* New York, NY: Van Nostrand Reinhold.

McLeroy, K. R., Bibeau, D., Steckler, A., & Glanz, K. (1988). An ecological perspective on health promotion programs. *Health Education Quarterly, 15*(4), 351–377. doi:10.1177/109019818801500401

McPheeters, M. L., Davis, A. M., Taylor, J. L., Brown, R. F., Potter, S. A., & Epstein, R. A., Jr. (2014). Transition care for children with special health needs [Technical Brief No. 15]. Rockville, MD: Agency for Healthcare Research and Quality. Retrieved from https://effectivehealthcare.ahrq.gov/sites/default/files/pdf/children-special-needs-transition_technical-brief.pdf

Minkler, M. (2005). Community-based research partnerships: Challenges and opportunities. *Journal of Urban Health, 82*(2 Suppl. 2), ii3–ii12. doi:10.1093/jurban/jti034

Mole, H. (2012). A US model for inclusion of disabled students in higher education settings: The social model of disability and universal design. *Widening Participation and Lifelong Learning, 14*(3), 62–86. doi:10.5456/wpll.14.3.62

Moscoso-Pooras, M. G., & Alvarado, G. F. (2018). Association between perceived discrimination and healthcare-seeking behavior in people with a disability. *Disability and Health Journal, 11*, 93–98. doi:10.1016/j.dhjo.2017.04.002

National Academies of Sciences, Engineering, and Medicine. (2018). *People living with disabilities: Health equity, health disparities, and health literacy: Proceedings of a workshop.* Washington, DC: National Academies Press. doi:10.17226/24741

National Association of County and City Health Officials. (n.d.). *NACCHO empowers local health departments to include people with disabilities in all activities.* Retrieved from https://insight.livestories.com/s/v2/health-and-disability-ta-program/8e69890c-d850-4ef7-b52d-bf3549ee2394

National Center on Health, Physical Activity and Disability. (n.d.). *Community health inclusion assessment tools.* Retrieved from https://www.nchpad.org/1261/6287/Community~Health~Inclusion~Assessment~Tools

National Council on Disability. (2009). *The current state of health care for people with disabilities.* Washington, DC: Author. Retrieved from https://www.ncd.gov/rawmedia_repository/0d7c848f_3d97_43b3_bea5_36e1d97f973d.pdf

National Institute on Minority Health and Health Disparities. (2019). *Notice of NIMHD's interest in research on disability in health disparity populations* (notice # NOT-MD-19-007). Retrieved from https://grants .nih.gov/grants/guide/notice-files/NOT-MD-19-007.html

Newman, L. (2005). Postsecondary education participation of youth with disabilities. In M. Wagner, L. Newman, N. Cameto, N. Garza, & P. Levine (Eds.), *After high school: A first look at the post-school experiences of youth with disabilities; A report from the National Transition Study-2 (NLTS-2)* (pp. 4-1-4-17). Menlo Park, CA: SRI International. Retrieved from https://files.eric.ed.gov/fulltext/ED494935.pdf

Nicolaidis, C., Raymaker, D., Katz, M., Oschwald, M., Goe, R., Leotti, S., ... Powers, L. E. (2015). Community-based participatory research to adapt health measures for use by people with developmental disabilities. *Progress in Community Health Partnerships, 9*(2), 157–170. doi:10.1353/cpr.2015.0037

Nicolaidis, C., Raymaker, D., McDonald, K., Dern, S., Ashkenazy, E., & Boisclair, C. (2011). Collaboration strategies in nontraditional community-based participatory research partnerships: Lessons from an academic community partnership with autistic self-advocates. *Progress in Community Health Partnerships, 5*(2), 143–150. doi:10.1353/cpr.2011.0022

Office of Disease Prevention and Health Promotion. (n.d.). *Disability and health*. Retrieved from https:// www.healthypeople.gov/2020/topics-objectives/topic/disability-and-health

Okoro, C. A., Hollis, N. D., Cyrus, A. C., & Griffin-Blake, S. (2018). Prevalence of disabilities and health care access by disability status and type among adults—United States, 2016. *Morbidity and Mortality Weekly Report, 67*(32), 882–887. doi:10.15585/mmwr.mm6732a2

Oliver, M. (1990). *The politics of disablement*. London, UK: Palgrave Macmillan.

Parks, R. (2014). The rise, critique, and persistence of the DALY in global health. *The Journal of Global Health*. Retrieved from http://www.ghjournal.org/the-rise-critique-and-persistence-of-the-daly-in-global-health

Perkins, E. A., & Moran, J. A. (2010). Aging adults with intellectual disabilities. *Journal of the American Medical Association, 304*(1), 91–92. doi:10.1001/jama.2010.906

Rios, D., Magasi, S., Novak, C., & Harniss, M. (2016). Conducting accessible research: Including people with disabilities in public health, epidemiological, and outcomes studies. *American Journal of Public Health, 106*(12), 2137–2144. doi:10.2105/ajph.2016.303448

Seekins, T., & Greiman, L. (2014). *Map facts: Disability in rural America* [Policy Brief]. Retrieved from https://scholarworks.umt.edu/ruralinst_independent_living_community_participation/8/

Shandra, C. L. (2018). Disability as inequality: Social disparities, health disparities, and participation in daily activities. *Social Forces, 97*, 157–192. doi:10.1093/sf/soy031

Story, M. F., Mueller, J. L., & Mace, R. L. (1998). *The universal design file: Designing for people of all ages and abilities*. Raleigh: Center for Universal Design, North Carolina State University.

Stough, L. M., Ducy, E. M., & Kang, D. (2017). Addressing the needs of children with disabilities experiencing disaster or terrorism. *Current Psychiatry Reports, 19*(24), 1–10. doi:10.1007/s11920-017-0776-8

University of Montana Rural Research & Training Center on Disability in Rural Communities. (2017). *Research that leads to solutions for rural Americans with disabilities*. Retrieved from http://rtc.ruralinstitute .umt.edu/www/wp-content/uploads/RTC-Rural_ResearchSummary_2017.pdf

U.S. Department of Health and Human Services. (2010). *The Secretary's Advisory Committee on National Health Promotion and Disease Prevention Objectives for 2020. Phase I report: Recommendations for the framework and format of Healthy People 2020. Section IV. Advisory Committee findings and recommendations*. Retrieved from https://www.healthypeople.gov/sites/default/files/PhaseI_0.pdf

U.S. Department of Health and Human Services. (2011a). *Assuring health equity for minority persons with disabilities: A statement of principles and recommendations*. Retrieved from http://minorityhealth.hhs.gov/ assets/pdf/checked/1/acmhhealthdisparitiesreport.pdf

U.S. Department of Health and Human Services. (2011b). *Implementation guidance on data collection standards for race, ethnicity, sex, primary language, and disability status*. Retrieved from http://aspe.hhs .gov/datacncl/standards/ACA/4302

U.S. Department of Health and Human Services. (2014). Healthy People 2020. Retrieved from http://www .healthypeople.gov

von Reichert, C., Greiman, L., & Myers, A. (2017). *The geography of disability in America: On rural-urban differences in impairment rates* [Fact Sheet]. Retrieved from https://scholarworks.umt.edu/ruralinst_independent_living_community_participation/7/

Web Accessibility in Mind. (n.d.). Retrieved from http://www.webaim.org

White, P. H., & Cooley, W. C. (2018). Supporting the health care transition from adolescence to adulthood in the medical home. *Pediatrics, 142*(5), e20182587. doi:10.1542/peds.2018-2587

Williams, A. S., & Moore, S. M. (2011). Universal design of research: Inclusion of persons with disabilities in mainstream biomedical studies. *Science Translational Medicine, 3*(82), 82cm12. doi:10.1126/scitranslmed.3002133

World Health Organization. (2001). *International Classification of Functioning, Disability and Health.* Geneva, Switzerland: Author.

World Health Organization. (2002). *Towards a common language for functioning, disability and health.* Geneva, Switzerland: Author. Retrieved from http://www.who.int/classifications/icf/training/icfbeginnersguide.pdf

World Health Organization. (2011). *World report on disability 2011.* Malta, Europe: Author. Retrieved from http://www.who.int/disabilities/world_report/2011/report.pdf

World Health Organization. (2013). *Guidance note on disability and emergency risk management for health.* Geneva, Switzerland: Author. Retrieved from https://apps.who.int/iris/bitstream/handle/10665/90369/9789241506243_eng.pdf;jsessionid=8591D4481FA347D48F79212233BA191C?sequence=1

World Health Organization. (2018). *Disability and health.* Retrieved from https://www.who.int/news-room/fact-sheets/detail/disability-and-health

17

ACHIEVING HEALTH EQUITY FOR CHILDREN

JUDITH PALFREY

LEARNING OBJECTIVES

- Discuss the ways in which children's health disparities differ from adult health disparities
- Describe the health disparities faced by children who are African American and/or Hispanic
- Articulate the ways in which disparities in asthma are closely related to social determinants of health
- Describe the importance of ensuring access to primary and preventive care in eliminating children's health disparities
- Summarize recommendations for improving children's health across diverse populations

INTRODUCTION

The past century and a half has witnessed remarkable achievements in child health in the United States. Since 1950, the infant mortality rate has been reduced fivefold (Hunt & Chenoweth, 1961). Vaccines and antibiotics have nearly eliminated major childhood illnesses, including diphtheria, tetanus, measles, rubella, polio, and hemophilus influenza disease (Orenstein & Ahmed, 2017). Young people with conditions such as cystic fibrosis, childhood cancer, sickle cell anemia, and Down's syndrome whose lives would have been cut short two to three decades ago are living well into adulthood (Berry, Bloom, Foley, & Palfrey, 2010). Unfortunately, the benefits of all of these advances have not been enjoyed in equal measure by children from different parts of the American society. Disparities exist for many health conditions because societal and environmental influences determine how children's bodies form and grow, and experience determines how they think and feel. Moreover, the roots of some conditions actually lie within the fabric of unhealthy communities (drug abuse, homelessness, hopelessness, interpersonal and intergroup violence) and add to the vulnerability of children and their health (Holman et al., 2016).

Children's health is exquisitely sensitive to external determinants such as community and family context, secular trends and developments, societal governance, priorities, and structure. This is in part because infants and young children are literally dependent on these external forces and in part because older children and adolescents have relatively little ability to influence the larger forces that affect their health and development. Older adolescents begin to have a greater ability to make their own decisions and to influence the structures around them, but are also constrained in just how much influence they can have.

In this chapter, we outline the contours of the problem of health inequity for children by delineating some statistics drawn from U.S. sources. We then illustrate the situation by giving an example of the path through which societal inequity leads to poor health and developmental outcomes in a child with asthma.

Despite what can look like a very distressing picture, all is not bleak. There are tried and true interventions that are working all over the United States, in cities, towns, and rural environments. We share some of these ideas and provide bibliographic references for the reader to dig deeper into learning about the causes of and interventions for addressing disparities in child health.

INTERSECTIONALITY IN CHILDREN'S HEALTH

The United States spends over 17.8% of the gross domestic product (GDP) on healthcare, and still the healthcare status of our people is below that of most of the Organization for Economic Cooperation and Development (OECD) countries (Centers for Disease Control and Prevention [CDC], n.d.-a; Vasilis et al., 2017). A recent World Health Organization (WHO) study offered a scathing summary of the state of health in the United States saying, "The USA has the highest child and maternal mortality, homicide rate and body-mass index of any high income country.... Not only does the USA have high and rising health inequalities, but also life expectancy has stagnated or even declined in some population groups" (Vasilis et al., 2017, p. 1334). The WHO report attributes the poor performance "at least partly…to high and inequitable mortality from chronic diseases and violence, and insufficient and inequitable health care" (Vasilis et al., 2017, p. 1334).

A disparity is said to exist "[i]f a health outcome is seen to a greater or lesser extent between populations" (U.S. Department of Health and Human Services, 2019, para. 1). Such populations can be defined on the basis of age, gender, race or ethnicity, gender identity, sexual orientation, disability, or socioeconomic status or geographic location. For children, many of the most glaring disparities are found for children with intersectional identities: specifically, along racial/ethnic and socioeconomic lines. It is occasionally difficult to disentangle racial and ethnic correlations with health outcome from socioeconomic connections. As can be seen in Figure 17.1, for children, race/ethnicity and poverty are tightly linked. Within the field of health equity, it is often a challenge to disentangle data on child health outcomes with precision because data are sometimes collected in great detail about racial/ethnic characteristics for one child health outcome, but for socioeconomic characteristics for another.

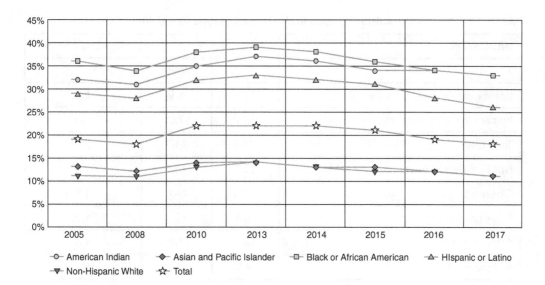

FIGURE 17.1 Children in poverty (100%) by age group and race and ethnicity in the United States.

SOURCE: Reproduced with permission from the Annie E. Casey Foundation, KIDS COUNT Data Center. (n.d.). *Children in poverty (100%) by age group and race and ethnicity in the United States*. Retrieved from https:// datacenter.kidscount.org/data/line/8447-children-in-poverty-100-by-age-group-and-race-and -ethnicity?loc=1&loct=1#1/any/false/871,870,573,869,36,133,35,16/asc/2757,4087,3654,3301,2322,2664l 140/17080

Some of the starkest child health disparities are related to differences in outcomes among children of different races. Table 17.1 presents the current differences in outcomes on a number of key child health indicators between non-Hispanic White and non-Hispanic Black children. Of grave concern is the wide gap in infant survival between Whites and Blacks. Why is it that Black babies are twice as likely to die before the first year of life than White babies? And how is it that the fruits of technologic advancement in obstetrics and newborn medicine have not been enjoyed by both racial/ethnic groups? We see this in the fact that 13.7% of non-Hispanic Black infants are born at low birth weight (LBW) as opposed to only 7.0% of non-Hispanic White babies (Martin, Hamilton, Osterman, Driscoll, & Drake, 2018). Moreover, teen births are often correlated with sociodemographic and ethnic factors. In 2016, the rate of births for non-Hispanic Black teens was 29.3 per 1,000 women, compared to 14.3 per 1,000 women for non-Hispanic White teens (Martin et al., 2018). These overall demographic trends in births and the contexts of those births have clear intersectional implications.

Beyond the newborn period, racial disparities in child health outcomes persist with higher rates of diseases such as asthma and obesity as well as higher rates of childhood death and significantly higher vulnerability to gun-related injuries and mortality. On the National Health Interview Survey, Black families sum all of these disparities up by reporting that their children are much more likely to be in fair or poor health than are White children (see Table 17.1).

TABLE 17.1 Health Disparities by Race in the United States: Black/White Differences

INDICATOR	RATE		BLACK/WHITE
	Black	White	Rate Ratio
Infant mortality[a]	11.4	4.9	2.3
Percent low birthweight[b]	13.7	7.0	2.0
Teen births[b]	29.3	14.3	2.0
Not in excellent or very good health[c]	21.1	13.6	1.6
Obesity (boys)[d]	19.0	14.6	1.3
Obesity (girls)[d]	25.1	13.5	1.9
Asthma currently[e]	12.8	7.9	1.6
Asthma mortality[e]	9.0	1.3	6.9
Gun-related deaths[f]	37.2	8.1	4.7

[a]Rate is per 1,000 live births in 2016; Centers for Disease Control and Prevention. (n.d.-b). *Infant mortality.* Retrieved from https://www.cdc.gov/reproductivehealth/maternalinfanthealth/infantmortality.htm

[b]Rates are percent of births and number of teen pregnancies (ages 15–19) per 1,000 women; Martin, J. A., Hamilton, B. E., Osterman, M. J. K., Driscoll, A. K., & Drake, P. (2018). *Births: Final data for 2016.* National Vital Statistics Reports, *67*(1), 1–55. Retrieved from https://www.cdc.gov/nchs/data/nvsr/nvsr67/nvsr67_01.pdf

[c]Percent replying child 0-18 is in good or fair/poor health; U.S. Department of Health and Human Services. (2018). *National health interview survey,* 2017. Retrieved from https://ftp.cdc.gov/pub/Health_Statistics/NCHS/NHIS/SHS/2017_SHS_Table_C-5.pdf

[d]Rate is percent of boys and girls from 2015 to 2016; Fryar, C. D., Carroll, M. D., & Ogden, C. L. (2018). *Prevalence of overweight, obesity, and severe obesity among children and adolescents aged 2–19 years: United States, 1963–1965 through 2015–2016.* Retrieved from https://www.cdc.gov/nchs/data/hestat/obesity_child_15_16/obesity_child_15_16.htm

[e]Rates are percent of children with asthma currently and number of deaths/million children attributed to asthma from 2004 to 2005; Akinbami, L. J., Moorman, J. E., Garbe, P. L., & Sondik, E. J. (2009). *Status of childhood asthma in the United States, 1980–2007* (Table 3). Retrieved from http://pediatrics.aappublications.org/content/123/Supplement_3/S131.long#F8. Table 3.

[f]Rate is deaths/100,000; Centers for Disease Control and Prevention, National Center for Injury Protection and Control. (n.d.). *WISQARS fatal injury reports, national, regional and state, 1981–2018.* Retrieved from https://webappa.cdc.gov/sasweb/ncipc/mortrate.html. Graph prepared by the AAP Research Department. Rate is deaths/100,000.

| CASE STUDY | ASTHMA |

To get a deeper look into the mechanisms at play in creating the kind of disparities in child health shown in the previously referenced tables and figures, we can look at the case of asthma: a highly prevalent condition that has been well-studied. There are several good theoretical frameworks about how social determinants play out for the outcome, providing the opportunity to more fully explore children's health equity through an applied lens. We begin with a composite vignette about a typical case of asthma.

Aidan is a 6-year-old boy who was born prematurely and spent several days in the newborn intensive care unit because of breathing problems. At age 2, he was diagnosed with asthma. He has "moderate persistent asthma," which means that he is sick much of the time with uncomfortable breathing, coughing at night, loss of sleep, and often loss of school and play. His parents are never 100% comfortable that he is "ok." His symptoms get much worse in the winter when it is wet and cold. Aidan lives in substandard housing with tight windows and a poorly functioning blown hot air heater. The neighborhood they live in is surrounded by industrial buildings, and there are few play spaces. His family is leery of him going outside anyway because there has been a high level of gang activity in the nearby open lots and side streets. After school, he mostly stays home and watches TV.

Aidan's parents do not own their apartment and have a very hard time getting the landlord to answer their calls for help with pest control. Also, there is peeling paint and a great deal of dust in the apartment. The family does not have a dog, but the neighbors do and Aidan loves to go by to play with Fuzzy.

For a long time, Aidan has been taking an inhaler of medicine when he gets symptoms. Sometimes it helps. Sometimes it does not, and his family have to ask a neighbor to help them get him to the local emergency department. This is hard because the neighbor works and they sometimes wait several hours for her to come home. When he gets to the emergency department, he often spends 4 or 5 hours under care. Fortunately, he has never had to be admitted to the hospital, but there have been a number of close calls where the doctors were considering putting him in the hospital for a day or 2. Whenever Aidan has an attack and an emergency department visit, he misses the next 2 or 3 days of school. His mother misses 2 to 3 days of pay from her work.

Fortunately, the family does have public medical insurance and have been able to receive the emergency care they need. They also have been able to obtain the medications that are prescribed by the doctors. They are grateful for this because they well remember when they could not get insurance for Aidan a few years ago and often had to put off filling his prescriptions because they did not have enough money to buy them.

Asthma is a disease of the breathing tubes that particularly affects children. Children are particularly prone to asthma because their bronchial tubes are small and narrow and very sensitive to outside stimulation from particulate matter in the air, allergens in the environment, smoke (including tobacco smoke), and from changing humidity levels when there are weather shifts. In Aidan's case, the most likely "triggers" for his asthma are coming largely from his home and neighborhood environment. Living near industrial plants, the air around his home is likely polluted with noxious particulate matter, and when the weather turns bad, the air pollutants hover closer to the streets and homes of the neighborhood. Inside, Aidan is also likely coming into contact with dust, mold, and, possibly, with cockroaches and rodents. While the family does not have a dog, Aidan may bring home some of Fuzzy's hairs on his clothing. All of these allergens very commonly bring on the tightening of the breathing tubes and cause the typical symptoms of wheezing, coughing, and shortness of breath.

Figure 17.2 shows the rate of asthma emergency department visits for 3-to 5-year-old children by neighborhood in Boston for the years 2012 to 2015. The disparity in neighborhoods is clearly delineated. Roxbury and Dorchester are neighborhoods with high housing density, numerous industrial and waste sites, and lower income levels than the city average. It is instructive to compare the emergency department visits in these neighborhoods with the other neighborhoods of Boston.

The other concern for children with asthma like Aidan is whether they have easy access to high-quality medical care as alluded to by the WHO statement mentioned earlier. While families

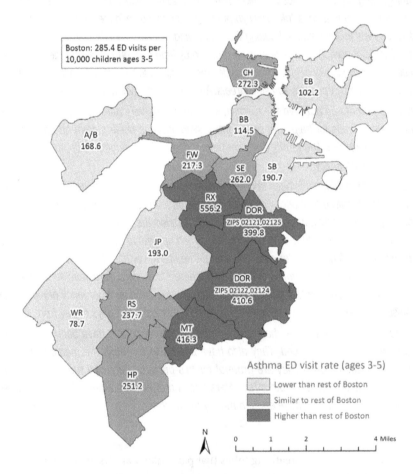

FIGURE 17.2 Asthma emergency department (ED) visits among 3- to 5-year-olds by Boston neighborhoods, 2012–2015.

NOTE: Four-year average annual rates per 10,000 children aged 3 to 5 years. "BB" includes Back Bay, Beacon Hill, Downtown, the North End, and the West End. "SE" includes the South End and Chinatown.
Data source: Acute hospital case-mix databases, Massachusetts Center for Health Information and Analysis.
SOURCE: Reproduced from Boston Public Health Commission Research and Evaluation Office. (2015). *Health of Boston 2014–2015* (Figure 8-15). Retrieved from http://www.bphc.org/healthdata/health-of-boston-report/Documents/11_C8_Chronic%20Dis_16-17_HOB_final-11.pdf

in cities like Boston theoretically have very good health insurance coverage and are surrounded by superb medical facilities—including a well-functioning community health center network—there continue to be access barriers for the kind of preventive and therapeutic health services that could benefit the children most. These barriers include lack of transportation, limited hours of primary care center appointments, difficulty with access to specialist care, language and cultural barriers, structural racism, and inadequate attention in medical facilities to inherent implicit bias toward groups who are poor or from a racial or ethnic group that is different from that of the professional staff. While some of these last barriers play out in subtle ways, they are very real and need serious attention. Sara Rosenbaum, one of the country's experts on Medicaid, wrote years ago about the high cost of being poor. She said that even if the financial access to healthcare was solved, poor families would still encounter "cost, poor services in poor communities, cultural and communications barriers, fear of the health system, and general overall problems in the relationships between patients and providers" (Rosenbaum, 2003, p. 665).

So, knowing all this, is anything happening to improve health equity for children?

Let's look again at the case of asthma to see what is happening. Dr. Laura Akinbami of the CDC has been closely monitoring the associations and trends in asthma in the United States for the past three decades, and she is beginning to see some welcome signs of improvement in racial disparities in asthma prevalence. Akinbami and her group have carefully followed the prevalence of asthma among children since 1980. They initially demonstrated a doubling of asthma prevalence from 1980 to 1995, with a period of slower increases from 2001 to 2010. Recently, they have shown that the asthma prevalence has reached a steady state with a suggestion of a slight decline. They have also demonstrated that the non-Hispanic Black–White disparity has stopped increasing because the prevalence among non-Hispanic Black children has "plateaued" (Akinbami, Simon, & Rossen, 2015).

These changes are not coming by accident, but rather by principled and practical approaches to the prevention and care of asthma. While some of the approaches are specific to asthma, many of them are generalizable and can transform the way much of child healthcare delivery is conducted.

BASIC SOLUTIONS TO PROMOTE HEALTH EQUITY (AND HOW THEY PLAY OUT IN ASTHMA)

All American Families Should Have High-Quality Health Insurance Coverage

The United States is the only OECD nation that excludes large percentages of people from the healthcare insurance system (Vasilis et al., 2017). Uninsured people suffer greater healthcare problems than insured people and cost the system more because they often need and use more costly care than do insured people. Multiple studies demonstrate significant improvement in access to quality healthcare when insurance coverage is assured (Szilagyi, Schuster, & Cheng, 2009). For families like Aidan's, it is critical that both he and his family are covered with health insurance. Through the Patient Protection and Affordable Care Act (ACA; and the activities that preceded its passage), for the most part, children in poverty have the right to healthcare insurance and, in most states, are seeing the benefits of access to Medicaid and Children's Health Insurance Program (CHIP). But some families who live just above the poverty line struggle to maintain adequate coverage and even may sacrifice a job opportunity because it means losing health insurance coverage for their children.

The expansion of Medicaid through the ACA has been a boon for millions of people like Aidan's parents, who can afford medical care when they are sick and access preventive health services to keep them well as long as this component of the ACA is kept intact. Without this coverage, families like Aidan's may need to make hard choices when they themselves are sick.

All Americans Should Have Access to Comprehensive Primary and Preventive Care

Most countries with advanced healthcare systems invest heavily in primary care. In the U.S., we have good proof of the effectiveness of primary care. Over the past decades, largely thanks to Medicaid, there has been steady progress and successes in the health and development of our children. Increasingly, providers in primary care settings are using more sophisticated tools that acknowledge the existence of the social determinants of health and add-in interventions to address issues like sub-standard housing, food insecurity, immigration status uncertainty, and lack of community resources for health and mental health promotion.

In the case of asthma, one particularly effective primary care innovation has been the development of the Asthma Action Plan (Simon & Akinbami, 2016). As Akinbami and her team have shown, Asthma Action Plans are being used increasingly as a powerful tool in the prevention of asthma attacks and the care for asthma exacerbations when they do occur. Initially conceived of as a protocol to ensure consistency of care across treatment sites through expert panel–generated guidelines, Asthma Action Plans have evolved to serve additional interrelated functions: education, trust-building, and empowerment.

Using a Green-Yellow-Red iconic schema, Asthma Action Plans provide a practical method and a common language for healthcare providers and families to understand and talk about the asthma status of the child. When the child is in the Green Zone, s/he may only need to have the family monitor how s/he is doing and keep an eye out to avoid common triggers; additionally, the child may be prescribed a rescue medicine to use if s/he starts to wheeze. A child may also be in the Green Zone if s/he remains symptom free on the combination of daily preventive medicines plus the use of occasional rescue medicine. The Yellow Zone denotes that the child's symptoms are worsening and that s/he may need more frequent administration of the rescue medicines or that a visit to the healthcare facility is in order. The child is in the Red Zone when s/he is extremely sick and needs emergent intense therapy. In this situation, the child will usually end up being admitted to the hospital. Working with the Asthma Action Plan and following the child's progress closely, the healthcare provider and family can determine if the child has mild, moderate, or severe asthma and if s/he is likely to have intermittent or persistent symptoms.

With the common language of the Asthma Action Plan, parents can formulate a clear understanding of how asthma affects their children, allowing them to become a very active participant in the monitoring and appropriate adjusting of medications. The medication regimen for asthma is confusing, and the various inhaled medications all look very much alike. The Asthma Action Plan educates parents through hands-on learning. By the nature of working on the plan together, the Asthma Action Plan breeds a stronger trusting relationship with families of their healthcare team. Finally, the Asthma Action Plan empowers families to engage fully in the care of their children, which, in turn, promotes a sense of self-efficacy. A key principle in health equity is that families are partners in the healthcare provision for their children. The Asthma Action Plan facilitates this partnership in a very practical way.

In her studies, Akinbami has found there are disparities in access to Asthma Action Plans based on insurance coverage (with privately insured children having a greater likelihood of having an Asthma Action Plan than children on public insurance). Somewhat unexpectedly, however, she found that non-Hispanic Black children are more likely to have Asthma Action Plans than non-Hispanic White children. This may be related to the fact that non-Hispanic Black children tend to get sicker with their asthma than non-Hispanic White children. Nonetheless, this is a positive sign that providers are identifying children who need the tool and are using it increasingly to aid in the care of children with asthma.

Another innovation in primary care that is targeted at increasing equity in healthcare for children is the use of specific screening tools to document unmet needs of families (Garg, Toy, Tripodis, Silverstein, & Freeman, 2015). These screening tools identify the social factors that determine child health outcomes if they are left unattended. Andrew Garg and his team have shown that a screener for social determinants, such as WE CARE, can identify unmet needs among children who are at risk of poor health and developmental outcomes. In a cluster randomized trial conducted in eight community health centers, Garg showed that the WE CARE screener identified two or more unmet needs among nearly 70% of the children. In the intervention arm of the study, the WE CARE team was able to provide specific services to the families, and in follow-up, the WE CARE families were more likely to have an employed mother and children in day-care placements. The WE CARE families were more likely than the control families to have received fuel assistance and less likely to be living in homeless shelters.

For decades, academic medical providers have written extensive papers about the impact of poverty on child health. The documentation was beneficial, but did little to fundamentally change anything for the families and children. Recently, under the championship of Benard Dreyer during his American Academy of Pediatrics presidential year, pediatricians have begun to address poverty not only as a correlate of bad health outcomes but as a direct cause of ill health and delayed development (Council on Community Pediatrics, 2016). With this reframing of poverty as a "pathogen," healthcare providers are now incorporating screening for social determinants into practice and using their role as healthcare providers to intervene directly in addressing social determinants. Of course, to do this, healthcare providers need to partner actively with social service providers, lawyers, community resource agencies, and, most importantly, with families themselves.

One of the best ways for healthcare providers to partner is to engage community health workers (CHWs) who are embedded in the children's home communities and have firsthand knowledge of both the potential obstacles that families face and the resources in the community that can be of real assistance to the families (community-based organizations, settlement groups, churches, youth-serving organizations, the park service officers, local police, day care, and school personnel). CHWs can greatly expand the role of the primary healthcare provider, especially in addressing a disease like asthma that is so deeply affected by home-based and neighborhood conditions. There is a growing body of literature that demonstrates the very valuable role that CHWs can play in combating childhood asthma (Bhaumik et al., 2019; Nicholas, Hutchinson, Ortiz, & Klighr-Beall, 2005). As CHW-based programs continue to expand, it will be important that equal access to such programs across intersectional identities—for example, immigrant, rural—is ensured.

As an example, researchers at Boston Children's Hospital using a CHW home-visiting model for asthma have been able to demonstrate healthcare cost–savings that more than cover the funds needed for the program (Bhaumik et al., 2019). An example of such a program is the innovative WIN for Asthma program, which is designed specifically to be time limited. There is the explicit goal of the program to spend 9 months to a year partnering with parents and providing them with all the tools and resources that they need to be in a position to "graduate" from the program. This graduation is a sign of confidence in the families and signals that the families are being respected as being on a similar plane with the healthcare team. Such an attitude is a building block of a more equitable approach to families and children.

DARE TO DREAM

Health equity for children is currently an aspiration—a dream. We know that there are still many challenges in a world where many families suffer from the effects of poverty, racism, and increasingly from the lack of strong political will in the federal government to attack the problems many families face. At the same time, we have examples of forward movement even in the face of adversity, and it is a time when people who are truly interested in health equity can put into place evidence-based practices that work for children and families.

The following principles can be helpful in working to increase health equity for children:

1. Recognize the importance of community, neighborhood, and home factors.

2. Identify unmet day-to-day needs for basic services, such as housing, food security, safety, education, and financial planning.

3. Partner with families in making plans for their children's health and listen attentively to their description of barriers and obstacles.

4. Identify resources in the community and local neighborhoods that can assist families.

5. Treat families and children with respect and work toward empowering families.

6. Health equity requires common language and attitudes and a shared dream for the children's health and well-being.

7. Dare to dream.

INTERSECTIONALITY SPOTLIGHT

Hispanic children are at high risk for disparities on many child health indicators, but despite high rates of poverty among Hispanic families, we do not see the same vulnerability around infant outcomes. The infant mortality rate for Hispanic babies is comparable to that of non-Hispanic Whites at 5.0% (see Figure 17.3), and LBW is equally in the same range as the LBW rate for non-Hispanic Whites. Many studies are now focusing on identifying the "protective" social factors in Hispanic communities that may explain these positive outcomes (both in children and adults; see Chapter 6, Health Equity in U.S. Latinx Populations). In addition, finer-grained analyses are being conducted with subgroups of "Hispanics." As an example, Mexican Americans and Puerto Rican families have different rates of infant mortality: the infant mortality rate among Mexican Americans is 5.5/1,000, compared to 8.2/1,000 for families from Puerto Rico (MacDorman & Mathews, 2008). Thus, when considering the role of intersectionality in children's health outcomes, it is important to consider variations that exist within health disparity populations as well as between them.

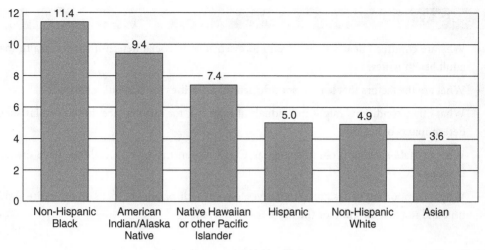

FIGURE 17.3 Infant mortality rates by race and ethnicity, 2016.

SOURCE: Centers for Disease Control and Prevention. (n.d.-b). *Infant mortality*. Retrieved from https://www.cdc.gov/reproductivehealth/maternalinfanthealth/infantmortality.htm

CURRENT EVENTS

SCHOOL-BASED HEALTH CENTERS

Nationally, school-based health centers (SBHCs, where fully functional doctors' offices are located on or adjacent to school grounds) have grown in popularity and presence. SBHCs allow students to go directly to a doctor's appointment without having to be transported and, in certain instances, without a parent or guardian present. While SBHCs do not replace school nurses, they help to expand upon the services of school nurses and provide direct access to care for many children who otherwise would not have access.

Discussion Question: How do SBHCs directly and indirectly address the social determinants of health that impact children's health disparities?

ANTI-VAXXERS

While the refusal to vaccinate one's child is something that has occurred as long as vaccinations themselves have existed, the anti-vaxxer movement in its current form is a relatively new phenomenon. Those who ascribe to anti-vaxxer rhetoric believe that vaccines are harmful and that ultimately they do more harm than good. The core issue with the anti-vaxxer movement is that it disrupts the delicate balance of herd immunity that protects children for whom vaccination is either unavailable or inaccessible—if too many children are voluntarily unvaccinated, there is no longer protection for those who are unable to get vaccines.

Discussion Question: How does a major shift in vaccination patterns have a disproportionate impact on children who are from a group impacted by disparities?

DISCUSSION QUESTIONS

- Why are children's health issues even more sensitive to social determinants of health than adult health issues?

- What are the factors that lead to specific health disparities for Hispanic children?

- What other conditions might individuals at high risk for asthma face due to similar social determinants of health?

- Why do state-specific programs such as CHIP not ensure that all children have medical insurance?

- Why is it important in designing initiatives to combat disparities to focus on the entire family unit and not just the child or the mother–child dyad?

REFERENCES

Akinbami, L. J., Moorman, J. E., Garbe, P. L., & Sondik, E. J. (2009). *Status of childhood asthma in the United States, 1980–2007*. Retrieved from http://pediatrics.aappublications.org/content/123/Supplement_3/S131.long#F8

Akinbami, L. J., Simon, A. E., & Rossen, L. M. (2015). Changing trends in asthma prevalence among children. *Pediatrics, 137*(1), e20152354. doi:10.1542/peds.2015-2354

Annie E. Casey Foundation, KIDS COUNT Data Center. (n.d.). *Children in poverty (100%) by age group and race and ethnicity in the United States*. Retrieved from https://datacenter.kidscount.org/data/line/8447-children-in-poverty-100-by-age-group-and-race-and-ethnicity?loc=1&loct=1#1/any/false/871,870,573,869,36,133,35,16/asc/2757,4087,3654,3301,2322,2664|140/17080

Berry, J., Bloom, S., Foley, S., & Palfrey, J. S. (2010). Health inequity in children and youth with chronic health conditions. *Pediatrics, 126*(s3), S111–S119. doi:10.1542/peds.2010-1466D

Bhaumik, U., Sommer, S. J., Lockridge, R. Penzias, R., Nethersole, S., & Woods, E. R. (2019). Community asthma initiative: Cost analyses using claims data from a Medicaid managed care organization. *Journal of Asthma*, 1–9. doi:10.1080/02770903.2019.1565825

Boston Public Health Commission Research and Evaluation Office. (2015). *Health of Boston 2014–2015*. Retrieved from http://www.bphc.org/healthdata/health-of-boston-report/Documents/11_C8_Chronic%20Dis_16-17_HOB_final-11.pdf

Centers for Disease Control and Prevention. (n.d.-a). *Health expenditures*. Retrieved from https://www.cdc.gov/nchs/fastats/health-expenditures.htm

Centers for Disease Control and Prevention. (n.d.-b). *Infant mortality*. Retrieved from https://www.cdc.gov/reproductivehealth/maternalinfanthealth/infantmortality.htm

Centers for Disease Control and Prevention/National Center for Injury Protection and Control. (n.d.). *WISQARS fatal injury reports, national, regional and state, 1981–2018*. Retrieved from https://webappa.cdc.gov/sasweb/ncipc/mortrate.html

Council on Community Pediatrics. (2016). Poverty and child health in the United States. *Pediatrics, 137*(4), e20160339. doi:10.1542/peds.2016-0339

Fryar, C. D., Carroll, M. D., & Ogden, C. L. (2018). *Prevalence of overweight, obesity, and severe obesity among children and adolescents aged 2–19 years: United States, 1963–1965 through 2015–2016*. Retrieved from https://www.cdc.gov/nchs/data/hestat/obesity_child_15_16/obesity_child_15_16.htm

Garg, A., Toy, S., Tripodis, Y., Silverstein, M., & Freeman, E. (2015). Addressing social determinants of health at well child care visits: A cluster RCT. *Pediatrics, 135*(2), e296–e304. doi:10.1542/peds.2014-2888

Holman, D. M., Ports, K. A., Buchanan, N. D., Hawkins, N. A., Merrick, M. T., Metzler, M., & Trivers, K. F. (2016). The association between adverse childhood experiences and risk of cancer in adulthood: A systematic review of the literature. *Pediatrics, 138*(s1), s81–s91. doi:10.1542/peds.2015-4268L

Hunt, E. P., & Chenoweth, A. D. (1961). Recent trends in infant mortality. *American Journal of Public Health*, *51*(2), 190–207. doi:10.2105/ajph.51.2.190

MacDorman, M. F., & Mathews, T. J. (2008). *Recent trends in infant mortality in the United States* (NCHS data brief, no. 9, pp. 1–8). Hyattsville, MD: National Center for Health Statistics. Retrieved from https://www.cdc.gov/nchs/data/databriefs/db09.pdf

Martin, J. A., Hamilton, B. D., Osterman, M. J. K., Driscoll, A. K., & Drake, P. (2018). Births: Final data for 2016. *National Vital Statistics Reports*, *67*(1), 1–55. Retrieved from https://www.cdc.gov/nchs/data/nvsr/nvsr67/nvsr67_01.pdf

Nicholas, S. W., Hutchinson, V. E., Ortiz, B., & Klighr-Beall, S. (2005). Reducing childhood asthma through community-based service delivery—New York City, 2001–2004. *Morbidity and Mortality Weekly Review*, *54*(1), 11–14. Retrieved from https://www.cdc.gov/mmwr/preview/mmwrhtml/mm5401a5.htm

Orenstein, W. A., & Ahmed, R. (2017). Simply put: Vaccination saves lives. *Proceedings of the National Academy of Sciences of the United States of America, 114*(16), 4031–4033. doi:10.1073/pnas.1704507114

Rosenbaum, S. (2003). Racial and ethnic disparities in health care: Issues in the design, structure, and administration of federal healthcare financing programs supported through direct public funding. In B. D. Smedley, A. Y. Stith, & A. R. Nelson (Eds.), *Unequal treatment: Confronting racial and ethnic disparities in health care*. Washington, DC: National Academies Press. Retrieved from https://www.nap.edu/read/12875/chapter/25

Simon, A. E., & Akinbami, L. J. (2016). Asthma action plan receipt among children with asthma 2–17 years of age, United States, 2002–2013. *Journal of Pediatrics, 171*, 283–289. doi:10.1016/j.jpeds.2016.01.004

Szilagyi, P. G., Schuster, M. A., & Cheng, T. L. (2009). The scientific evidence for child health insurance. *Academic Pediatrics, 9*(1), 4–6. doi:10.1016/j.acap.2008.12.002

U.S. Department of Health and Human Services. (2018). *National health interview survey, 2017*. Retrieved from https://ftp.cdc.gov/pub/Health_Statistics/NCHS/NHIS/SHS/2017_SHS_Table_C-5.pdf

U.S. Department of Health and Human Services. (2019). *Disparities*. Retrieved from https://www.healthypeople.gov/2020/about/foundation-health-measures/Disparities

Vasilis, K., Bennett, J. E., Mathers, C. D., Li, G., Foreman, K., & Ezzati, M. (2017). Future life expectancy in 35 industrialised countries: Projections with a Bayesian model ensemble. *Lancet, 389*(10076), 1323–1335. doi:10.1016/S0140-6736(16)32381-9

THE PATH FORWARD

THE ROLE OF CULTURAL COMPETENCE AND CULTURAL HUMILITY IN ACHIEVING HEALTH EQUITY

ERIC K. SHAW

LEARNING OBJECTIVES

- Distinguish between the concepts of cultural competence and cultural humility
- Describe the components of the BELIEF and LEARN models
- Describe Purnell's model of cultural competence
- Contrast the Developmental Model of Intercultural Sensitivity and the Process of Cultural Competence in the Delivery of Healthcare Services Model
- Describe various models for improving cultural competence within the clinical education setting

INTRODUCTION

In this chapter, I focus on two concepts—cultural competency and cultural humility—as they relate to achieving health equity. Ultimately, this chapter is about the complexities of human interaction and social dynamics and is, therefore, relevant not only to medical professionals and "health equity agents" but to all persons who inevitably interact with diverse populations. I begin by (a) discussing key definitions and why cultural competence matters; (b) presenting a higher level way of understanding cultural competence; (c) discussing several models/frameworks; and (d) presenting contemporary evidence-based solutions for achieving cultural competency and humility in healthcare by focusing on several contexts (medical education, mental/behavioral health, and Lesbian, Gay, Bisexual, Transgender, Queer/Questioning [LGBTQ]).

What Is Cultural Competence and Cultural Humility?

The origins of cultural competence date back to the 1960s and 1970s when growing civil rights tensions were prompting new understandings of cultural diversity and greater attention to racial and ethnic inequalities in the U.S. The work of Cross, Bazron, Dennis, and Isaacs (1989) was fundamental in developing a philosophical framework of cultural competence that also incorporated practical application for improving certain healthcare services. Here, "cultural competence" was defined as "a set of congruent behaviors, attitudes, and policies that come together in a system, agency, or among professionals and enable that system, agency, or those professionals to work effectively in cross-cultural situations" (Cross et al., 1989, p. 13). Although Cross et al.'s early framework has been valuable in the development of cultural competency, many have noted its flawed underlying assumptions. As their title indicates, their work aimed at improving services to minority children who were severely emotionally disturbed. It was posited that new approaches or communication tools would help overcome cultural differences between the assumed "non-colored" clinician and the "colored" child (Paul, Ewen, & Jones, 2014). This early work influenced how cultural competence training and education was developed and implemented in the U.S. with underlying assumptions about who the learners are (e.g., White, male, heterosexual) and what they need to learn about the cultures of "different" (minority ethnic or other) groups (Rajaram & Bockrath, 2014). Critics have noted that these early definitions and underlying principles failed to address structural origins of societal inequalities and the systems of power and privilege that contribute to health disparities (Kumagai & Lypson, 2009; Powell Sears, 2012; Thackrah & Thompson, 2013).

More recent shifts in the conceptualization and enactment of cultural competency have addressed many of these earlier shortcomings by including many intersecting identities (e.g., race, ethnicity, sexual orientation, gender, religion, disability status, immigration status, education, age, socioeconomic status) that encompass an individual's culture (Notaro, 2012). Moreover, the focus has incorporated "the administration and bureaucracy of healthcare systems, systems of prejudice, stereotyping, the social determinants of health, and the impact to communities and systems within communities" (Notaro, 2012, p. 265). With these new developments in cultural competence, multiple definitions have emerged, still with most focusing on examining personal biases, understanding the worldview of others, and improving effective communication skills in cross-cultural encounters (Notaro, 2012). See Table 18.1 for definitions of cultural competency and other key terms used in this chapter.

Cultural humility is "the ability to maintain an interpersonal stance that is other-oriented (or open to the other) in relation to aspects of cultural identity that are most important to the [person]" (Hook, Davis, Owen, Worthington Jr, & Utsey, 2013, p. 2). Self-reflection "of one's own multidimensional and multiethnic identities, backgrounds, and an examination of biases and patterns of intentional and unintentional racism, classism, and homophobia" (Rajaram & Bockrath, 2014, p. 83) is paramount for developing cultural humility[1].

Why Cultural Competence Matters

Multiple data points indicate that the population of the U.S. is increasingly diverse. For example, in 1950, U.S.-born, non-Hispanic Whites comprised about 90% of the U.S. population. By 2010,

TABLE 18.1 Definitions of Key Concepts

CONCEPT	DEFINITION
Culture	Culture has been defined as an integrated pattern of learned beliefs and behaviors that can be shared among groups. It includes thoughts, styles of communicating, ways of interacting, views on roles and relationships, values, practices, customs, etc. Culture serves as a roadmap for both perceiving and interacting with the world. Iceberg theory of culture (see Penstone, 2011): The iceberg depicts the areas of culture that we can see manifest in the physical sense such as "visible" elements that include things such as music, dress, dance, architecture, language, food, gestures, greetings, and behaviors. They are shown as cultural characteristics above the water line—the tip of the iceberg. There are many other habits, assumptions, understandings, values, and judgments that we know but do not or cannot articulate that are depicted as hidden on the bottom side of the iceberg, the invisible side. When thinking about culture, the bottom of the iceberg will include things such as religious beliefs, worldviews, rules of relationships, approaches to the family, and motivations.
Cultural competence	Cultural competence "entails understanding the importance of social and cultural influences on patients' health beliefs and behaviors; considering how these factors interact at multiple levels of the health care delivery system (e.g., at the level of structural processes of care or clinical decision-making); and, finally, devising interventions that take these issues into account to assure quality health care delivery to diverse patient populations" (Betancourt, Green, Carrillo, & Ananeh-Firempong, 2003, p. 297). The NCCC of Georgetown University defines cultural competence of an organization as "a set of values and principles, and demonstrate[d] behaviors, attitudes, policies, and structures that enable them to work effectively cross-culturally" (n.d.-a, National Center for Cultural Competence, 1998).
Cultural humility	"A process that requires humility as individuals continually engage in self-reflection and self-critique as lifelong learners and reflective practitioners. It is a process that requires humility in how physicians bring into check the power imbalances that exist in the dynamics of physician–patient communication by using patient-focused interviewing and care" (Tervalon & Murray-García, 1998, p. 118).
Health disparities	Healthy People 2020 defines *health disparities* as "a particular type of health difference that is closely linked with social, economic, and/or environmental disadvantage. Health disparities adversely affect groups of people who have systematically experienced greater obstacles to health based on their racial or ethnic group; religion; socioeconomic status; gender; age; mental health; cognitive, sensory, or physical disability; sexual orientation or gender identity; geographic location; or other characteristics historically linked to discrimination or exclusion" (ODPHP, n.d.-a, para. 6).

(continued)

TABLE 18.1 Definitions of Key Concepts (*continued*)

CONCEPT	DEFINITION
Health equity	Healthy People 2020 defines *health equity* as the "attainment of the highest level of health for all people. Achieving health equity requires valuing everyone equally with focused and ongoing societal efforts to address avoidable inequalities, historical and contemporary injustices, and the elimination of health and health care disparities" (ODPHP, n.d.-a, para. 5). Health equity may involve "removing obstacles to health such as poverty, discrimination, and their consequences, including powerlessness and lack of access to good jobs with fair pay, quality education and housing, safe environments, and health care" (Braveman, Arkin, Orleans, Proctor, & Plough, 2017, p. 2).
Racism: three levels	"*Institutionalized racism* is defined as differential access to the goods, services, and opportunities of society by race. ... It is structural, having been codified in our institutions of custom, practice, and law." "*Personally mediated* racism is defined as prejudice and discrimination ... (it) can be unintentional, and it includes acts of commission as well as acts of omission." "*Internalized racism* is defined as acceptance by members of the stigmatized races of negative messages about their own abilities and intrinsic worth" (Jones, 2000, pp. 1212–1213).
Bias	The tendency among humans to make decisions based on cognitive factors instead of evidence. Bias becomes a concern when it interferes with how humans make impartial decisions.
Stereotype	A cognitive structure that contains the perceiver's knowledge, beliefs, and expectations about a group of people. Stereotypes are reflected in the preconceptions that one person has about another dependent on membership of a specific group. Stereotypes are common strategies that humans use to process and store information in a noncomplex manner. A stereotype is "a widely held image of a group of people through which individuals are perceived or the application of an attitude set based on the group or class to which the person belongs" (van Ryn & Burke, 2000, p. 814).
Unconscious or implicit bias	The unintentional activation of prejudicial attitudes toward a group based on stereotypes that have receded from consciousness overtime and have become invisible to the holder. These attitudes represent "overlearned associations with a strong affective basis that are difficult to completely overwrite with recent experiences or acquired values" (Dovidio & Fiske, 2012, p. 948). Unconscious or implicit biases result in an automatic reaction.
Discrimination	"Differential behavior or conduct of one person or group toward another person or group that is based on individual prejudice or societal norms that have institutionalized prejudicial attitudes" (NCCC, n.d.-b, "Discrimination")

NCCC, National Center for Cultural Competence; ODPHP, Office of Disease Prevention and Health Promotion.

the percentage of non-Hispanic Whites had decreased to about 69% (Laveist, 2014). By 2050, it is estimated that 50% of the U.S. population will consist of racial and ethnic minorities (Nair & Adetayo, 2019).

The landmark Institute of Medicine (IOM) report *Unequal Treatment: Confronting Racial and Ethnic Disparities in Healthcare* (Smedley, Stith, & Nelson, 2002) presented findings on inequities in healthcare quality among racial and ethnic minority patients. Predominately, these inequities were not due to lack of insurance or access to healthcare; rather some evidence pointed to healthcare providers' biases and prejudices (see also Laveist, 2014; Nelson, 2002). Since 2002, health equity agents have developed and implemented various efforts aimed at achieving greater health equity across not only racial groups but other groups that have faced their own forms of unequal healthcare treatment (e.g., LGBTQ, obese populations, persons with disabilities). Cultural competence training has been one of the key ways to address health and healthcare disparities (Rajaram & Bockrath, 2014).

Additionally, there is ample empirical evidence showing the value of cultural competence:

- Patients are less likely to comply with treatment if they do not understand it (Coleman-Miller, 2000; Vermeire, Hearnshaw, Van Royen, & Denekens, 2001) or if they have conflicting health beliefs (Vermeire et al., 2001).

- Members of "minority communities" or "communities of color" often perceive higher levels of discrimination in healthcare; this perception can lead to patient mistrust, which causes provider disengagement and results in less vigorous treatment.

- Being culturally competent as a physician and having a culturally competent healthcare organization can have administrative and operational efficiencies, reduced malpractice costs, compliance with legal requirements, and a more positive image in the community.

- Higher cultural competency scores predicted higher quality of care for children with asthma (Lieu et al., 2004).

- A group provided with a culturally competent smoking cessation intervention adapted for African Americans had a significantly higher rate of smoking cessation than the standard group (Orleans, Strecher, Schoenbach, Salmon, & Blackmon, 1989).

- Physicians self-reporting more culturally competent behaviors had patients who reported higher levels of satisfaction and were more likely to share medical information (Paez, Allen, Beach, Carson, & Cooper, 2009).

A 30,000 FOOT VIEW

This section takes a "30,000 foot view" of some key concepts from the scientific literature on social psychology in order to lay the groundwork for understanding current theory and research on cultural competence.

When's the last time you went to a restaurant and ordered a plate of bat … or dog … or horse? I will assume you answered "never." And if forced to eat one of those dishes, it's possible you would literally feel sick to your stomach. But there may be some groups who eat these foods regularly and enjoy doing so. Why is it that most Americans would deem these inedible while others may not share in these same "food rules"? In social psychology, the concepts of "lumping" and "splitting" provide valuable insights. Lumping is the mental process of "grouping 'similar' things together in distinct clusters" and splitting "involves perceiving 'different' clusters as separate from one another" (Zerubavel, 1996, p. 421; see Figure 18.1). In this example, we lump certain types of animal meat into a group that we have been socialized to accept as "edible," even though there is great variation in the kinds of animal meat that is included here. As we lump these various "edible" animals together, we (cognitively) highlight certain similarities and downplay or ignore differences. The complementary cognitive act of splitting, then, entails designating other animals as being in this other group deemed "inedible." Whereas lumping is done at the *intra*categorical level, splitting is done at the *inter*categorical level, whereby we highlight the differences and separateness of these mental clusters (such as edible vs. inedible meats). Now think for a moment about the ubiquitous ways in which we carve up the world into various clusters: everything from "strangers and acquaintances, fiction and nonfiction, business and pleasure, normal and perverse" (Zerubavel, 1996, p. 421) or the way we draw lines between types of music genres (classical or pop) or movies (drama vs. comedy vs. romantic comedy) or between political parties or racial identities.

We (re)create, live with, and use many, many of these categories every day. For example, we often hear or use phrases such as the Black community, LGBTQ community, Latinx community, etc. Why don't we hear political pundits talk about a blue-eyed community or the obese community? We have been socialized to lump members of a (e.g., Black) racial category into a "community" and cognitively split that community from other racial "communities." In this process of lumping and splitting, we are making assumptions that particular aspects of one's identity (e.g., skin color, hair type/color) are important for identifying/understanding the person *and* we assume that people who share these characteristics are similar—perhaps in terms of their values, beliefs, and behaviors. We do this, even though there are numerous similarities across racial groups and many variations within particular racial groups.

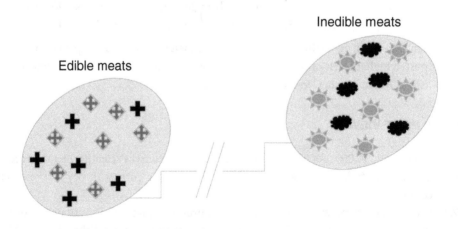

FIGURE 18.1 Lumping and splitting.

There is a tension we face whenever there is something that is both unique and also has commonalities with other things. As human beings, we are both unique individuals and also members of particular social environments, families, groups, and communities. Sue (2001) provides a useful framework for exploring personal identity. At the universal level, we all share certain biological and physical similarities (e.g., bleed when cut), common life experiences (birth, death, laughter, sadness, etc.), and have a level of self-awareness and an ability to use symbols (such as language; p. 793). The group level of personal identity encompasses the numerous categories to which we belong (race/ethnicity, religion, sexual orientation, disability status, etc.) that may be ascribed at birth or chosen or ascertained over one's life course. Some group-level categories may be more fluid and changeable than others. Lastly, at the individual level, "our unique genetic endowment guarantees that no two individuals are identical" (Sue, 2001, p. 794).

There is no one in the world the same as you, but if I met you for the first time, I would immediately (in micro-seconds) perceive certain features about you: your gender, age, skin color, hair type/style, height, clothing, etc. And I would use these, consciously or unconsciously, to start forming impressions about you, to understand you. Now, of course, we know we can't fully know a person based on a handful of these exterior cues, but we still use these—they are shortcuts that help us make the many social interactions we have manageable. These shortcuts can be helpful, but they can be problematic. Our perceptions may be misleading. And our assumptions about a particular individual based on group-level categories we think they belong to may be wrong. Such is the basis for stereotyping.

MODELS AND FRAMEWORKS

Multiple models and frameworks on cultural competence have been developed. Virtually all share some common elements (in accordance with the core definitional components as specified previously, see Table 18.1). However, there are differences in comprehensiveness across these models/frameworks. Therefore, I have *lumped and split* these into three categorical types: those that focus on or address elements at a micro-level, at a meso-level, or at a macro-level.

Micro-Level Models

There are a variety of models represented here typically developed using memorable acronyms. These tend to be geared towards practicing healthcare professionals and focus mainly on providing practical steps or strategies to better communicate in cross-cultural dyadic interactions (see Boxes 18.1 and 18.2).

Macro-Level Model

At the opposite end of this spectrum are models that aim to provide a more comprehensive and holistic understanding of cultural dynamics at multiple levels (e.g., individual, family, societal) and that can be used across disciplines and settings. The primary example at this level is Purnell's Model for Cultural Competence (Purnell, 2005, 2019).

BOX 18.1

THE BELIEF MNEMONIC

(Health) **B**eliefs: "What do you believe has caused your problem?"
Explanation: "Why do you think your illness/problem occurred at this time?"
Learn from the patient: "Help me understand what you feel/believe about this problem."
Impact: "What impact is this illness/problem having on you?"
Empathy
Feelings: "How are you feeling about this?"

BOX 18.2

THE LEARN MNEMONIC

Listen to and understand the patient's perception of the problem.
Explain your perceptions of the problem and your strategy of treatment.
Acknowledge and discuss the differences and similarities between these perceptions.
Recommend treatment while remembering the patient's cultural parameters.
Negotiate agreement. It is important to understand the patient's explanatory modes so that medical treatment fits in their cultural framework.

Purnell conceptualizes the development of cultural competence along an upward curve of learning and practice. An increasing level of achievement of competence views the practitioner moving through four levels: (a) from a stage of unconscious incompetence to (b) conscious incompetence, followed by (c) conscious competence, and finally (d) unconscious competence.

Purnell's model of cultural competence consists of two sets of factors that are described as the macro-aspects and micro-aspects. The macro aspects include the following:

- *Global Society*. Worldwide systems of politics, communication systems, commerce and economics, technologies and events, and the way these global systems shape the individual's or group's worldview form the global society.

- *Community*. A community is a group of people having a common interest or identity; goes beyond the physical environment to include the social and symbolic characteristics that cause people to connect.

- *Family*. Two or more people who are emotionally involved, whether they live together or not, may constitute a family. Family structure and roles vary.

- *The Person*. The person is conceptualized as "a biopsychosociocultural human being who is constantly adapting" (Purnell, 2005, p. 13).

The micro-aspects include Overview/Heritage, Communication, Family Roles and Organization, Workforce Issues, Biocultural Ecology, High-Risk Health Behaviors, Nutrition, Pregnancy and Childbearing Practices, Death Rituals, Spirituality, Healthcare Practices, and Healthcare Practitioners.

Overall, the model should be understood as a framework for thinking about one's cultural competency. This needs to be a conscious process in which the individual (over time):

- Develops an awareness of one's own culture and environment.

- Gains understanding of the patients' culture, health-related needs, and meanings of health and illness.

- Accepts and respects cultural differences.

- Does not assume that the healthcare provider's beliefs and values are the same as the patient's.

- Resists judgmental attitudes.

- Is open to cultural encounters.

- Adapts care to be congruent with the patient's culture.

Meso-Level Models

At this midrange level, we find models that fall between the micro- and macro-levels or reveal connections between the micro- and macro-levels. One example is Bennett's *Developmental Model of Intercultural Sensitivity* (DMIS; Bennett, 2004).

Developmental Model of Intercultural Sensitivity

Like Purnell's model, the DMIS depicts a developmental process: in this case, movement from *ethnocentrism* ("the experience of one's own culture as 'central to reality' ") to *ethnorelativism* ("the experience of one's own beliefs and behaviors as just one organization of reality among many viable possibilities"; Bennett, 2004). Additionally, Bennett depicts a typology of six different experiences that occur during the personal development process. The three ethnocentric stages of development include:

Stage 1: Denial—disinterest in cultural difference and denies that cultural differences exist;
Stage 2: Defense—acknowledges the existence of cultural differences, but "one's own culture is experienced as the only viable one—the most 'evolved' "; consequently, other cultures are considered threatening to his/her sense of self;
Stage 3: Minimization—"elements of one's own cultural worldview are experienced as universal" (Bennett, 2004); consequently, one may acknowledge cultural differences, but downplays them, believing that human similarities outweigh human differences (Ware, 2012).

As an individual progresses through the previous stages (though not necessarily in linear fashion), the next three ethnorelative stages include:

Stage 4: Acceptance—recognizes and values cultural differences and thus recognizes others as different but "equally human";
Stage 5: Adaptation—"the experience of another culture yields perception and behavior appropriate to that culture"; "one's worldview is expanded to include relevant constructs from

other cultural worldviews"; unlike "assimilation," adaptation "involves the extension of your repertoire of beliefs and behavior, not a substitution of one set for another";

Stage 6: Integration—"one's experience of self is expanded to include the movement in and out of different cultural worldviews."

As a point of emphasis, the DMIS reflects changes in one's *worldview* and, therefore, does not assert that merely gaining more knowledge about a culture or greater skill in communicating with someone from a different culture will necessarily lead to progression of the stages. Moreover, Bennett (2004) disavows the idea that "more interculturally sensitive people are generally *better* people." Rather, the model posits that those who have achieved an ethnorelativistic worldview are "better at experiencing cultural differences than are more ethnocentric people and therefore are probably better at adapting to those differences in interaction."

EVIDENCE-BASED SOLUTIONS

With the immense growth of writing and research on cultural competence, this section provides evidence-based solutions—including insights from what has worked and has not worked well—within several specific contexts. While there are important insights that may transcend any particular context, these are organized as medical education, mental/behavioral health, and LGBTQ contexts.

Medical Education

Cultural competence training for health providers has focused largely on patient–provider or other types of interpersonal dynamics related to health and healthcare. A recent systematic literature review showed there to be low quality of evidence in studies that have assessed the impact of cultural competence education on health outcomes (Horvat, Horey, Romios, & Kis-Rigo, 2014). Some research has shown that few cultural competence education programs explicitly mentioned or dealt with racism, bias, or discrimination, prompting calls for new efforts to incorporate content on social justice and advocacy (Sauaia, 2014) and to address the underlying determinants of healthcare disparities (Paul et al., 2014). New curricular innovations started within the past 5 years have attempted to address these and other shortcomings. Three case studies are presented.

Structural Competency: Vanderbilt University

Aiming to extend cultural competency educational efforts beyond individual clinical interactions, Metzl and Hansen (2014) developed a new conceptual model they call "structural competency" (www.structuralcompetency.org). This new educational paradigm seeks to systematically train healthcare professionals to think about larger structural contexts as well as variables of race, social class, gender, religion, sexual orientation, or other markers of difference. Structural competency overlaps in some ways with the emerging conceptual framework called "syndemic vulnerability," which is developing new ways of understanding how diseases or health conditions that arise in populations are exacerbated by social, economic, environmental, and political structures (Hart & Horton, 2017; Singer, Bulled, Ostrach, & Mendenhall, 2017; Tsai, Mendenhall, Trostle, & Kawachi, 2017). As Metzl and Hansen (2014) note, "clinicians require skills that help them treat persons that come to clinics as patients and at the same time recognize how social and economic determinants, biases, inequities, and blind spots shape health and illness long before doctors or patients enter examination rooms" (p. 128).

Their conceptual model includes five intersecting core structural competencies (Metzl & Hansen, 2014):

1. Recognizing the structures that shape clinical interactions: promotes recognition of how economic, physical, and socio-political forces impact medical decision

2. Developing an extra-clinical language of structure: helps clinicians begin to articulate how the persons, diseases, and attitudes that appear before them can be better understood as the product of social structures interacting with biologies

3. Rearticulating "cultural" presentations in structural terms: provides a more constructive alternative (to culture) because it allows medical classrooms to emphasize how "cultural" barriers arise when structural forces manifest themselves in patterns of interpersonal communication and institutional practices

4. Observing and imagining structural intervention: moves trainees toward real-world application by asking students to analyze structural interventions and then propose interventions that address health infrastructures

5. Developing structural humility: helps students demonstrate a critical awareness of medical education's realistic goals and end points

The pre-health major in medicine, health, and society (MHS) at Vanderbilt University is one of the earliest examples of a structural competency educational program in a prehealth undergraduate setting (Metzl & Petty, 2017; Metzl, Petty, & Olowojoba, 2018; Petty, Metzl, & Keeys, 2017). In 2005, the new MHS major combined course work in health sciences, humanities, and social sciences. The curriculum was revised for 2013, which used structural competency as a central unifying rubric. This revised 36-credit-hour major offered various interdisciplinary courses on (e.g.) racial and ethnic health disparities, structural aspects of mental health, economic determinants of health, politics of health, health activism, disability studies, and critical perspectives on global health (Metzl & Petty, 2017). One marker of success for this major is based on tremendous growth in student enrollment: from 40 students the first year to 500+ in 2015. Early analyses of student impact showed that students were more adept and comfortable analyzing relationships between structural factors and health outcomes and held more nuanced understandings of structures underlying various health outcomes (Metzl & Petty, 2017; Metzl et al., 2018). They concluded that their

> data suggests that structural competency is a skill set that develops from training; and, that improving awareness about structural equity and well-being results, not just from challenging students' implicit biases or sensitivities, but from imparting analytic skills . . .. Our study . . . suggest[s] that teaching students about the 'social' foundations of health needs to begin sooner in the educational process, during the baccalaureate years, when access to interdisciplinary pedagogies remains accessible. (Metzl et al., 2018, p. 199)

Teaching Social Determinants of Health: Baylor University

Recognizing that students typically receive minimal formal preclinical training that incorporates evidence-based understanding of nonbiomedical factors that contribute to their patients' health, a group from Baylor College of Medicine developed an innovative curriculum for first-year medical students during orientation (Song, Poythress, Bocchini, & Kass, 2018). Faculty facilitators led group discussions with about 10 students per group in 1-hour sessions. Students worked through interactive learning exercises focused on various topics, including food insecurity; immigrant and refugee health, LGBT health; human trafficking; race and ethnicity; and women's health (Song et al., 2018). Based on assessments of the first year of implementation, they saw marked improvements in the following:

- Student comfort level with discussing these topics
- Student knowledge of these topics
- Student familiarity with particular terminology associated with the social determinants of health

Lessons learned from the first-year implementation yielded several recommendations for other institutions: (a) contact and coordinate with faculty facilitators at least 3 months in advance, (b) faculty facilitators should expect to spend at least 2 to 3 hours preparing for the small discussion groups using the included facilitator guides, (c) implement a site visit opportunity (to local nonprofits, etc.) to foster longitudinal student interest in their communities and social disparities, and (d) revisit these subjects in other mandatory courses throughout medical school (Song et al., 2018).

Racial/Ethnic Health Disparities: A Pharmacy Elective

Although hospitals and other anchor healthcare institutions have implemented cultural competence trainings, pharmacy has not always been a participant in these efforts (Avant & Gillespie, 2019). To combat this deficit, a group at the University of Cincinnati developed a pharmacy elective focused on the causation of health disparities, such as poverty, public policies, discrimination, and structural racism (Avant & Gillespie, 2019). This three-credit course dealt specifically with structural inequalities in the first part of the course and personal awareness as it relates to cultural competence in the second part. All students were also required to complete a final project that prompted students to use and master core concepts learned throughout the semester. Facilitators led self-discovery discussions and used active-learning activities rather than dictating terms/concepts in a typical lecture format. Moreover, facilitators used innovative learning tools and techniques. For example, students engaged in "social identity mapping" that prompted discussion and learning about one's own marginalized/subordinated identities, as well as their privileged/superordinated identities (Avant & Gillespie, 2019).

Initial reports show that the course achieved its primary aims. A qualitative analysis of student reflections yielded important insights regarding its success:

1. The need for a welcoming and inclusive learning environment: this included setting some "rules of engagement" on Day 1 to establish a tone of respect

2. The importance of experiential learning for personal awareness and knowledge expansion: this pedagogical approach enhanced students' ability to "identify their intersectional positions within systems of inequality" (Avant & Gillespie, 2019, p. 385) and made the teachings relatable to their own personal stories

3. Incorporating intergroup diversity helped to empower learners to create change: this included intentionally designing small group discussions so that "students could listen

to classmates describe their lived experiences" (Avant & Gillespie, 2019, p. 385) and prompted students to shift away from binary thinking regarding complicated issues

4. Anticipate and acknowledge emotions: unlike traditional didactic courses, this experiential learning environment brought out a range of emotions from learning new perspectives, recognizing/acknowledging one's own biases, or hearing about others' lived experiences (Efforts must be made to ensure a safe environment so that emotional dialogue facilitates the learning process.)

5. The value of students writing a final self-reflection paper: this "assignment provided students the ability to connect lessons learned to practice, space for closure, a chance to offer feedback to the facilitator, and an opportunity to provide future directions for the course" (Avant & Gillespie, 2019, p. 386)

Mental/Behavioral Health

Important developments in addressing mental and behavioral health from a cultural competency standpoint include (a) the development of integrated primary and behavioral/mental health services to better address the needs of individuals with mental health and substance use conditions, and (b) the development of a mental health practitioner guide using a knowledge-to-action (KTA) process.

Integration of Primary and Behavioral/Mental Health Services

Although Cartesian notions of a separate mind and body provided a foundation for the biomedical model in medicine (Mehta, 2011), critiques of this dualism have led to major changes in how we view human beings and practical applications that are founded on a more robust understanding of the inseparability of behavioral/mental and physical health (Farber, Ali, Van Sickle, & Kaslow, 2017). "Integrated healthcare, particularly primary care and behavioral health integration, is an evidence-based healthcare strategy designed to improve healthcare outcomes among individuals with multiple healthcare needs through the systematic coordination of services, such as those for physical and behavioral health" (McGregor, Belton, Henry, Wrenn, & Holden, 2019, p. 359).

Integration occurs along a continuum of collaboration and integration, and development of a recent framework includes six levels (Heath, Wise Romero, & Reynolds, 2013).

Coordinated care

- ■ Level 1—*Minimal collaboration*
  Behavioral health and primary care providers work at separate facilities and have separate systems. Providers communicate rarely about cases. When communication occurs, it is usually based on a particular provider's need for specific information about a mutual patient.

- ■ Level 2—*Basic collaboration at a distance*
  Behavioral health and primary care providers maintain separate facilities and separate systems. Providers view each other as resources and communicate periodically about shared patients. These communications are typically driven by specific issues. For example, a primary care physician may request copy of a psychiatric evaluation to know if there is a confirmed psychiatric diagnosis. Behavioral health is most often viewed as specialty care.

Co-located care

■ Level 3—*Basic collaboration onsite*
Behavioral health and primary care providers are co-located in the same facility, but may or may not share the same practice space. Providers still use separate systems, but communication becomes more regular due to close proximity, especially by phone or email, with an occasional meeting to discuss shared patients. Movement of patients between practices is most often through a referral process that has a higher likelihood of success because the practices are in the same location. Providers may feel like they are part of a larger team, but the team and how it operates are not clearly defined, leaving most decisions about patient care to be done independently by individual providers.

■ Level 4—*Close collaboration with some system integration*
There is closer collaboration among primary care and behavioral healthcare providers due to colocation in the same practice space, and there is the beginning of integration in care through some shared systems. A typical model may involve a primary care setting embedding a behavioral health provider. In an embedded practice, the primary care front desk schedules all appointments, and the behavioral health provider has access and enters notes in the medical record. Often, complex patients with multiple healthcare issues drive the need for consultation, which is done through personal communication. As professionals have more opportunity to share patients, they have a better basic understanding of each other's roles.

Integrated care

■ Level 5—*Close collaboration approaching an integrated practice*
There are high levels of collaboration and integration between behavioral and primary care providers. The providers begin to function as a true team, with frequent personal communication. The team actively seeks system solutions as they recognize barriers to care integration for a broader range of patients. However, some issues, such as the availability of an integrated medical record, may not be readily resolved. Providers understand the different roles team members need to play, and they have started to change their practice and the structure of care to better achieve patient goals.

■ Level 6—*Full collaboration in a transformed/merged practice*
The highest level of integration involves the greatest amount of practice change. Fuller collaboration between providers has allowed antecedent system cultures (whether from two separate systems or from one evolving system) to blur into a single transformed or merged practice. Providers and patients view the operation as a single health system treating the whole person. The principle of treating the whole person is applied to all patients, not just targeted groups (Heath et al., 2013).

A growing body of research has shown that integrating behavioral/mental health and primary care produces improved clinical outcomes and can help reduce mental health service disparities, although it is not well established what variations exist at the different levels of integration (Farber et al., 2017), and there is limited research exploring how cultural considerations may impact physical and behavioral health outcomes among racial/ethnic minorities or other marginalized groups in integrated settings (McGregor et al., 2019). As Farber et al. (2017) emphasize,

Integrated care stands to benefit individuals from diverse medically underserved groups who are vulnerable to adverse health outcomes at the intersection of the physical, psychological, social, and cultural aspects of health.... It can enhance health provider ability to develop integrative diagnoses of physical, behavioral, sociocultural, and systemic aspects of health and illness; assess for psychological disorders; address modifiable health behavior practices; offer timely initiation of mental health treatment; and promote patient empowerment, adherence and retention in care. Integrated care can increase focus on the intersection of health care delivery practices with contextual social and cultural dimensions that influence patient experiences of health and illness, patient health behavior practices, and patient-health provider communication and relationships. (pp. 31–32)

To improve cultural competence efforts in integrated care settings, McGregor et al. (2019) provide valuable recommendations.

Cultural competence training initiatives for integrated care settings must leverage the work of coalitions and governmental agencies (e.g., Substance Abuse and Mental Health Services Administration (SAMHSA) that can provide technical assistance resources and expert advice and guidance that will encourage adoption by providers and staff. (p. 362)

Proficiency in culturally competent care especially in an integrated care setting requires monitoring and assessment of provider knowledge, skills, and efficacy.... (and) must be incentivized to accomplish its goals.... As metrics for success in culturally competent care in integrated care settings are not well elucidated, monitoring healthcare provider well-being and burnout rates is also vital to the sustainability to culturally competent care. Providers who are unprepared to provide effective, quality healthcare to patients in a culturally responsive way may experience frustration with communication barriers and patient dissatisfaction. (pp. 363–364)

Translating Research Using a Knowledge-to-Action Process

In 2001, the report *Mental Health: Cultural, Race, and Ethnicity: A Supplement to Mental Health* documented striking racial/ethnic disparities in mental health services (Office of the Surgeon General, 2001). Since then, a growing body of research has described these persistent disparities; however, the translation of research into action has been slow. A recent approach using the knowledge-to-action process sheds new light on solutions that can enable effective translation of research knowledge to community practice (Valdez et al., 2019). Knowledge translation is defined as "the synthesis, exchange, and application of knowledge by relevant stakeholders to accelerate the benefits of global and local innovation in strengthening health systems and improving people's health" (WHO, 2005).

As Valdez et al. (2019) write, their efforts to translate knowledge into action are founded on social justice principles, "which include(s) the equitable distribution of resources, physical and psychological safety and security of all members of society, and empowerment of individuals and communities" (p. 127).

Within the knowledge creation phase, knowledge producers (e.g., researchers, content experts), and knowledge users (e.g., practitioners) collaborate on creating and tailoring relevant knowledge by building a knowledge base, synthesizing relevant knowledge, and then creating tools and products emerging directly from this knowledge creation process. Working in parallel, the action phase involves a series of reciprocal activities needed for knowledge application. Action may begin with the identification and clarification of the problem, the adaptation of knowledge to a specific context, an assessment and understanding of barriers to the utilization of knowledge, and the tailoring and implementation of specific interventions, followed by efforts to monitor use and evaluate outcomes in order to sustain use of knowledge. (pp. 128–129)

Using the KTA process, this group developed a guide for psychologists and other mental health providers titled, "Addressing the Mental Health Needs of Racial and Ethnic Minority Youth – A Guide for Practitioners" (Valdez et al., 2019). In the first phase of the KTA process, core members of the development group (a) hosted discussion groups with psychologists to better understand their target audience and (b) assembled content experts (e.g., psychologists) to solidify content for the guide, and subsequently, they (c) designed the guide. In the discussion groups, a prominent theme emerged on system-level barriers that impacted their work with racial/ethnic minority youth, notably restrictive organizational policies regarding no-shows/termination, lack of assessment of social determinants of health, and limited collaboration across agencies (p. 130). Solutions to be included in the guide to address system-level barriers included providing mental health services within schools and implementing routine assessments of social determinants of health. To address provider-level barriers, the group included information on how to address disparities during the clinical encounter as well as other contexts (p. 131).

After this first phase of "knowledge creation" (which included problem identification and solution generation), they moved to the action phase. New stakeholders who had extensive experience conducting research or providing psychological services to racial/ethnic minority youth were now brought into the process. Over a series of meetings, this group finalized the content and format of the practitioner guide and discussed strategies to disseminate the guide. Consistent with the action phase of the KTA process, this group provided recommendations regarding which knowledge to prioritize, how to simplify uptake of knowledge, and which interventions to include in the guide (p. 132).

The final guide is available on the Children Youth and Families page of the American Psychological Association website (www.apa.org/pi/families/resources/mental-health-needs.pdf). The guide is structured around (a) mechanisms leading to disparities in mental health outcomes among racial/ethnic minority youth, (b) factors that protect against negative mental health outcomes, (c) determinants of mental healthcare use, (d) strategies that practitioners can use within their clinical practice, and (e) potential roles of practitioners to address disparities outside the clinical encounter (p. 132).

The value of this work comes not only from the final product—the practitioner's guide—but also to the development process that was used by this working group. Utilizing the KTA process, important insights were gained from stakeholder groups to identify broader points of emphasis regarding mental health as well as context-dependent needs as they relate to mental health among racial/ethnic minority youth. Moreover, this process illustrates the inner workings of translating research into practice. Based on lessons learned, the authors note that "having practicing psychologists' voices 'at the table' should be a priority" (Valdez et al., 2019, p. 133). They did recognize some of their own gaps and limitations, including limited expertise representing Asian Americans (and other groups). This gap needs to be addressed in future efforts. Finally, the authors prompt future developmental work to extend beyond psychologists and to collaborate across multiple mental health practitioners, including social workers, psychiatrists, and mental health counselors (p. 133).

LGBTQ Contexts[2]

Although sexual and gender identity have long been viewed as constructs with binary categories, current and more nuanced understandings have revealed their complexity and the ways in which cultural and social contexts shape these constructs. As Fredrikson-Goldsen et al. (2014) write,

Sexuality encompasses at least three key components: sexual identity, sexual attraction, and sexual behavior. Sexual identity is an individual's own perception of his or her overall sexual self.... Gender refers to the behavioral, cultural, or psychological traits that a society associates with male and female sex. Transgender generally refers to people whose gender identity is at odds with the gender they were assigned at birth according to their sex and physiological characteristics of their bodies. (pp. 653–654)

Extensive research has focused on health and healthcare of LGBTQ people; however, it was not until the report Health People 2020 that LGBTQ people were identified in U.S. health priorities as an at-risk population (Fredriksen-Goldsen et al., 2014; Office of Disease Prevention and Health Promotion, n.d.-b). And while much of this research has focused on interpersonal and individual factors (such as fear of being stigmatized or provider bias) that negatively impact the health of LGBTQ individuals, emerging research developments have honed in on structural factors (Donald, DasGupta, Metzl, & Eckstrand, 2017; Fredriksen-Goldsen et al., 2014).

In this section, I review the Health Equity Promotion model—a framework oriented toward LGBTQ people—and present a case study from Veterans Affairs (VA) Boston Healthcare System on their initiatives to enhance LGBTQ cultural competency at the organizational, structural, and clinical levels.

Health Equity Promotion Model

According to Fredriksen-Goldsen et al. (2014), this model

integrates a life course development perspective within a health equity framework to highlight how (a) social positions (socio-economic status, age, race/ethnicity) and (b) individual and structural and environmental context (social exclusion, discrimination, and victimization) intersect with (c) health-promoting and adverse pathways (behavioral, social, psychological, and biological processes) to influence the continuum of health outcomes in LGBT communities. (p. 655)

Recognizing a dearth of research on heterogeneity within LGBTQ populations, and little exploration of how multiple intersecting social positions impact LGBTQ health, Fredriksen-Goldsen et al. (2014) emphasize the need to attend to "the potential for synergistic disadvantage or advantage based on multiple statuses" (p. 656). For example, health researchers should consider the experience of an LGBTQ person who came of age when homosexuality was considered a psychiatric disorder or if they live in a country/region marked by overt LGBTQ discrimination compared with a 20-year-old LGBTQ adult living in a politically/environmentally LGBTQ-friendly country/region. Likewise, the intersection of one's LGBTQ identity and one's racial identity or immigration status or disability status matters for understanding their health and healthcare. This work reinforces the earlier discussion on *lumping and splitting* and shows how the ways in which we categorize people is often too simplistic.

Most LGBTQ cultural competency efforts have focused on the individual level—improving healthcare professionals' knowledge base of the unique health concerns affecting LGBTQ people and improving their attitudes toward LGBTQ people (including explicit and implicit bias; Radix & Maingi, 2018). But "structural and contextual factors create a context of marginalization and oppression, including laws and policies that unfairly treat sexual and gender minorities as well as cultural and institutional oppressions, widespread societal stigma, and religious intolerance and persecution" (Fredriksen-Goldsen et al., 2014, p. 657). For example, LGBTQ patients may have less access to healthcare when needed and transgender individuals frequently postpone healthcare (Fredriksen-Goldsen et al., 2013, 2014). Moving beyond a deficit-oriented approach to understanding health and healthcare of LGBTQ people, the Health Equity Promotion model seeks to include sexual and gender identity–specific strengths and resources in current conceptions and investigations (Fredriksen-Goldsen et al., 2014).

Enhancing LGBTQ Cultural Competency: VA Boston Healthcare System

The following case study described by Ruben et al. (2017) provides firsthand accounts and insights into innovative LGBTQ cultural competency efforts in the VA Boston Healthcare System. The findings and recommendations can be utilized by other healthcare systems interested in developing LGBT health initiatives.

First, this case study reflects a valuable point of intersectionality that is not often addressed: that of sexual/gender identity and military status. Ruben et al. (2017) note that while there is a growing literature on health disparities among LGBTQ veterans, changing regulations (e.g., employment nondiscrimination laws) and policies (e.g., "Don't Ask, Don't Tell" or the ban on transgender military service) impact veteran health disparities "and have cultural repercussions for LGBT veterans seeking care at VA hospitals" (p. 1413).

Predominantly, when cultural competence has focused on sexual and gender minority patients, it has tended to deal with individual and/or interpersonal factors. Larger system-level issues are rarely dealt with explicitly. Ruben et al. (2017) note that this individualized focus is tied to the use of Meyer's (1995, 2003) minority stress theory as a framework for understanding health disparities. This theory posits that "sexual and gender minority individuals experience chronic stress related to ongoing stigma, discrimination, and general lack of acceptance and understanding, contributing to internalized negative feelings toward the self, chronic worry of rejection, and actual and/or perceived negative experiences, which in turn increase risk and rates of physical and mental health problems" (Ruben et al., 2017, p. 1417). While this theory is useful for understanding individual-level factors, new concepts and methodologies must be employed that take into consideration larger structures.

Ruben et al. (2017) use Betancourt, Green, Carrillo, and Ananeh-Firempong's (2003) cultural competence framework because it allowed them to specify key steps that were taken at the organizational, structural, and clinical levels. At the organizational level, they had a group of committed clinicians and researchers who spearheaded a grassroots effort to develop specific committees and policies. Important insights gleaned from these early developmental stages included (a) ensuring LGBTQ staff's voices were represented; (b) creating a psychologically safe place to discuss sensitive issues; and (c) having organizational support—in this case, from the Medical Center Director's Office. At the structural level, the authors note the importance of how national policy changes may impact organizational culture and policies. In this case, in 2011, the Offices of Patient Care Services and Mental Health created the Transgender Directive that "established a policy of respectful delivery of healthcare to transgender and intersex veterans enrolled in the VA healthcare system or those eligible for VA care" (Ruben et al., 2017, p. 1420). This proved to be an important first step "as it mandated treatment (and pronoun use) based on self-identified gender identity" and "assured that VA staff would provide care to transgender patients without discrimination in a manner consistent with care and management of all veteran patients" (p. 1420).

This case study—which reported multiple challenges and setbacks but also many successes—highlights the importance of larger contextual/structural factors. Policy changes within the Department of Defense (e.g., repeal of "Don't Ask Don't Tell) and organizational factors created an environment that was conducive for a group of passionate individuals to start discussing LGBTQ healthcare and to take appropriate action steps. Also, "significant resources were developed, devoted, and staffed regarding LGBT clinical competence, including (a) the creation of and time devoted by multiple diversity committees, (b) an LGBT Health Fellowship position, and (c) the acquisition of training materials and the time of knowledgeable staff who were willing to train others" (Ruben et al., 2017, p. 1424). The authors' final recommendations include making concerted efforts to better understand local cultural and community resources, conduct an organizational self-study (such as the Healthcare Equality Index) to assess your strengths and weaknesses in current delivery of healthcare to LGBTQ patients, and empower a group of passionate individuals to tackle one problem/issue at a time (pp. 1425–1426).

CONCLUSION

In 2012, Dr. Paul Farmer—anthropologist, physician, and founder of Partners in Health—gave a commencement speech at Northwestern University where he emphasized that the graduates must "try to counter failures of imagination." In one example, his ambitious efforts to build a hospital in the rural mountains of Haiti reflected this directive in his own life (Farmer & Weigel, 2013). With decades of hands-on experience across the world, Dr. Farmer lamented that "the great majority of global public health experts and others who seek to attack poverty are hostages to (such) failures of imagination" (p. 59). Indeed, the problems evident in almost daily news cycles of newly-diagnosed cancer patients seeking financial help through online crowdfunding (e.g., GoFundMe.com) or citizens choosing between paying for insulin or rent, or deadly medical errors, leave many exasperated, wondering how they can make a difference. As any remarkable commencement speech should, Dr. Farmer did not leave the graduates with a distressing story. Rather, he implored the new graduates to tackle the most difficult health and development problems "with innovation and resolve and a bolder vision" (Farmer & Weigel, 2013, p. 64).

This chapter has explored the complexities of cultural competence and cultural humility. I implore readers to keep in mind the big picture: global health equity. If we assume that amazing healthcare across the world is not in our purview, do we have a failure of imagination? At the heart of cultural competence and cultural humility is the human being making concerted efforts—in a lifelong process—to become more self-reflective, self-aware, understanding of others, appreciative of differences, caring. But we are also all part of larger social groups (our families, schools, organizations, nationalities, etc.). And there are institutionalized systems of practice that we create and recreate on a daily basis through our actions, norms, and policies. Thus, efforts to achieve health equity must also extend beyond individual-level changes and incorporate larger, systemic changes. There are no "magic bullets" or quick-fixes. But new understandings of our diverse world and evidence-based action will make a difference.

DISCUSSION QUESTIONS

- Should the concept of cultural humility replace that of cultural competence, or do they both serve a conceptual purpose?
- Why is it important to utilize models and frameworks for communication when engaging in cross-cultural interactions?
- How does Purnell's Model of Cultural Competence interconnect with the Social Ecological Model (see Chapter 3, Health Equity Frameworks and Theories)?
- Why is a movement from ethnocentrism to ethnorelativism critical to ensure cultural competence in cross-cultural interactions?
- How could the models developed for clinical cultural competency training be adapted to meet the needs of public health professionals?

NOTES

1 Although there are valuable debates in using the concepts of cultural competence or cultural humility (or even new conceptions that literally combine the two), I maintain that these concepts can and should operate synergistically in a lifelong process of improvement. With this understanding, the term "cultural competence" is used as the main descriptor throughout this chapter.

2 The naming of lesbian, gay, bisexual, transgender, and queer and/or questioning (LGBTQ) people has changed over time; I use this full acronym unless referencing others' work that may use LGBT or another variant.

REFERENCES

Avant, N. D., & Gillespie, G. L. (2019). Pushing for health equity through structural competency and implicit bias education: A qualitative evaluation of a racial/ethnic health disparities elective course for pharmacy learners. *Currents in Pharmacy Teaching & Learning, 11*(4), 382–393. doi:10.1016/j.cptl.2019.01.013

Bennett, M. J. (2004). Becoming interculturally competent. In J. S. Wurzel (Ed.), *Toward multiculturalism: A reader in multicultural education.* Newton, MA: Intercultural Resource Corporation.

Betancourt, J. R., Green, A. R., Carrillo, J. E., & Ananeh-Firempong, O. (2003). Defining cultural competence: A practical framework for addressing racial/ethnic disparities in health and health care. *Public Health Reports, 118*(4), 293. doi:10.1093/phr/118.4.293

Braveman, P., Arkin, E., Orleans, T., Proctor, D., & Plough, A. (2017). *What is health equity? And what difference does a definition make?* (pp. 1–20). Princeton, NJ: Robert Wood Johnson Foundation. Retrieved from https://www.rwjf.org/en/library/research/2017/05/what-is-health-equity-.html

Coleman-Miller, B. (2000). A physician's perspective on minority health. *Health Care Financing Review, 21*(4), 45–56. Retrieved from https://www.ncbi.nlm.nih.gov/pmc/articles/PMC4194640

Cross, T. L., Bazron, B. J., Dennis, K. W., & Isaacs, M. R. (1989). *Towards a culturally competent system of care: A monograph on effective services for minority children who are severely emotionally disturbed.* Washington, DC: Child and Adolescent Service System Program Technical Assistance Center.

Donald, C. A., DasGupta, S., Metzl, J. M., & Eckstrand, K. L. (2017). Queer frontiers in medicine: A structural competency approach. *Academic Medicine, 92*(3), 345–350. doi:10.1097/ACM.0000000000001533

Dovidio, J. F., & Fiske, S. T. (2012). Under the radar: How unexamined biases in decision-making processes in clinical interactions can contribute to health care disparities. *American Journal of Public Health, 102*(5), 945–952. doi:10.2105/AJPH.2011.300601

Farber, E. W., Ali, M. K., Van Sickle, K. S., & Kaslow, N. J. (2017). Psychology in patient-centered medical homes: Reducing health disparities and promoting health equity. *American Psychologist, 72*(1), 28–41. doi:10.1037/a0040358

Farmer, P., & Weigel, J. (2013). *To repair the world: Paul Farmer speaks to the next generation.* Berkeley: University of California Press.

Fredriksen-Goldsen, K. I., Emlet, C. A., Kim, H. J., Muraco, A., Erosheva, E. A., Goldsen, J., & Hoy-Ellis, C. P. (2013). The physical and mental health of lesbian, gay male, and bisexual (LGB) older adults: The role of key health indicators and risk and protective factors. *Gerontologist, 53*(4), 664–675. doi:10.1093/geront/gns123

Fredriksen-Goldsen, K. I., Simoni, J. M., Kim, H.-J., Lehavot, K., Walters, K. L., Yang, J., … Muraco, A. (2014). The health equity promotion model: Reconceptualization of lesbian, gay, bisexual, and transgender (LGBT) health disparities. *American Journal of Orthopsychiatry, 84*(6), 653–663. doi:10.1037/ort0000030

Georgetown University National Center for Cultural Competence. (n.d.). *Defining bias.* Retrieved from https://nccc.georgetown.edu/bias/module-1

Hart, L., & Horton, R. (2017). Syndemics: Committing to a healthier future. *Lancet, 389*(10072), 888–889. doi:10.1016/S0140-6736(17)30599-8

Heath, B., Wise-Romero, P., & Reynolds, K. (2013). *A standard framework for levels of integrated healthcare and update throughout the document.* Washington, DC: Substance Abuse and Mental Health Services Administration-Health Resources and Services Administration Center for Integrated Health Solutions. Retrieved from http://www.integration.samhsa.gov/integrated-care-models/A_Standard_Framework_for_Levels_of_Integrated_Healthcare.pdf

Hook, J. N., Davis, D. E., Owen, J., Worthington Jr, E. L., & Utsey, S. O. (2013). Cultural humility: Measuring openness to culturally diverse clients. *Journal of Counseling Psychology, 60*(3), 353.

Horvat, L., Horey, D., Romios, P., & Kis-Rigo, J. (2014). Cultural competence education for health professionals. *Cochrane Database of Systematic Reviews,* (5), CD009405. doi:10.1002/14651858.CD009405.pub2

Jones, C. P. (2000). Levels of racism: A theoretic framework and a gardener's tale. *American Journal of Public Health, 90*(8), 1212–1215. doi:10.2105/ajph.90.8.1212

Kumagai, A. K., & Lypson, M. L. (2009). Beyond cultural competence: Critical consciousness, social justice, and multicultural education. *Academic Medicine, 84*(6), 782–787. doi:10.1097/ACM.0b013e3181a42398

Laveist, T. (2014). Expanding the evidence base for health equity. *Frontiers of Health Services Management, 30*(3), 38–42. doi:10.1097/01974520-201401000-00005

Lieu, T. A., Finkelstein, J. A., Lozano, P., Capra, A. M., Chi, F. W., Jensvold, N., … Farber, H. J. (2004). Cultural competence policies and other predictors of asthma care quality for Medicaid-insured children. *Pediatrics, 114*, E102–E110. doi:10.1542/peds.114.1.e102

McGregor, B., Belton, A., Henry, T. L., Wrenn, G., & Holden, K. B. (2019). Commentary: Improving behavioral health equity through cultural competence training of health care providers. *Ethnicity & Disease, 29*, 359. doi:10.18865/ed.29.S2.359

Mehta, N. (2011). Mind-body dualism: A critique from a health perspective. *Mens Sana Monographs, 9*(1), 202–209. doi:10.4103/0973-1229.77436

Metzl, J. M., & Hansen, H. (2014). Structural competency: Theorizing a new medical engagement with stigma and inequality. *Social Science & Medicine, 103*, 126–133. doi:10.1016/j.socscimed.2013.06.032

Metzl, J. M., & Petty, J. (2017). Integrating and assessing structural competency in an innovative prehealth curriculum at Vanderbilt University. *Academic Medicine, 92*(3), 354–359. doi:10.1097/ACM.0000000000001477

Metzl, J. M., Petty, J., & Olowojoba, O. V. (2018). Using a structural competency framework to teach structural racism in pre-health education. *Social Science & Medicine, 199*, 189–201. doi:10.1016/j.socscimed.2017.06.029

Meyer, I. H. (1995). Minority stress and mental health in gay men. *Journal of Health and Social Behavior, 36*(1), 38–56. doi:10.2307/2137286

Meyer, I. H. (2003). Prejudice, social stress, and mental health in lesbian, gay, and bisexual populations: Conceptual issues and research evidence. *Psychological Bulletin, 129*(5), 674–697. doi:10.1037/0033-2909.129.5.674

Murray-García, J., & Tervalon, M. (2014). The concept of cultural humility. *Health Affairs, 33*(7), 1303. doi:10.1377/hlthaff.2014.0564

Nair, L., & Adetayo, O. A. (2019). Cultural competence and ethnic diversity in healthcare. *Plastic and Reconstructive Surgery, Global Open, 7*(5), e2219. doi:10.1097/GOX.0000000000002219

National Center for Cultural Competence, Georgetown University. (n.d.-a). *Definitions of cultural competence.* Retrieved from https://nccc.georgetown.edu/curricula/culturalcompetence.html

National Center for Cultural Competence, Georgetown University. (n.d.-b). *Definitions realted to disparate treatment, health status, and health care.* Retrieved from https://nccc.georgetown.edu/bias/module-1/1.php

Nelson, A. (2002). Unequal treatment: Confronting racial and ethnic disparities in health care. *Journal of the National Medical Association, 94*(8), 666–668. Retrieved from https://www.ncbi.nlm.nih.gov/pmc/articles/PMC2594273/pdf/jnma00325-0024.pdf

Notaro, S. R. (2012). *Health disparities among under-served populations: Implications for research, policy and praxis.* Bingley, UK: Emerald Group Publishing.

Office of Disease Prevention and Health Promotion. (n.d.-a). *Disparities.* Retrieved from https://www.healthypeople.gov/2020/about/foundation-health-measures/Disparities

Office of Disease Prevention and Health Promotion. (n.d.-b). *Lesbian, gay, bisexual, and transgender health.* Retrieved from https://www.healthypeople.gov/2020/topics-objectives/topic/lesbian-gay-bisexual-and-transgender-health#top

Office of the Surgeon General. (2001). *Mental health: Culture, race and ethnicity—A supplement to mental health: A report of the surgeon general.* Rockville, MD: Substance Abuse and Mental Health Services Administration. Retrieved from https://www.ncbi.nlm.nih.gov/books/NBK44243

Orleans, C. T., Strecher, V. J., Schoenbach, V. J., Salmon, M. A., & Blackmon, C. (1989). Smoking cessation initiatives for Black Americans: Recommendations for research and intervention. *Health Education Research, 4*(1), 13. doi:10.1093/her/4.1.13

Paez, K. A., Allen, J. K., Beach, M. C., Carson, K. A., & Cooper, L. A. (2009). Physician cultural competence and patient ratings of the patient–physician relationship. *Journal of General Internal Medicine, 24*(4), 495–498. doi:10.1007/s11606-009-0919-7

Paul, D., Ewen, S. C., & Jones, R. (2014). Cultural competence in medical education: Aligning the formal, informal and hidden curricula. *Advances in Health Sciences Education, 19,* 751–758. doi:10.1007/s10459-014-9497-5

Penstone, J. (2011). *Visualizing the iceberg model of culture.* Retrieved from http://opengecko.com/interculturalism/visualising-the-iceberg-model-of-culture

Petty, J., Metzl, J. M., & Keeys, M. R. (2017). Developing and evaluating an innovative structural competency curriculum for pre-health students. *Journal of Medical Humanities, 38*(4), 459–471. doi:10.1007/s10912-017-9449-1

Powell Sears, K. (2012). Improving cultural competence education: The utility of an intersectional framework. *Medical Education, 46*(6), 545–551. doi:10.1111/j.1365-2923.2011.04199.x

Purnell, L. (2005). The Purnell model for cultural competence. *The Journal of Multicultural Nursing & Health, 11*(2), 7–15. doi:10.1007/978-3-030-21946-8_2

Purnell, L. (2019). Update: The Purnell theory and model for culturally competent health care. *Journal of Transcultural Nursing, 30*(2), 98–105. doi:10.1177/1043659618817587

Radix, A., & Maingi, S. (2018). LGBT cultural competence and interventions to help oncology nurses and other health care providers. *Seminars in Oncology Nursing, 34*(1), 80–89. doi:10.1016/j.soncn.2017.12.005

Rajaram, S. S., & Bockrath, S. (2014). Cultural competence: New conceptual insights into its limits and potential for addressing health disparities. *Journal of Health Disparities Research & Practice, 7*(5), 82–89. Retrieved from https://digitalscholarship.unlv.edu/jhdrp/vol7/iss5/6

Ruben, M. A., Shipherd, J. C., Topor, D., AhnAllen, C. G., Sloan, C. A., Walton, H. M., … Trezza, G. R. (2017). Advancing LGBT health care policies and clinical care within a large academic health care system: A case study. *Journal of Homosexuality, 64*, 1411–1431. doi:10.1080/00918369.2017.1321386

Sauaia, A. (2014). *The quest for health equity*. New York, NY: Nova Science.

Singer, M., Bulled, N., Ostrach, B., & Mendenhall, E. (2017). Syndemics and the biosocial conception of health. *Lancet, 389*(10072), 941–950. doi:10.1016/S0140-6736(17)30003-X

Smedley, B. D., Stith, A. Y., & Nelson, A. R. (Eds.). (2002). *Unequal treatment: Confronting racial and ethnic disparities in health care*. Washington, DC: National Academies Press.

Song, A. Y., Poythress, E. L., Bocchini, C. E., & Kass, J. S. (2018). Reorienting orientation: Introducing the social determinants of health to first-year medical students. *Mededportal: The Journal of Teaching and Learning Resources, 14*, 10752–10752. doi:10.15766/mep_2374-8265.10752

Sue, D. W. (2001). Multidimensional facets of cultural competence. *The Counseling Psychologist, 29*, 790–821. doi:10.1177/0011000001296002

Tervalon, M., & Murray-García, J. (1998). Cultural humility versus cultural competence: A critical distinction in defining physician training outcomes in multicultural education. *Journal of Health Care for the Poor and Underserved, 9*(2), 117–125. doi:10.1353/hpu.2010.0233

Thackrah, R. D., & Thompson, S. C. (2013). Refining the concept of cultural competence: Building on decades of progress. *Medical Journal of Australia, 199*(1), 35–38. doi:10.5694/mja13.10499

Tsai, A. C., Mendenhall, E., Trostle, J. A., & Kawachi, I. (2017). Co-occurring epidemics, syndemics, and population health. *Lancet, 389*(10072), 978–982. doi:10.1016/S0140-6736(17)30403-8

Valdez, C. R., Rodgers, C. R. R., Gudiño, O. G., Isaac, P., Cort, N. A., Casas, M., & Butler, A. M. (2019). Translating research to support practitioners in addressing disparities in child and adolescent mental health and services in the United States. *Cultural Diversity and Ethnic Minority Psychology, 25*(1), 126–135. doi:10.1037/cdp0000257

van Ryn, M., & Burke, J. (2000). The effect of patient race and socio-economic status on physicians' perceptions of patients. *Social Science & Medicine, 50*(6), 813–828. doi:10.1016/s0277-9536(99)00338-x

Vermeire, E., Hearnshaw, H., Van Royen, P., & Denekens, J. (2001). Patient adherence to treatment: Three decades of research. A comprehensive review. *Journal of Clinical Pharmacy & Therapeutics, 26*(5), 331–342. doi:10.1046/j.1365-2710.2001.00363.x

Ware, M. (2012). *Everything you need to know about culturally competent health care*. Newmarket, ON: BrainMass.

World Health Organization. (2005). *Bridging the "know-do" gap: Meeting on knowledge translation in global health*. Retrieved from https://www.measureevaluation.org/resources/training/capacity-building-resources/high-impact-research-training-curricula/bridging-the-know-do-gap.pdf

Zerubavel, E. (1996). Lumping and splitting: Notes on social classification. *Sociological Forum, 11*(3), 421–433. doi:10.1007/BF02408386

THE FUTURE OF HEALTH EQUITY

K. BRYANT SMALLEY ■ JACOB C. WARREN ■ M. ISABEL FERNÁNDEZ

INTRODUCTION

We hope that the preceding chapters have provided a comprehensive and informative view of the design, implementation, and impact of efforts to achieve health equity, as well as the theories that underlie health equity practice. In this concluding chapter, we offer our final thoughts on key areas we believe will be critical to achieving health equity moving forward.

INVESTIGATING, NOT JUST ACKNOWLEDGING, INTERSECTIONALITY

As discussed within nearly every chapter of this text, the importance of intersectionality in understanding and intervening in health disparity processes cannot be overstated. Unfortunately, for the most part, the field of health equity has largely focused on *acknowledging* rather than specifically *investigating* the impact of intersectional identities on health outcomes and health interventions. There are several reasons for this, not the least of which is the methodological complexity associated with extracting and quantifying the impact of multiple identities within the same individual. A core challenge is achieving an adequate sample size to conduct within-group analyses. For example, to fully investigate the effect of intersectionality on a rural, African American, transgender woman, one would have to investigate the outcome/process of interest in every combination of geographic, racial/ethnic, and gender identity (e.g., at its simplest, urban vs. rural, African American vs. Caucasian vs. Hispanic, cisgender vs. transgender). Achieving an adequate sample size is very prohibitive, and unfortunately, funding agencies are not always attuned to the immense need for sufficiently powered studies to investigate the impact of intersectionality. This leaves researchers having to compare results across studies of different groups (e.g., comparing a study of minority transgender women to a study of cisgender nonminority women), introducing several opportunities for both error and bias in conclusions. This directly inhibits the ability to draw meaningful, translational conclusions regarding intersectionality.

The impact of intersectionality is not merely academic. As discussed throughout this book, the role of identity—be it racial/ethnic, gender, sexual orientation, geographic, etc.—in developing, maintaining, and intervening in health decision-making is a critical area of inquiry that continually produces results supporting the importance of at minimum acknowledging and ideally embracing identity factors in delivery of health interventions. Without fully understanding how these roles intersect and potentially even conflict with each other, identity-based interventions will not fully achieve their potential. Future research must begin to truly describe and integrate the influence of intersectionality on health equity rather than passively, and often off-handedly, acknowledging it.

INCREASING FUNDING STREAMS FOR HEALTH EQUITY WORK

Historically, funding for health equity–related work has lagged far behind its pressing need. However, funders recently seem to be increasingly aware of the need to expand funding opportunities specifically focused on health equity research, and this trend must continue for health equity to be achieved. Although the National Institutes of Health's (NIH) National Institute on Minority Health and Health Disparities (NIMHD) and its predecessor agencies have served as a focal point for federal health disparities work for nearly 30 years, to truly achieve health equity, all federal agencies and sub-branches need to be cognizant of the ways in which disparities impact their individual focus areas. They also need to specifically solicit and support health equity–focused work—not just express an overall interest that may or may not translate into study section, project officer, and advisory council recommendations. Beyond NIMHD, several NIH institutes and centers have focal points for their health equity work—for example, the Eunice Kennedy Shriver National Institute of Child Health and Human Development (NICHD) has its own Office of Health Equity (OHE) to ensure NICHD is optimally addressing and eliminating health disparities. Similarly, the Health Resources and Services Administration (HRSA) has an OHE charged with reducing health disparities nationwide and advancing health equity efforts across HRSA's bureaus. The impact of HRSA's OHE can be seen in the numerous disparities-focused initiatives across the agency, including the national Healthy Start initiative (focused on eliminating disparities in maternal and infant mortality) and the federal government's Office of Rural Health Policy. Ensuring continuing and expanded focus on health equity within agencies is critical to long-term change.

While these organizing functions are important and should continue to be supported, until health equity work is emphasized and prioritized even *outside* the context of disparities-specific funding opportunities, we will continue to underrepresent minority health concerns and populations in biomedical research. While NIH has attempted to increase the representation of diverse populations within its clinical research (through documentation of inclusion of women and minorities in research), this approach is largely passive and subject to interpretation by individual applicants and grant reviewers. Further, it has a focus on *documenting* what is proposed rather than actively *encouraging* diversity within studies. Active, strategic funding in key health disparities areas is needed from all federal funders to truly achieve change. In addition, it is vital that all funding agencies support changes to policies (including innovations such as implicit bias training for grant reviewers) that will increase both the diversity of research being supported and the diversity of the researchers conducting the work (for additional discussion of the importance of diversification of the biomedical research workforce, see later discussion in this chapter).

ENGAGING COMMUNITIES IN HEALTH EQUITY RESEARCH

Another theme that has repeated throughout this text is the critical importance of the involvement—and ideally the leadership—of communities impacted by health disparities in the design, execution, interpretation, and dissemination of health equity research. This is not to say that investigator-driven research is not important to the development of solutions to health equity issues; however, community-driven research methodologies such as community-based participatory research are widely recognized as one of the most successful and impactful methods for creating scalable, sustainable solutions to health equity issues (Berge, Mendenhall, & Doherty, 2009; Israel, Schulz, Parker, & Becker, 1998; Wallerstein & Duran, 2006, 2010). The core strength of community-partnered approaches is that they inherently ensure the voice of the community is at the forefront of the initiative. This helps not only to counteract the mistrust of the medical and research communities held by many populations impacted by health disparities, it also helps to ensure the wisdom and lived experiences of the community are brought to the research process.

While it is nearly universally viewed as a powerful vehicle for promoting health equity, for academic-based researchers, engaging in community-based participatory research (CBPR) and similar approaches can present challenges. CBPR requires a significant time investment that may take years to produce "traditional" research products, such as peer-reviewed journal articles or successfully funded grants. Particularly for new investigators facing pressures of tenure and/or promotion, this investment may seem risky. However, the long-term benefits of establishing a trusted relationship directly with the community impacted by an individual's research far outweigh any initial perceived risk. Once established, CBPR partnerships provide opportunities for large-scale research that would be exceedingly difficult to accomplish without the existing relationships in place. For example, the CBPR partnerships of two of the editors (Smalley and Warren) have been in place for over a decade, and the trust built within those relationships provides opportunities to pursue projects within historically difficult-to-access populations (e.g., school children) at a large scale (in one instance, across seven contiguous counties) because of the existing relationships with key stakeholders (e.g., superintendents and principals). Another challenge for researchers engaging in CBPR is that the variety of topics on which a community may be interested in focusing may either extend beyond the academic researcher's own knowledge base or may lead to a CV with a perceived "lack of focus." It is important for supervisors and promotion/tenure committees to be made aware of the nature of community-based research and the impact (and scientific evidence base) behind it.

SUPPORTING THE DEVELOPMENT OF RESEARCHERS FROM BACKGROUNDS UNDERREPRESENTED IN THE BIOMEDICAL RESEARCH WORKFORCE

There is a well-documented and persistent lack of diversity within the biomedical research workforce that plays an undeniable role in limiting the ability of the scientific community to meet the needs of groups impacted by health disparities. As stark evidence of this, less than 5% of science and engineering–based doctoral degrees are awarded to both women and men from under-represented minority groups (National Science Foundation, 2017). This lack of diversity among biomedical researchers led the national academies to specifically identify a critical need to diversify the biomedical research workforce in order to bring "an intensified focus on understanding and eradicating health disparities" (Hahm & Ommaya, 2006). In line with this call, numerous training programs exist to promote diversity of students entering research careers, such as the NIMHD's Minority Health Research Training Program. This diversification is critical to the advancement of all realms of health research, but has particular relevance for work focused on health equity.

Unfortunately, even after achieving a doctoral degree in the biomedical sciences, inequities remain. African American researchers are 10% less likely to receive NIH research project grant (R01) funding when compared to Caucasian researchers; strikingly, this difference persists even when controlling for score-driving factors, such as educational background, country of origin, training, previous funding, publication record, and employer characteristics (Ginther et al., 2011). Therefore, it is important to establish not only pipeline programs that support the diversity of researchers entering the workforce but also programs that support researchers once they have entered their research careers. This ensures the full pipeline is in fact supported.

To be optimally impactful, programs designed to increase the diversity of the biomedical research workforce should provide a full range of training necessary for exploring a career focused on health equity and provide support from before the selection of a career all the way through the establishment of an independent research career. In doing so, programs must be responsive to the growing evidence that groups underrepresented in biomedical research careers respond differently to "traditional" mentoring models and that newer, more inclusive mentoring approaches should be considered. Specifically, models that incorporate multiple simultaneous mentors (also known as "multiple mentoring") and the use of peer mentoring have been widely supported in the literature as particularly impactful for groups underrepresented in biomedical research careers (including racial/ethnic minority groups and women), but such programs remain relatively uncommon (Burlwe, 1991; Chandler, 1996; Chesler & Chesler, 2013; Darwin & Palmer, 2009; Etzkowitz, Kemelgor, & Uzzi, 2000; McGee, Saran, & Krulwich, 2012; Portillo, 2018). An inherent challenge in establishing such programs is that they require an intentional approach to mentoring that may differ from the ways in which program faculty were themselves trained. In practice, mentoring programs tend to default to a traditional mentoring model because, for the most part, those running the programs were themselves mentored in a traditional manner. Calls for establishing new pipeline and mentoring programs should be cognizant of these factors and encourage the use of innovative mentoring approaches.

ADVANCING PUBLIC AWARENESS AND UNDERSTANDING OF HEALTH EQUITY

Unfortunately, there is still a lack of general public awareness, understanding, and, in certain circles, even fundamental support of the importance of health equity. Health disparities are, by definition, associated with social injustices and imbalances in power, and the factors that drive the genesis and maintenance of health disparities (e.g., discrimination and marginalization) also impede the field of health equity as a whole.

While the elimination of health disparities has been an organizing focus of the Healthy People initiative (that purportedly guides all the Department of Health and Human Service [DHHS] investments in health) since the launch of Healthy People 2010, studies conducted in that same year revealed that "the majority of Americans [were] uninformed about health care disparities" (Lillie-Blanton, Brodie, Rowland, Altman, & McIntosh, 2000, p. 218). Research conducted 10 years later revealed that while the majority of the public was now aware that health outcomes differed between socioeconomic statuses, the majority of the public remained unaware that African Americans faced health disparities in comparison to their Caucasian counterparts (Booske, Robert, & Rohan, 2011). This lack of awareness extended even into communities impacted by disparities—for instance, a 2011 study found that nearly 80% of Hispanic Americans were unaware of the HIV/AIDS disparity between Hispanics and Caucasians in the U.S. (Benz, Espinosa, Welsh, & Fontes, 2011).

This lack of awareness also extends into elected leadership. Recent studies investigating awareness among key local policy makers (e.g., mayors and health commissioners) reveal that those in key positions to influence related policy remain unaware even today of the effects of health disparities—less than half of mayors and only 60% of health commissioners strongly agree that health disparities exist in their own communities (Purtle et al., 2018). This creates obvious barriers to implementation of health equity initiatives and requires health equity workers to "take a step back" and work on conveying basic knowledge of health disparities prior to engaging in the work necessary to actually eliminate them.

To have the highest level of impact, efforts to achieve health equity must recognize and work to counteract the broader context in which the disparities occur—even at the fundamental level of ensuring communities and policy makers are aware that the disparities even exist.

CONCLUSION

In conclusion, while there is immense need, there is also immense opportunity to make a difference in the field of health equity, and a tremendous diversity of populations and focal areas in need of motivated and determined mentors, activists, educators, researchers, and public health professionals. As we become more aware both of additional needs within communities and of additional communities in need of support, opportunities for innovative work are continually expanding.

The time for change is now, and the power for change lies in each of us.

REFERENCES

Benz, J. K., Espinosa, O., Welsh, V., & Fontes, A. (2011). Awareness of racial and ethnic disparities has improved only modestly over a decade. *Health Affairs, 30*(10), 1860–1867. doi:10.1377/hlthaff.2010.0702

Berge, J., Mendenhall, T. J., & Doherty, W. J. (2009). Using community-based participatory research (CBPR) to target health disparities in families. *Family Relations, 58*(4), 475–488. doi:10.1111/j.1741-3729.2009.00567.x

Booske, B. C., Robert, S. A., & Rohan, A. M. K. (2011). Awareness of racial and socioeconomic health disparities in the United States: The National Opinion Survey on Health and Health Disparities, 2008–2009. *Preventing Chronic Disease, 8*(4), A73. Retrieved from http://www.cdc.gov/pcd/issues/2011/jul/10_0166.htm

Burlew, L. D. (1991). Multiple mentor model: A conceptual framework. *Journal of Career Development, 17*(3), 213–221. doi:10.1007/BF01322028

Chandler, C. (1996). Mentoring and women in academia: Reevaluating the traditional model. *National Women's Studies Association Journal, 8*(3), 79–100. doi:10.2979/NWS.1996.8.3.79

Chesler, N. C., & Chesler, M. A. (2013). Gender-informed mentoring strategies for women engineering scholars: On establishing a caring community. *Journal of Engineering Education, 91*(1), 49–55. doi:10.1002/j.2168-9830.2002.tb00672.x

Darwin, A., & Palmer, E. J. (2009). Mentoring circles in higher education. *Higher Education Research and Development, 28*(2), 125–136. doi:10.1080/07294360902725017

Etzkowitz, H., Kemelgor, C., & Uzzi, B. (2000). *Athena unbound: The advancement of women in science and technology*. London, UK: Cambridge University Press.

Ginther, D. K., Schaffer, W. T., Schnell, J., Masimore, B., Lie, F., Haak, L. L., & Kington, R. (2011). Race, ethnicity, and NIH research awards. *Science, 333*(6045), 1015–1019. doi:10.1126/science.1196783

Hahm, J., & Ommaya, A (Eds.).. (2006). *Opportunities to address clinical research workforce diversity needs for 2010*. Washington, DC: National Academies Press. Retrieved from https://www.ncbi.nlm.nih.gov/books/NBK20280/

Israel, B. A., Schulz, A. J., Parker, E. A., & Becker, A. B. (1998). Review of community-based research: Assessing partnership approaches to improve public health. *Annual Review of Public Health, 19*, 173–202. doi:10.1146/annurev.publhealth.19.1.173

Lillie-Blanton, M., Brodie, M., Rowland, D., Altman, D., & McIntosh, M. (2000). Race, ethnicity, and the health care system: Public perceptions and experiences. *Medical Care Research and Review, 57*(1), 218–235. doi:10.1177/1077558700057001S10

McGee, R., Saran, S., & Krulwich, T. A. (2012). Diversity in the biomedical research workforce: Developing talent. *Mt. Sinai Journal of Medicine, 79*(3), 397–411. doi:10.1002/msj.21310

National Science Foundation. (2017). *Women, minorities, and persons with disabilities in science and engineering*. Arlington, VA: Author. Retrieved from https://ncses.nsf.gov/pubs/nsf19304/digest

Portillo, S. (2018). Mentoring minority and female students: Recommendations for improving mentoring in public administration and public affairs programs. *Journal of Public Affairs Education, 13*(1), 103–113. doi:10.1080/15236803.2007.12001470

Purtle, J., Henson, R. M., Carroll-Scott, A., Kolker, J., Joshi, R., & Diez Roux, A. V. (2018). US mayors' and health commissioners' opinions about health disparities in their cities. *American Journal of Public Health, 108*(5), 634–641. doi:10.2105/AJPH.2017.304298

Wallerstein, N. B., & Duran, B. (2006). Using community-based participatory research to address health disparities. *Health Promotion Practice, 7*(3), 312–323. doi:10.1177/1524839906289376

Wallerstein, N. B., & Duran, B. (2010). Community-based participatory research contributions to intervention research: The intersection of science and practice to improve health equity. *American Journal of Public Health, 100*(s1), S40–S46. doi:10.2105/AJPH.2009.184036

AFTERWORD: COVID-19 AND HEALTH INEQUITIES

As this text approaches publication, we find ourselves in a strange, new world where the very fabric of society has been turned on end by a virus that is 120 nm in size, but seismic in its impact. Strangers and loved ones have become potential vectors, groceries are potential fomites, and we are physically shielding ourselves from the outside world to a degree no one alive has ever seen.

At the same time COVID-19 has changed the world, it has also further entrenched many of the issues discussed throughout this book. The headlines that are grabbing attention worldwide are not new to anyone in the field of health equity, and many of us knew the day would come where the dire inequities discussed throughout this text revealed themselves in newly disturbing ways as a result of the pandemic. As we go to press, we are only beginning to see the magnitude of disparities in outcomes, with initial state reports showing African American populations facing double, sometimes even triple, the risk of dying in comparison to their White counterparts. Major media outlets are covering this disparity as if it were some new horror inflicted upon the United States, but it is just the latest manifestation of health inequities.

While the full ways in which COVID-19 has exacerbated inequities will not be known for many years—if ever—there are already marked issues that have emerged. Many states now acknowledge that minority populations are much more likely to die from COVID-19. One of the current prevailing theories maps back to everything discussed in these pages: The social determinants of health that lead to inequities in outcomes ranging from cancer to heart disease bear out in the same way with this new pandemic. Lack of transportation, higher rates of uninsurance, poverty, lack of a primary care provider—all of these factors place minority communities at particular risk for negative outcomes. In addition, the cumulative impact of these inequities—for instance, diabetes and hypertension—are in and of themselves risk factors. So the virus reveals what many of us have seen for years: individual health inequities compounding to create accumulative, synergistic inequities of even higher magnitude. For instance, we know that maternal mortality rates are up to five times higher for African American women, with factors ranging from social determinants of health to disparities in underlying health status contributing to this massive level of risk. The same applies to COVID-19: A population already facing an increased likelihood of nearly every identified risk factor for negative COVID-19 outcome (e.g., asthma, heart conditions, obesity, diabetes, chronic kidney disease, liver disease) will inevitably face a higher mortality risk than those not facing the same risk factors and preexisting conditions.

At the same time, members of minority groups not directly infected with COVID-19 are still unequally impacted by it. Minority groups are disproportionately represented among numerous categories of essential workers, including grocery store and supermarket clerks, convenience store workers, and food processing plant workers. These high-touch and close-proximity jobs not only placed workers at higher risk for being exposed to COVID-19 prior to shutdown and shelter-in-place ordinances, the subsequent designation of their jobs (understandably) as essential requires them to continue to place themselves at risk for the "benefit of society." Thus, the nature of employment is inherently increasing risk for minority Americans.

The impact is deeper, however, as even the designated actions to prevent spread further reveal the depth of privilege in the United States. Minority populations are less represented in managerial and professional occupations that lend themselves to telecommuting and are less likely to have access to the home broadband necessary to telecommute even if it is an option. This impacts not only work-from-home capabilities but also access to telehealth and home-based education for children. While figures have not been published as of this text going to press, because of these factors, it is highly likely that unemployment claims will include a disproportionate representation of minority residents, and the financial fallout could have years—if not decades—of impact. This will only worsen the already dire inequities that exist and will likely result in even more pronounced health inequities moving forward unless decisive action is taken.

Issues with discrimination are also becoming more prominent. Even early in the outbreak, Asian Americans reported increased numbers of verbal and even physical attacks due to their heritage. The effects of racism in the age of COVID-19 can also be more sinister and emerge in ways that further heighten risk for minority groups. For example, the control strategy of wearing a mask in public further reveals privilege as African American men in particular recount multiple instances of profiling and even harassment for following federal guidelines of wearing masks in public. Many news stories have spotlighted minority men who are electing not to wear masks in light of this, which further increases their risk. Thus, experiences of discrimination are not only becoming more frequent, the effects of racism are also directly increasing risk of infection.

Finally, in states that have begun reopening strategies, the industries initially released often include a high relative proportion of minority workers—for example, barbershops, hair salons, and nail salons. Some officials have even described opening these industries as test cases, despite the known disproportionate impact these actions will have on minority groups. It is unclear what effect this will have on continuing the inequities in COVID-19 outcomes that are already being revealed, but it is difficult to see how things will not worsen.

We are in strange times, and these times are highlighting and exacerbating the factors discussed throughout this text. We can only hope that as a country we seek to find solutions that will lessen, rather than heighten, the impact of health inequities.

INDEX

CPSIA information can be obtained
at www.ICGtesting.com
Printed in the USA
BVHW022018240723
667724BV00002B/10